Essential

Health Skills
for Middle School

by

Catherine A. Sanderson, PhD
Professor of Psychology
Amherst College
Amherst, Massachusetts

Mark Zelman, PhD
Associate Professor of Biology
Aurora University
Aurora, Illinois

Pedagogy Developers

Lindsay Armbruster
Health Education Teacher
Burnt Hills-Ballston Lake Central
    School District
Burnt Hills, New York

Mary McCarley
Health and Physical Education Teacher
Hawthorne Academy High School
Charlotte, North Carolina

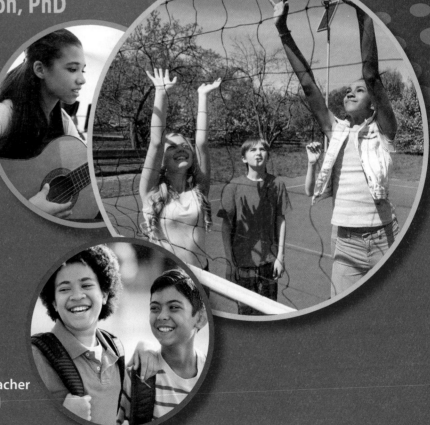

Publisher
The Goodheart-Willcox Company, Inc.
Tinley Park, IL
www.g-w.com

Introduction

We wrote this exciting new textbook for middle school health and wellness classes based on our experiences as professors of psychology (Catherine Sanderson) and biology (Mark Zelman), and as the accomplished authors of high school and college-level textbooks. Our backgrounds give us a deep well of knowledge of the most current scientific theory and research to draw from.

Perhaps the most valuable experience we had in preparing us to write this book is our roles as parents to a combined total of seven children, ages 8 through 22. After all, in writing this book, we both reflected frequently on our experiences as parents and our goal of ensuring that our own children maintain excellent physical, emotional, intellectual, and social health.

This book includes all of the standard topics found in middle school health and wellness books—including nutrition, physical fitness, substance use and abuse (including tobacco, alcohol, and drugs), stress management, disease prevention, and healthy relationships. We wanted our book to give middle school students the most current health information, presented in an engaging writing style so students would enjoy reading the book. Additionally, we included a focus on practical health skills that young people can use to develop and promote good health and wellness habits throughout their lives.

As the authors of high school and college-level textbooks, we felt confident in our research and writing abilities, but felt that the pedagogy was better left to master teachers. We would like to thank Middle School Health Education teachers Lindsay Armbruster, of Burnt Hills-Ballston Lake Central School District in Burnt Hills, New York, and Mary McCarley, of Hawthorne Academy High School in Charlotte, North Carolina, for developing the skills-based questions, activities, and features that are a vital part of this course. We are delighted with the final product, and wish all readers of this book a lifetime of good health.

Cathi A. Sanderson

Mark Zelman

About the Authors

Textbook Authors

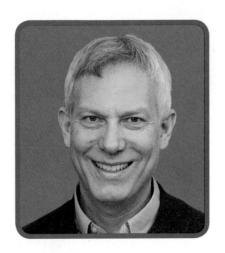

Catherine A. Sanderson is the James E. Ostendarp Professor of Psychology at Amherst College, Amherst, Massachusetts. She received a bachelor's degree in psychology, with a specialization in health and development, from Stanford University, and received both a master's and a doctoral degree in psychology from Princeton University. Professor Sanderson's research examines how personality and social variables influence health-related behaviors, such as safer sex and disordered eating. She also studies the development of persuasive messages, interventions to prevent unhealthy behavior, and the predictors of relationship satisfaction. Professor Sanderson's research has received grant funding from the National Science Foundation and the National Institutes of Health. She has published over 25 journal articles and book chapters in addition to three college textbooks and a popular-press book on parenting. In 2012, she was named one of the country's top 300 professors by the Princeton Review.

Mark Zelman is an Associate Professor of Biology at Aurora University, Aurora, Illinois. He received a bachelor's degree in biology at Rockford College, with minors in chemistry and psychology. He received a PhD in microbiology and immunology at Loyola University of Chicago, where he studied the molecular and cellular mechanisms of autoimmune disease. During his postdoctoral research at the University of Chicago, he studied aspects of cell physiology pertaining to cell growth and cancer. Dr. Zelman supervises undergraduate research on streptococcal and staphylococcal infections, and mechanisms of antibiotic resistance. He also teaches in the science education graduate program for biology and chemistry high school teachers. He has published articles on microbiology, infectious disease, autoimmune disease, and biotechnology, and he has written two college texts on human diseases and infection control. Dr. Zelman is an officer of the Illinois State Academy of Sciences.

Pedagogy Developers

Lindsay Armbruster experiences, on a daily basis, the impact that positivity and happiness can have on a class, an individual, and on students' health behaviors. As a result, her teaching focuses on strengths and possibilities and is highly influenced by the theories of skills-based health education and positive psychology. Lindsay has been teaching Health Education since 2004, ranging all grade levels—kindergarten through twelfth grade—with most of her experience occurring at the middle school level. Lindsay received her bachelor's degree in school and community health education from the State University of New York College at Brockport and her master's degree in instructional design and educational technology from the University at Albany, while also completing coursework toward a master's degree in Public Health at the George Washington University. She is an award winner of the New York State Association for Health, Physical Education, Recreation and Dance (NYSAHPERD) Health Teacher of the Year award and the Society of Health & Physical Educators (SHAPE) America Eastern District Health Teacher of the Year award. Lindsay is a frequent presenter at local, state, and regional conferences.

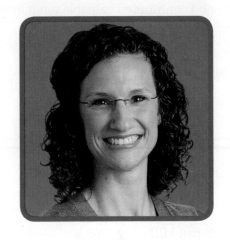

Mary McCarley is a health and physical education teacher at Hawthorne Academy High School in Charlotte, North Carolina. She has 14 years of teaching experience and excels at creating an engaging, student-centered environment with a focus on real-world learning based on personal interest and self-exploration. Mary graduated from UNC-Chapel Hill with an Exercise and Sports Science degree and East Carolina University with a Master of Arts in Education in Health Education. She is a National Board Certified Teacher in Health Education. In addition, Mary is the 2016 North Carolina High School Teacher of the Year for Health Education and the 2016 High School Southern District Teacher of the Year for the Advancement of Health Education. Mary presents at conferences and for school districts on various health education topics locally and nationally.

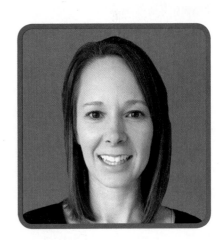

Reviewers

Goodheart-Willcox Publisher would like to thank the following teachers who reviewed selected chapters and contributed valuable input into the development of *Essential Health Skills for Middle School.*

Gwyneth Aldridge
Randolph Middle School
Charlotte, North Carolina

Lynnea Allen
Wayzata East Middle School
Plymouth, Minnesota

Lindsay Armbruster
Burnt Hills-Ballston Lake
    Central School District
Burnt Hills, New York

Kelsey Baker
Aliamanu Middle School
Honolulu, Hawaii

Heather Berlin
Harmon Middle School
Aurora, Ohio

Dawn Blevins
San Fernando Middle
    School
San Fernando, California

Scott Borowicz
Normandin Middle School
New Bedford, Massachusetts

Corbin Bray
Banks Trail Middle School
Fort Mill, South Carolina

Tammi Conn
Valley View School District
Romeoville, Illinois

Julie Connor
Wydown Middle School
Clayton, Missouri

Anita Dunham
Lexington Junior High School
Cypress, California

Cheryl Friske
Vernon Verona Sherrill
    Middle School
Verona, New York

Kim Gillick
Greenwich Middle School
Greenwich, Connecticut

Dwayne Hamlette
Amherst Middle School
Amherst, Virginia

Cathy Hawkins
Tri-North Middle School
Bloomington, Indiana

Emily Hill
Southern Hills Middle
    School
Boulder, Colorado

Diane Jones
Fairfield Middle School
Henrico, Virginia

Mike Kruse
Gilbert Middle School
Gilbert, Iowa

Sheila Leamer
Chittenango CSD
Chittenango, New York

Ben Leven
Twin Groves Middle School
Buffalo Grove, Illinois

Sarah Lewis
Van Hoosen Middle School
Rochester Hills, Michigan

Charlie Means
Scott Middle School
Denison, Texas

Matthew Nichols
Lopez Middle School
San Antonio, Texas

Pam Nitsche
Madison Middle School
Trumbull, Connecticut

Judith R. Peters
School District of Philadelphia
Philadelphia, Pennsylvania

Marla Rickard
Suzanne Middle School
Walnut, California

Pam Riddle
Wayland Middle School
Wayland, Massachusetts

Jamie Rucci
Solon Middle School
Solon, Ohio

Shannon Todd
Lake Oswego Junior
    High School
Lake Oswego, Oregon

Craig Walter
Upper Moreland
    School District
Hatboro, Pennsylvania

Susie Woerner
Hinsdale Middle School
Hinsdale, Illinois

Brief Contents

Contents

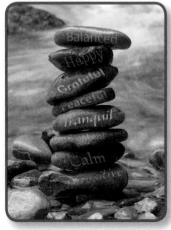

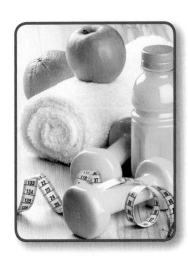

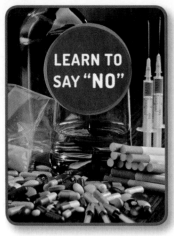

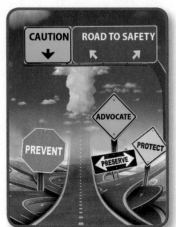

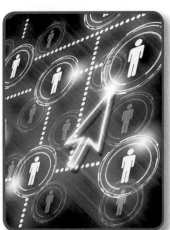

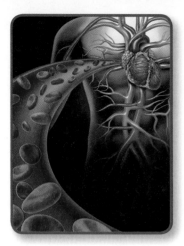

Features

CASE STUDIES

BUILDING Your Skills

Infographics

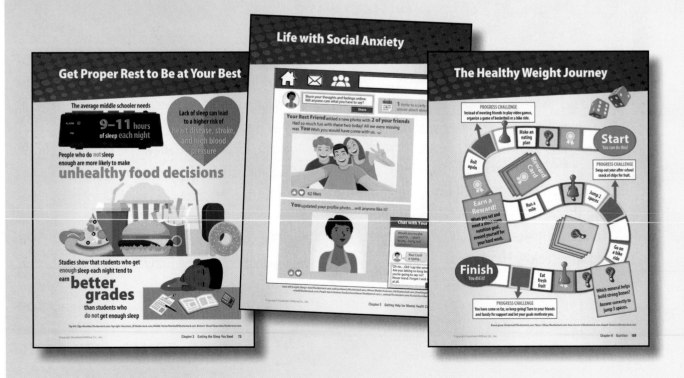

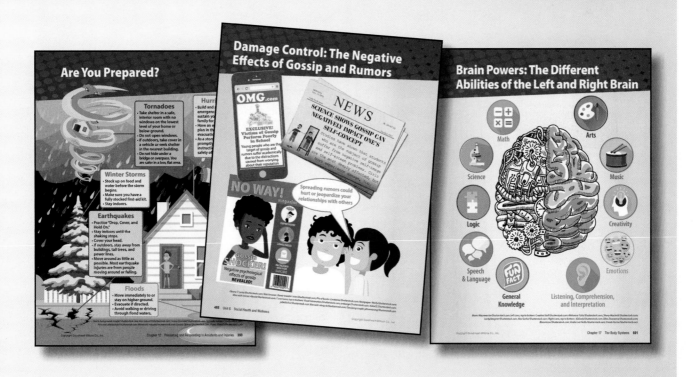

How Healthy Are You?

To the Student

The best way to learn and develop your skills is not just to read, but to organize and apply the information you see. Getting ready to read and taking frequent breaks to complete activities can make reading seem less daunting. It can also help you remember information longer and understand it better. That is why this textbook does more than just *present* the information you need to know. It also contains features and activities to help you *understand* and *apply* what you learn. Knowing how to use these features will help you learn more quickly and effectively. To learn how best to use this textbook, join us on a walkthrough of a typical unit, chapter, and lesson.

Start with the Unit Opener

1. Read the unit number and title.

2. See what chapters are included in the unit. Think about what information you are excited to learn.

3. Complete the **Warm-Up Activity**. Some Warm-Up Activities ask you to come back to them after reading the chapters in the unit, so do not throw away your completed activity. Keep it so you can revisit it after reading the unit.

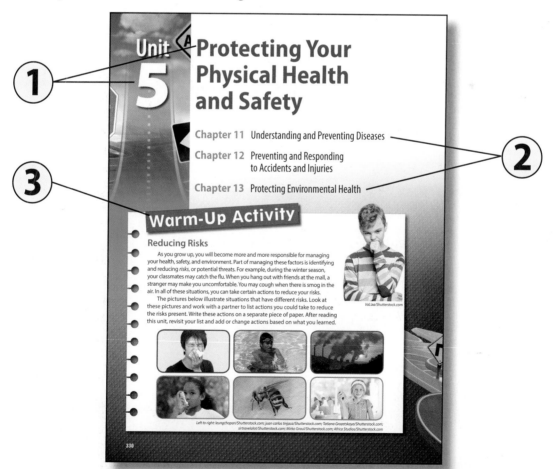

Read the Chapter Opener

1. Read the chapter number and title.

2. Consider the **Essential Question**. You can discuss the question with your classmates and talk about related information you want to learn.

3. See what lessons are included in the chapter. Think about questions you have that relate to each lesson.

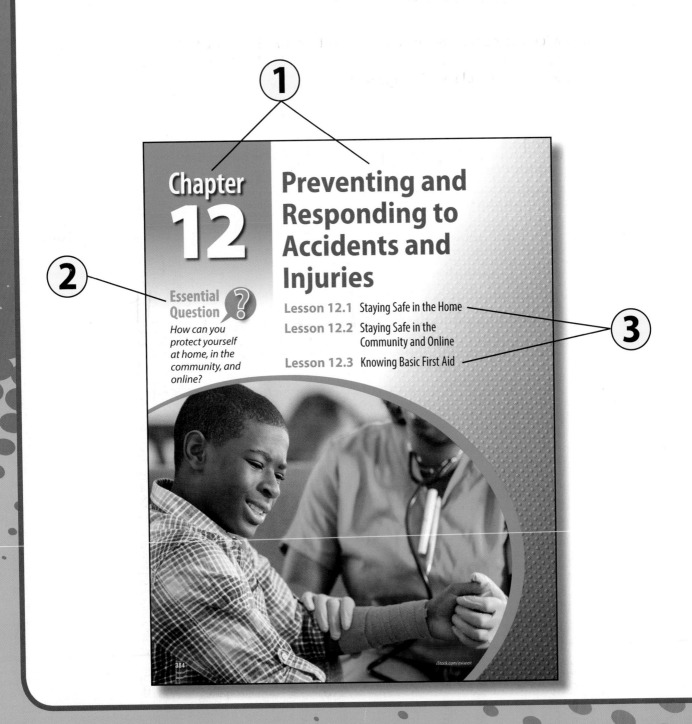

Chapter

12

Preventing and Responding to Accidents and Injuries

Essential Question ❓
How can you protect yourself at home, in the community, and online?

Lesson 12.1 Staying Safe in the Home

Lesson 12.2 Staying Safe in the Community and Online

Lesson 12.3 Knowing Basic First Aid

384

iStock.com/asiseeit

Complete the Chapter Opener Activities

1. Complete the **Reading Activity**. The Reading Activity will help you understand and remember what you learn in the chapter.

2. Assess your own health habits using the **How Healthy Are You?** quiz. Answer "Yes" or "No" to each question and count your "Yes" or "No" responses. Use your answers to think about how you can improve your overall health.

3. Click on the activity icon or go to the G-W Learning Companion Website to complete the assessment online.

4. Take a look at the activities you can complete on the G-W Learning Companion Website. For each lesson, you can use flash cards to remember key terms, print the graphic organizer, and complete online quizzes and assessments.

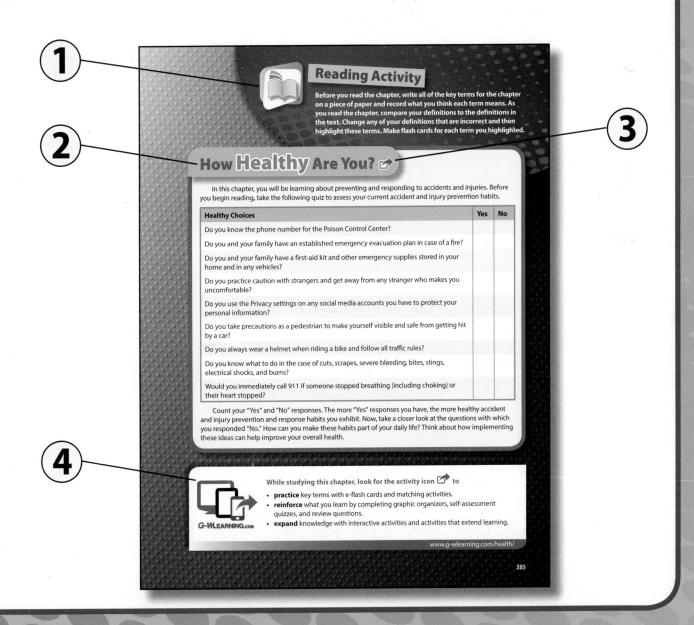

1

Reading Activity

Before you read the chapter, write all of the key terms for the chapter on a piece of paper and record what you think each term means. As you read the chapter, compare your definitions to the definitions in the text. Change any of your definitions that are incorrect and then highlight these terms. Make flash cards for each term you highlighted.

3

2

How Healthy Are You?

In this chapter, you will be learning about preventing and responding to accidents and injuries. Before you begin reading, take the following quiz to assess your current accident and injury prevention habits.

Healthy Choices	Yes	No
Do you know the phone number for the Poison Control Center?		
Do you and your family have an established emergency evacuation plan in case of a fire?		
Do you and your family have a first-aid kit and other emergency supplies stored in your home and in any vehicles?		
Do you practice caution with strangers and get away from any stranger who makes you uncomfortable?		
Do you use the Privacy settings on any social media accounts you have to protect your personal information?		
Do you take precautions as a pedestrian to make yourself visible and safe from getting hit by a car?		
Do you always wear a helmet when riding a bike and follow all traffic rules?		
Do you know what to do in the case of cuts, scrapes, severe bleeding, bites, stings, electrical shocks, and burns?		
Would you immediately call 911 if someone stopped breathing (including choking) or their heart stopped?		

Count your "Yes" and "No" responses. The more "Yes" responses you have, the more healthy accident and injury prevention and response habits you exhibit. Now, take a closer look at the questions with which you responded "No." How can you make these habits part of your daily life? Think about how implementing these ideas can help improve your overall health.

4

G-WLEARNING.com

While studying this chapter, look for the activity icon to

- **practice** key terms with e-flash cards and matching activities.
- **reinforce** what you learn by completing graphic organizers, self-assessment quizzes, and review questions.
- **expand** knowledge with interactive activities and activities that extend learning.

www.g-wlearning.com/health/

385

Prepare to Read Each Lesson

1. Read the lesson number and title.
2. See what topics are covered in the lesson by reading the **Learning Outcomes**.
3. Look at the **Key Terms** in the lesson and read their definitions. You will learn more about these terms in the lesson. You will also see these definitions again in the **English and Spanish Glossary** in the back of the textbook.
4. Click on the activity icon or go to the G-W Learning Companion Website to use e-flash cards to review the terms.
5. Use the **Graphic Organizer** to take notes. You will need a separate piece of paper to create the organizer. Keep the organizer to help you study for the test.
6. Click on the activity icon or go to the G-W Learning Companion Website to find and print the organizer online.

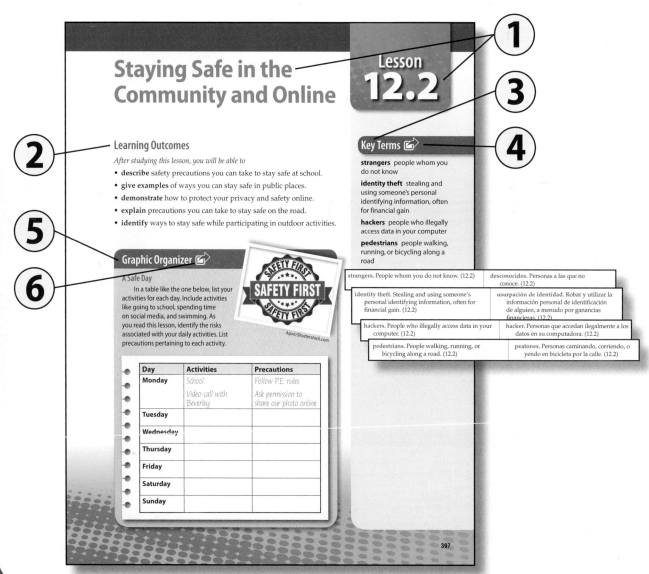

Staying Safe in the Community and Online

Lesson 12.2

Learning Outcomes

After studying this lesson, you will be able to

- **describe** safety precautions you can take to stay safe at school.
- **give examples** of ways you can stay safe in public places.
- **demonstrate** how to protect your privacy and safety online.
- **explain** precautions you can take to stay safe on the road.
- **identify** ways to stay safe while participating in outdoor activities.

Key Terms

strangers people whom you do not know
identity theft stealing and using someone's personal identifying information, often for financial gain
hackers people who illegally access data in your computer
pedestrians people walking, running, or bicycling along a road

Graphic Organizer

A Safe Day

In a table like the one below, list your activities for each day. Include activities like going to school, spending time on social media, and swimming. As you read this lesson, identify the risks associated with your daily activities. List precautions pertaining to each activity.

Aquir/Shutterstock.com

Day	Activities	Precautions
Monday	School	Follow P.E. rules
	Video-call with Beverley	Ask permission to share our photo online
Tuesday		
Wednesday		
Thursday		
Friday		
Saturday		
Sunday		

strangers. People whom you do not know. (12.2)	desconocidos. Personas a las que no conoce. (12.2)
identity theft. Stealing and using someone's personal identifying information, often for financial gain. (12.2)	usurpación de identidad. Robar y utilizar la información personal de identificación de alguien, a menudo por ganancias financieras. (12.2)
hackers. People who illegally access data in your computer. (12.2)	hacker. Personas que accedan ilegalmente a los datos en su computadora. (12.2)
pedestrians. People walking, running, or bicycling along a road. (12.2)	peatones. Personas caminando, corriendo, o yendo en bicicleta por la calle. (12.2)

397

Remember to Read the Captions and Features

1. Click on the activity icon or go to the G-W Learning Companion Website to play the animation or complete the activity.

2. As you are reading a lesson, do not forget to read the captions and features. Sometimes, captions have caption questions that you can answer to check your knowledge.

3. **Building Your Skills** features are activities that will help you act on the health skills you are learning.

4. **Case Study** features present lifelike scenarios in which young people have to make decisions about their health.

5. After reading each Case Study, complete the **Thinking Critically** questions. Discuss your answers with your classmates.

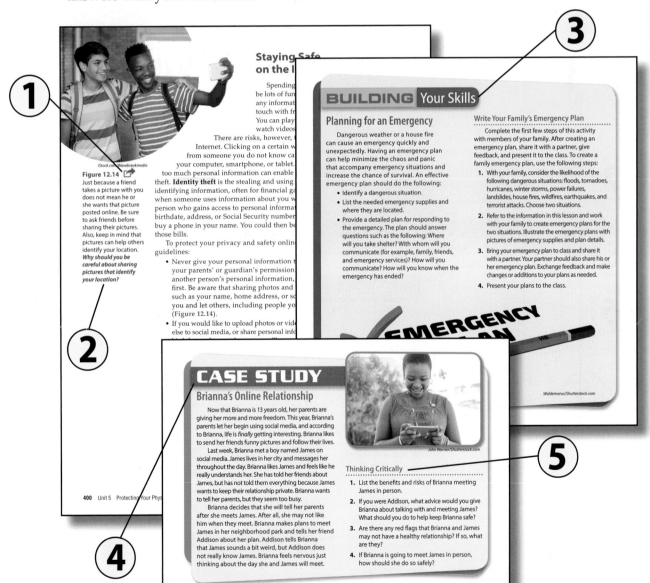

Staying Safe on the I...

Spending...
be lots of fun...
any informat...
touch with fr...
You can play...
watch videos...
There are risks, however, t...
Internet. Clicking on a certain w...
from someone you do not know ca...
your computer, smartphone, or tablet...
too much personal information can enable...
theft. **Identity theft** is the stealing and using...
identifying information, often for financial ga...
when someone uses information about you w...
person who gains access to personal informa...
birthdate, address, or Social Security number...
buy a phone in your name. You could then be...
those bills.

To protect your privacy and safety online...
guidelines:

- Never give your personal information t...
  your parents' or guardian's permission...
  another person's personal information...
  first. Be aware that sharing photos and...
  such as your name, home address, or so...
  you and let others, including people yo...
  (Figure 12.14).

- If you would like to upload photos or vide...
  else to social media, or share personal info...

Figure 12.14
Just because a friend takes a picture with you does not mean he or she wants that picture posted online. Be sure to ask friends before sharing their pictures. Also, keep in mind that pictures can help others identify your location. *Why should you be careful about sharing pictures that identify your location?*

iStock.com/Wavebreakmedia

400 Unit 5 Protecting Your Phys...

BUILDING Your Skills

Planning for an Emergency

Dangerous weather or a house fire can cause an emergency quickly and unexpectedly. Having an emergency plan can help minimize the chaos and panic that accompany emergency situations and increase the chance of survival. An effective emergency plan should do the following:

- Identify a dangerous situation.
- List the needed emergency supplies and where they are located.
- Provide a detailed plan for responding to the emergency. The plan should answer questions such as the following: Where will you take shelter? With whom will you communicate (for example, family, friends, and emergency services)? How will you communicate? How will you know when the emergency has ended?

Write Your Family's Emergency Plan

Complete the first few steps of this activity with members of your family. After creating an emergency plan, share it with a partner, give feedback, and present it to the class. To create a family emergency plan, use the following steps:

1. With your family, consider the likelihood of the following dangerous situations: floods, tornadoes, hurricanes, winter storms, power failures, landslides, house fires, wildfires, earthquakes, and terrorist attacks. Choose two situations.

2. Refer to the information in this lesson and work with your family to create emergency plans for the two situations. Illustrate the emergency plans with pictures of emergency supplies and plan details.

3. Bring your emergency plan to class and share it with a partner. Your partner should also share his or her emergency plan. Exchange feedback and make changes or additions to your plans as needed.

4. Present your plans to the class.

Waldemarus/Shutterstock.com

CASE STUDY

Brianna's Online Relationship

Now that Brianna is 13 years old, her parents are giving her more and more freedom. This year, Brianna's parents let her begin using social media, and according to Brianna, life is *finally* getting interesting. Brianna likes to send her friends funny pictures and follow their lives.

Last week, Brianna met a boy named James on social media. James lives in her city and messages her throughout the day. Brianna likes James and feels like he really understands her. She has told her friends about James, but has not told them everything because James wants to keep their relationship private. Brianna wants to tell her parents, but they seem too busy.

Brianna decides that she will tell her parents after she meets James. After all, she may not like him when they meet. Brianna makes plans to meet James in her neighborhood park and tells her friend Addison about her plan. Addison tells Brianna that James sounds a bit weird, but Addison does not really know James. Brianna feels nervous just thinking about the day she and James will meet.

John Warner/Shutterstock.com

Thinking Critically

1. List the benefits and risks of Brianna meeting James in person.

2. If you were Addison, what advice would you give Brianna about talking with and meeting James? What should you do to help keep Brianna safe?

3. Are there any red flags that Brianna and James may not have a healthy relationship? If so, what are they?

4. If Brianna is going to meet James in person, how should she do so safely?

Answer Questions About Each Lesson

 1. A **Lesson Review** follows each lesson. Read the Lesson Review number.

2. Click on the activity icon or go to the G-W Learning Companion Website if you want to complete the review online and submit your answers to your teacher.

3. Answer the first four questions, which will test your knowledge of what you learned in the lesson.

4. The fifth **Critical thinking** question will have you think more deeply about what you learned. Take some time to consider and write an answer to this question. Discuss your answer with your classmates.

5. Complete the **Hands-On Activity**, which will ask you to put your learning into practice. Many Hands-On Activities ask you to work with your classmates.

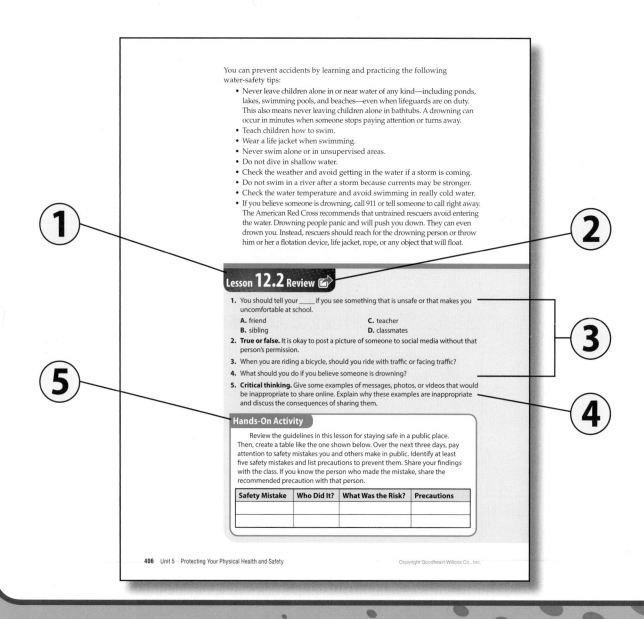

You can prevent accidents by learning and practicing the following water-safety tips:
- Never leave children alone in or near water of any kind—including ponds, lakes, swimming pools, and beaches—even when lifeguards are on duty. This also means never leaving children alone in bathtubs. A drowning can occur in minutes when someone stops paying attention or turns away.
- Teach children how to swim.
- Wear a life jacket when swimming.
- Never swim alone or in unsupervised areas.
- Do not dive in shallow water.
- Check the weather and avoid getting in the water if a storm is coming.
- Do not swim in a river after a storm because currents may be stronger.
- Check the water temperature and avoid swimming in really cold water.
- If you believe someone is drowning, call 911 or tell someone to call right away. The American Red Cross recommends that untrained rescuers avoid entering the water. Drowning people panic and will push you down. They can even drown you. Instead, rescuers should reach for the drowning person or throw him or her a flotation device, life jacket, rope, or any object that will float.

Lesson 12.2 Review

1. You should tell your _____ if you see something that is unsafe or that makes you uncomfortable at school.
   A. friend
   B. sibling
   C. teacher
   D. classmates
2. **True or false.** It is okay to post a picture of someone to social media without that person's permission.
3. When you are riding a bicycle, should you ride with traffic or facing traffic?
4. What should you do if you believe someone is drowning?
5. **Critical thinking.** Give some examples of messages, photos, or videos that would be inappropriate to share online. Explain why these examples are inappropriate and discuss the consequences of sharing them.

Hands-On Activity

Review the guidelines in this lesson for staying safe in a public place. Then, create a table like the one shown below. Over the next three days, pay attention to safety mistakes you and others make in public. Identify at least five safety mistakes and list precautions to prevent them. Share your findings with the class. If you know the person who made the mistake, share the recommended precaution with that person.

Safety Mistake	Who Did It?	What Was the Risk?	Precautions

Recall What You Learned

1. Each chapter ends with a three-page **Review and Assessment**. Start by reading the chapter number and heading.

2. Read each lesson number and title.

3. Review the **Summary** for each lesson. While reading the bullets, look at your notes and add any information you missed.

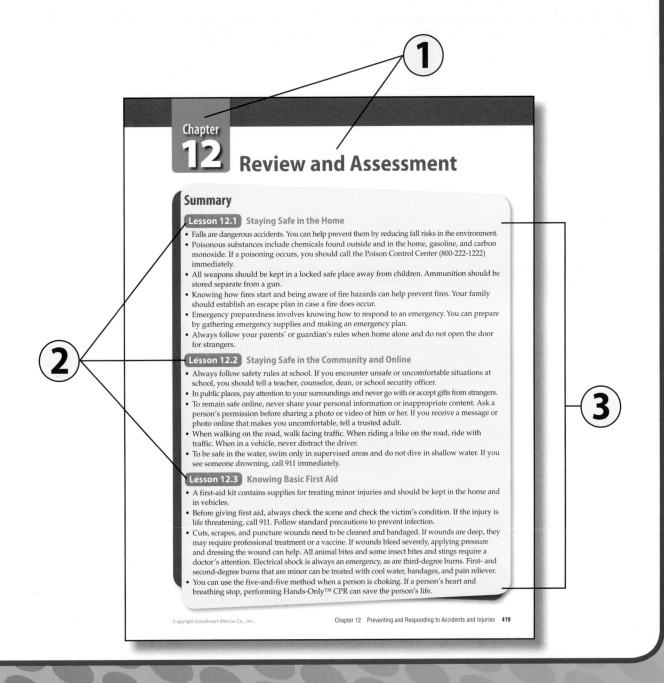

1

Chapter 12 Review and Assessment

Summary

Lesson 12.1 Staying Safe in the Home

- Falls are dangerous accidents. You can help prevent them by reducing fall risks in the environment.
- Poisonous substances include chemicals found outside and in the home, gasoline, and carbon monoxide. If a poisoning occurs, you should call the Poison Control Center (800-222-1222) immediately.
- All weapons should be kept in a locked safe place away from children. Ammunition should be stored separate from a gun.
- Knowing how fires start and being aware of fire hazards can help prevent fires. Your family should establish an escape plan in case a fire does occur.
- Emergency preparedness involves knowing how to respond to an emergency. You can prepare by gathering emergency supplies and making an emergency plan.
- Always follow your parents' or guardian's rules when home alone and do not open the door for strangers.

Lesson 12.2 Staying Safe in the Community and Online

- Always follow safety rules at school. If you encounter unsafe or uncomfortable situations at school, you should tell a teacher, counselor, dean, or school security officer.
- In public places, pay attention to your surroundings and never go with or accept gifts from strangers.
- To remain safe online, never share your personal information or inappropriate content. Ask a person's permission before sharing a photo or video of him or her. If you receive a message or photo online that makes you uncomfortable, tell a trusted adult.
- When walking on the road, walk facing traffic. When riding a bike on the road, ride with traffic. When in a vehicle, never distract the driver.
- To be safe in the water, swim only in supervised areas and do not dive in shallow water. If you see someone drowning, call 911 immediately.

Lesson 12.3 Knowing Basic First Aid

- A first-aid kit contains supplies for treating minor injuries and should be kept in the home and in vehicles.
- Before giving first aid, always check the scene and check the victim's condition. If the injury is life threatening, call 911. Follow standard precautions to prevent infection.
- Cuts, scrapes, and puncture wounds need to be cleaned and bandaged. If wounds are deep, they may require professional treatment or a vaccine. If wounds bleed severely, applying pressure and dressing the wound can help. All animal bites and some insect bites and stings require a doctor's attention. Electrical shock is always an emergency, as are third-degree burns. First- and second-degree burns that are minor can be treated with cool water, bandages, and pain reliever.
- You can use the five-and-five method when a person is choking. If a person's heart and breathing stop, performing Hands-Only™ CPR can save the person's life.

2

3

Review Your Learning and Vocabulary

1. Answer the **Check Your Knowledge** review questions.
2. Click on the activity icon or go to the G-W Learning Companion Website if you want to answer the questions online and submit your answers to your teacher.
3. Read the list of terms in the **Use Your Vocabulary** section.
4. Complete the vocabulary activities to review the meanings of the terms.
5. Click on the activity icon or go to the G-W Learning Companion Website to complete additional vocabulary activities online.

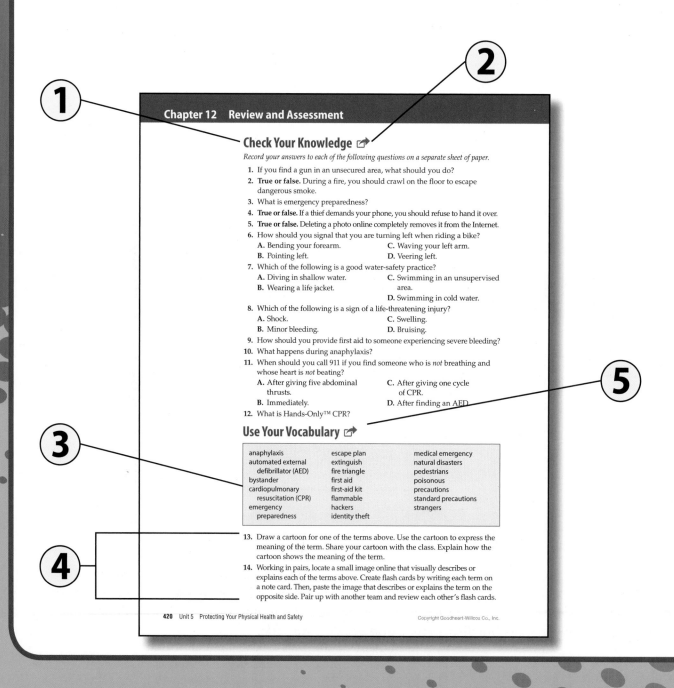

Chapter 12   Review and Assessment

Check Your Knowledge

Record your answers to each of the following questions on a separate sheet of paper.

1. If you find a gun in an unsecured area, what should you do?
2. **True or false.** During a fire, you should crawl on the floor to escape dangerous smoke.
3. What is emergency preparedness?
4. **True or false.** If a thief demands your phone, you should refuse to hand it over.
5. **True or false.** Deleting a photo online completely removes it from the Internet.
6. How should you signal that you are turning left when riding a bike?
   - A. Bending your forearm.
   - B. Pointing left.
   - C. Waving your left arm.
   - D. Veering left.
7. Which of the following is a good water-safety practice?
   - A. Diving in shallow water.
   - B. Wearing a life jacket.
   - C. Swimming in an unsupervised area.
   - D. Swimming in cold water.
8. Which of the following is a sign of a life-threatening injury?
   - A. Shock.
   - B. Minor bleeding.
   - C. Swelling.
   - D. Bruising.
9. How should you provide first aid to someone experiencing severe bleeding?
10. What happens during anaphylaxis?
11. When should you call 911 if you find someone who is *not* breathing and whose heart is *not* beating?
    - A. After giving five abdominal thrusts.
    - B. Immediately.
    - C. After giving one cycle of CPR.
    - D. After finding an AED.
12. What is Hands-Only™ CPR?

Use Your Vocabulary

anaphylaxis	escape plan	medical emergency
automated external defibrillator (AED)	extinguish	natural disasters
bystander	fire triangle	pedestrians
cardiopulmonary resuscitation (CPR)	first aid	poisonous
emergency preparedness	first-aid kit	precautions
	flammable	standard precautions
	hackers	strangers
	identity theft	

13. Draw a cartoon for one of the terms above. Use the cartoon to express the meaning of the term. Share your cartoon with the class. Explain how the cartoon shows the meaning of the term.
14. Working in pairs, locate a small image online that visually describes or explains each of the terms above. Create flash cards by writing each term on a note card. Then, paste the image that describes or explains the term on the opposite side. Pair up with another team and review each other's flash cards.

Act On What You Learned

✐ 1. The **Think Critically** questions ask you to think more deeply about what you learned in the chapter. Consider the questions and answer them. Some questions may need to be discussed with a partner or in small groups.

✐ 2. Complete the **Develop Your Skills** activities, which will help you improve your health and wellness skills. The type of skill the activity reinforces is bold and purple. Some activities involve working in groups and interacting with teachers and the community.

①

②

Think Critically

15. Cause and effect. What are the consequences of being unprepared for an emergency? Give examples of consequences for at least three emergency situations.
16. Draw conclusions. In a small group, discuss whether a middle school student is old enough and responsible enough to stay home alone.
17. Compare and contrast. Compare and contrast a safe and unsafe school environment. Give examples of how the school environment can positively or negatively impact a middle-school student's physical and emotional health.
18. Identify. What are some ways that middle school students can have fun on social media without putting their personal safety at risk?

DEVELOP Your Skills

19. Access information and communication skills. Talk with your parents or guardian about expectations and rules for staying home alone. Create a *Guide to Staying Home Alone* that lists at least five safety rules for staying home alone. Use pictures to illustrate each rule and display your guide in a visible place in your home.

20. Refusal and communication skills. Imagine that you are flirting with someone you met on social media. You have been talking with this person for three weeks and enjoy your online relationship. One day, this person sends the following message to you. How would you respond to protect your personal safety?

> You are amazing. Tell me more about yourself. I want to know everything about you.

21. Decision-making skills. Imagine that you are seeing a movie with two friends. The movie is not very good, so you and your friends decide to walk to the mall 10 blocks away. To save time, your friends plan to walk behind buildings and on side streets. When you reach the lobby

of the theater, however, you notice how dark it is outside. List the pros and cons of each decision you could make and write a summary describing the pros and cons, safety risks and precautions, and what you would do.

22. Advocacy. Think about the personal safety threats that endanger students in your school and create a personal safety flyer highlighting one safety threat. Include at least five safety tips related to the threat and at least two pictures to support your content. If you have permission, hang your flyer on a wall in your school.

23. Teamwork and technology skills. As a class, divide into three groups and assign each group one lesson in this chapter. In your group, review your assigned lesson and outline the most important ideas and safety practices. Ask your teacher if you are not sure which ideas and safety practices are most important. Create a multimedia presentation that uses text, photos and illustrations, and music to summarize the main points in the lesson. Present your interactive summary to the class and answer any questions your classmates have.

Now that you understand how to use this textbook, you are ready to begin your study of health and wellness skills. If you are ever not sure how to use a feature of the textbook, revisit this walkthrough. Remember to take advantage of the activities in this textbook. They will help you not only know information, but also apply it and use it in your life.

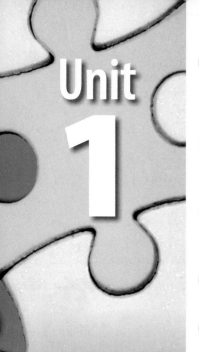

Unit 1

Taking Charge of Your Health and Wellness

Warm-Up Activity

Health Advice: Ask Avalon

Avalon is the regular advice columnist for your middle school newspaper. She has asked you to respond to the following letter she received from someone asking for advice:

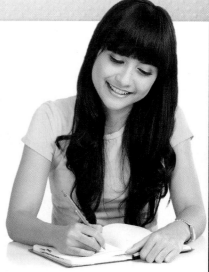

Odua Images/Shutterstock.com

> Dear Avalon,
>
> My dad has been in the hospital for the last two days. I overheard the doctor tell my mom that he would be okay, but needs to live a healthier life. While I'm only 13, I want to be healthy, too. I know it is important to take care of my health, but I'm not sure how to do it. Can you give me some advice on how to be healthy today and as I age?
>
> Thanks,
> Anonymous

When asked a difficult question, even an advice columnist will seek the help of a friend. Work with a partner to respond to Anonymous. Give at least four suggestions on how to be healthy. Include information on physical, mental and emotional, and social health. Give a detailed response and provide examples. Begin your response with "Dear Anonymous."

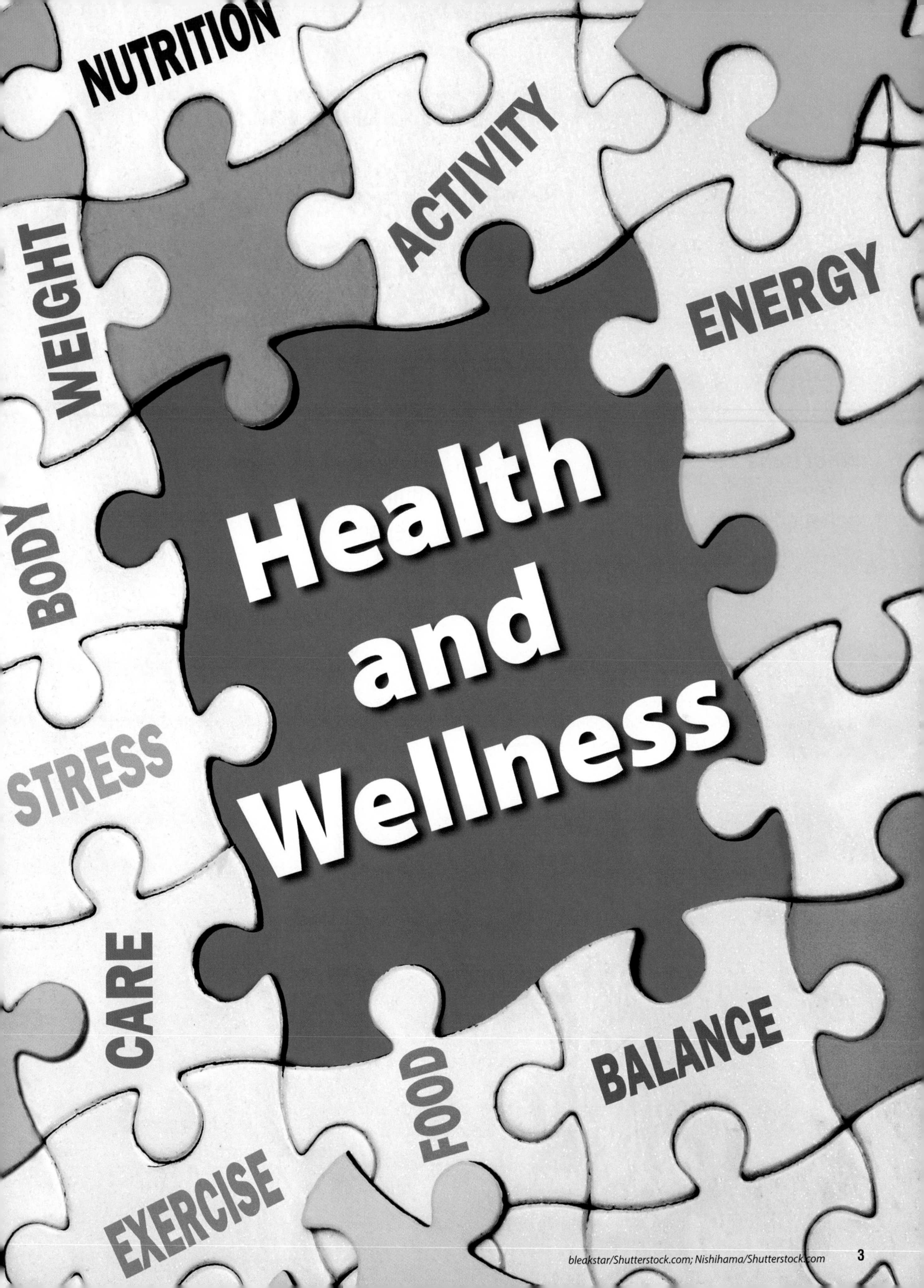

NUTRITION
ACTIVITY
WEIGHT
ENERGY
BODY
Health and Wellness
STRESS
CARE
BALANCE
FOOD
EXERCISE

bleakstar/Shutterstock.com; Nishihama/Shutterstock.com

Chapter 1

Understanding Your Health and Wellness

Lesson 1.1 Defining Health and Wellness

Lesson 1.2 Recognizing Factors That Affect Health and Wellness

Lesson 1.3 Building Skills for Health and Wellness

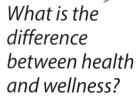

Essential Question

What is the difference between health and wellness?

Video
Access the Chapter 1 video to start thinking about chapter topics.

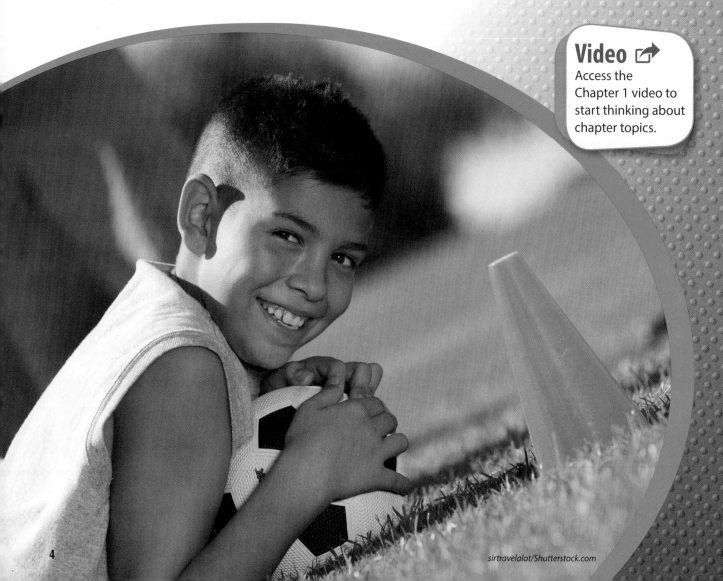

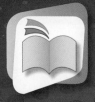

Reading Activity

List the chapter headings to create an outline for taking notes during reading and class discussion. Under each heading, list any key terms. Finally, write two questions you expect to have answered by reading the chapter. After completing the chapter, ask your teacher any questions you still have about this chapter's information.

How **Healthy** Are You?

In this chapter, you will be learning about health and wellness. Before you begin reading, take the following quiz to assess your current health and wellness habits.

Healthy Choices	Yes	No
Do you regularly set short-term and long-term goals that are specific, measurable, achievable, relevant, and timely?		
Do you set a series of short-term goals to help you meet a long-term goal?		
Do you assume responsibility for your personal health behaviors?		
Do you avoid spending time with friends or family who engage in harmful behaviors like smoking or bullying?		
Can you maintain mature relationships by respecting and valuing others and yourself?		
Do you cope well with stress?		
Can you identify reliable sources of health-related information?		
Do you clearly and honestly communicate your thoughts and feelings to others?		
Do you refuse to do things that go against your values and beliefs, regardless of what your friends and family do or say?		
Do you consider the impact of your decisions on others?		
Are you confident in your ability to learn and apply new knowledge, viewing learning as a chance to continually improve yourself?		

Count your "Yes" and "No" responses. The more "Yes" responses you have, the more habits you exhibit for promoting health and wellness. Now, take a closer look at the questions with which you responded "No." How can you make these healthy habits part of your daily life? Think about how implementing these ideas can help improve your overall health and wellness.

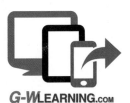

G-WLEARNING.com

While studying this chapter, look for the activity icon to

- **practice** key terms with e-flash cards and matching activities.
- **reinforce** what you learn by completing graphic organizers, self-assessment quizzes, and review questions.
- **expand** knowledge with interactive activities and activities that extend learning.

www.g-wlearning.com/health/

Defining Health and Wellness

Key Terms

health absence of physical illness and disease

wellness balance of all aspects of health—physical, mental and emotional, and social

physical health aspect of health that refers to how well a person's body functions

mental and emotional health aspect of health that has to do with a person's thoughts and feelings

social health aspect of health that involves interacting and getting along with others in positive, healthy ways

well-being state of health and wellness in which people generally feel good about their present conditions

healthcare treatment and prevention of illnesses, injuries, or diseases to improve wellness

preventive healthcare going to the doctor when you are well to help you stay healthy; involves getting an annual physical exam, regular checkups, and screenings for conditions like hearing or vision loss

primary care physician regular doctor who provides checkups, screenings, treatments, and prescriptions

Learning Outcomes

After studying this lesson, you will be able to

- **define** the terms *health* and *wellness*.
- **identify** the aspects of health and wellness.
- **describe** how the aspects of health are interrelated.
- **explain** how people in a state of well-being generally feel.
- **summarize** the connection between healthcare and wellness.

Graphic Organizer

The Health Triangle

Write *Health and Wellness* in the center of a triangle like the one shown. Then, add *physical*, *mental and emotional*, and *social* in the remaining sections of the triangle. As you read this lesson, write what you learn about each aspect of health in the appropriate sections of the triangle. After reading, review your notes and highlight what you think are the most important points.

march.photo/Shutterstock.com

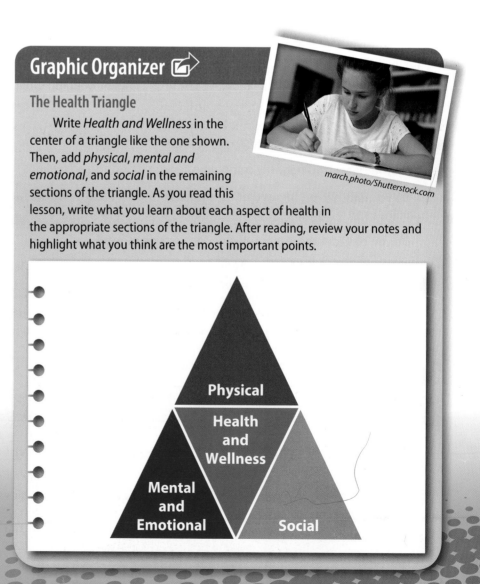

Physical

Health and Wellness

Mental and Emotional

Social

According to her doctor, 13-year-old Hannah passed her physical exam with flying colors and is the picture of health. At home, however, Hannah is often under stress and gets so anxious that she cannot sleep or focus on her schoolwork. She is frequently tired and eats on the go. She quit the soccer team and took up smoking with her boyfriend and his friends. Hannah avoids making decisions and planning for her future. Instead, she prefers to "go with the flow."

Aiden, also 13, was born with a breathing condition that makes running and playing most sports difficult. He manages his condition by following his doctor's orders. He takes his medicine, makes sure to eat well, and gets plenty of sleep. He also gets a moderate amount of physical activity. He does not smoke or drink. Aiden's positive attitude attracts other people to him, so he has many friends. He sets goals for his future, and is confident that he will succeed if he works hard.

So who do you think is healthier—Hannah or Aiden? Is Hannah healthier because her doctor said she is in good physical health? Is Aiden healthier because he seems to take better care of himself overall?

In this lesson, you will learn about the different aspects of health and wellness and overall well-being. You will also discover the connections between healthcare and wellness.

Aspects of Health and Wellness

What do the terms *health* and *wellness* mean? The term **health** usually refers to the absence of physical illness and disease. There is more to health and wellness, however, than just physical health. **Wellness** is a balance of all aspects of health—physical, mental and emotional, and social (**Figure 1.1**). To maintain wellness, you need to focus on all aspects of your health equally.

Figure 1.1
A combination of all aspects of health is necessary to form overall wellness.

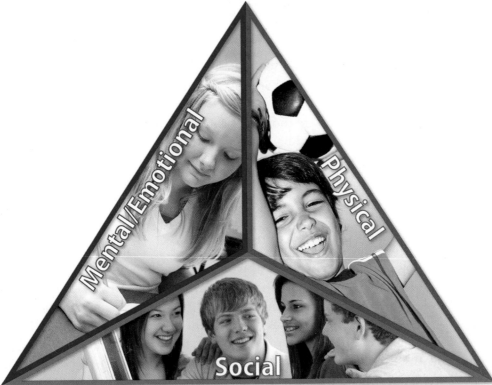

Left: Lisa F. Young/Shutterstock.com; Right: Anna Om/Shutterstock.com; Bottom: Monkey Business Images/Shutterstock.com

Physical Health

Physical health is the aspect of health that refers to how well your body functions. If you have a physically healthy body, you are not slowed by disease. Your body functions well. You are able to engage in the activities of daily life. You can also cope with the stresses of disease, injury, aging, and an active lifestyle. In other words, being physically healthy enables you to do more than walk to school or lift a bag of books. You can recover from a sprained ankle, fight off the flu, and have the energy to cope with daily stresses.

Mental and Emotional Health

Your **mental and emotional health** has to do with your internal life—your thoughts and feelings. When you have good mental and emotional health, you can think clearly and critically. You can express your thoughts and feelings. You can cope well with stress. You can also realize your own skills and have a positive attitude and willingness to adapt, learn, and grow.

Sometimes people do not recognize declines in their mental and emotional health. For example, you might experience ongoing feelings of sadness or worry that are not healthy. These feelings harm your mental and emotional health and can keep you from doing well in school or joining in your favorite activities. Poor mental and emotional health can also affect your sleep, diet, and activity level, and prevent you from forming friendships. The good news is that mental and emotional health issues can get better.

Social Health

Can you imagine your life with no human interaction? Living without contact from others is unhealthy. Humans are social animals who must interact and communicate with one another. **Social health** refers to how well you get along with other people.

Being socially healthy means having enjoyable and supportive relationships with others. In healthy relationships, you talk openly and honestly with family and friends. You trust others and others trust you. These are important parts of healthy relationships.

Unhealthy relationships are those that cause harm or make you feel bad about yourself. Social skills and healthy relationships give you the support you need to enjoy life and meet its challenges. Healthy relationships are among your most valuable resources.

Overall Well-Being

Well-being is a state of health and wellness in which people generally feel good about their present conditions. People in a state of well-being have a sense of fulfillment and engage in behaviors that promote health. They have a positive mood, are happy, and enjoy life. They get along well with others. They also have a sense of purpose and are productive at school, work, and home. In other words, personal well-being depends on good physical, mental and emotional, and social health.

Ways to Maintain Good Mental Health

Stay Connected to Others
Having fun with friends and family is a great way to fight loneliness and promote happiness.

Help Others
Making others feel good is a rewarding activity that will help you to feel good, too!

Get Professional Help If Needed
Talking to a professional about your troubles can help you to resolve them.

Stay Active
Exercise reduces stress and creates a chemical in the brain that causes feelings of happiness.

Sleep Properly
Sleep gives your mind and body time to rest and recharge so that you are ready to take on the day.

Manage Your Stress
By organizing your time and responsibilities properly, you can save yourself from feelings of panic or anxiety.

The aspects of your health are *interrelated*, meaning they all interact with and affect each other (**Figure 1.2**). Decline in one aspect of your health may lead to decline in another. Likewise, an improvement in one aspect of your health may lead to improvements in other aspects. Any changes in your health can affect your well-being.

For example, suppose someone who is overweight eats healthier, gets more activity, and becomes physically fit. Improvement in physical health can also affect all other aspects of health. Becoming more physically fit can improve how you feel about yourself and help you face challenges with a positive outlook (mental and emotional health). Being more active might result in participating in new activities with friends (social health). These positive changes can improve your overall health and well-being.

The Healthcare and Wellness Connection

Healthcare directly relates to wellness. **Healthcare** involves the treatment and prevention of illnesses, injuries, or diseases to improve wellness. Focusing on wellness means that you do not only go to the doctor to receive treatment when you are sick. You also go to the doctor when you are well to help you stay healthy (called *preventive healthcare*). **Preventive healthcare** involves getting an annual physical exam, regular checkups, and screenings for conditions like hearing or vision loss.

In the United States, healthcare comes in many forms, takes place in different settings, and is delivered by many types of professionals. The following sections will introduce you to different types of healthcare services and settings, and explore how people pay for healthcare.

Figure 1.2
Your physical health, mental and emotional health, and social health are all interrelated. *What does the term interrelated mean?*

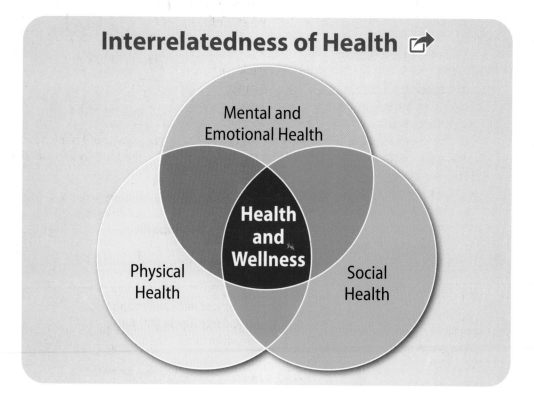

Interrelatedness of Health

Mental and Emotional Health

Physical Health

Health and Wellness

Social Health

Healthcare Services

The healthcare field employs more people than any other type of business in the United States. The field is diverse and includes many types of professions and healthcare services. Some professions provide highly specialized services.

People usually see their **primary care physician** (regular doctor) to get routine checkups, diagnosis of conditions, and receive medical treatment. Physician assistants and nurse practitioners also provide primary care.

The *physician assistant* works under the supervision of physicians. He or she usually provides the same types of healthcare services as a physician. A *nurse practitioner* has an advanced nursing education and can provide many of the same services as a doctor. Today, many people receive their primary care from physicians, physician assistants, and nurse practitioners.

CASE STUDY

A Day in the Life of Sarah

Next year, Sarah will be off to high school and almost old enough to get a job. Her mom works so hard, but there never seems to be enough money. As the oldest, it is Sarah's responsibility to take care of her younger siblings when her mom is at work. Sarah is an amazing big sister! She works so hard to take care of everyone else that she often does not take time to care for herself.

Sarah learned in school about the importance of eating healthy and being physically active to promote good health. Sarah is always so busy, though. She finds it a lot easier to grab some fast food at the restaurant down the street or some snacks at the nearby gas station on her way home from school. Sarah recently noticed that she has gained some weight.

Due to her mom's work schedule, Sarah cannot remember the last time she visited a doctor for a yearly check, until today that is. Sarah had to see the doctor because she has been thirsty and tired all the time, and her vision is blurred. The doctor informed Sarah's mother that Sarah's blood work indicated that she has type 2 diabetes and she needs to eat better to improve her health. She also has to take medicine now and check the level of sugar in her blood every day.

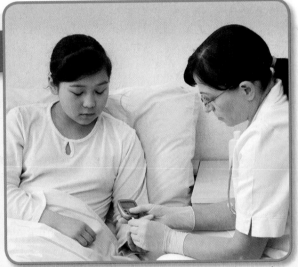

anetta/Shutterstock.com

Thinking Critically

1. How could preventive care have decreased the likelihood of Sarah's diagnosis of type 2 diabetes?

2. How might Sarah's life be different if Sarah and her mother received the guidance of a healthcare provider, such as a pediatrician?

3. If you were Sarah's doctor, what advice would you give Sarah and her mom to improve Sarah's health? Consider Sarah's obstacles to healthy eating and exercise.

4. How could Sarah's poor physical health affect her social and emotional health?

Primary care physicians may also refer their patients to *specialists* who possess extra training and experience with certain types of diseases and disorders. **Figure 1.3** shows the common types of specialists and the care they provide.

Healthcare Settings

Healthcare workers work in inpatient and outpatient facilities. *Inpatient facilities* are hospitals where patients stay while they receive diagnosis, treatment, surgery, and therapy. *Outpatient facilities* treat patients who live in the community and who do not require a hospital. Most healthcare in the United States is delivered in outpatient settings. These settings include the following:

- doctors' offices and private healthcare clinics that provide checkups, physical therapy, outpatient surgery, counseling, addiction treatment, and eye and dental care
- hospital emergency rooms
- urgent care or walk-in clinics
- health clinics and counseling centers in high schools and colleges
- county public health clinics

Health Insurance

How do people pay for healthcare? A three-day hospital stay costs an average of $30,000 and the cost to fix a broken leg is about $7,500. One medicine may cost more than $100 each month. A visit with a counselor can cost more than $100 for one hour each week. Healthcare is expensive, and most people cannot afford to pay the full cost of services.

Instead, people must buy insurance to help pay for healthcare costs. Most people get this insurance through their employers. Employers offer health insurance to full-time employees as a benefit. Many employers split the cost of an insurance plan with their employees. The two main types of insurance plans are the *health maintenance organization (HMO)* and the *preferred provider organization (PPO)*. **Figure 1.4** shows some of the differences between these two plans.

Figure 1.3
Each type of physician specialist has been expertly educated and trained in his or her particular field.
What type of specialist is a dermatologist?

Physician Specialists	
Specialist	**Treatment of...**
Cardiologist	heart disease
Dermatologist	skin conditions
Gastroenterologist	diseases and disorders of the digestive system
Neurologist	diseases and disorders of the brain, nerves, and spinal cord
Oncologist	cancer
Orthopedist	bones, joints, and muscle conditions
Pediatrician	medical conditions of children from infancy through adolescence
Psychiatrist	mental illnesses and disorders
Pulmonologist	breathing problems and lung diseases
Rheumatologist	diseases of the joints, such as arthritis
Surgeon	surgical problems, such as gallbladder or appendix removal
Urologist	urination problems

HMOs Versus PPOs	
HMO	**PPO**
• Must have a primary care physician (PCP) in network • PCP referral needed to see a specialist • Lower cost • Will not cover nonemergency out-of-network physician or hospital costs	• Do not need to have a primary care physician (PCP) • Referral is not needed to see a specialist • Higher monthly premiums • Will cover in-network or out-of-network costs (costs may be higher for out-of-network services)

Figure 1.4
Understanding the differences between a PPO and an HMO can help people choose the best plan to meet their needs. *Which type of plan—a PPO or an HMO—is most likely to have a lower monthly premium?*

The United States government funds some types of health insurance, such as Medicare and Medicaid. *Medicare* is insurance made available for people 65 years of age and older. Medicare is also available for people younger than 65 who are unable to work due to a disability. *Medicaid* pays healthcare costs of people living in poverty who have no way to pay for insurance or medical expenses. Medicaid receives part of its funding through the individual states.

Although insurance can help some people afford healthcare services, other individuals still cannot access healthcare. Barriers to accessing healthcare may include a lack of availability, high cost, and lack of insurance coverage. Without adequate healthcare, people cannot receive the care they need. As a result, they are more likely to have poor health status.

Lesson **1.1** Review

1. Describe the difference between health and wellness.
2. **True or false.** Focusing on wellness means that you go to the doctor to receive treatment only when you are sick.
3. The regular doctor patients see for routine checkups and medical treatment is a(n) _____.
4. What is the term for hospitals where patients stay while they receive diagnosis, treatment, surgery, and therapy?
5. **Critical thinking.** Explain how a decline in mental and emotional health can affect the other aspects of health.

Hands-On Activity

Working in groups of three, create a digital or paper collage that includes at least five pictures of healthy behaviors for each aspect of health: physical, mental and emotional, and social. Add captions to your photos as needed to clarify pictures. Display the completed collages throughout the classroom. Remaining in your group, conduct a gallery walk to view all of the collages and pick one, other than your own, that your group likes the best. Discuss your choice with the rest of the class, explaining why this collage is your favorite.

Recognizing Factors That Affect Health and Wellness

genes segments of DNA that determine the structure and function of a person's cells and affect his or her development, personality, and health

family history record of a disease's presence and impact within a family

risk factors aspects of people's lives that increase the chances that they will develop a disease or disorder

environment circumstances, objects, or conditions that surround a person in everyday life

physical environment places where a person spends his or her time, such as school, home, or workplace; the region in which a person lives; the air a person breathes; and the water a person drinks

social environment people with whom a person interacts, such as family members, friends, peers, teachers, coaches, neighbors, and coworkers

peers people who are similar in age to one another

culture beliefs, values, customs, and arts of a group of people

economic environment person's level of education and income level

Learning Outcomes

After studying this lesson, you will be able to

- **identify** factors that can increase or reduce your level of health and wellness.
- **describe** actions you can take to help prevent genetically linked diseases and disorders.
- **give examples** of risk factors within a person's physical, social, and economic environments.
- **evaluate** how the lifestyle choices you make now can affect your health and wellness in the future.

Graphic Organizer ↪

Health and Wellness Risk Factors

While you are reading this lesson, think about the important facts you discover and areas you still question. After you finish reading, fill in a T-chart like the one below.

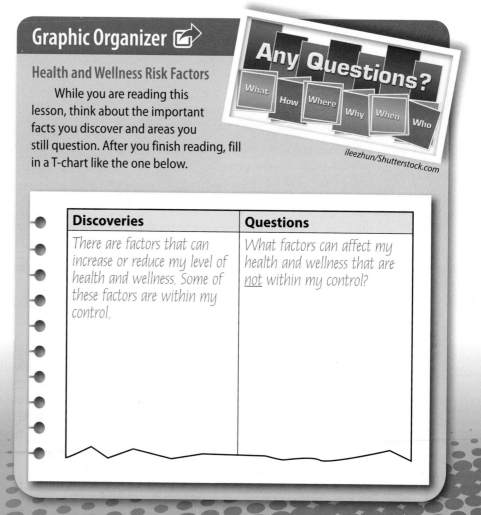

ileezhun/Shutterstock.com

Discoveries	Questions
There are factors that can increase or reduce my level of health and wellness. Some of these factors are within my control.	What factors can affect my health and wellness that are <u>not</u> within my control?

How would you describe your current health status? Are you in excellent health, or are you in poor health? Do you fall somewhere in between? If you have *optimal health*, you have the best health possible. You are in a state of excellent health and wellness in all areas of your life. This includes your physical, mental and emotional, and social health. A person's health status normally lies somewhere between the extremes of poor and excellent. This is because most people experience one or more problems that put their health status somewhere in the middle of the health and wellness spectrum.

Recall the examples of Hannah and Aiden from Lesson 1.1. Hannah passed her physical exam, but her health is far from excellent. Factors such as her stress, anxiety, and smoking habit negatively impact her health. On the other hand, Aiden has some physical health issues, but he does not smoke or drink, and he has a positive outlook on life. Hannah and Aiden each fall somewhere in the middle of the health and wellness spectrum.

As you can see in **Figure 1.5**, there are factors that can increase or reduce your level of health and wellness. Some of these factors, such as genetic factors, are not within your control. Many of the factors, however, are within your control. For example, a person who smokes can increase his or her level of health and wellness by quitting smoking. The choices you make now largely determine your level of health and wellness, both today and in the future.

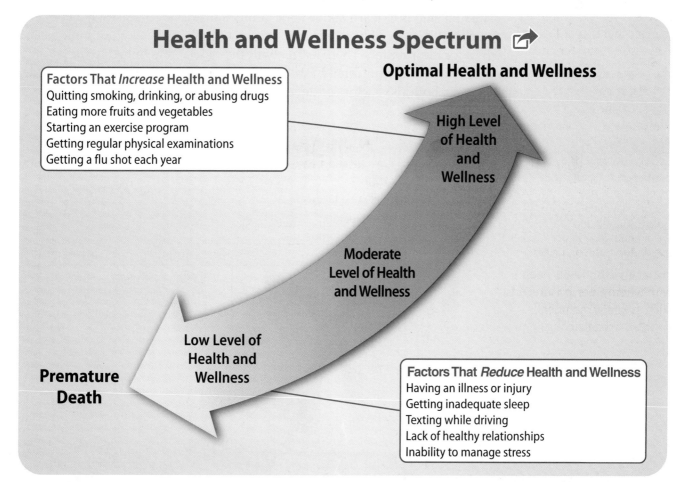

Health and Wellness Spectrum

Optimal Health and Wellness

Factors That *Increase* Health and Wellness
Quitting smoking, drinking, or abusing drugs
Eating more fruits and vegetables
Starting an exercise program
Getting regular physical examinations
Getting a flu shot each year

High Level of Health and Wellness

Moderate Level of Health and Wellness

Low Level of Health and Wellness

Premature Death

Factors That *Reduce* Health and Wellness
Having an illness or injury
Getting inadequate sleep
Texting while driving
Lack of healthy relationships
Inability to manage stress

Figure 1.5 Your level of health and wellness can be plotted on a spectrum. The choices you make largely determine where you are on the spectrum. *What kind of health do you have if you are at the top of the health and wellness spectrum?*

Genetic Risk Factors

The term *genetic* relates to your genes. Your **genes** are present in every cell in your body and contain the blueprint for the structure and function of your cells. Genes direct how you grow and develop, influence your personality, and affect your health. Humans have 20,000 to 25,000 genes, which are composed of a chemical often referred to as *DNA*.

Located in a cell's nucleus, genes are bundled in packages called *chromosomes* (**Figure 1.6**). Humans inherit half of their chromosomes from each parent. The unique combination of genes from your parents determines many of your body's characteristics. For example, perhaps the shape of your nose is the same as the shape of your father's nose. Maybe your hair is red and wavy, just like your mother's hair. Perhaps you have blue eyes like your parents.

The genes you receive from your parents can affect your health and wellness by putting you at risk for developing certain diseases, such as heart disease. In this way, your family influences your health. To determine a person's genetic *risk factors* for developing a disease, doctors study a person's **family history**, the record of disease within a family. **Risk factors** are aspects of people's lives that increase the chances that they will develop a disease or disorder. Although you are "stuck" with the genes you receive, there are actions you can take to reduce the risk factors for developing genetically linked diseases and disorders.

The first step is to learn about your family's history of diseases. Do you have a family history of heart disease, cancer, or diabetes? Ask your biological relatives for information. Then, learn about the risk factors linked to the diseases that run in your family. For example, leading an inactive lifestyle and smoking are both risk factors of developing heart disease.

Figure 1.6
Each cell in your body contains a total of 46 chromosomes (23 pairs), which hold about 20,000 to 25,000 genes. One set of 23 chromosomes is inherited from your biological mother and the other set of 23 is from your biological father.

Cell Structure

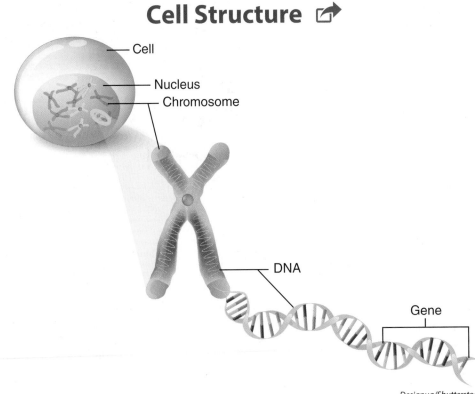

- Cell
- Nucleus
- Chromosome
- DNA
- Gene

Designua/Shutterstock.com

Preventable Risk Factors

INACTIVITY

increases risk for high blood pressure, stroke, diabetes, obesity, and heart disease

NEW PLAYER   START

Excessive Alcohol Consumption
can cause liver disease, pancreatitis, brain damage, heart issues, ulcers, and immune disorders

Warning
Smoking can cause lung disease and cancer and worsen asthma

Nutrition Facts
An unhealthy diet can lead to obesity, heart disease, and diabetes

Screen and game control: 4zevar/Shutterstock.com; Bottle and glass: Vector Goddess/Shutterstock.com; Cigarettes: VikiVector/Shutterstock.com; Nutrition label: LinGraphics/Shutterstock.com; French fries: supirloko89/Shutterstock.com

Once you have this information, you can try to eliminate or reduce your risk factors for these diseases. Eliminating extra risk factors for a certain disease will lower your chances of getting that disease. Reducing these risk factors is just another way you can improve your health and wellness.

Environmental Risk Factors

A person's environment can greatly impact his or her health. Your **environment** includes the circumstances, objects, or conditions that surround you in your everyday life. It consists of your physical, social, and economic environment.

In general, your environment is probably a safe place. Every environment, however, has risk factors that can affect health and wellness. The more you are exposed to risk factors within your environment, the more likely those factors are to reduce your level of health and wellness.

Physical Environment

Your **physical environment** consists of the places where you spend your time, such as your school, home, or workplace. Physical environment also consists of the region in which you live, the air you breathe, and the water you drink.

Risk factors within your physical environment differ from region to region, home to home, and school to school (**Figure 1.7**). Some hazards may include weather conditions, pollution, violence, unsafe drinking water, and other unsafe conditions. Certain hazards may depend on the policies at your school or in your community. To reduce the risk factors in your physical environment, you must first identify any hazards and unsafe conditions. Then, you can develop a plan of action to make your environment a safer place.

Figure 1.7
Your environment impacts your health and wellness. *Give some examples of how environmental risk factors can vary from one person to the next.*

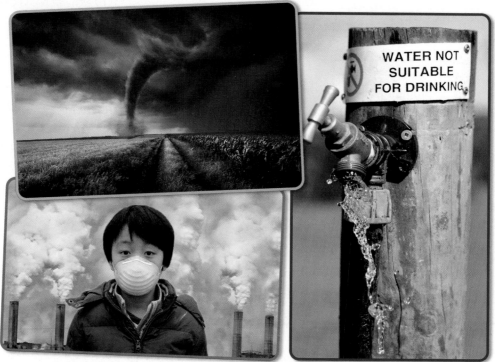

Clockwise from upper left: Rasica/Shutterstock.com; ChameleonsEye/Shutterstock.com; Hung Chung Chih/Shutterstock.com

Social Environment

The people around you make up your **social environment**. Your social environment may include family members, friends, **peers** (people similar in age to you), teachers, coaches, neighbors, and coworkers. The people you interact with on social media sites are a part of your social environment, too.

BUILDING Your Skills

The Power of Social Media to Inspire

How often do you spend time on social media sites? What kinds of messages do you receive in your online social community? Do the people within your social media network promote positive, healthy behaviors or negative, risky behaviors?

Social media can be a powerful tool to inspire healthy behaviors. It can also influence you to engage in risky behaviors, such as smoking, alcohol usage, or sexual activity. Just as peer pressure from your friends and classmates can impact the decisions you make regarding your health, so can the content you view on social media.

If the social network that you see on a day-to-day basis promotes unhealthy eating habits, doing drugs, or bullying, you may feel more pressured to participate in these activities yourself. Exposure to posts by your classmates with mean comments or embarrassing photographs, for example, might make you think you need to do this too in order to fit in with the group.

Pay attention to how these posts impact the way you might think about risky behaviors. Carefully choose who you follow on social media based on how their messages could impact the way you view your own health and wellness. Surround yourself with a social network that cultivates a respectful, safe, and overall healthy lifestyle. In addition, inspire others to live this kind of lifestyle too, through the content you post on social media.

Inspire a Healthy Life

In this activity, you will create an inspiring digital representation of a social media post that encourages a healthy behavior. The materials you need depend on how you want to create your visual representation. You may choose to use a social media template or a paper representation using poster board or construction paper. To create your digital representation, complete the following steps:

1. Identify a healthy behavior that is meaningful and relevant to you, your classmates, or your friends. Topic examples may include green living, healthy eating, antismoking, physical activity, or other topics of interest. The healthy behavior you choose should positively affect a person's physical, mental and emotional, or social health.

2. Create a representation on the social media platform of your choice to raise awareness of this healthy behavior. Your digital representation may include infographics, pictures with captions to illustrate this behavior, famous quotes, and a hashtag or other link to a larger health community. Add other details as needed to make your representation inspiring, informative, creative, and visually appealing.

3. With permission, display these social media healthy posts around the classroom or throughout the school to inspire your peers. You may also want to post your message on a social media site, with permission, to get feedback from your online social community.

Antonio Francois/Shutterstock.com

In addition to the people in your life, your **culture** (the beliefs, values, customs, and arts of a group of people) is also a part of your social environment. The cultural practices and behaviors of your social group affect your health and wellness. Cultural practices that may affect your social environment can include food and taste preferences and eating patterns. Religious or spiritual practices, activity preferences, and medical treatment and customs are other examples.

The risk factors in your social environment depend on the practices and behaviors of those in your group and their influences on you. If your parents practice healthy eating habits, you are more likely to practice them as well. If your friends smoke or drink and pressure you to do so, your risk of engaging in these harmful behaviors increases, too. To reduce the risk factors within your social environment, maintain healthy relationships with others and focus on engaging in healthy behaviors.

Economic Environment

Your **economic environment** includes your level of education and income level. Through different studies, scientists have linked higher education and higher income to better health. Exactly how this works is unclear. Perhaps people with more education have access to more information about nutrition and physical activity. More education may also enable people to earn more money and, therefore, have access to better healthcare. If this is true, focusing on education is key to reducing risk factors in a person's economic environment.

Lifestyle Risk Factors

The way you choose to live your life can greatly affect your health and wellness (**Figure 1.8**). For example, what you choose to eat and drink affects your health. How active or inactive you are makes a difference in your level of health, too.

Figure 1.8
Often, the habits we form as children, such as eating healthy foods and being physically active, impact our lifestyle choices as we get older.

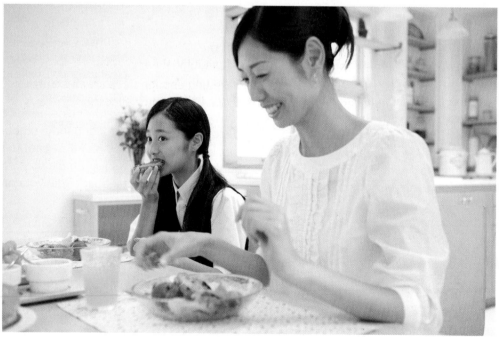

TAGSTOCK1/Shutterstock.com

How much sleep you get each night can also have an impact on your health and wellness. Engaging in risky behaviors, such as drinking, smoking, or doing drugs, can reduce your level of health and wellness. Texting while driving is also an example of a risky behavior that can be a hazard to your health.

Some behaviors have an immediate impact on health and wellness. If you did not get enough sleep last night, you may lack energy and have trouble focusing. Other behaviors have both short-term and long-term effects. Sun exposure is just one example. Spending too much time in the sun can result in the short-term effect of sunburn. Regularly spending too much time in the sun without using sunscreen can increase your risk of developing skin cancer.

Many of the lifestyle choices you make and behaviors you develop begin in childhood and adolescence. Oftentimes, these behaviors continue into adulthood and can affect your health for years to come. If you have an inactive lifestyle as a child, you are more likely to become physically inactive as an adult. Inactive adults have a higher risk of developing high blood pressure and heart disease.

Parents and culture often influence lifestyle choices and behaviors that begin in childhood and adolescence. If your parents stay up late on a regular basis, you are more likely to stay up late as well. If your culture does not believe in taking medication, you will likely feel the same way. Your parents and culture may be a strong influence on you when you are young.

Making healthy lifestyle choices and practicing healthy behaviors promote your personal health and wellness today and in the future. Even if you do not make healthy lifestyle choices now, you have the power to change your behavior and take charge of your health and wellness.

Lesson 1.2 Review

1. What is the record of disease from within your biological family called?
2. Name the three types of environments that can affect a person's health and wellness.
3. **True or false.** Risk factors in your social environment depend on the practices and behaviors of those in your group and their influences on you.
4. Eating unhealthy foods, smoking, and not getting enough sleep are all examples of _____ that can negatively impact your health and wellness.
5. **Critical thinking.** Give an example of a cultural practice that influences your family's health and wellness. Is this an example of a positive influence or a negative influence?

Hands-On Activity

In small groups, create a role play and script that shows the importance of making healthy lifestyle choices today to promote personal health and wellness in the future. Your role play may include preventive actions young people can take to avoid peer pressure to engage in unhealthy behaviors or it can focus on how to change an unhealthy behavior. Practice your role play and present it to the rest of the class.

Building Skills for Health and Wellness

decision-making skills tools a person uses to make good choices about health and wellness

collaborate work together

goal plan of action that will guide someone in achieving something he or she wants to reach

SMART goals plan of action that is specific, measurable, achievable, relevant, and timely

refusal skills strategies you can use to stand up to pressures and influences that want you to engage in unhealthy behaviors

conflict resolution skills strategies that can help you deal with arguments in a positive, respectful way to promote healthy relationships

mediation method of resolving conflict that involves a third, neutral party

mediator neutral third party who helps resolve conflicts by listening carefully to each person's point of view

health literacy person's ability to locate, interpret, and apply information as it relates to his or her health

advocate support or recommend

Learning Outcomes

After studying this lesson, you will be able to

- **demonstrate** decision-making and goal-setting skills.
- **describe** how refusal skills help people avoid unhealthy behaviors.
- **identify** conflict management strategies.
- **demonstrate** how to access and evaluate health-related information.
- **explain** how to communicate about health topics.

Graphic Organizer 📲

Health and Wellness Skills

Each section of this organizer represents a set of skills necessary to achieve and maintain your health and wellness. As you read the lesson, record what you have learned by filling in the graphic organizer with techniques for mastering these skills.

Duncan Andison/Shutterstock.com

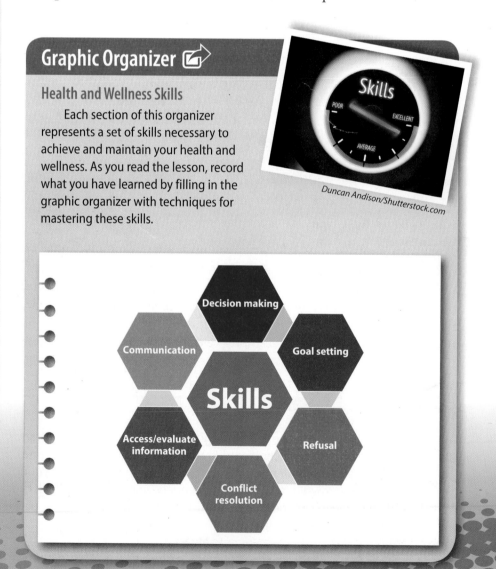

What is the best way to control asthma, muscle cramps, or acne? What can you do to manage the stress in your life? How can you help a friend who is going through a crisis? Do you know how you would find answers to these questions—good, reliable answers? You would not want answers based on rumors or unreliable sources of information.

Knowledge is power. Health knowledge gives you the power to prevent disease and promote your well-being. Consider Hannah and Aiden's situations, as described in the previous lessons. Hannah might improve her mental and emotional health if she researched counseling resources in her area. Aiden must be careful to get the best possible information about his breathing condition. With the right skills and resources, you can apply that knowledge and successfully take charge of your own health and wellness.

Making Decisions and Setting Goals

Decision-making skills are tools you can use to make choices about your health and wellness. Decision-making and goal-setting skills will help you move closer to and maintain optimal health and wellness. These skills will serve you well in all aspects of your life.

Making Healthy Decisions

You make decisions each day that affect your health and wellness. For instance, should you stay up late playing video games, or should you get a good night's sleep? Should you exercise on a painful knee? Should you eat that second piece of pie? Many everyday situations offer you healthy and unhealthy options (**Figure 1.9**). Choosing the healthy option is important to avoid injury or health risks.

Being able to make healthy decisions involves skill. Some decisions you make will be easy, while others will be much more difficult. Deciding whether to eat an apple or a piece of apple pie is a relatively easy decision when you want to be healthy. Deciding what course of action to take in a health crisis, however, requires much more thought.

Your personal needs, wants, values, and priorities are factors that will influence the decisions you make. Your *needs* are the things you must have to live, such as air, water, sleep, food, clothing, and housing. Your *wants* are the things you desire or would like to have. *Values* are the things that are important to you in life. Examples of values include family, peers, culture, health, and happiness. The things you value the most become your *priorities*.

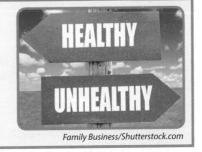

Healthy or Unhealthy Choices

1. Interact positively with others on social media.
2. Eat fast food when you are stressed or in a rush.
3. Get enough sleep every night.
4. Frequently go to a tanning bed.
5. Spend time with people who make you doubt your self-esteem.
6. Honestly communicate your feelings to others.

Family Business/Shutterstock.com

Figure 1.9
Each of these examples of lifestyle choices is either healthy or unhealthy. *Which of these choices are healthy and which are unhealthy?*

How you approach making a decision is important. Sometimes you may make a decision on your own. Other times, you may **collaborate** (work together) with others to make a group decision. Collaborating with others can give you options you may not have considered otherwise. Still other times, you may want to seek the advice of your family or friends. When you do ask others for their opinions, consider how their advice aligns with your values and priorities. In this way, you are more likely to make a good decision.

Making good decisions involves skill. You can use the decision-making process in **Figure 1.10** as a guide to help you make good, healthy decisions.

Setting and Reaching Goals

Goals are important for many aspects of life, including your health. Therefore, learning the skills you need to set and work toward goals is important. A **goal** is a plan of action that will guide you in achieving something you want to reach. A goal often involves adopting, maintaining, or improving a health practice. Do you have goals regarding your physical, mental, or social wellness?

Goals can be short-term or long-term. A *short-term goal* is a goal you want to accomplish in the near future, or within days or weeks. A *long-term goal* requires more time—months or years—to achieve. Reaching a long-term goal may involve achieving a series of short-term goals. Effective goals are **SMART goals**. SMART stands for *specific, measurable, achievable, relevant,* and *timely* (**Figure 1.11**).

Remember that not all goals are appropriate for all people. Before you set a goal, determine your values, or what is important to you, and assess your current situation. Your goals may change as your priorities change and you learn new abilities. Mastering goal-setting skills will enable you to continually grow and improve yourself, your health, and your overall well-being.

Using Refusal Skills

Refusal skills are strategies you can use to stand up to pressures and influences that want you to engage in unhealthy behaviors. These skills can help you respond to peer influences and conflicting messages without compromising your own goals, values, and health.

Figure 1.10
Using the decision-making process can help you choose the healthy path for even the most difficult decisions. *What is it called when you work with others to make a group decision?*

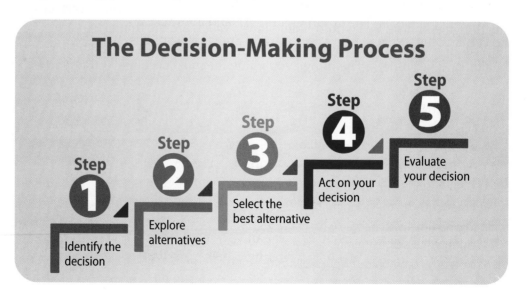

The Decision-Making Process

Step **1** Identify the decision

Step **2** Explore alternatives

Step **3** Select the best alternative

Step **4** Act on your decision

Step **5** Evaluate your decision

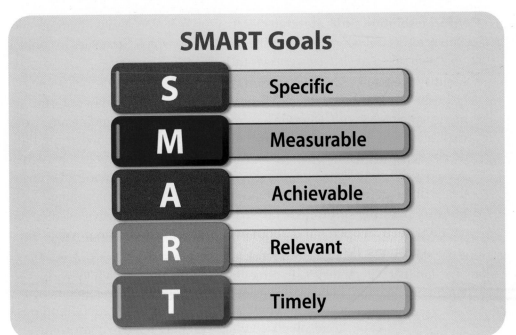

SMART Goals

S Specific

M Measurable

A Achievable

R Relevant

T Timely

Figure 1.11 Short-term SMART goals should add up to help you reach one or more long-term SMART goals.

For example, you might be pressured to use drugs, cigarettes, or alcohol. You could be pressured to engage in an activity that is illegal, inappropriate, or unhealthy. Your peers might pressure you into these activities, or you might see these behaviors modeled in television shows and movies you watch. You may think that this is what all young people are doing. These influences can make saying *no* difficult.

Using refusal skills helps you take responsibility for your health behaviors. By using refusal skills, you ensure that no one is responsible for your health but you. Practicing strong refusal skills will also help you avoid or reduce health risks. Behaviors such as smoking or drinking increase your risk of certain health issues. Refusing to engage in these behaviors helps you avoid the health risks associated with them.

Refusal skills help you make independent, informed decisions despite messages you may receive from peers, society, and the media. The tips in **Figure 1.12**, and information throughout this text, will help you learn and apply refusal skills to resist pressure.

Resolving Conflicts

As people interact with one another, *conflicts* (disagreements) are bound to arise. Conflicts can occur when people have different opinions or priorities. You may even have conflicts with your family or friends. Conflicts are a normal part of life. Some conflicts can be healthy, letting you see another person's point of view and even build relationships. Conflicts that are unhealthy cause stress and put strain on relationships.

Tips for Resisting Pressure

- Watch your body language—stand up straight and make eye contact.
- Say how you feel—use a firm voice to say *no*.
- Be honest and do not make excuses—your friends should accept your response when you say, "No, I don't want to." Remember, you have the right not to give a reason.
- Suggest something else to do—if your friends do not want to do another activity, find another friend who does.
- Stick up for yourself—be prepared to walk away to get out of the situation.

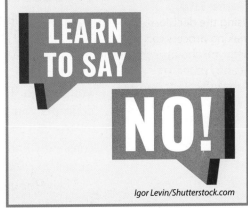

Igor Levin/Shutterstock.com

Figure 1.12 Pressure from others can be difficult to resist, but you have a right to say "no" and walk away from the situation.

Conflict resolution skills are strategies that can help you deal with arguments in a positive, respectful way to promote healthy relationships. Strategies in conflict resolution (also called *conflict management*) include the following:

- **Identify the issue.** Have each person who is part of the conflict state what he or she thinks is the problem. Listen carefully to what the other person has to say. Share your feelings in a calm manner and avoid getting angry or frustrated, which can make a conflict worse. State your opinions firmly, but do not demand that the other person agree with you. Remember that each person is different. There is nothing wrong with someone having an opinion that is different from yours. Differences make people more interesting.
- **Identify possible solutions.** Have each person think of ways to solve the conflict. Keep an open mind about everyone's ideas and do not rule out any suggestions. Be creative.

- **Begin the negotiation process.** *Negotiation* involves calmly discussing an issue to reach an agreement that is acceptable to all parties involved. Oftentimes, to resolve a conflict, you may have to compromise. A *compromise* is a solution in which each side of a disagreement gives in a little (**Figure 1.13**).
- **Carry out the decision.** Be sure everyone follows through on what he or she agreed to during the negotiation process. If for some reason the solution is not working, you may need to renegotiate.

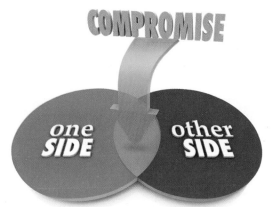

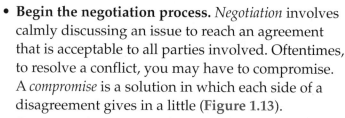

iQoncept/Shutterstock.com

Figure 1.13 Compromise is all about finding the middle ground between the disagreeing parties. *Why is it important to deal with arguments in a positive, respectful way?*

In some cases, a conflict is too serious or too difficult for the people directly involved to manage by themselves. In this situation, an outside individual with a neutral perspective can help the people or groups find a good solution.

Mediation is a strategy for resolving difficult conflicts by involving a neutral third party, or **mediator**. During mediation, both parties in the conflict separately share their perspective of the conflict with the mediator. The mediator then brings the two parties together to share their views and tries to help them reach an agreement.

Accessing and Evaluating Health Information and Services

As you learn about health-related terms, concepts, and facts, you will develop the ability to locate, interpret, and apply information as it relates to your health. This is **health literacy**. Your health literacy builds on basic facts and concepts you learn at home and at school.

As you learn about health and wellness, you will discover that researchers are constantly finding out new information about the human body and its health. This means you will need to keep learning about health and wellness throughout your life.

Developing health literacy means you can also evaluate health-related products and services. Health literacy helps you analyze advertisements for products (**Figure 1.14**). With health literacy skills, you can find out whether various products actually promote health. Health literacy can help you determine which health services are right for you.

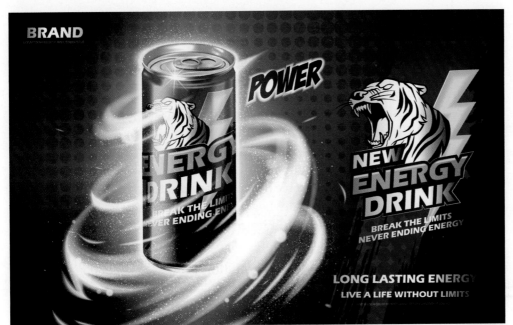

Figure 1.14
Health literacy helps you to analyze advertisements, such as this one. *What health claim is being made in this advertisement?*

Technology can influence your health literacy. By using the Internet and a few key search words, you can find lots of health-related information. Just because health information is on the Internet, however, does not make it accurate or true. Developing health literacy can help you locate reliable health-related information on the Internet and evaluate health claims.

Locating Reliable Information

Your health and wellness depend on your use of reliable information. You need to be able to tell information grounded in science from health claims based on rumors, opinions, and theories. *Science* is a body of knowledge regarding the natural world, based on observation and experimentation. Science poses questions and proposes explanations about the natural world—including the human body, human health, and diseases. Scientists test these explanations repeatedly to prove or disprove them as factual. Therefore, science-based information is reliable, unlike opinions and theories that have not been tested and verified as fact (**Figure 1.15**).

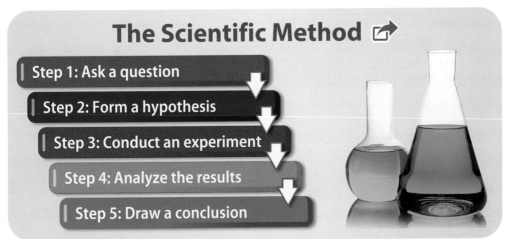

The Scientific Method

Step 1: Ask a question
Step 2: Form a hypothesis
Step 3: Conduct an experiment
Step 4: Analyze the results
Step 5: Draw a conclusion

Figure 1.15
To find reliable health-related information, always try to find evidence provided by the scientific method. *What is the name of the ability to locate, interpret, and apply health-related information?*

When using the Internet to answer questions about your health, you will see several websites. How do you decide which source you should trust? In general, you can find reliable information from agencies or organizations whose main mission is education, research, or providing direct healthcare. Safe or reliable URL stems generally include *.gov*, *.edu*, and *.org*.

Websites of businesses that earn profits from the healthcare industry are often not trustworthy. The main goal of a business is to make money by selling the product or service it provides. Information from a business may play up the benefits of the product or service and play down or omit any negative information. Locating reliable information can help you locate reliable health-related products and services as well.

When searching for information, begin with a reliable, general source such as one of the agencies or websites in **Figure 1.16**. When in doubt, ask your school librarian or doctor about a reliable media source to find information about health and wellness. Librarians specialize in finding and evaluating sources, which means you can rely on their advice should questions arise.

Evaluating Health Claims

"Get six-pack abs in two weeks!"
"You will catch a cold if you go outside with wet hair."
"The bumps on your skull reveal your character."
"Cell phones cause brain cancer."
"Caffeinated energy drinks will make you perform better on exams."

These are some examples of the thousands of health claims you can find in magazines, on websites, and in advertisements. Claims such as these are not supported by science. What is at stake if you believe health claims not

Figure 1.16
These websites from reputable government and health agencies are a great place to start when looking for accurate health-related information. ***What are three examples of safe or reliable URL stems?***

Health and Safety Information	
Sources of Information	**URLs**
Academy of Nutrition and Dietetics	www.eatright.org
American Academy of Pediatrics	www.aap.org
American Cancer Society	www.cancer.org
American Heart Association	www.heart.org
American Red Cross	www.redcross.org
Centers for Disease Control and Prevention (CDC)	www.cdc.gov
Mayo Clinic	www.mayoclinic.org
MedlinePlus® (U.S. National Library of Medicine, National Institutes of Health)	www.nlm.nih.gov/medlineplus/
National Highway Traffic Safety Administration	www.nhtsa.gov
National Institute of Mental Health	www.nimh.nih.gov
National Institute on Drug Abuse	www.drugabuse.gov
Office of the Surgeon General	www.surgeongeneral.gov
Tufts University Health & Nutrition Letter	www.nutritionletter.tufts.edu
United States Consumer Products Safety Commission	www.cpsc.gov
United States Department of Agriculture	www.choosemyplate.gov
United States Department of Health and Human Services	www.healthfinder.gov
United States Food and Drug Administration	www.fda.gov
World Health Organization	www.who.int

based in science? You can waste money and time, and you can harm your health. This is why carefully evaluating health-related information is so important.

Refer to the information in **Figure 1.17** to learn more about evaluating health websites. You can also use the following tips to help you evaluate specific health-related articles in print or online. Remember, if a health claim sounds too good to be true, it probably is.

- The information is in a news story, not in an opinion piece or editorial.
- The story refers to research published by medical scientists.
- The story gives the names of the researchers and the journal in which the original work is published.
- You can find other stories with the same results.
- The newspaper, magazine, or website is not produced by a company that manufactures or sells medicine or medical devices.

Evaluating Health Websites

Checklist for Evaluating Web Pages	Hints
• Is the sponsor a respectable organization? If there is an author, is he or she an expert in the field?	• The organization or sponsor should be visible in the header. The author name is typically listed at the top of each article.
• When was the web page created? When was it last updated?	• The publication and update dates should be in the headers or footers of resources.
• Does the URL end in *.gov*, *.edu*, or *.org*?	• *.net* and *.com* websites are less likely to be reliable health-related information sources.
• Does the resource cite the sources for all statistics, data, or other health claims?	• All sources should be listed at the bottom of articles as footnotes.
• Are any digital sources correctly linked to active web pages?	• Broken links (to pages that no longer exist or have been moved) can indicate incorrect or outdated information.

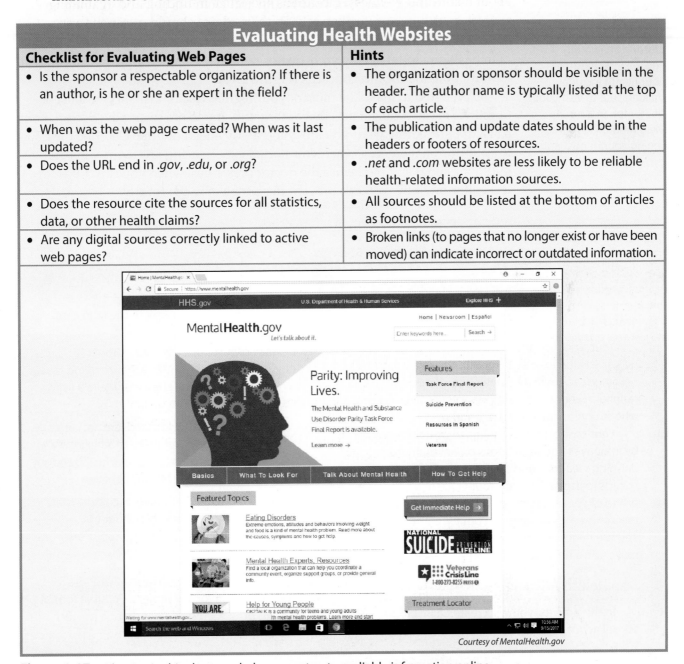

Courtesy of MentalHealth.gov

Figure 1.17   The tips in this chart can help you sort out unreliable information online.

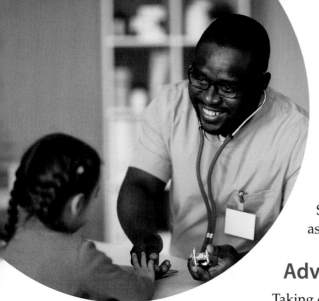

Pressmaster/Shutterstock.com

Figure 1.18
Starting at a young age, taking charge of your health includes making sure to visit your doctor for an annual examination as well as seeing your dentist and eye doctor regularly.

Communicating About Health

When you tell someone you are not feeling well, you are communicating about your health. If you encourage a family member to choose a healthy behavior, you are using your communication skills to enhance the health of others. You can use your communication skills to spread awareness of health-related issues in your community. Sometimes you must also use your communication skills to ask for help as you try to lead a healthy life.

Advocating for Personal Health

Taking charge of your health and wellness involves playing an active role in your healthcare and advocating for your personal health. To **advocate** is to support or recommend something publicly. Supporting your own health includes seeing your doctor regularly for checkups, which can help identify potential health concerns (**Figure 1.18**).

Be prepared to make the most of your regular doctor visits. Write a list of questions in case you get nervous or forgetful. If you are seeing the doctor about a health issue, know what you are going to say ahead of time. Describe the issue to your doctor, including when you started experiencing any symptoms. Ask questions about any medicines the doctor prescribes, when you can expect to feel better, and how you can prevent this problem in the future.

BUILDING Your Skills

Your School Environment

Your school environment can have a positive or a negative influence on your health. Unhealthy food and beverage choices in the cafeteria can diminish student nutrition. School counseling services can help students who struggle with their mental and emotional health.

Your school environment can be influenced by initiatives and regulations on anything from banning weapons and alcohol to building speed bumps in the parking lot. Your voice or a collective group of voices has the power to change a school environment. Speaking up about your health needs and the needs of those around you is what can make you a health advocate in your community.

Be a Health Advocate at School

In this activity, you will create an inspiring school advocacy project for a new health initiative.

To create your initiative, complete the following steps:

1. In small groups, discuss your school environment and what actions are being taken to encourage healthy students. Make a list of these positive actions.

2. Next, discuss which health needs are not currently being met at your school. Make another list of the actions not being taken to improve health and any actions that discourage healthy behavior.

3. Identify one school initiative or change that would improve the health of students.

4. Create a plan to gather student awareness and support to create this change.

5. Create a product to help raise awareness for your school advocacy project. Possible formats for this product include handmade posters, social media posts, and petitions.

Advocating for Family Health

In addition to advocating for your own health, you can also advocate for the health of your family members. Just as your family influences your health, you can influence the health of your family members. Hearing you advocate for their health may cause family members to change unhealthy behaviors.

For example, if your mother smokes, consider encouraging her to try quitting. Smoking causes many health issues, and quitting can help reduce a person's risk for those issues. You can research the health risks of smoking and present the information to your mother. You can tell her that you love her, and that you want her to be around for a long time. If your mother decides to quit smoking, support her as she goes through the process of quitting.

Advocating for family health may also include spreading health information to those who cannot use technology. The Internet can be a helpful source of health information. Some older individuals, however, may not know how to access this information (**Figure 1.19**). If your grandparents have health-related questions, you can help them by researching the topic on the Internet. You can give them this information in a format they are more likely to understand.

Advocating for Community Health

As you learned in Lesson 1.2, your environment influences your health. Your environment includes the policies that exist in your community. Advocating for your personal health may mean advocating for the health of your community.

For example, suppose your state has a high rate of obesity. To advocate for your state's health, you could write to your elected officials about supporting a healthy eating program. On a local level, you could start a fitness club at school. You could also attend community meetings and speak up about health issues that concern you.

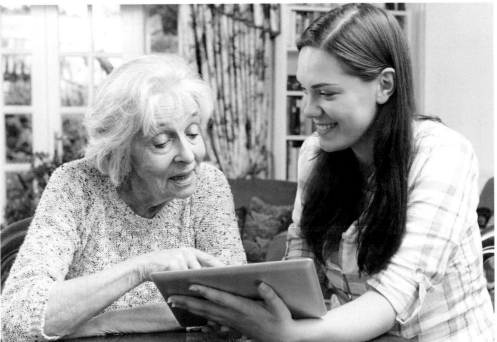

Figure 1.19
Many elderly family members may be unable to use new digital devices or to find health-related information on the Internet. Helping them do so is one way of advocating for your family's health.

SpeedKingz/Shutterstock.com

Advocating for your community may also include spreading awareness of health issues. You can make posters explaining the hazards of unhealthy behaviors, such as smoking and underage drinking. Display these posters at your school to help educate your fellow students.

Asking for Assistance

Everyone needs help sometimes. Health issues can be complicated, and you may need help to handle them. If you want more information about a health issue, you can ask a healthcare professional for help. Perhaps you feel sick and need to ask for help in getting treatment. If you are worried about a friend who is engaging in unhealthy behaviors, you can ask a school counselor how to help your friend.

Sometimes advocating for personal, family, or community health requires a group effort. You might ask your siblings to help you talk with a parent about his or her smoking habit. You might ask for your friends' help to create health awareness posters. Collaborating with others can increase your personal ability to advocate for health.

Lesson 1.3 Review

1. What are the five steps to making a good, healthy decision?
2. What are SMART goals?
3. To stand up to pressures and influences toward unhealthy behaviors, you can build _____ skills.
4. Health _____ is the ability to locate, interpret, and apply information as it relates to your health.
5. **Critical thinking.** Give an example of a long-term goal and the series of short-term goals involved in achieving it. Make sure that your goals are SMART.

Hands-On Activity

Imagine that the following text messages were sent to you during this school year:

> My mom cooked. LOL Want to walk to McDonald's?

> Nobody is home tonight. Want to come over and get drunk?

> Hey, can we play video games today instead of going to the park?

On a separate sheet of paper, respond to the text messages using refusal skills and conflict resolution skills. With a partner, share how you responded to the text messages and discuss how refusing these offers would help maintain good health and wellness.

Review and Assessment

Summary

Lesson 1.1 Defining Health and Wellness

- The term *health* usually refers to the absence of physical illness and disease. *Wellness* is a balance of all aspects of health—physical, mental and emotional, and social.
- *Well-being* is a state of health and wellness in which you generally feel good about your present condition.
- Personal well-being depends on good physical, mental and emotional, and social health. These aspects of your health are *interrelated*, meaning they all interact with and affect each other.
- Focusing on wellness means that you not only go to the doctor to receive treatment when you are sick, you also go to the doctor when you are well to help you stay healthy.

Lesson 1.2 Recognizing Factors That Affect Health and Wellness

- *Risk factors* are aspects of your life that increase the chances you will develop a disease or disorder. Some risk factors, such as genetic factors, are not within your control. Many environmental and lifestyle risk factors, however, are within your control.
- Your *environment* includes the circumstances, objects, or conditions that surround you in everyday life and affect your health and wellness. This includes your physical, social, and economic environments.
- Your *physical environment* consists of the places where you spend your time, the region in which you live, the air you breathe, and the water you drink. Your *social environment* includes the people in your life and your culture (the beliefs, values, customs, and arts of a group of people). Your *economic environment* includes your level of education and income level.
- Making healthy lifestyle choices and practicing healthy behaviors promote your personal health and wellness today and in the future.

Lesson 1.3 Building Skills for Health and Wellness

- Decision-making skills involve identifying a decision, exploring alternatives, selecting the best alternative, acting on your decision, and evaluating your decision.
- A *goal* is a plan of action that will guide you in achieving something you want to reach. Effective goals are *SMART goals*—specific, measurable, achievable, relevant, and timely.
- When peers or family members attempt to influence you to engage in unhealthy behaviors, refusal skills can help you respond without compromising your goals, values, or health.
- Conflict resolution skills, which involve negotiation and compromise, help you resolve arguments in a way that promotes healthy relationships.
- The ability to locate, interpret, and apply information as it relates to your health is called *health literacy*.
- Taking charge of your health and wellness involves playing an active role in your healthcare and advocating for your personal health.

Check Your Knowledge ↗

Record your answers to each of the following questions on a separate sheet of paper.

1. **True or false.** Health and wellness are both terms that refer to the absence of physical illness and disease.
2. Identify the aspects of your health. How are these aspects interrelated?
3. Which type of healthcare involves getting an annual physical exam, regular checkups, and screenings?
4. How do most people pay for the expensive cost of healthcare services?
5. The _____ you receive from your parents can affect your health and wellness by putting you at risk for developing certain diseases, such as heart disease.
6. **True or false.** Your school and home are part of your economic environment.
7. Food and taste preferences and eating patterns are examples of _____ practices that may affect your social environment.
   - **A.** peer
   - **B.** physical
   - **C.** cultural
   - **D.** economic
8. Identify three risky behaviors that can be a hazard to your health.
9. Using _____ skills can help you make good choices about health and wellness.
10. Which of the following URL stems is *not* generally a reliable source of health-related information?
    - **A.** *.gov*
    - **B.** *.org*
    - **C.** *.edu*
    - **D.** *.com*
11. What is at stake if you believe health claims that are *not* based in science?
12. Helping your grandfather research health information on the Internet is an example of _____ for family health.

Use Your Vocabulary ↗

advocate	goal	physical health
collaborate	health	preventive healthcare
conflict resolution skills	healthcare	primary care physician
culture	health literacy	refusal skills
decision-making skills	mediation	risk factors
economic environment	mediator	SMART goals
environment	mental and emotional health	social environment
family history		social health
genes	peers	well-being
	physical environment	wellness

13. Working in pairs, locate a small image online that visually describes or explains each of the terms above. Create flash cards by writing each term on a note card. Then paste the image that describes or explains the term on the opposite side.
14. With a partner, create a T-chart. Write each of the terms above in the left column. Write a *synonym* (a word that has the same or similar meaning) for each term in the right column. Discuss your synonyms with the class.

Think Critically

15. **Predict.** How can a change in a student's social health, such as being the victim of bullying, also affect his or her physical and mental and emotional health?

16. **Identify.** What are three reasons young people may be tempted by risky behaviors? Explain why this group in particular is vulnerable.

17. **Draw conclusions.** In what ways do your friends have a positive impact on your health?

18. **Determine.** Does a young person have the power to change family health? Give a detailed explanation.

DEVELOP Your Skills

19. **Communication.** Imagine that you are in the following scenario: As a middle school student, life is pretty good. You have great friends, school is going well, and your family is a lot of fun. Last week, however, your grandma died and you are struggling to cope with the loss. You are sad, lack interest in everyday activities and friendships, and do not have much of an appetite. Write an essay reflecting on the following questions:
    - If you continue struggling with the loss of your grandma, how could it impact your physical and social health?
    - What would you do in this situation?
    - Who would you talk to, and how would you begin the conversation?
    - What self-help strategies could be helpful in coping?

20. **Goal setting.** Reflect on the parts of your health that you think could use more development. What improvements would you like to see in your health and wellness? Establish three or more long-term personal health goals. For each long-term goal, create three or more short-term goals. Your short-term goals should act as stepping stones for each of your long-term goals. Make sure to follow the SMART goal guidelines to make the most effective goals for you. Make a creative product that will serve as a reminder of your goals.

21. **Analyze influences.** Analyze a social media post, image, or web page that could potentially have a negative influence on a young person's physical, mental and emotional, or social health. Write a short paragraph about how this post, image, or web page could negatively affect a teenager's behavior or health. Share your reflection with the class. Include the post, image, or web page for the class to view during your presentation.

22. **Advocacy.** Imagine that your family has a history of a health condition, such as diabetes, heart disease, cancer, or obesity. Despite this, your family continues to make poor lifestyle decisions and you are worried about their health across the life span. Write a letter to your family talking about their current lifestyle choices and offer a plan to improve family health. This plan should include the big and small lifestyle changes that you would want to make with your family. It should also include a way to hold each other accountable for achieving these goals, such as a rewards system.

Chapter 2

Developing Good Personal Hygiene

Lesson 2.1 Caring for Your Skin, Hair, and Nails

Lesson 2.2 Keeping Your Mouth, Eyes, and Ears Healthy

Essential Question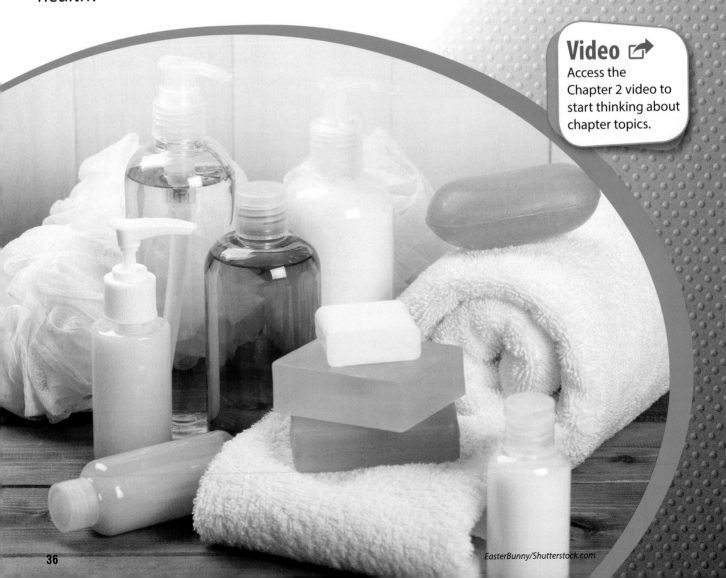

Which aspects of good hygiene are important to your health?

Video ↗

Access the Chapter 2 video to start thinking about chapter topics.

EasterBunny/Shutterstock.com

Reading Activity

Write a short dialogue in which friends discuss personal hygiene concerns. As you read the chapter, note any concerns your dialogue did not address. Write a paragraph detailing what might happen if the friends addressed only the concerns you originally noted.

How Healthy Are You?

In this chapter, you will be learning about personal hygiene. Before you begin reading, take the following quiz to assess your current personal hygiene habits.

Healthy Choices	Yes	No
Do you wear deodorant and regularly wash your face, body, and hair?		
Do you drink plenty of water to keep your skin hydrated?		
Do you wash your face (and rinse well) twice a day to prevent acne?		
Do you avoid tanning beds, tanning booths, and sunlamps?		
Do you follow the cleanliness guidelines for any piercings you may have?		
Do you use sunscreen every time you go out in the sun?		
Do you avoid listening to music at a high volume, especially when using headphones?		
Do you wear a mouth guard during activities that can result in broken teeth, such as basketball or ice hockey?		
Do you floss after meals and brush your teeth at least twice a day?		
When spending time outdoors, do you wear sunglasses that block at least 99 percent UVB and UVA rays, or provide UV 400 protection?		
Do you keep your nails dry and clean and regularly trim your fingernails?		
Do you avoid exposure to very high levels of noise, like construction sites or rock concerts?		

Count your "Yes" and "No" responses. The more "Yes" responses you have, the more healthy personal hygiene habits you exhibit. Now, take a closer look at the questions with which you responded "No." How can you make these healthy habits part of your daily life? Think about how implementing these ideas can help improve your overall health.

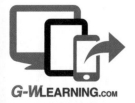

G-WLEARNING.com

While studying this chapter, look for the activity icon to

- **practice** key terms with e-flash cards and matching activities.
- **reinforce** what you learn by completing graphic organizers, self-assessment quizzes, and review questions.
- **expand** knowledge with interactive activities and activities that extend learning.

www.g-wlearning.com/health/

Caring for Your Skin, Hair, and Nails

Key Terms 🔗

epidermis outermost layer of the skin

dermis middle layer of the skin, which contains hair follicles

hypodermis innermost layer of the skin, which contains fat, blood vessels, and nerve endings; attaches to underlying bone and muscle

deodorant product designed to cover up body odor

antiperspirant product designed to stop or dry up sweat

acne skin condition in which inflamed, clogged hair follicles cause pimples

eczema chronic condition that causes swollen, red, dry, and itchy patches of skin on one or more parts of the body

body art permanent decorations that are applied to the body; examples include tattoos and piercings

dandruff dead skin that flakes off the scalp due to dryness, infrequent shampooing, or irritation

lice tiny insects that attach to hair and feed on human blood

Learning Outcomes

After studying this lesson, you will be able to

- **describe** the three distinct layers of skin.
- **demonstrate** ways to care for the skin.
- **give examples** of conditions that affect the skin.
- **identify** strategies to keep hair healthy and looking good.
- **practice** effective nail care.

Graphic Organizer 🔗

Grooming Routines

Grooming tasks are a normal part of people's daily routines. Consider your grooming routines that involve taking care of your skin, hair, and nails. In a chart like the one shown below, list these grooming routines or activities and indicate how often you perform them.

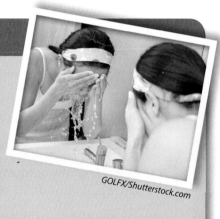

GOLFX/Shutterstock.com

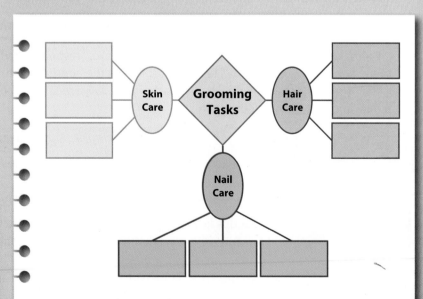

Twelve-year-old Gabriela spends much more time on her grooming than ever before. On days when she has basketball practice, she showers and applies deodorant twice a day. Her face seems to get oily all the time, so she washes it every morning and night. Gabriela knows this grooming routine is necessary to keep her skin healthy.

Levi is 11 years old and likes to hang out with his friends outside. They enjoy playing soccer, riding their bikes around the neighborhood, and swimming in Levi's backyard pool. To avoid sunburns, Levi applies sunscreen every few hours and reminds his friends to do the same.

Taking care of your personal hygiene is hard work, but Gabriela and Levi know that caring for their bodies by keeping them clean will keep them healthy. In this lesson, you will learn some basic steps to ensure that your body is healthy and clean and that you present your best self to the world. The good personal hygiene skills you develop now can help to promote your health and wellness throughout your life.

Skin

The skin, which is the largest organ of the human body, is the outer covering of the entire body. Your skin plays a very important role in keeping you healthy. First, the skin protects everything inside the body. This includes muscles, bones, and other organs, such as the brain, heart, and liver. The skin serves as a barrier for keeping bacteria and viruses from entering your body. Your skin also plays an important role in regulating your body temperature.

Layers of the Skin

The skin has three distinct layers (**Figure 2.1**). The outermost layer of the skin is the **epidermis**. The epidermis, which consists of five layers of its own, is the thinnest layer of the skin. The function of the epidermis is to protect the body from infection by stopping foreign substances from entering into the body.

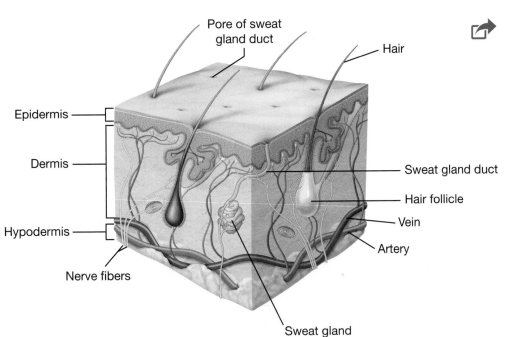

Pore of sweat gland duct

Hair

Epidermis

Dermis

Hypodermis

Nerve fibers

Sweat gland duct

Hair follicle

Vein

Artery

Sweat gland

Figure 2.1
This diagram shows the three distinct layers of skin and the locations of your nerves, hair follicles, sweat glands, pores, and arteries and veins. *Which layer of skin is the outermost layer?*

© Body Scientific International

The epidermis also contains cells, called *melanocytes*, which produce the skin's pigment, or *melanin*. People who have a darker complexion have more melanin in their skin than people with fairer skin.

The middle layer of the skin is the **dermis**. This layer contains *hair follicles* (small tubes that hold the hair roots). These follicles determine what your hair looks like—whether it is curly, straight, thick, or thin. As hair grows, it pushes out of the follicle and through the skin. Once it passes through the skin, the cells of the hair are no longer alive. Every follicle is attached to a gland that produces oil. When these glands produce too much oil, a person's skin or hair may look greasy.

The dermis contains sweat glands, blood vessels, and nerve endings. This layer also includes two proteins: *collagen* and *elastin*. These proteins provide support to the skin and give skin the ability to stretch and return to its normal shape. With age, the body creates less of these proteins, which leads to the appearance of wrinkles and sagging skin (**Figure 2.2**). The dermis also contains the nerve endings that allow you to feel pain, pressure, and temperature.

The innermost layer of the skin is the **hypodermis**. This layer consists of fat, blood vessels, and nerve endings. It also connects the skin to the bone and muscle underneath.

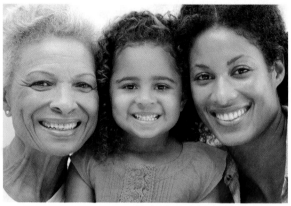

Monkey Business Images/Shutterstock.com

Figure 2.2 As you age, your skin loses its elasticity and hydration and gains wrinkles and age spots. *Which two proteins provide support to the skin and keep it looking young?*

Care of the Skin

Keeping your skin healthy requires care. Taking a bath or shower every day will keep your skin clean and prevent body odor. When bathing or showering, use a mild soap and warm water to rid your skin of dirt and oil. After bathing, applying a lotion or moisturizer can keep skin from becoming too dry. Also, applying a deodorant or antiperspirant will prevent body odor. A **deodorant** covers up the odor of sweat, while an **antiperspirant** actually stops or dries up sweat.

In addition to these basic skin care steps, caring for your skin also involves making healthy lifestyle choices. Eating healthy foods, such as fruits and vegetables, and drinking lots of water can help keep your skin looking its best. Getting enough sleep each night, managing your stress, and avoiding smoking are all choices that can also keep your skin looking healthy.

Because spending too much time in the sun can damage your skin, applying sun protection whenever you go outside is very important. A sunscreen protects the skin by absorbing, reflecting, or scattering ultraviolet (UV) light. *Ultraviolet (UV) light* is an invisible kind of radiation that comes from the sun, tanning beds, and sunlamps. UV light can seriously damage your skin.

Skin Conditions

People may experience several common types of skin conditions. Examples of conditions that affect the skin include acne, eczema, and sunburn. Body decorations, such as tattoos and body piercings, may also cause skin problems.

In the following sections, you will learn about these skin conditions. You will also learn how to prevent or treat them.

CASE STUDY

Malcolm: Changes in Hygiene

Malcolm feels like the typical sixth-grade boy in many ways. He likes school, but would rather play with his friends. His favorite times of the school day are recess, PE, lunch, and reading. He loves to read science fiction novels!

Lately, however, everything is changing so quickly for him. Malcolm has grown taller, which he hoped for, but he is not excited about other changes in his body. Malcolm did not notice how bad he smelled until his mom told him. He wears deodorant, but he is not sure how well it is working for him.

Malcolm has noticed his face getting very oily, and he does not know why. Pimples have started to develop on his nose and forehead. He has noticed them on his friends' faces, which helps him feel less awkward. The oil is not only on Malcolm's face though. It is in his hair, too. He should not be surprised because he does not do a great job of shampooing and he often skips showers altogether.

Malcolm knows that changes will continue to happen to him as he gets older. He just hopes the next set of changes will make him happier.

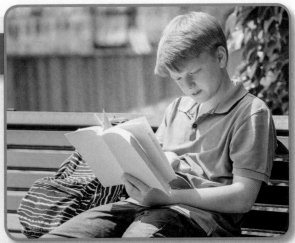

Thinking Critically

1. How can changes in one's appearance and personal hygiene affect self-esteem?

2. Of the changes that are happening to Malcolm, which ones can he control by taking better care of his personal hygiene?

3. What advice would you give to Malcolm to improve his personal hygiene?

4. What are other ways that Malcolm can take care of his personal hygiene to prevent future problems and insecurities?

Acne

Acne, a skin condition characterized by pimples, commonly develops during adolescence. Acne occurs when the oil glands produce too much oil and clog the *pores*, which are hair follicles under the skin. The excess oil mixes with dead skin cells and creates a blockage in the pore. Over time, oil and bacteria leak into the skin surrounding this pore. This causes infection and inflammation, including redness, swelling, and pus.

A pimple called a *whitehead* gets its name from the whitish pus inside a clogged pore that has only a tiny opening to the skin's surface. In contrast, a *blackhead* is a yellow or blackish bump inside a clogged pore that is more open to the air. When air gets inside the follicle, it causes the oil inside the follicle to become darker (**Figure 2.3**).

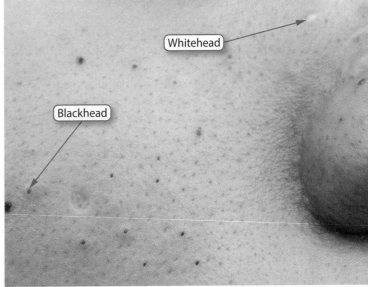

Figure 2.3 Pimples are common among adolescents and can be treated and prevented. *What are pores?*

Fortunately, there are steps you can take to prevent and treat acne breakouts. The following strategies can help:

- Wash your face gently twice a day. After washing your face, rinse well so that the soap does not stay on your skin.
- Do not squeeze pimples. Doing so can lead to permanent acne scars.
- Avoid touching your face with your fingers, which can spread bacteria and cause inflammation and irritation to other parts of your face or body.
- Make sure anything that touches your face is clean, including glasses, headbands, and hats. Keep your hair clean and pulled away from your face.
- Protect your skin from sunburn, which can make acne appear even worse.
- Wash any makeup off your skin before going to sleep. Throw away old makeup as it can contain bacteria.
- Shave your face lightly, and not too frequently, to avoid accidentally cutting a skin blemish.
- Use over-the-counter acne medication to clear and prevent acne. For serious cases of acne, consult a *dermatologist* (doctor who is a skin specialist). A dermatologist can give you useful information about caring for your skin type, and prescribe medication, if necessary.

BUILDING Your Skills

Health in the Media

Mass media messages aim to directly affect people's health behaviors. Some media messages, such as those that focus on antismoking and heart disease prevention, are positive and encourage healthy behaviors. Other media messages focus on behaviors that can have harmful effects on people's health, such as drinking alcohol or eating foods that are high in fat and low in nutrients. Additionally, only some media messages tell the truth. False advertising is common in health products—from "no sugar added" foods to "anti-aging" skin creams.

Browsing skin care or hair care products can be daunting. The options seem endless, and the products all look the same. Most advertisements say the same things. How do you know which products are scams? What will work best for you?

You must be able to analyze how messages from media and labels on products may influence your purchases. You also need to be able to evaluate which products will improve your health and which ones will not.

Evaluating Skin and Hair Care Products

The best way to fight against false advertising for health claims on skin care and hair care products is to do your research. Evaluate the scientific studies done on that brand, product, and any ingredients used.

Working in groups of four, choose two skin care products and two hair care products to evaluate. For each product, research and record your answers to the following questions. Share your group's findings with the rest of the class.

1. Was this product tested on human subjects? Tests conducted on animals or tissue samples can have different effects.

2. What are the ingredients in the product? Can any of these ingredients be harmful to your skin or hair? Can they cause any side effects?

3. Are any health claims of this product backed by scientific research? All true health claims will have scientific data in multiple studies to back them up.

4. Do the products contain added colors, preservatives, or fragrances? Large amounts of these may irritate sensitive skin.

Eczema

Eczema, or *dermatitis*, is a condition that causes swollen, red, dry, and itchy patches of skin on one or more parts of the body (**Figure 2.4**). Eczema is a chronic disease, which means it typically reoccurs over time. Colds or other minor illnesses, irritating substances, and stress may all trigger eczema flare-ups. Eczema is not contagious, meaning you cannot catch it from someone else.

You can often treat symptoms of eczema using over-the-counter products. To relieve the dryness and itching of eczema, apply a lotion or cream when the skin is damp, such as after bathing or washing your hands. This locks in moisture and can help reduce itching. Avoid scratching any patches of eczema. Doing so may cause an infection.

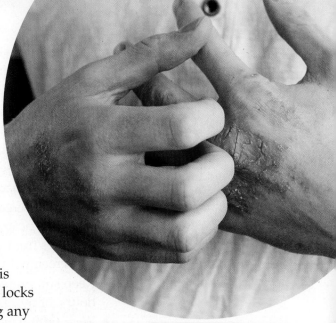

Ternavskaia Olga Alibec/Shutterstock.com

Figure 2.4
Eczema patches can occur anywhere on the body, but are commonly found on the hands, feet, face, and creases of the elbows and knees. *Is eczema contagious?*

Suntans, Sunburns, and Skin Cancer

Spending too much time in the sun's UV rays can damage your skin. Suntans and sunburns are both indicators of damage to the skin because of too much time in the sun. Scientific evidence suggests that overexposure to UV rays and damage to the skin can lead to skin cancer.

There are three main types of skin cancer (**Figure 2.5**). Two of these types—*basal cell carcinoma* and *squamous cell carcinoma*—are common and curable. *Melanoma* is the most dangerous type of skin cancer because it spreads rapidly throughout the body, sometimes before the initial skin cancer is recognized.

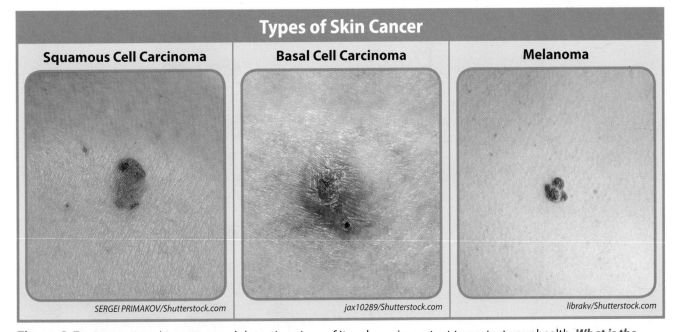

Types of Skin Cancer

| Squamous Cell Carcinoma | Basal Cell Carcinoma | Melanoma |

SERGEI PRIMAKOV/Shutterstock.com   *jax10289/Shutterstock.com*   *librakv/Shutterstock.com*

Figure 2.5 Preventing skin cancer and detecting signs of it early are important to protect your health. *What is the most dangerous type of skin cancer?*

To protect your skin and prevent skin damage, which can lead to skin cancer, reduce intentional UV exposure and increase sun protection. Other ways to protect your skin include the following:

- Avoid outdoor activities during the midday hours when the sun's rays are the strongest.
- Wear a hat with a large brim to protect your face, head, ears, and neck. Wear sunglasses to protect your eyes.
- Stay in the shade whenever possible.
- Apply sunscreen to all exposed areas of skin. The higher the *sun protection factor (SPF)* of a sunscreen, the greater the protection it provides from UV rays. For the best protection against UV rays, use sunscreen with a sun protection factor of at least 15.
- Keep sun protection handy and reapply sunscreen at least every two hours, or more often if you sweat or swim.
- Wear tightly woven clothing that protects any skin exposed to the sun's UV rays. Certain fabrics have built-in SPF protection.
- Avoid tanning beds, tanning booths, and sunlamps. The UV rays these machines produce are just as dangerous as the sun's UV rays, and are just as likely to cause skin cancer.
- Monitor your skin for possible signs of skin cancer. Use the ABCDE method to note any unusual changes in the skin (**Figure 2.6**).

Figure 2.6
Early treatment of skin cancer can help prevent it from spreading or getting worse. The ABCDE method can help you spot possible signs of skin cancer on your skin. ***What does ABCDE stand for?***

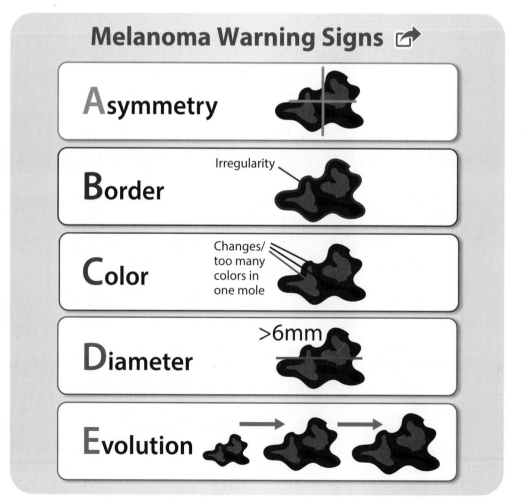

Melanoma Warning Signs

Asymmetry

Border — Irregularity

Color — Changes/ too many colors in one mole

Diameter — >6mm

Evolution

Sun Safety Tips

Wear a Hat to protect face and eyes

Wear Sunscreen

SPF 30

reapply every 2 hours

Seek Some Shade

Stay Hydrated to replace fluids lost from sweat

Wear Sunglasses to protect eyes from harmful UV rays

Tattoos and Piercings

Since ancient times, people have chosen to decorate their bodies in permanent ways. Two of the most common types of body decoration, or **body art**, are tattoos and piercings. These types of body decorations can potentially impact health.

Tattoos are designs on the skin made by using a needle to insert colored ink under the skin. *Body piercing* involves the use of a needle to make a hole in the skin to insert jewelry. The most common body piercing is to the earlobe. Other pierced body parts often include ear cartilage, the belly button, the nose, and the tongue.

In most states, people are required to be at least 18 years of age or have written permission by a legal guardian to get a tattoo or body piercing. To reduce the risk of complications from tattoos or piercings, people should have them done at clean, safe, and well-regarded facilities by licensed professionals (**Figure 2.7**). Following the care instructions closely can help decrease the possibility of infection.

Although getting a tattoo or a body piercing may seem harmless, it is a big decision—and a permanent one. People should think carefully about the risks involved with these procedures before making a decision. Health problems can occur whenever inserting needles into the body. This is especially true if the needles are not sterilized, or clean. Serious infections may result. Some people with body art can also experience an allergic reaction, typically to the jewelry worn in the pierced area, or to the tattoo ink.

Sometimes, tattoos and piercings may affect jobs or relationships. For example, some businesses do not allow their employees to have visible tattoos or piercings. If a worker has a tattoo, he or she may be required to cover it up while on the job. It is possible to have a tattoo removed, but this is a painful, expensive, and time-intensive process. Removal of a tattoo often leaves scarring, too.

Figure 2.7
Licensing regulations vary state by state, but all body art professionals should follow similar standards for sanitation, including the use of gloves and sterile instruments.

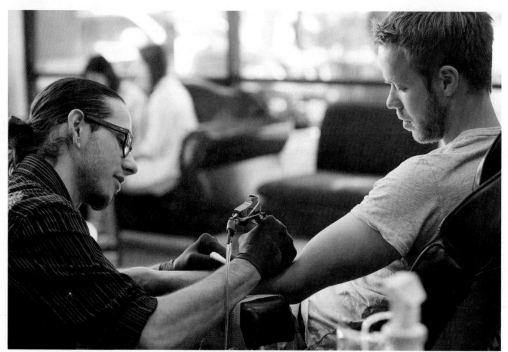

Monkey Business Images/Shutterstock.com

Hair

Although you have more than 100,000 hairs on your head, you lose about 50 to 100 hairs every day through normal activities such as washing, brushing, or combing your hair. These hairs are replaced by new hairs, which grow from the same follicles. Practicing good hair care will help you keep your hair looking clean and healthy (**Figure 2.8**). Maintaining the health of your hair can be easy when you understand common hair conditions and know how to prevent and treat them.

Understanding Common Hair Conditions

A common hair condition many people experience is having oily hair. This is especially true for teenagers who are going through puberty. Every hair follicle is attached to a gland that produces oil. When these glands produce too much oil, such as during puberty, a person's hair may look greasy.

Another common hair condition people may experience is **dandruff**, which is the flaking of dead skin cells from the scalp. A common cause of dandruff is having dry skin. People who have dandruff because of dry skin often notice white flakes of dead skin in their hair and on their shoulders (**Figure 2.9**). Dandruff is usually worse in the fall and winter, when indoor heating can dry out skin. Infrequent shampooing, which allows oils and skin cells from the scalp to build up, is another common cause of dandruff. Shampooing too often or using too many hair care products may irritate the scalp and lead to dandruff, too.

A highly contagious hair condition some people may contract is lice. **Lice** are tiny insects that attach to the hair and feed on human blood. Lice can transmit easily from one person to another through direct head-to-head contact or if people share combs, brushes, or hats. Although lice do not cause any major health conditions, they are very itchy and uncomfortable.

ESUN7756/Shutterstock.com

Figure 2.8
Getting your hair cut on a regular basis can keep the ends healthy and strong. *Approximately how many hairs do you lose every day?*

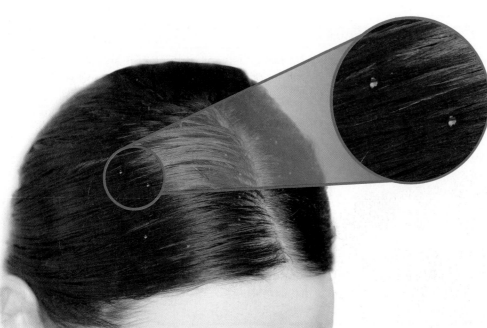

Figure 2.9
White flakes of dead skin cells on the scalp are the result of a common hair condition called *dandruff*. *What is one possible cause of dandruff?*

lavizzara/Shutterstock.com

Preventing and Treating Hair Conditions

Following are some strategies you can use to keep your hair healthy and looking good:

- Wash and condition your hair regularly to keep it clean and prevent it from becoming too dry.
- Eat a healthful diet (**Figure 2.10**). Some hair conditions are caused in part by a lack of certain vitamins and fats.
- If you have dandruff, try using a medicated shampoo. If the dandruff continues, see your doctor or dermatologist.
- Avoid sharing items that have touched your hair with other people.
- If you become infected with lice, use a medicated shampoo to kill the lice and their eggs (or *nits*). You also need to wash all bedding, towels, and other items that have touched your hair in hot water.

Nails

Fingernails and toenails are made up of layers of a hard protein called *keratin*. This hard substance protects the sensitive tissues on the tips of your fingers and toes. Nails grow out from the area at the base of the nail. As new cells continuously grow, older cells are pushed out.

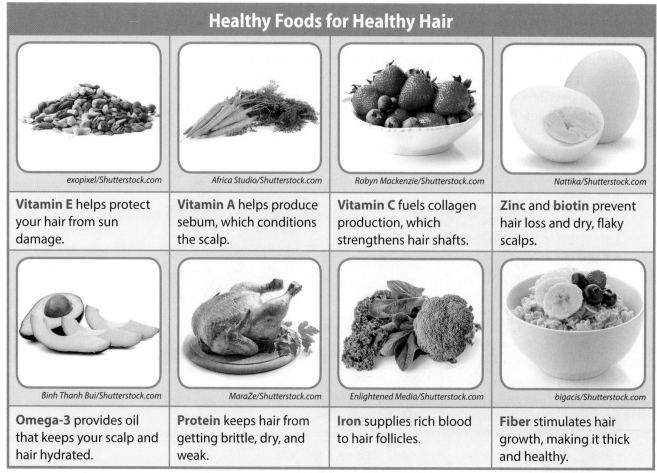

Healthy Foods for Healthy Hair

exopixel/Shutterstock.com	*Africa Studio/Shutterstock.com*	*Robyn Mackenzie/Shutterstock.com*	*Nattika/Shutterstock.com*
Vitamin E helps protect your hair from sun damage.	**Vitamin A** helps produce sebum, which conditions the scalp.	**Vitamin C** fuels collagen production, which strengthens hair shafts.	**Zinc** and **biotin** prevent hair loss and dry, flaky scalps.
Binh Thanh Bui/Shutterstock.com	*MaraZe/Shutterstock.com*	*Enlightened Media/Shutterstock.com*	*bigacis/Shutterstock.com*
Omega-3 provides oil that keeps your scalp and hair hydrated.	**Protein** keeps hair from getting brittle, dry, and weak.	**Iron** supplies rich blood to hair follicles.	**Fiber** stimulates hair growth, making it thick and healthy.

Figure 2.10   Hair is made up of protein and is kept long, full, healthy, and strong by the nutrients we eat.

Healthy fingernails and toenails are smooth, free of spots or discoloration, and consistent in color. Some irregularities in the nails, such as white spots or vertical ridges, are normal. Other conditions, however, such as nail discoloration, curled nails, or redness and swelling around the nail, can sometimes indicate health concerns.

Fortunately, it is relatively easy to keep your nails strong and healthy. First, keep your nails dry and clean to prevent bacteria and other organisms from growing under them. If you must soak your hands, such as while washing dishes, or if you must use harsh chemicals, wear gloves. Be sure to trim your fingernails regularly using clippers, manicure scissors, or a nail file (**Figure 2.11**).

In addition, moisturize your hands regularly, including your fingernails and cuticles. Do not bite your fingernails, pick at your cuticles, or pull off your hangnails. Doing so can cause infections.

Before using the services of a salon for nail care, make sure the salon and the nail technician are licensed. All tools should be properly sterilized between customers to avoid spreading infections.

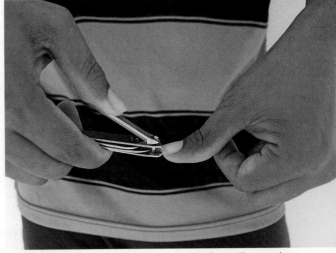

chittakorn59/Shutterstock.com

Figure 2.11 Trimming your fingernails and toenails regularly is a great way to keep your nails clean, strong, and healthy.

Lesson 2.1 Review 📲

1. Name the three distinct layers of skin.

2. What is the difference between a deodorant and an antiperspirant?

3. **True or false.** Your diet, sleeping patterns, and water intake have a big impact on how healthy your skin looks.

4. Swollen, red, dry, and itchy patches of skin on one or more parts of the body describes a skin condition called _____.

5. **Critical thinking.** Name three different hair conditions and describe different ways to prevent and treat them.

Hands-On Activity

In small groups, create an advertisement on how to take care of the skin, hair, or nails. Include the following information in your advertisement:

- conditions or problems due to poor hygiene
- products needed for good personal hygiene
- tips to taking care of this region of the body

Possible formats for your advertisement include posters, videos, and social media posts. Present your advertisement to the class.

Keeping Your Mouth, Eyes, and Ears Healthy

Key Terms ☞

plaque sticky, colorless film that coats the teeth and dissolves their protective enamel surface

cavities holes in the teeth that occur when plaque eats into a tooth's enamel

gingivitis inflammation of the gums

periodontitis infection caused by bacteria getting under the gum tissue and destroying the gums and bone

orthodontist dental specialist who prevents and corrects teeth misalignments

nearsightedness condition in which objects close to the eye appear clear, while objects farther away appear blurry

farsightedness condition in which distant objects are seen more clearly than nearby objects

astigmatism condition in which the eye does not focus light evenly onto the retina; objects appear blurry and stretched out

presbyopia condition beginning in middle age in which the lens of the eye loses its elasticity and it becomes harder to see close objects clearly

tinnitus pain or ringing in the ears after exposure to excessively loud sounds

Learning Outcomes

After studying this lesson, you will be able to

- **summarize** common mouth problems people may experience.
- **list** strategies to prevent some of the most common mouth and teeth problems.
- **identify** parts of the eye and their functions.
- **describe** common vision problems.
- **identify** parts of the ear and their functions.
- **describe** common hearing problems.

Graphic Organizer ☞

Mouth, Ear, and Eye Health

Create a KWL chart like the one below. Before reading this lesson, write what you know and what you want to know about mouth, eye, and ear health in the appropriate columns. After studying the lesson, write what you have learned.

WHAT HAVE YOU LEARNED?

Krasimira Nevenova/Shutterstock.com

K What I Know	W What I Want to Know	L What I Have Learned
I should brush and floss my teeth at least twice a day.	What are different events that can cause ear damage?	The colored part of the eye is the iris.

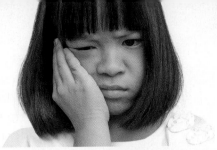

The mouth, teeth, ears, and eyes are important parts of the body that help people live their lives to the fullest (**Figure 2.12**). Do you remember how Levi and Gabriela, from the previous lesson, took such good care of their skin?

Levi went to the dentist for his regular checkup last month and was told that he has a cavity. Levi sometimes forgets to brush his teeth and almost never flosses. His dentist also tells Levi's dad that he should consider taking Levi to an orthodontist to get braces.

Gabriela loves listening to music and always seems to be wearing her headphones. She plays the music as loud as she can. She sometimes has a ringing in her ears when she takes off her headphones. Gabriela also has a hard time reading the board when she sits in the back of the classroom. She does not want to tell her parents, however, because she does not want to wear glasses. What can Levi and Gabriela do to improve how they take care of their mouth, teeth, eyes, and ears?

In this lesson, you will read about some common health concerns relating to your mouth, teeth, eyes, and ears. You will also learn ways to help you keep them in good working condition.

Figure 2.12
Having a toothache can affect other parts of your health. For example, the pain can prevent you from focusing in school or wanting to spend time with friends.

The Mouth and Teeth

Having good oral health is important to your overall health. *Oral health* refers to your mouth, teeth, and gums. Did you know that many bacteria live in your mouth? If you do not take good care of your mouth and teeth, bacteria can grow to dangerous levels that result in infections or diseases.

One of the primary functions of the mouth is to take in food and break it down for digestion. Through chewing, teeth help break down large pieces of food into smaller ones. The mouth also produces *saliva*, which is a clear liquid that contains substances that help you chew and swallow food. After swallowing food, it travels through the esophagus and into the stomach. Regularly brushing your teeth and flossing after meals helps keep the bacteria in your mouth under control.

Teeth consist of three distinct parts (**Figure 2.13**). The *crown* is the visible portion of the tooth. It is protected by a hard, white substance made of calcium, called *enamel*.

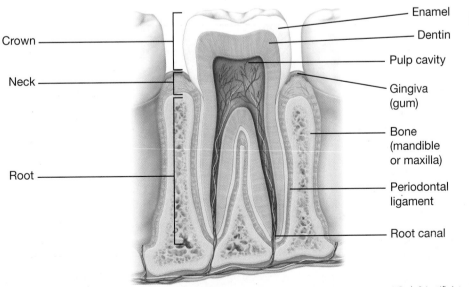

Crown
Neck
Root

Enamel
Dentin
Pulp cavity
Gingiva (gum)
Bone (mandible or maxilla)
Periodontal ligament
Root canal

© Body Scientific International

Figure 2.13
The structure of a tooth.
What substance protects the crown of a tooth?

The *neck* connects the crown to the root of the tooth at the gum line. The *root* contains blood vessels and nerve endings that connect the tooth to the jaw.

A normal adult mouth contains 32 teeth. Different types of teeth have different shapes, locations in the jaw, and functions (**Figure 2.14**). These types include the following:

- incisors (8 total)—the four teeth at the very front of the mouth on the upper and lower jaws
- canines (4 total)—the pointy teeth right beside the incisors
- premolars (8 total)—teeth between the canines and the molars
- molars (8 total)—flat teeth in the rear of the mouth
- wisdom teeth (4 total)—the teeth at the very back of the mouth, which are the last permanent teeth to come in, usually between 17 and 21 years of age

Common Mouth and Teeth Problems

Many people experience problems with their mouths at some point. These problems can interfere with important daily life functions such as chewing, swallowing, and even talking. Some of the common mouth problems people may experience include tooth decay, gum disease, teeth misalignment, cold sores, bad breath, and teeth grinding.

Figure 2.14
Deciduous teeth are more commonly known as "baby teeth," and are eventually replaced by permanent teeth. *How many teeth does a normal adult mouth contain?*

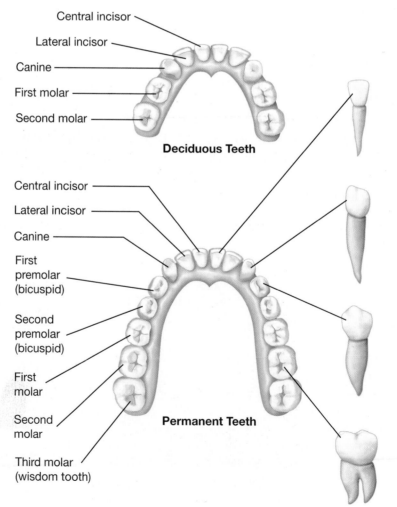

Central incisor
Lateral incisor
Canine
First molar
Second molar

Deciduous Teeth

Central incisor
Lateral incisor
Canine
First premolar (bicuspid)
Second premolar (bicuspid)
First molar
Second molar
Third molar (wisdom tooth)

Permanent Teeth

© *Body Scientific International*

Tooth Decay

When you eat or drink something, a substance in your saliva breaks down the food particles and sugars for digestion. This process turns everything you eat or drink into a type of acid. When this acid combines with the bacteria in your mouth, as well as saliva and small food particles, it forms plaque. **Plaque** is a sticky, colorless film that coats the teeth and dissolves their protective enamel surface. If plaque is not removed, it mixes with minerals to become tartar, a harder substance. Tartar removal requires professional cleaning.

If you do not brush and floss your teeth daily, food particles remain in your mouth and promote bacterial growth (**Figure 2.15**). This results in tooth decay. Over time, tooth decay causes **cavities**, or holes in the teeth that occur when plaque eats into a tooth's enamel. Cavities are also known as *dental caries*. As the decay continues, the hole gets deeper and eventually reaches the nerve layer under the enamel known as the *dentin*. This causes painful nerve damage. The *death of the tooth* occurs when the decay reaches the deepest layer of the tooth (the *pulp cavity*).

Rob Marmion/Shutterstock.com

Figure 2.15 Brushing your teeth at least twice a day, especially after eating or drinking something sticky or high in sugar, can help prevent cavities. *What is another name for cavities?*

Gum Disease

Your *gums* consist of the pinkish tissue that surrounds your teeth. The gums lie on top of the bones of the jaw, and cover the entire root of each tooth. The gums help keep your teeth in place.

Gum disease occurs when plaque and tartar build up on the teeth (**Figure 2.16**). The bacteria in plaque cause toxins to form in the mouth, which irritates the gums. Over time, this irritation can lead to **gingivitis**, an inflammation of the gums. It can also lead to periodontitis. **Periodontitis**, or *periodontal disease*, is an infection caused by bacteria getting under the gum tissue and destroying the gums and bone. Early signs of gum disease include swelling and bleeding of the gums. If gum disease goes untreated, it can damage the gums and jawbone.

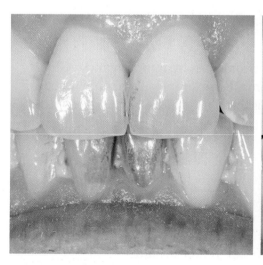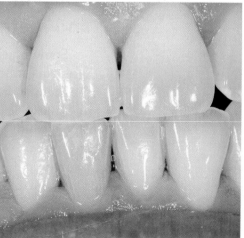

Figure 2.16 Brushing your teeth can help remove plaque, but it can also be removed professionally at the dentist. *If you do not remove plaque buildup on your teeth, what conditions can occur?*

Lighthunter/Shutterstock.com

Teeth Misalignment and Impacted Wisdom Teeth

A misalignment (incorrect position) of the upper teeth and the lower teeth may result in an overbite or underbite. An *overbite* is a condition in which the upper teeth extend significantly over the lower teeth. An *underbite* is a condition in which the lower teeth extend significantly past the upper teeth.

Wisdom teeth may become stuck under the gum tissue, or may only be able to partially come through the gums. This can be caused by lack of room in the jaw. When this occurs, the condition is called *impacted wisdom teeth*. In this case, the teeth may need to be removed because they can become infected or displace other teeth.

Cold Sores

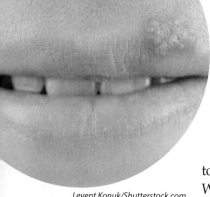

Levent Konuk/Shutterstock.com

Figure 2.17
Painful blisters, called *cold sores*, are contagious through saliva, such as through sharing a beverage or a utensil. *How long do cold sores last?*

Cold sores, or *fever blisters*, are small blisters that appear on the lips and inside the mouth (**Figure 2.17**). These blisters are red, swollen, and painful, especially when touched. Cold sores typically last several days, but can last as long as two weeks. Cold sores are caused by a virus spread from person to person through passing saliva in some way, such as sharing a utensil.

Bad Breath and Teeth Grinding

Bad breath, or *halitosis*, can be caused by poor oral hygiene. Bad breath is also caused by gum disease, cavities, trapped food particles, and certain medical conditions. For example, respiratory tract infections, diabetes, and chronic bronchitis can all cause bad breath. The best way to fight bad breath is to practice good oral hygiene and see the dentist every six months for checkups.

Teeth grinding occurs when a person repeatedly clenches and grinds his or her teeth. This problem may be caused by stress or anxiety, having an abnormal bite, or missing or crooked teeth. Many people who grind their teeth are unaware they do it because it often occurs during sleep. They may learn from other people that they grind their teeth. Although teeth grinding is usually harmless, persistent teeth grinding can lead to tooth damage, a sore jaw, headaches, and even hearing loss. A dentist can determine whether you are grinding your teeth. If you do grind your teeth, the dentist may suggest that you wear a mouth guard during sleep to protect your teeth.

Preventing and Treating Mouth and Teeth Problems

Sometimes people can treat mouth and teeth problems at home. For example, a person with bad breath may brush and floss more often to keep teeth and gums clean and free of food particles. To treat other mouth problems, people need to see a dentist for treatment. For example, tooth sensitivity may indicate a cavity in the tooth, which requires professional treatment. Similarly, many teenagers wear devices such as braces, which an orthodontist applies. An **orthodontist** is a dental specialist who prevents and corrects teeth misalignments (**Figure 2.18**).

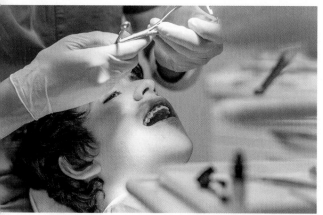

GoneWithTheWind/Shutterstock.com

Figure 2.18 Braces are applied by dental specialists called *orthodontists*.

Take Charge of Your Personal Hygiene

Are you taking charge of your personal hygiene to treat current health issues or prevent future problems? Practicing good personal hygiene can boost self-confidence and help you stay healthy. Examples of good personal hygiene tasks include the following:

- bathing or showering regularly
- washing your face daily
- applying lotion to your skin
- using deodorant or antiperspirant
- brushing and flossing your teeth
- keeping your nails dry, clean, and trim
- eating healthy foods
- drinking plenty of water
- getting enough sleep

- managing stress
- wearing sunglasses outside
- avoiding loud noises

Setting Personal Hygiene Goals

If you are currently skipping any healthy personal hygiene habits, you may want to set some personal hygiene goals. Remember to write SMART (specific, measurable, achievable, relevant, and timely) goals. After developing your goals, create a *Personal Hygiene Goal Chart* like the one below to monitor daily and weekly progress. If you are successful in meeting your goal for the day, add a smiley face in your chart.

Based on your results, what changes, if any, should you make to your goals? Continue to adjust your goals each week as needed until these healthy habits are part of your lifestyle.

Personal Hygiene Goal Chart

Goals	Monday	Tuesday	Wednesday	Thursday	Friday	Saturday	Sunday
Floss							
Turn my music down							
Sleep for 9 hours							
Wash my face							

Many common problems with the mouth and teeth result from the choices people make. You have some control over whether you develop these problems, and these problems tend to be easier to fix. The following are strategies you can use to prevent some of the most common mouth and teeth problems:

- Brush your teeth, including your tongue, at least twice a day. Use a soft-bristle brush and toothpaste that contains fluoride.
- Get a new toothbrush when the bristles wear out, which is usually about every three months.
- Floss your teeth every day to help remove food particles that remain stuck between your teeth after brushing.
- Avoid using any type of tobacco, including cigarettes and chewing tobacco.
- Eat healthful foods, such as fruits and vegetables. Avoid eating sticky foods that are high in sugar and starch, such as candy, cakes, and soda. If you do eat these types of foods, brush your teeth as soon as possible afterward.
- If you have bad breath and you brush and floss regularly, use an antiseptic mouth-rinse, which reduces the bacteria that cause bad breath.
- See your dentist twice a year. Your dentist will catch mouth problems early on, when they can be more easily treated.
- Wear a mouth guard during activities that can result in broken teeth, such as football or ice hockey.
- If cold sores are painful, treat them using a skin cream or ointment that will speed up the healing and help ease the pain.

Eyes

Most people rely on their sense of vision more than their other senses. You need good vision for many activities in your daily life, from kicking a soccer ball and taking a photograph to riding a bicycle. Keeping your eyes healthy is important. How do your eyes let you see the world? What are some good strategies for keeping them healthy?

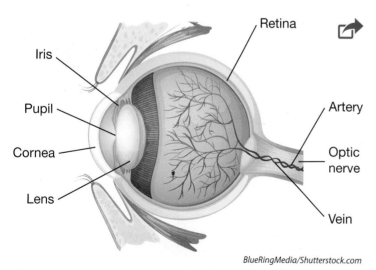

BlueRingMedia/Shutterstock.com

Figure 2.19 The cornea, iris, pupil, lens, and retina work together in the eye to give you vision. *What is the name of the opening in the middle of the iris?*

Understanding Vision

Many different parts of your eyes must work together to show you the world (**Figure 2.19**). The light you see first passes through the *cornea*, a clear tissue that covers the front of the eye.

Next, light reaches the *iris*, which is the colored part of the eye. Light passes into the inner eye through a small opening in the middle of the iris—the *pupil*. The pupil changes size, which influences the amount of light that can enter the inner eye. In bright light, the pupil is small and lets in relatively little light. In dim light, the pupil is large and considerable light enters the eye.

After the light moves through the pupil, it reaches the *lens*, a clear part of the eye. The lens focuses the light onto the *retina*. The retina is a light-sensitive tissue that contains millions of specialized cells called *rods* and *cones*. Rods and cones convert light into nerve impulses or electrical signals. These nerve impulses travel from the retina to the brain through the optic nerve. The brain interprets these impulses into the color images you see.

Because the eyes and brain work together to convert light into color, people may experience slight differences in the way they see colors. People who see colors very differently from the way others see colors have color blindness. People with *color blindness* are not aware of differences among colors. The most common form of color blindness is an inability to distinguish red from green (**Figure 2.20**). Another form is blue-yellow color blindness. A complete lack of color vision is *total color blindness*, which is very rare.

Common Vision Problems

For many people, especially young people, vision works well. Other people, however, experience vision problems. For example, in some people, the shape of the eyeball is such that light does not focus where it needs to focus—on the retina (**Figure 2.21**). People whose parents have vision problems are also more likely to have vision problems themselves. Vision problems are more common in older people because aging can cause changes in parts of the eye.

eveleen/Shutterstock.com

Figure 2.20 A common test to check for red-green color blindness is shown here. *What are the two most common forms of color blindness?*

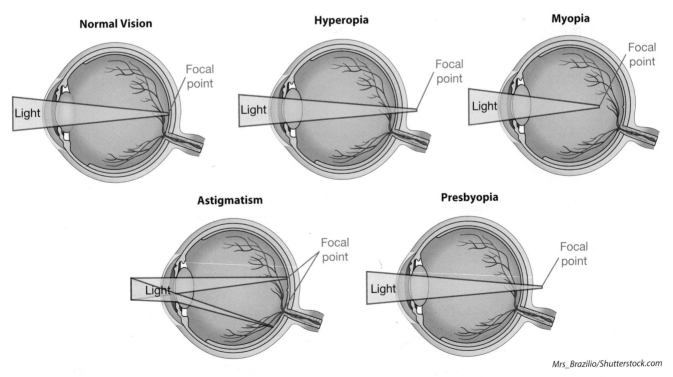

Normal Vision **Hyperopia** **Myopia**

Light — Focal point

Light — Focal point

Light — Focal point

Astigmatism **Presbyopia**

Light — Focal point

Light — Focal point

Mrs_Brazilio/Shutterstock.com

Figure 2.21 Common vision problems include hyperopia (farsightedness), myopia (nearsightedness), astigmatism, and presbyopia. *Where is the focal point of light in a person with normal vision?*

The following are the most common vision problems:

- **Nearsightedness** (or *myopia*) is a condition in which objects close to the eye appear clear, while objects farther away appear blurry. In the eye of someone who is nearsighted, light focuses in front of the retina instead of on the retina.
- **Farsightedness** (or *hyperopia*) is a condition in which distant objects are seen more clearly than nearby objects. In the eye of someone who is farsighted, light focuses behind the retina instead of on the retina.
- **Astigmatism** is a condition in which the eye does not focus light evenly onto the retina. As a result, objects appear blurry and stretched out.
- **Presbyopia** is a condition that affects adults beginning in middle age. In this condition, the lens of the eye loses its elasticity. It becomes harder to see close objects clearly.

Fortunately, these problems can usually be corrected with glasses or contact lenses. Surgery can also correct, or at least improve, some vision problems. LASIK (or *laser in-situ keratomileusis*) is a surgery that works by reshaping the cornea, which allows light to reach the retina, and helps improve vision.

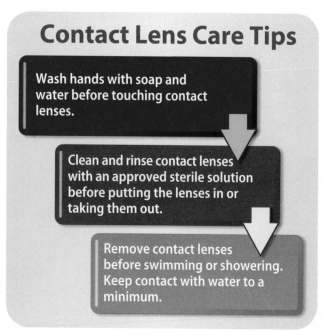

Figure 2.22 Proper care of contact lenses is essential to eye health.

Protecting Your Eyes

There are several simple strategies to help you keep your eyes as healthy as possible throughout your lifetime. Wear protective eyewear when playing contact sports or doing activities that can create flying debris that could hit the eyes. When spending time outdoors, wear sunglasses to block harmful UV rays. If you wear contact lenses, care for your lenses properly to avoid infection (**Figure 2.22**). Perhaps the simplest step you can take to protect your eyes is to get regular eye exams.

Ears

What do the following activities have in common: target shooting, woodworking, playing in a band, attending rock concerts, and using a leaf blower? All of these activities can contribute to hearing loss. Many teenagers regularly expose themselves to loud noises, often through headphones. The sense of hearing allows you to listen to music you enjoy, talk with friends, and be alerted to approaching cars and other dangers. Did you know your ears also play a role in helping you keep your balance?

In the following sections, you will learn about parts of the ear and their functions. You will also learn about common hearing problems and strategies for maintaining your hearing.

Parts of the Ear

The ear has three main parts, and each serves a different, but important, role (**Figure 2.23**). The outer ear, which is called the *pinna*, is the large part of the ear that people can see. The main job of the pinna is to help bring sounds into the ear. Sounds then enter the *auditory canal*, the part of the ear that extends inward. The ear canal is where earwax is produced. This part of the ear also *amplifies* (increases the volume of) sounds so they can be clearly heard and interpreted.

After sound is gathered by the outer ear and sent through the ear canal, it reaches the middle ear. The middle ear includes the *eardrum*, which vibrates when sounds reach it. This part of the ear also includes three small bones—the hammer, the anvil, and the stirrup.

The inner ear converts sound vibrations produced in the middle ear into neural impulses that the brain recognizes as sound. This part of the ear includes the *cochlea*, which is a spiral tube. The cochlea is covered with nerve cells, which pick up different vibrations. These vibrations are then sent to the brain through the auditory nerve. The inner ear also includes the *semicircular canals*, which are attached to the cochlea. These canals are filled with fluids that move when you move, helping you to keep your balance.

Anatomy of the Ear

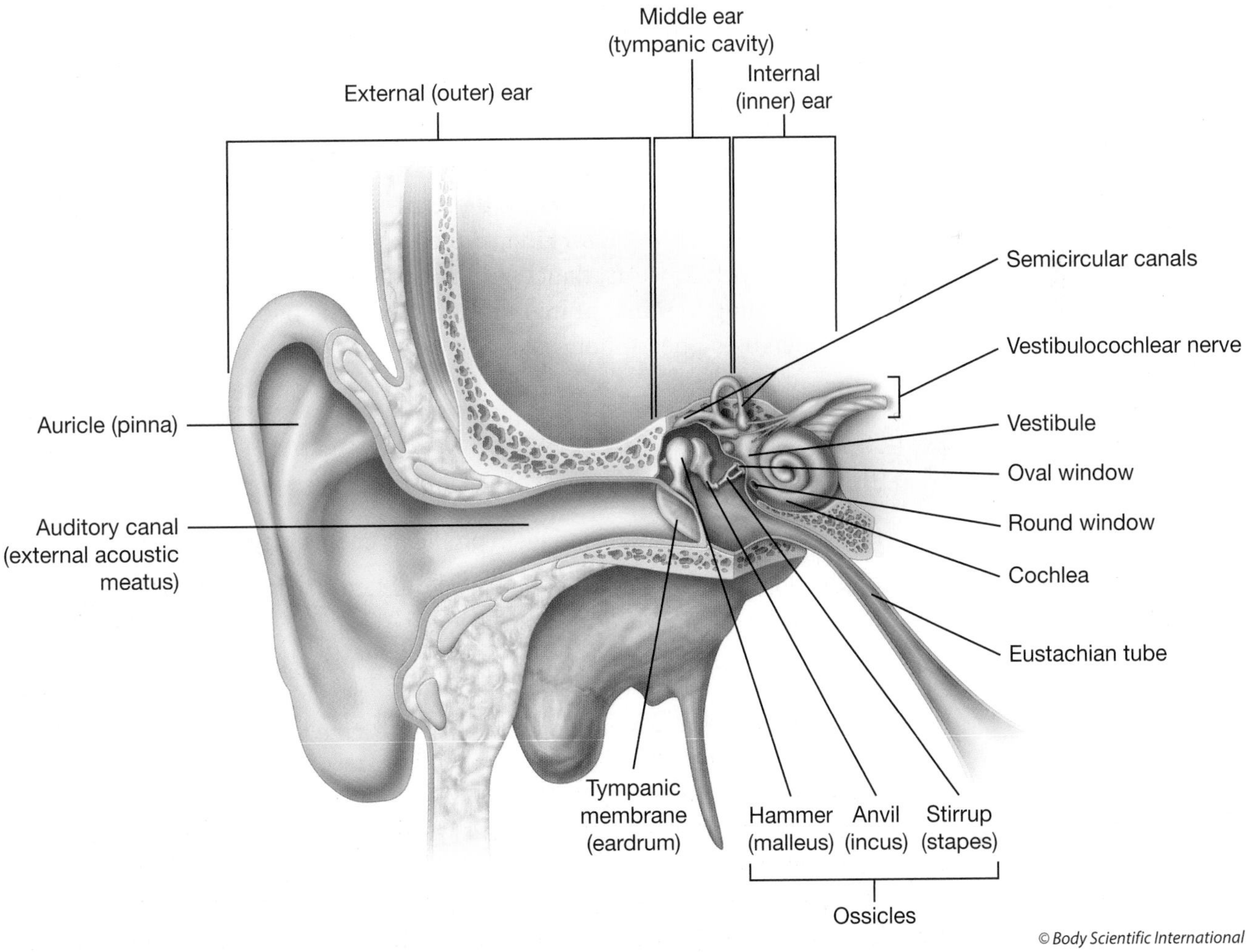

© Body Scientific International

Figure 2.23 This diagram shows the anatomy of the ear. *Where in the ear is earwax produced?*

Common Hearing Problems

The most serious health problem associated with the ears is permanent loss of hearing. Hearing loss is typically caused by damage to the inner ear. This damage is often the result of repeated exposure to excessively loud sounds, which can cause damage to the nerve cells in the cochlea. This may mean exposure to loud music through headphones (**Figure 2.24**).

Sound *intensity*, or loudness, is measured in units called *decibels*. You can experience hearing loss by listening to sounds at or above 85 decibels over an extended period of time. The louder the sound, the less time it takes for hearing damage to occur.

Hearing loss can also be caused more suddenly by a ruptured eardrum. This may occur as a result of loud blasts of noise, sudden changes in pressure, insertion of an object into the ear, or an infection. In fact, just one exposure to a very loud sound, blast, or impulse (at or above 120 decibels) can cause hearing loss.

Unfortunately, many people do not notice that they are losing their hearing because damage from noise exposure is usually gradual. By the time they notice, they have substantial symptoms of permanent hearing loss. Early signs of hearing damage include the following:

- difficulty hearing relatively soft sounds, such as doorbells
- difficulty understanding speech during telephone conversations or in noisy environments
- pain or ringing in the ears, or **tinnitus**, after exposure to excessively loud sounds

Protecting Your Hearing

Once hearing is lost, it cannot be brought back completely, but hearing aids can help improve hearing. Fortunately, there are several simple ways to protect your ears and avoid hearing loss. First, avoid exposure to very high levels of noise, such as at rock concerts, dances, or construction sites, whenever possible. Next, avoid listening to music at high volume levels (above 85 decibels), especially when using headphones.

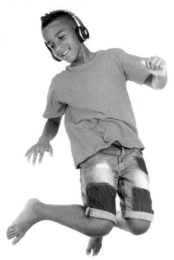

Samuel Borges Photography/ Shutterstock.com

Figure 2.24
One recent study found that 12.5 percent of children and teenagers (6 to 19 years of age) experience hearing loss caused by using headphones or earbuds at too high a volume. *What level of sound intensity can cause hearing damage?*

Lesson 2.2 Review

1. Name two common mouth and teeth problems people may experience.
2. You should brush and floss your teeth at least _____ a day.
3. The colored part of the eye is called the _____.
4. **Critical thinking.** Name the parts of the ear and describe the function of each part.

Hands-On Activity

In small groups, create a life-size guide to personal hygiene. To begin, have a group member lie down to allow the others to trace his or her body on paper. Outside the outline, draw arrows from various body parts to the following information: personal hygiene tips to care for this area, hygiene products to care for it, and the benefits to using the product.

Review and Assessment

Summary

Lesson 2.1 Caring for Your Skin, Hair, and Nails

- *Personal hygiene* is the act of caring for and cleaning your body. Taking a bath or shower and applying deodorant or antiperspirant every day will help prevent body odor.
- Eating healthy foods, drinking lots of water, and getting enough sleep can help your skin look and stay healthy.
- Spending too much time in the sun, or in tanning beds, can damage skin and possibly lead to skin cancer. Take precautions such as applying sunscreen with a minimum of 15 SPF to protect yourself when outdoors.
- *Acne* is a skin condition commonly developed during adolescence. It occurs when glands produce too much oil and clog pores. Washing your face gently twice a day can help treat and prevent acne.
- A condition that causes swollen, red, dry, and itchy patches of skin on one or more parts of the body is *eczema*, or dermatitis. Eczema is not contagious and is often treatable with over-the-counter products.
- Getting a tattoo or a body piercing is a permanent decision. People should think carefully about the risks involved with these procedures before making a decision.
- Having oily hair or dandruff are common conditions during puberty. Regularly washing your hair and eating a diet of healthy foods will help keep your hair healthy.
- To care for your nails, keep them dry, clean, and trimmed. Wear gloves when using harsh chemicals.

Lesson 2.2 Keeping Your Mouth, Eyes, and Ears Healthy

- *Oral health* refers to your mouth, teeth, and gums. If you have poor oral hygiene, bacteria can cause infections or disease.
- You should brush and floss your teeth at least twice a day to prevent cavities and plaque from forming. Plaque can harm the enamel surface of your teeth and lead to gingivitis in the gums.
- Poor oral hygiene, gum disease, cavities, trapped food particles, and certain medical conditions can cause bad breath.
- Certain mouth and teeth problems can be treated at home while others need to be treated by a dentist or orthodontist.
- Common vision problems can be corrected with glasses, contact lenses, or surgery (like LASIK). Protect your eyes with eyewear during contact sports or in construction areas and with sunglasses when outdoors.
- Exposure to loud sound through headphones can damage the inner ear and cause hearing loss. The louder the sound, the less time it takes to inflict hearing damage. Hearing loss can also be caused by a ruptured eardrum from changes in pressure, insertion of an object into the ear, or an infection.
- Get regular vision and hearing exams to treat any conditions before they get worse.

Check Your Knowledge

Record your answers to each of the following questions on a separate sheet of paper.

1. **True or false.** You can damage your skin with exposure to UV light from the sun, tanning beds, and sunlamps.
2. Which of the following strategies will help prevent and treat acne breakouts?
   A. Cover up existing acne with makeup.
   B. Pop pimples on your skin.
   C. Avoid touching dirty glasses, headbands, and hats to your face.
   D. Cover pimples with your hair.
3. A doctor who specializes in skin conditions is called a(n) _____.
4. The higher the _____, the more a sunscreen will protect skin from UV rays.
5. What are the two most common types of body art?
6. Which hair condition can be the result of either dry or irritated skin or infrequent shampooing?
7. **True or false.** Irregularities in toenails and fingernails, such as redness and swelling, discoloration, or curled nails, are normal.
8. List the three distinct parts of a tooth.
9. **True or false.** Plaque helps protect teeth and gums from diseases caused by small food particles or bacteria in the mouth.
10. What are two potential causes of bad breath?
11. Which of the following types of specialists helps prevent and correct teeth misalignments?
    A. Dentist.
    B. Dermatologist.
    C. Orthodontist.
    D. Cardiologist.
12. **True or false.** You should brush your teeth at least twice a day, and especially after eating foods that are sticky or high in starch and sugar.
13. What are the four most common vision problems?
14. The three main parts of the ear are the _____, _____, and _____.

Use Your Vocabulary

acne	dermis	nearsightedness
antiperspirant	eczema	orthodontist
astigmatism	epidermis	periodontitis
body art	farsightedness	plaque
cavities	gingivitis	presbyopia
dandruff	hypodermis	tinnitus
deodorant	lice	

15. In small groups, brainstorm different topics or categories for the terms above and classify as many of the terms as possible. Then, share your ideas with the remainder of the class.
16. Choose one of the terms from the list above. Then, use the Internet to locate photos that visually show the meaning of the term you chose. Print the photo with a caption that explains the term. Share the photo and meaning of the term in class. Ask for clarification if necessary.

Think Critically

17. **Analyze.** Are there differences in the rules and expectations of personal hygiene between different races, cultures, and religions? Give a detailed answer.

18. **Determine.** How can a child's environment and family impact his or her desire to get a tattoo or body piercing?

19. **Identify.** What are some reasons someone would not take care of his or her personal hygiene?

20. **Cause and effect.** How can personal hygiene affect how someone feels about himself or herself and his or her relationships with others?

DEVELOP Your Skills

21. **Advocacy and teamwork skills.** In small groups, create three flyers to raise awareness of personal hygiene issues that affect the students at your school. Choose three personal hygiene issues in this chapter to research. For each issue, create one flyer that provides important health information about the topic. The flyers should provide accurate information and be colorful and creative. With permission, hang these flyers in the school bathrooms to help raise awareness about these issues among people your age.

22. **Access information and technology skills.** Choose a personal hygiene issue commonly affecting middle school students. Search reliable health resources online to learn more about some of the hygiene products suggested for people in your age group to treat or prevent this issue. Evaluate two different products. Were the products scientifically tested? Are they safe and effective? Compare and contrast these products. Is one product more expensive, healthy, or useful than the other? Which one would you recommend to your peers? Create a presentation highlighting the information learned. Present your findings to the class.

23. **Technology and communication skills.** Imagine your best friend confesses her insecurities about her personal hygiene in the following text message. Write a response with respectful, encouraging words and honest feedback. What advice can you share? Should your friend speak to a trusted adult about Devon?

> PE was horrible today. We had to run three miles! My armpits were so sweaty and Devon made fun of me. I smelled horrible and now I have two pimples on my nose.

24. **Decision-making skills.** Imagine your family has to cut back on basic hygiene products such as deodorant, soap, floss, toothpaste, and hair and skin products due to financial problems. In addition, you have less access to water to bathe and wash your clothes. As a result, your clothes are not being washed regularly and you shower less often. Recently, you have begun to notice an increase in body odor. Lastly, your teeth have a film and yellow stain on them. Write a short essay about how you would respond to a situation like this. What would you do? What resources are available to you? Who would you go to for guidance? What would you say to begin the conversation?

Chapter 3

Getting the Sleep You Need

Lesson 3.1 Understanding Sleep

Lesson 3.2 Common Sleeping Problems

Lesson 3.3 Developing Strategies for Getting Enough Sleep

Essential Question ?

What health benefits accompany getting enough sleep?

Video ↗
Access the Chapter 3 video to start thinking about chapter topics.

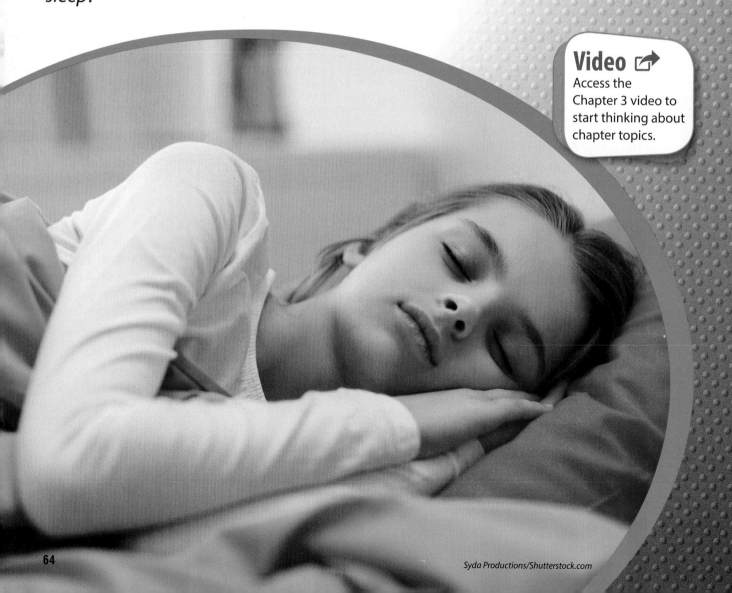

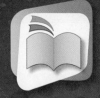

Using reliable online resources, find an article discussing strategies for getting quality sleep. Take notes as you read the article and then this chapter. Compare your notes on the article and the chapter and assess how the article is similar to or different from this chapter. Write a summary of your findings.

How Healthy Are You?

In this chapter, you will be learning about sleep. Before you begin reading, take the following quiz to assess your current sleep habits.

Healthy Choices	Yes	No
Do you get 8½ to 9½ hours of sleep every night?		
If you suffer from a sleep disorder, like sleep apnea or nightmares, have you sought out forms of treatment?		
Do you go to bed at approximately the same time each night and get up at approximately the same time each morning?		
Do you follow the same sleeping pattern on weekends as throughout the week?		
Do you exercise for 20 to 30 minutes a day?		
Do you avoid caffeine in food or drinks in the hours leading up to your bedtime?		
Do you practice relaxation techniques like reading a book or taking a warm shower to wind down before bed?		
Have you created a cool, dark, and quiet environment in which you can sleep?		
Do you minimize the time you spend in front of a television, computer, or phone screen near the end of the day?		
Do you avoid napping for too long or too close to your bedtime, so you do not disrupt your normal sleep cycle?		

Count your "Yes" and "No" responses. The more "Yes" responses you have, the more healthy sleep habits you exhibit. Now, take a closer look at the questions with which you responded "No." How can you make these healthy habits part of your daily life? Think about how implementing these ideas can help improve your overall health.

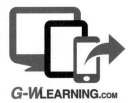

G-WLEARNING.com

While studying this chapter, look for the activity icon to

- **practice** key terms with e-flash cards and matching activities.
- **reinforce** what you learn by completing graphic organizers, self-assessment quizzes, and review questions.
- **expand** knowledge with interactive activities and activities that extend learning.

www.g-wlearning.com/health/

Understanding Sleep

Key Terms ⏩

sleep deprived term used to describe a person who gets inadequate amounts of sleep

short sleepers people who can function well on less sleep than other people

sleep deficit condition that occurs when people frequently get less sleep than they should

circadian rhythms naturally occurring physical, behavioral, and mental changes in the body that typically follow the 24-hour cycle of the sun

sleep-wake cycle pattern of sleeping in a 24-hour period

melatonin hormone that increases feelings of relaxation and sleepiness and signals that it is time to go to sleep

jet lag fatigue that people feel after changing time zones when they travel

REM sleep active stage of sleep during which your breathing changes, your heart rate and blood pressure rise, and your eyes dart around rapidly

Learning Outcomes

After studying this lesson, you will be able to

- **understand** why sleep is important.
- **describe** the sleep needs of each age group.
- **explain** the science of sleep, the stages of sleep, and dreams.
- **determine** the consequences of not getting enough sleep.

Graphic Organizer ⏩

The Importance of Sleep

In a graphic organizer like the one shown below, write five to six statements about the importance of sleep to your health. As you read the lesson, add any health benefits of sleep that you did not previously know.

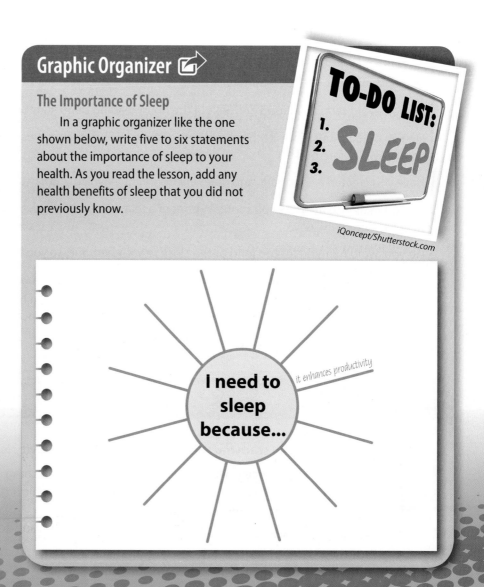

iQoncept/Shutterstock.com

it enhances productivity

I need to sleep because...

Sanjay is 12 years old and rarely gets 10 to 11 hours of sleep, the recommended amount for his age group. He has to wake up at 5:30 a.m. to get to school on time. He also likes to stay up late at night because this is when his favorite TV shows air. When he tries to go to bed, it takes him a long time to fall asleep. Sanjay knows he is sleep deprived. He has a hard time paying attention in class and maintaining his energy during football practice. He has been getting sick more often, too.

Sleep is an important process that his body needs each night. Without sleep, Sanjay's body is unable to heal or rest after performing daily activities. This can pose serious risks to his health and lifestyle.

In this lesson, you will learn why sleep is so important to your overall health and wellness, and how much sleep you need based on your age. You will also learn about the processes in your body that influence sleep. Finally, you will learn about the effects of not getting enough sleep.

Why You Need Sleep

How did you feel when you woke up this morning? Did you spring out of bed to face the new day, feeling completely refreshed and rested? Did you hit the snooze button a few times before crawling out of bed, dragging yourself to school, and nearly nodding off in class? How much sleep you get can affect your overall health and wellness (**Figure 3.1**).

If you felt completely refreshed, you likely got an *adequate* amount of sleep. This means that you got enough sleep to function properly throughout the day. If you find yourself falling asleep in class, however, you likely got an *inadequate* amount of sleep. This means you did not get enough sleep to function. *Insufficient* is another term for inadequate. A person who is **sleep deprived** gets inadequate amounts of sleep.

Sleep is a complex process. During sleep, the body is *unconscious*, or inactive, but the brain remains very active. Some scientists think that your brain sorts through stress and information, replaces chemicals, and solves problems during sleep.

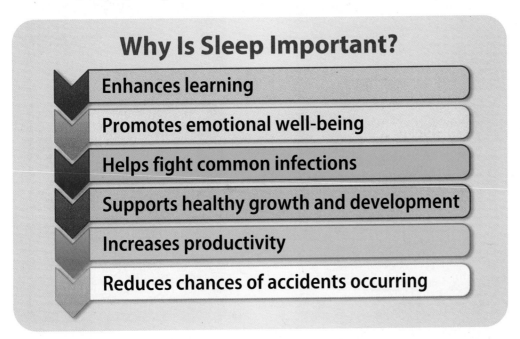

Why Is Sleep Important?

- Enhances learning
- Promotes emotional well-being
- Helps fight common infections
- Supports healthy growth and development
- Increases productivity
- Reduces chances of accidents occurring

Figure 3.1
Regularly getting enough sleep can benefit your health and wellness in many ways. *What is the term for a person who gets inadequate amounts of sleep?*

Why do your body and brain require an adequate amount of sleep? Scientists do not know the true purpose of sleep (**Figure 3.2**). It is clear, however, that getting an adequate amount of sleep helps the body heal, rest, and *rejuvenate* itself. The term *rejuvenate* means to refresh and feel more energetic. Getting an inadequate amount of sleep can result in feeling cranky, being unable to think clearly, and getting into arguments more easily.

Although scientists do not know exactly why people need sleep, you are likely to notice the benefits of a good night's sleep. After getting an adequate amount of sleep, you likely feel refreshed and ready to tackle a new day. If you go without sleep, you may not feel like yourself. It is important to get an adequate amount of sleep each night so your body and brain can function properly each day.

Sleep Needs and Age

The amount of sleep that a person needs depends on his or her age. Infants, children, and teens need considerably more sleep than adults need. Young people need more sleep because their bodies and brains are still developing. Sleep encourages the development process and helps young people grow.

Figure 3.2
Scientists may not know the true purpose of sleep, but there are many facts about sleep that they do know to be true. Some might surprise you because of persisting myths about sleep.

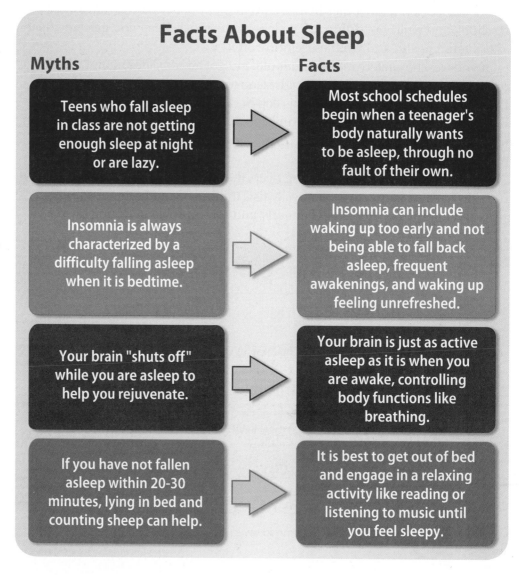

Facts About Sleep

Myths	Facts
Teens who fall asleep in class are not getting enough sleep at night or are lazy.	Most school schedules begin when a teenager's body naturally wants to be asleep, through no fault of their own.
Insomnia is always characterized by a difficulty falling asleep when it is bedtime.	Insomnia can include waking up too early and not being able to fall back asleep, frequent awakenings, and waking up feeling unrefreshed.
Your brain "shuts off" while you are asleep to help you rejuvenate.	Your brain is just as active asleep as it is when you are awake, controlling body functions like breathing.
If you have not fallen asleep within 20-30 minutes, lying in bed and counting sheep can help.	It is best to get out of bed and engage in a relaxing activity like reading or listening to music until you feel sleepy.

Figure 3.3 shows general sleep requirements for different age groups. Keep in mind, however, that each person may need more or less sleep. For example, some people are **short sleepers**, meaning they can function well on less sleep. These people often feel fully awake after sleeping for only 4 to 6 hours. Other people may need more than 9 hours of sleep to feel fully rested.

Many people in each age group experience a **sleep deficit**. This means that they frequently get less sleep than they should. Think about how much sleep you usually get each night. Do you get enough sleep according to the amounts identified in Figure 3.3? Not meeting these sleep requirements causes people to experience a sleep deficit. People might experience a sleep deficit for a variety of reasons. They may go to sleep too late based on when they have to wake up in the morning. Over time, a sleep deficit can result in health concerns.

The Science of Sleep

The body and brain are very active during sleep, and this activity is essential to staying healthy. This healing activity cannot occur unless you sleep. Systems in your body help you get this necessary rest. Certain *mechanisms*, or processes, in the body control when you feel tired and when you feel awake. These mechanisms include circadian rhythms and the release of hormones such as melatonin.

Circadian rhythms are naturally occurring physical, behavioral, and mental changes in the body that typically follow the 24-hour cycle of the sun (**Figure 3.4** on the next page). For example, the body's temperature drops during the night and rises during the day. Most circadian rhythms are controlled by the body's master biological "clock." This "clock" controls circadian rhythms such as the sleep-wake cycle, body temperature, hormone levels, and brain wave activity.

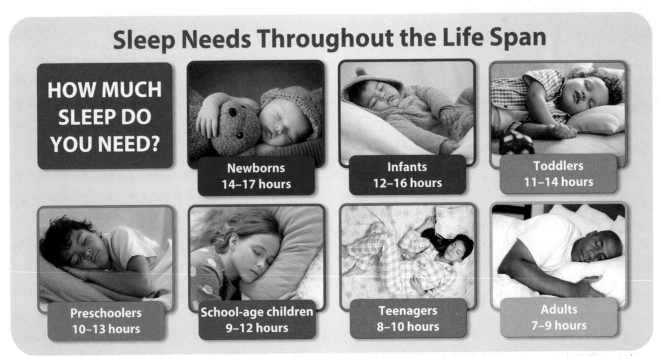

Clockwise from top left: Ramona Heim/Shutterstock.com; Durganand/Shutterstock.com; g-stockstudio/Shutterstock.com; JPC-PROD/Shutterstock.com; Ruslan Guzov/Shutterstock.com; Ariwasabi/Shutterstock.com; pixelheadstudio digitalskillet/Shutterstock.com

Figure 3.3 Sleep needs are not the same for every person across the life span. As you grow, you require fewer hours of sleep each night.

Figure 3.4
The body automatically adjusts to specific times, providing better coordination and alertness during the day and deepest sleep at night. *When does the body start secreting melatonin to help encourage sleep?*

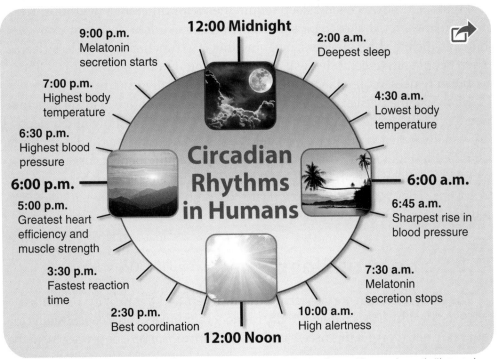

Circadian Rhythms in Humans

12:00 Midnight

9:00 p.m.
Melatonin secretion starts

7:00 p.m.
Highest body temperature

6:30 p.m.
Highest blood pressure

6:00 p.m.

5:00 p.m.
Greatest heart efficiency and muscle strength

3:30 p.m.
Fastest reaction time

2:30 p.m.
Best coordination

12:00 Noon

10:00 a.m.
High alertness

7:30 a.m.
Melatonin secretion stops

6:45 a.m.
Sharpest rise in blood pressure

6:00 a.m.

4:30 a.m.
Lowest body temperature

2:00 a.m.
Deepest sleep

Clockwise from top: kdshutterman/Shutterstock.com; Sanit Fuangnakhon/Shutterstock.com; estherpoon/Shutterstock.com; sihy/Shutterstock.com

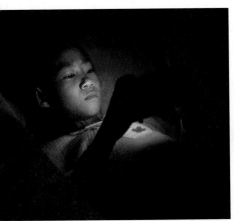

My Life Graphic/Shutterstock.com

Figure 3.5 A person's body will only produce melatonin when the person is in an environment that is dark or dimly lit. Sunlight and bright indoor lighting can prevent the release of melatonin. *What is the body's physical reaction to the hormone melatonin?*

A person's **sleep-wake cycle** is his or her pattern of sleeping in a 24-hour period. The biological clock regulates the sleep-wake cycle in two ways. First, it monitors the amount of light in the environment. If it senses light, the biological clock sends signals in the body that result in activity. If there is less light, the biological clock can send signals to make the body less active. The biological clock also causes a gland located in the brain to release the hormone **melatonin** when it gets dark (**Figure 3.5**). Melatonin increases feelings of relaxation and sleepiness and signals that it is time to go to sleep.

When the natural circadian rhythm is disrupted, the body's biological clock takes a while to readjust. This explains **jet lag**, which is a fatigue that people feel after changing time zones when they travel. When people travel by plane from California to New York, their bodies feel like they "lost" three hours. When their alarms ring the next morning at 7 a.m., they are tired because it is only 4 a.m. according to their biological clocks. Jet lag, however, is not the only possible disruption of the sleep-wake cycle. Working night shifts, adjusting the clock for daylight savings, or simply using electric lights late into the night can trick your body into an unnatural circadian rhythm.

Stages of Sleep

Each night, you usually pass through five distinct stages of sleep (**Figure 3.6**). A complete sleep cycle—from Stage 1 through Stage 5—lasts about 90 to 110 minutes. Over the course of a night, you go through this sleep cycle three to five times, depending on how long you sleep. The amount of time you spend in each stage of sleep, however, changes considerably as the night progresses.

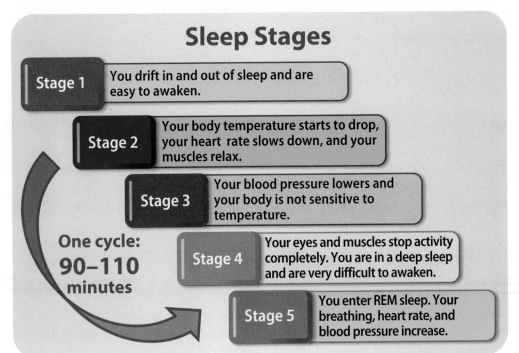

Sleep Stages

Stage 1 You drift in and out of sleep and are easy to awaken.

Stage 2 Your body temperature starts to drop, your heart rate slows down, and your muscles relax.

Stage 3 Your blood pressure lowers and your body is not sensitive to temperature.

One cycle: 90–110 minutes

Stage 4 Your eyes and muscles stop activity completely. You are in a deep sleep and are very difficult to awaken.

Stage 5 You enter REM sleep. Your breathing, heart rate, and blood pressure increase.

Figure 3.6
You should cycle through all five stages of sleep multiple times each night, experiencing noticeable changes in the body's temperature, movement, and systems. *During which stage of sleep does your blood pressure lower?*

The first period of REM sleep usually occurs about 70 to 90 minutes after you fall asleep. **REM sleep** is an active stage of sleep during which a person's breathing changes and becomes irregular, shallow, and more rapid. Heart rate and blood pressure also rise. A person's eyes dart about rapidly under the eyelids (REM stands for *rapid eye movement*), and muscles are temporarily paralyzed.

The first sleep cycles of the night contain relatively short REM periods and long periods of deep sleep (Stage 4). The periods of REM sleep get longer with each sleep cycle, while the deep sleep periods get shorter.

There are smartphone apps available which track users' sleep cycle patterns (**Figure 3.7**). These apps can identify if the user is getting enough good quality sleep, and offer techniques and tools for falling and staying asleep. They can also wake the user at the ideal time, while entering the first stage of sleep. It is important to note, however, that many sleep experts do not believe that a sleep app can provide reliable, accurate data regarding a person's quality of sleep.

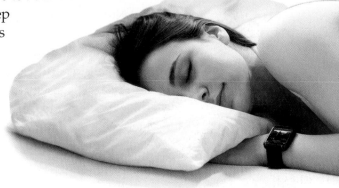

Andrey_Popov/Shutterstock.com

Figure 3.7
Smartphone apps can connect to devices, such as smart watches, which will record heart rate, blood pressure, and more to track the sleep patterns of the user.

Dreaming

Even though you may not remember your dreams, you do dream every night. On most nights, people spend more than two hours dreaming. Many of these dreams will last between 5 and 20 minutes. What a person dreams about, however, may change a lot from night to night. Sometimes dreams may closely relate to what is going on in someone's daily life. At other times, dreams may appear bizarre and unreal.

Although most dreams occur during REM sleep, they can also occur during other sleep stages (**Figure 3.8**). Dreams that occur during REM sleep—when the brain is particularly active—are very vivid. People who wake up at the end of a REM sleep period are more likely to remember their dreams.

How dreams influence a person's well-being is unclear because it is difficult to study dreams. This difficulty is because people often forget most of their dreams. Some sleep researchers believe that dreams play a valuable role in daily life. They believe dreams help people remember information, resolve conflicts, and regulate their moods. Dreams may provide important information about a person's deepest feelings, thoughts, and motives.

The Impact of Insufficient Sleep

Getting enough sleep is just as important to good health as eating well or exercising. Unfortunately, there is no way to train your body to function well on less sleep. Getting insufficient sleep on a regular basis can lead to health conditions, accidents, and poor performance in both school and athletics.

Health Conditions

Not getting enough sleep can have a negative effect on a person's health in many different ways. People who do not get enough sleep are more likely to get colds and other types of infections. Inadequate sleep on a regular basis can result in serious health conditions, such as diabetes, high blood pressure, and heart disease. Children who do not get enough sleep might not grow at the expected rate. A person's memory and learning can also be affected by lack of sleep.

Figure 3.8
These fun facts about dreaming explore this body function that people do not fully understand. *During which stage of sleep does dreaming typically occur?*

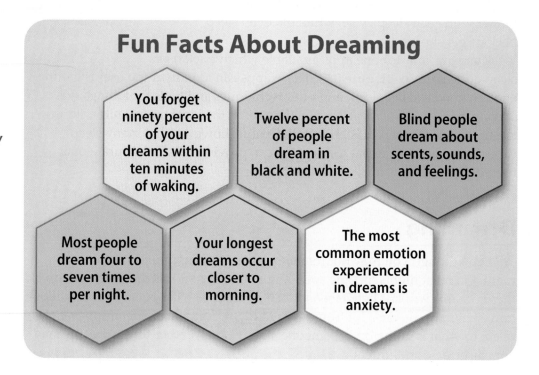

Fun Facts About Dreaming

You forget ninety percent of your dreams within ten minutes of waking.

Twelve percent of people dream in black and white.

Blind people dream about scents, sounds, and feelings.

Most people dream four to seven times per night.

Your longest dreams occur closer to morning.

The most common emotion experienced in dreams is anxiety.

Get Proper Rest to Be at Your Best

The average middle schooler needs

9–11 hours of sleep each night

Lack of sleep can lead to a higher risk of heart disease, stroke, and high blood pressure

People who do not sleep enough are more likely to make

unhealthy food decisions

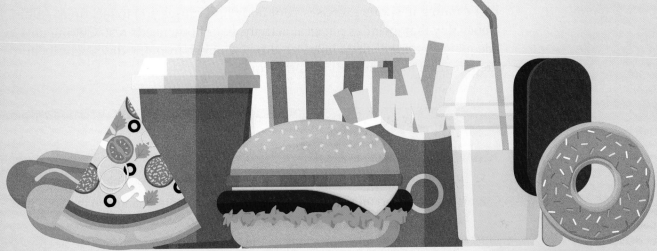

Studies show that students who get enough sleep each night tend to earn **better grades** than students who do not get enough sleep

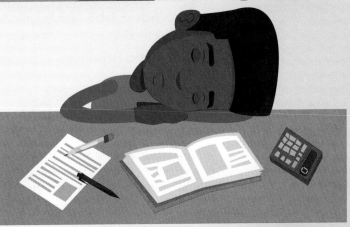

Top left: Olga Kovalska/Shutterstock.com; Top right: Anastasia_B/Shutterstock.com; Middle: VectorPlotnikoff/Shutterstock.com; Bottom: Visual Generation/Shutterstock.com

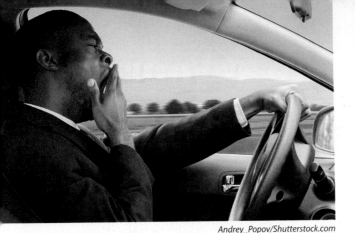

Andrey_Popov/Shutterstock.com

Figure 3.9 People who drive while drowsy are just as likely to have an accident as those who drive while drunk. *How can sleep deprivation lead to accidents?*

Accidents

People who are sleep deprived often have trouble paying attention, concentrating, and reacting quickly. This can result in accidents that may cause serious injuries and even death. For example, driving while tired is very dangerous (**Figure 3.9**). A drowsy driver could miss a stop sign or a red light and cause an accident. In some cases, sleepy drivers fall asleep at the wheel and drive off the road. Some people may drink coffee or sodas with caffeine to try to stay awake while driving. These substances do not make up for lack of sleep, however.

Poor School and Athletic Performance

Students who do not get enough sleep often have problems concentrating, paying attention, solving problems, and remembering information. They may even fall asleep during class. If students are too tired to focus on their studies, they may get bad grades. Over time, not getting enough sleep can lead to lower grades. It is important to get an adequate amount of sleep each night if you want to learn and maintain good grades in school.

Insufficient sleep can also affect a young person's athletic performance. Participating in sports exercises your body and causes you to feel tired. After a busy day that includes physical activity, your body needs rest. Getting an adequate amount of sleep helps your body refresh from the day's activity and prepare itself for more activity tomorrow.

Lesson 3.1 Review

1. How much sleep do school-age children and teens need each night?
2. The naturally occurring physical, behavioral, and mental changes in the body that typically follow the 24-hour cycle of the sun are known as _____ _____.
3. The body releases the hormone _____ in the late evening to encourage sleep.
4. **True or false.** People typically go through the sleep cycle once over the course of a night.
5. **Critical thinking.** List three negative impacts lack of sleep can have on your health.

Hands-On Activity

Explore starting and ending times of middle schools in and surrounding your community. What impact do start and end times have on students' sleep and performance in school and activities? If needed, recommend an appropriate adjustment to your school's schedule and support your recommendation with information about sleep needs of people your age.

Common Sleeping Problems

Learning Outcomes

After studying this lesson, you will be able to

- **explain** symptoms of delayed sleep phase syndrome and insomnia.
- **describe** common types of parasomnia.
- **understand** the symptoms of and treatment for sleep apnea.
- **explain** the symptoms of narcolepsy.

Key Terms

delayed sleep phase syndrome (DSPS) condition that results from a delay in the sleep-wake cycle that affects a person's daily activities

insomnia trouble falling or staying asleep

parasomnia term for sleep disorders that occur when people are partially, but not completely, awoken from sleep

sleep apnea potentially serious disorder in which a person stops breathing for short periods of time during sleep

narcolepsy disorder that affects the brain's ability to control the sleep-wake cycle

Graphic Organizer

Sleep Disorders

In a table like the one shown below, list all the sleep disorders you know about and include a list of possible causes for each one. If multiple disorders have possible causes in common, highlight each repeated cause in a different color.

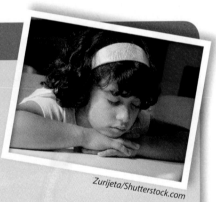

Zurijeta/Shutterstock.com

Sleep Disorders	Possible Causes

75

Have you ever spent an hour or more trying and failing to fall asleep? Have you had nightmares or experienced sleepwalking? Remember the example from Lesson 3.1. Sanjay stays up late watching TV at night and has a hard time falling asleep, which is causing him not to get enough sleep. His sleep deficit is causing him to get sick more often and to struggle to pay attention and work hard in class and at football practice.

Common sleep problems such as these may cause you to lose sleep, but they are usually not serious. Long-term sleep disorders, however, can cause problems at school and in your life. Most importantly, sleep disorders have health consequences. Fortunately, most sleep disorders can be treated once the person recognizes the problem and seeks help. In this lesson, you will learn about some common sleep disorders, as well as available treatments.

Delayed Sleep Phase Syndrome

A common sleep disorder that affects a person's sleep-wake cycle is **delayed sleep phase syndrome (DSPS)**, also called *"night owl" syndrome*. DSPS is a disorder that results in a person being unable to fall asleep until very late at night and naturally not waking up until much later in the morning.

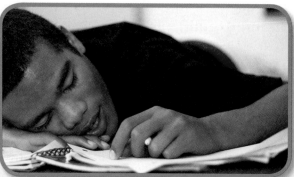

Arieliona/Shutterstock.com

CASE STUDY

Time to Wake Up, Beckett!

Beckett lies in his bed, unable to fall asleep. He keeps rolling over to check the time—10:30 p.m., 11 p.m., 11:30 p.m., 12 a.m., 12:30 a.m. Beckett is starting to worry because he isn't falling asleep and he knows that he needs to get up early in the morning to catch his school bus.

Beckett's alarm goes off at 6:30 a.m., but he hits the snooze button. He knows he has to wake up, but he can't keep his eyes open. He just feels so tired. Maybe if he gets five more minutes of sleep.

The next thing Beckett hears is his dad yelling from the kitchen for him to get up. *Oh man, that must mean it's after 7 a.m.* His dad gets so angry every time he has to wake up Beckett on school days. Beckett realizes his dad just thinks he is being lazy or is sleeping in on purpose or something. He is running late now and will not have time to eat breakfast. Beckett barely has time to get dressed and brush his teeth before the bus arrives.

The extra 30 minutes of sleep Beckett got this morning does not seem to help at all. He still falls asleep during Math, which is his first subject of the

day. Beckett's teacher gently shakes him awake and Beckett can tell that his teacher is annoyed. Mad at himself, Beckett promises himself that tonight he *will* go to sleep at 10:00 p.m. No matter what!

Thinking Critically

1. Consider what you know about sleep among adolescents. Is Beckett's experience common? Why or why not?

2. What sleep disorder may explain Beckett's inability to fall asleep and wake up early?

3. If this happens to Beckett again, what strategies could help him fall asleep?

4. What could Beckett adjust in his life to prevent this from happening again?

DSPS can affect anyone, but is most common during the teenage years. This is because teenagers' bodies are going through many changes as part of the normal growth process. One of these changes is the body's release of melatonin later in the night than normal. This means teens are unable to fall asleep earlier in the evening. As a result, teenagers often do not get enough sleep because they go to bed late, but must still get up early to go to school.

The most common treatment method for DSPS is slowly changing the time a person goes to bed. People with DSPS can try to go to sleep a few minutes earlier each night until they reach the desired bedtime. Once they reach the desired time, the next step is to stick to that new time. If a person stays up late just one night, even on the weekend, his or her sleep-wake cycle can reset to an unhealthy pattern.

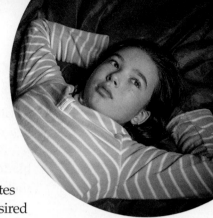

Oleg Golovnev/Shutterstock.com

Figure 3.10
People who have insomnia do not get adequate amounts of sleep. This often affects their ability to function the next day at work or school. *Why is long-term use of sleeping pills to combat insomnia discouraged?*

Insomnia

Almost everyone experiences **insomnia**, which is trouble falling asleep or staying asleep. Some people with insomnia lay awake for hours at night without being able to fall asleep. Others wake up several hours early and are unable to go back to sleep. Having insomnia can negatively affect all aspects of a person's health and well-being (**Figure 3.10**).

Insomnia may be a short-term, temporary problem that is a result of changes in a person's normal routine. For example, if you are going on a family vacation tomorrow, you may not be able to fall asleep on time the night before you leave. Insomnia like this usually goes away on its own.

Long-term insomnia is more serious than short-term insomnia. Long-term insomnia lasts a month or longer. It is often a symptom or side effect of another problem, such as a medical condition, substance abuse, or a sleep disorder. People with long-term insomnia can get help from a doctor, therapist, or counselor.

The most common cause of insomnia is stress. This stress may be a result of issues in a person's life. The stress could even be about the insomnia. Worrying about being unable to fall asleep or about being tired the next day can make insomnia worse.

Insomnia may be treated in many ways. Treatment can include sleeping pills, which are a type of medication that helps people sleep. Long-term use of sleeping pills is discouraged, however, because using them can interfere with good sleeping habits.

Parasomnia

Parasomnia is a term for sleep disorders that occur when people are partially, but not completely, awoken from sleep. Parasomnia occurs more commonly in young people because their brains are still developing. These disorders can occur when people first fall asleep, when they are between sleep stages, or when they awaken from sleep. There are five common types of parasomnia (**Figure 3.11**).

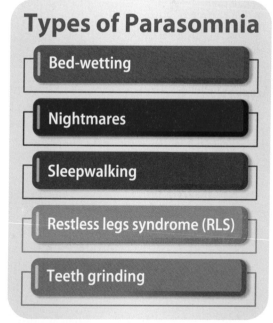

Types of Parasomnia

- Bed-wetting
- Nightmares
- Sleepwalking
- Restless legs syndrome (RLS)
- Teeth grinding

Figure 3.11 Bed-wetting, nightmares, sleepwalking, RLS, and teeth grinding are common parasomnia disorders.

Bed-wetting

Bed-wetting occurs when a person unintentionally urinates (pees) at night during sleep. This condition is very common in children younger than five years of age, but older children and adults even wet the bed sometimes.

Bed-wetting may occur in young children because they have small bladders or they do not yet have full bladder control. It may occur because they sleep too deeply to be woken up by the need to use the bathroom. Some children continue to wet the bed until their teen years. Doctors do not know what causes bed-wetting to continue or why it eventually stops. Adults who wet the bed often do so because of underlying medical issues. They should see a doctor if bed-wetting occurs.

To reduce or avoid instances of bed-wetting, it may help to drink more liquid during the day and less at night, and go to the bathroom immediately before bedtime. If these methods do not work, however, other treatments exist. These include bed-wetting alarms to awaken a person if he or she begins wetting the bed, bladder training, and some medicines.

What Causes Nightmares?

- Daily life stresses or major life changes
- Trauma, such as an accident or injury
- Reading books and watching television programs or movies, especially right before bed
- Eating right before bed, which can cause an increase in energy and brain activity
- Lack of sleep and sleep disorders
- Illness, especially a fever
- Alcohol, illegal drugs, and some types of medications

Figure 3.12 No single factor causes nightmares, and they can occur due to multiple factors at once. *What do young people typically have nightmares about?*

Nightmares

Have you ever woken up terrified after being chased by someone who wanted to do you harm? Perhaps you have dreamt that your teeth fell out or that you forgot about a big test in school. These are some common nightmare scenarios.

Nightmares are scary dreams associated with negative feelings, such as anxiety, fear, and sadness. These dreams are common and often seem real. They may cause people to wake up and have difficulty falling asleep again. Nightmares usually occur during the last hours of sleep in a given night. **Figure 3.12** shows factors that may cause nightmares.

Children often have nightmares about monsters or scary scenarios. The scary images or scenarios are sometimes based on something they saw on television or read about immediately before going to bed. Young people typically have nightmares that focus on fears about their daily lives, such as problems at school or at home.

Having nightmares or being afraid of having nightmares can cause some people to develop a fear of going to sleep. People who have this problem should talk to a doctor.

Sleepwalking

Sleepwalking is a sleep disorder in which people get out of bed and walk around while they are in a state of deep sleep. Sleepwalking typically occurs during stages three and four of the sleep cycle. Sleepwalking runs in families, and it most often affects young people. A person may sleepwalk when he or she is sick, has a fever, is not getting enough sleep, or is experiencing stress.

Sleepwalking may look different for each person. A person who is sleepwalking may walk slowly around a bedroom. Another person may run around the house. While sleepwalking, people may speak in gibberish.

Daytime Issues That Can Cause Nightmares

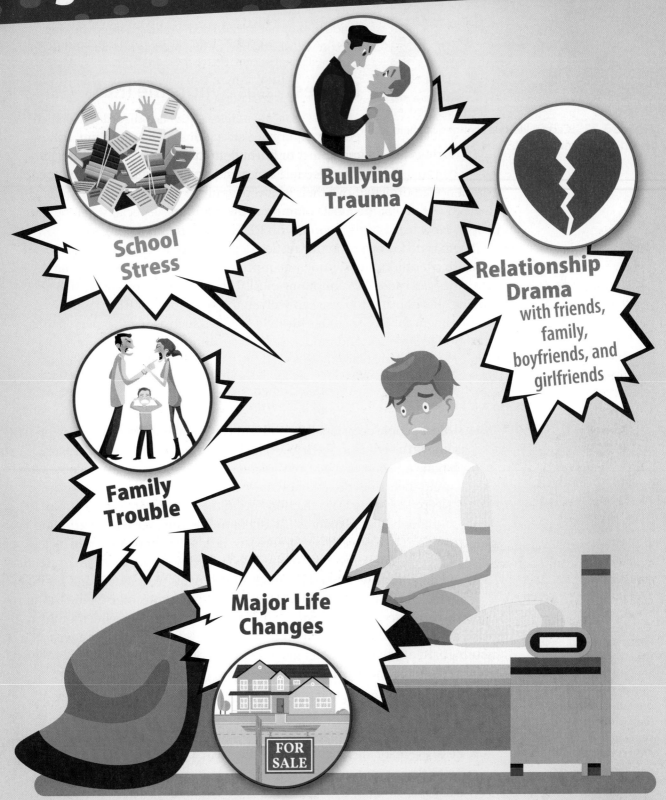

School Stress

Bullying Trauma

Relationship Drama with friends, family, boyfriends, and girlfriends

Family Trouble

Major Life Changes

FOR SALE

Middle: CharacterFamily/Shutterstock.com; Speech bubbles: Fourleaflover/Shutterstock.com; Clockwise from top left: Iconic Bestiary/Shutterstock.com; L-astro/Shutterstock.com; Martial Red/Shutterstock.com; sivVector/Shutterstock.com; Orkidia/Shutterstock.com

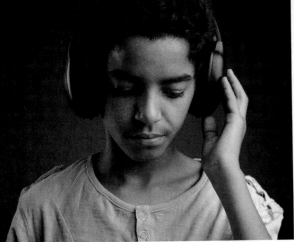
Stokkete/Shutterstock.com

Figure 3.13 Certain lifestyle changes can help lessen the symptoms of RLS.

Although a sleepwalking person's eyes are typically open, he or she will not respond to questions. The affected person will also not remember sleepwalking.

Sleepwalking is not usually a serious problem. A person who is sleepwalking will often find his or her way back to bed. If you find a person sleepwalking, gently guide him or her back to bed. Waking a sleepwalking person will startle him or her, but it is not harmful to do so.

Restless Legs Syndrome (RLS)

Restless legs syndrome (RLS) is a disorder in which people experience sensations such as tingling, itching, cramping, or burning in their legs. People with RLS may also feel aches and pains in their legs. These people experience an urge to move their legs constantly to make these sensations go away. RLS is one of the most common sleep disorders, especially among older people. Not surprisingly, people with RLS have difficulty falling sleep.

There is no known cause for restless legs syndrome. Another disease or health condition, such as anemia or pregnancy, may cause RLS. Some medicines can cause the symptoms of RLS. In addition, substances such as caffeine, alcohol, and tobacco can worsen the symptoms of RLS.

Treatment for RLS includes lifestyle changes such as regular sleep habits, relaxation techniques, and moderate exercise during the day (**Figure 3.13**). Certain medicines can also help lessen the symptoms of these conditions.

Teeth Grinding

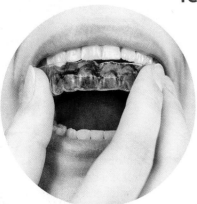
vvoe/Shutterstock.com

Figure 3.14
Wearing a mouth guard at night, such as the one shown here, can help prevent the effects of teeth grinding. *What are some long-term health effects of bruxism?*

Most people occasionally grind and clench their teeth. This behavior is known as *bruxism*. Teeth grinding can be caused by stress or anxiety, having an abnormal bite, or missing or crooked teeth. Many people who grind their teeth do not know they do it because it often occurs during sleep. They may learn that they grind their teeth from other people. Although this behavior is usually harmless, long-term teeth grinding can lead to tooth damage, a sore jaw, headaches, and even hearing loss.

Fortunately, effective treatment methods exist for bruxism. A dentist can determine whether a person is grinding his or her teeth and may suggest wearing a mouth guard during sleep to protect the teeth. A mouth guard, also called a *night guard*, is a piece of plastic similar to the mouth guard athletes wear to protect their teeth (**Figure 3.14**). A person can wear the mouth guard at night to protect his or her teeth and prevent bruxism. A dentist may also recommend the following:

- Avoid chewing on pencils, pens, or gum, which accustoms the jaw muscles to more clenching.
- Focus on relaxing the teeth and jaw while awake.
- Place the tip of the tongue between the teeth to help prevent teeth clenching.
- Relax the jaw muscles before going to sleep by pressing a warm washcloth to the side of the face, or by massaging and stretching the jaw to help it relax.

Since stress can lead to bruxism, other treatment methods focus on reducing overall stress. For example, starting an exercise program can help manage stress. People who experience bruxism should also reduce their consumption of caffeinated foods and drinks, which tend to increase teeth grinding. Drinking more water can be helpful since *dehydration*, or a loss of fluid in the body, may also increase teeth grinding. In severe cases of bruxism, doctors may recommend a prescription medication to prevent the symptoms.

Sleep Apnea

Sleep apnea is a potentially serious disorder in which a person stops breathing for short periods of time during sleep. This disorder is usually associated with loud snoring, but not everyone who snores has this disorder. Many people have sleep apnea, but do not know it, or have not been diagnosed. Sleep apnea is most common among older people, and it is more common in men than in women. There are two types of sleep apnea (**Figure 3.15**).

People with sleep apnea can suffer numerous side effects due to inadequate sleep and a lack of oxygen in their blood. These side effects include the following:

- excessive daytime sleepiness
- irritability or depression
- morning headaches
- decline in mental functioning
- high blood pressure
- irregular heartbeats
- increased risk of heart attack and stroke
- accidents, including car accidents

Once a doctor diagnoses someone with obstructive sleep apnea, he or she will suggest possible treatments. One common treatment for sleep apnea is continuous positive airway pressure (CPAP) therapy. CPAP therapy consists

Types of Sleep Apnea	
Obstructive sleep apnea	Occurs when a person's airway is *obstructed*, or blocked. Obstructive sleep apnea follows a cycle that may repeat hundreds of times a night. First, the sleeping person's effort to inhale air creates suction that collapses the airway. This blocks the airflow for 10 seconds to a minute while the sleeping person struggles to breathe. When the level of oxygen in the person's blood falls, the brain responds by awakening the person enough to tighten the upper throat muscles and open the airway. The person may snort or gasp, and then resume snoring.
Central sleep apnea	Occurs when the brain fails to send the right signals to the muscles that control breathing. This type of sleep apnea may be caused by other medical conditions, such as heart failure and stroke, or by sleeping at a high altitude. Central sleep apnea is less common than obstructive sleep apnea.

Figure 3.15
The two types of sleep apnea, obstructive and central, are caused by different factors. *What is the most common treatment for sleep apnea?*

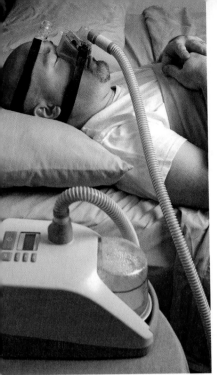

Amy Walters/Shutterstock.com

Figure 3.16 A CPAP machine consists of either a mask that covers the nose and mouth or prongs inserted into the nose to deliver oxygen. *What does CPAP stand for?*

of a special machine that increases air pressure in the throat and keeps the airway open to help a person breathe. Someone with sleep apnea may wear a CPAP machine while sleeping (**Figure 3.16**).

Narcolepsy

Narcolepsy is a disorder that affects the brain's ability to control the sleep-wake cycle. People with narcolepsy have frequent *sleep attacks* at various times of the day, even if they have had a normal amount of nighttime sleep.

During a sleep attack, a person falls asleep suddenly for several seconds or even more than 30 minutes. Strong emotions, such as fear, stress, or excitement, may trigger sleep attacks. These sleep attacks can be embarrassing and dangerous. They may occur when people are walking, driving, or performing other forms of physical activity.

Symptoms of narcolepsy typically appear first between the ages of 10 and 25, but diagnosis may not occur right away. The causes of narcolepsy are still unclear. This disorder tends to run in families. People whose parents have narcolepsy are more likely to develop it themselves. Narcolepsy may also be caused by brain damage resulting from a head injury or brain-related disease.

Narcolepsy can be treated with medications that help control the symptoms. People with narcolepsy can also make lifestyle changes to treat their symptoms. These changes include taking short naps, maintaining a regular sleep schedule, avoiding caffeine or alcohol before bedtime, exercising daily, and avoiding eating large meals before bedtime.

Lesson 3.2 Review

1. What age group is most commonly affected by "night owl" syndrome?
2. **True or false.** Young people typically have nightmares about events in their daily lives, such as at home or at school.
3. What are the two types of sleep apnea?
4. Which sleep problem involves having sleep attacks at various times of the day?
   A. Delayed sleep phase syndrome.
   B. Insomnia.
   C. Sleep apnea.
   D. Narcolepsy.
5. **Critical thinking.** Name three of the treatment methods available for bruxism and explain why these methods might help.

Hands-On Activity

Make a list of resources (print, online, and personal) that could help someone who is dealing with difficult or abnormal sleep. Rank the list in order from easiest to most difficult to access. Which resources would you be most comfortable accessing? Which resources do you think are the best? Is there a difference? Why or why not?

Developing Strategies for Getting Enough Sleep

Learning Outcomes

After studying this lesson, you will be able to

- **create** a sleep schedule based on your needs.
- **explain** the best way to take naps.
- **demonstrate** how exercise can help you sleep better.
- **describe** which substances interfere with sleep.
- **understand** how relaxing before bedtime can help you sleep.
- **demonstrate** how to create a comfortable sleep environment.
- **explain** how to control exposure to light before bedtime.

Graphic Organizer

Sleep Tips

Write the phrase *Improving Sleep* in the middle of a graphic organizer like the one shown below. As you read this lesson, brainstorm and write what you learn about techniques for improving sleep in the surrounding circles.

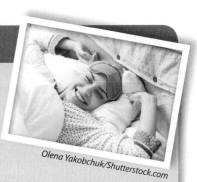

Olena Yakobchuk/Shutterstock.com

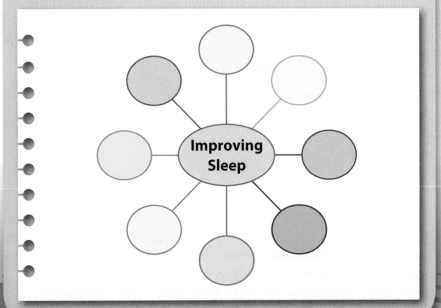

Improving Sleep

Key Terms

sleep-wake schedule routine for going to bed at about the same time each night and getting up at about the same time each morning

caffeine substance that produces a temporary increase in activity in the body, making it difficult to sleep

tryptophan substance that helps the body make chemicals that help you sleep

night-light small lamp, often attached directly to an electrical outlet, that provides dim light during the night

Getting enough sleep is an essential part of staying healthy. You need plenty of sleep to help protect your physical, social, and mental-emotional health and well-being. While you are sleeping, your brain is gearing up for the next day. Your body is getting the rest it needs to function well and be productive throughout the day.

Sanjay, the boy from the previous lessons, rarely gets enough sleep. It negatively affects his health and well-being, hurting his abilities in school and sports and making him more vulnerable to getting sick. What strategies can Sanjay use to improve his sleep habits?

Keep in mind that different sleep strategies work best for different people. The strategies that work best for Sanjay may be different from the strategies that work best for his parents, siblings, or friends. They may also be different from the strategies that work best for you. In this lesson, you will learn some sleep strategies that may help you get adequate amounts of sleep.

Set (and Follow) a Schedule

Setting and following a sleep-wake schedule is one of the best ways to make sure you get enough sleep. When you follow a **sleep-wake schedule**, you go to bed at about the same time each night and get up at about the same time each morning. Maintaining this schedule creates a sleep-wake pattern for your body to follow (**Figure 3.17**).

Use the same schedule every day of the week—not just Monday through Friday. Many people get too little sleep during the week and then try to "catch up" on the weekend. Sleeping in for two or three extra hours on Saturday and Sunday disrupts your body clock. This makes it more difficult to get up early again on Monday morning.

There may be times when you want to change your sleep schedule. For example, you may be able to sleep later than usual during your summer vacation. You can help your body adjust to a new sleep schedule by changing the time you go to bed and the time you wake up by a few minutes each day. Going to bed and waking up just 15 or 20 minutes later each day helps you reset your biological clock to the new time and get better sleep.

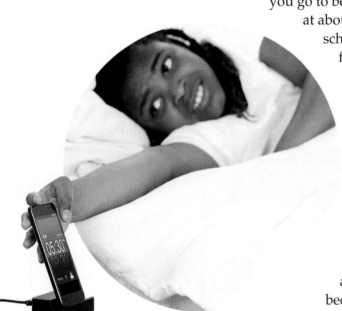

Andrey_Popov/Shutterstock.com

Figure 3.17
The predictable pattern of a sleep-wake schedule makes it easier for the body to fall asleep and wake up. *What is a common reason it is difficult to wake up on Monday morning?*

Take Naps

If you have a younger brother or sister, you have probably seen a caregiver tucking in your sibling for a nap in the afternoon. It may surprise you to learn that naps are not just for your younger brother or sister. Taking naps is a better way of catching up on sleep than sleeping in late on the weekends. Taking naps during the day can help you get some extra sleep without disrupting your regular sleep schedule.

BUILDING Your Skills

Setting and Following a Sleep-Wake Schedule

Busy lives can make it difficult to fall asleep on time. After you get home from sports practice or another after-school program, you may still need to finish your homework. After you finish your homework and relax with a book, you may be falling asleep late. The next night, you may not have any after-school programs and not much homework, meaning that you get to sleep earlier. Having an irregular sleep-wake schedule like this can mean that you get an inadequate amount of sleep.

As with any health behavior change, getting enough sleep starts with understanding where you are right now. Start the process of getting enough sleep by tracking your sleep habits for the next week using a chart similar to the one below.

After a week, look at your log to review your sleep-wake cycle. Are you going to bed and waking up at consistent times each day? Are you getting 8–10 hours of sleep each night? If not, it is time to set a sleep-wake schedule. Remember, the sleep-wake schedule you set has to work for you, and this option may be different from what works for a friend.

If you discover that you need to fall asleep earlier, start by adjusting your bedtime to five minutes earlier than usual. After you are comfortable with this new bedtime, set it another five minutes earlier. Once you are comfortable with this new bedtime, set it yet another five minutes earlier. Do this as many times as needed to get to your goal bedtime. Another way to increase your total sleep is by gradually setting your morning alarm clock five minutes later each week. Five minutes may not seem like a huge deal, but over time it adds up.

Writing down your sleep-wake schedule and discussing it with someone who can help you follow it is likely to make you more successful. Review your progress regularly in following your sleep-wake schedule and make adjustments to your schedule as needed.

Sleep-Wake Schedule							
	Day 1	Day 2	Day 3	Day 4	Day 5	Day 6	Day 7
Last night, I went to bed at:							
Last night, I fell asleep around:							
This morning, I woke up at:							
Total number hours slept:							
Notes about the day: (include mood, activity level, naps, etc.)							

Naps have other benefits as well. People who take even a short nap—for 20 to 30 minutes—feel more alert, find it easier to learn new skills, and are better able to use their memory. They are also more creative. If you choose to take naps during the day, remember the strategies in **Figure 3.18**.

Exercise Regularly

Have you noticed that you feel more tired on nights when you have sports practice or spend time outside with your friends? This is because your body uses up energy during physical activity, and it has to rest to get that energy back. Engaging in physical activity has many benefits, such as helping you get an adequate amount of sleep.

Generally, young people should try to get at least 60 minutes of exercise each day. Exercising for as little as 20 to 30 minutes a day, however, can help people get to sleep—and stay asleep. Find ways to add at least this much exercise to your day in whichever way feels best for you. You can exercise in a variety of ways, as you will learn in Chapter 7.

Remember that you do not need to do the 20 to 30 minutes of exercise all at once. Sometimes it can be easier to find smaller periods of time for exercise. Fortunately, exercising for five to ten minutes several times during the day will still help you get to sleep at night.

Try to schedule your exercise so that you finish at least three hours before you plan to go to sleep. Too much activity in the evening can make it difficult to fall asleep. It is best to exercise in the morning or afternoon if you can.

Avoid Substances That Interfere with Sleep

You may have seen your dad make a cup of tea before bedtime. If you asked him what kind of tea he was making, he would likely say that it was herbal tea with no caffeine. **Caffeine** is a substance that produces a temporary increase in activity in the body, making it difficult to sleep.

Figure 3.18
If you use the napping strategies listed at the right, you can get a small amount of extra sleep without disrupting your regular sleep-wake cycle.

Napping Strategies

- **Set an alarm.** Naps that are longer than 30 minutes can prevent you from getting adequate sleep at night. Short naps are best because they refresh you during the day while allowing you to get a full night's sleep.
- **Nap in the early afternoon.** Your body's biological clock tells your body it is time to rest in the early afternoon. Listening to your biological clock can help you get the most out of naps.
- **Do not nap after dinner.** This can disrupt your regular sleep schedule. If you are drowsy after dinner, do something active to avoid falling asleep.

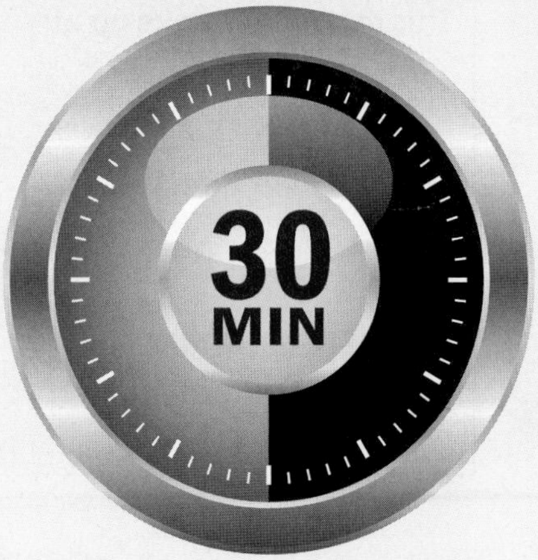

30 MIN

Arcady/Shutterstock.com

Try to avoid any drink or food that contains caffeine, especially near bedtime (**Figure 3.19**).

Your eating habits also influence how well you sleep. It is particularly important to avoid eating large meals or snacks right before bedtime. A light snack before bed, however, can promote sleep for some people. Eating foods that contain **tryptophan** may help calm the brain and allow you to sleep better. Tryptophan is a substance that helps the body make chemicals that help you sleep. Examples of foods containing tryptaphan include turkey, cheese, yogurt, poultry, fish, and eggs. You might consider experimenting with foods to determine evening meals and snacks that help you sleep.

Relax Before Bedtime

At the end of the day, people may focus on stressful experiences or worry about upcoming events. For example, you may feel worried about a test in one of your classes. You may feel stressed about a big assignment that is due, or feel angry about an argument you had with a friend. Thinking about these things at the end of a busy day is natural, but worries can cause you not to get enough sleep.

Fortunately, there are ways to clear your mind of stressful thoughts. One of the easiest and most effective ways is to create a bedtime routine. A peaceful bedtime routine sends a powerful signal to your brain that it is time to relax and let go of the day's stresses. Practicing relaxation techniques before bed is also a great way to wind down, calm the mind, and prepare for sleep (**Figure 3.20** on the next page).

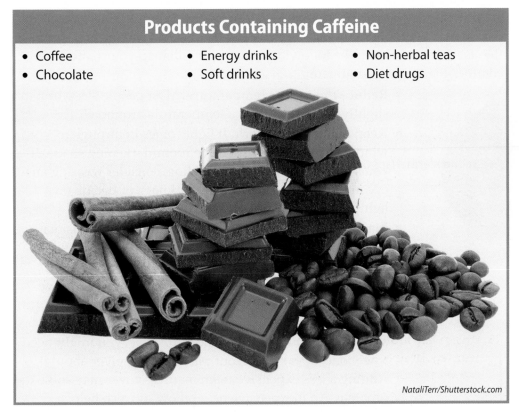

Products Containing Caffeine

- Coffee
- Chocolate
- Energy drinks
- Soft drinks
- Non-herbal teas
- Diet drugs

NataliTerr/Shutterstock.com

Figure 3.19
Coffee and energy drinks are not the only drinks that contain caffeine. Some foods do, too. *What substance could you consume to help you sleep?*

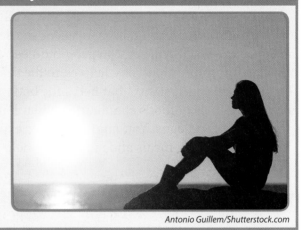

Relaxation Techniques

- Take slow, deep breaths.
- Relax all of the muscles in your body, starting at your toes and working up to your head.
- Think about being in a peaceful, calm place, such as a warm beach or a lush forest.
- Read a book or magazine or listen to an audiobook.
- Write in a journal to help your mind stop thinking about the day.
- Take a warm bath or shower.
- Listen to quiet music.
- Perform gentle stretches or meditate to relax your body and mind.

Antonio Guillem/Shutterstock.com

Figure 3.20   Creating a relaxed and peaceful bedtime routine through various relaxation techniques helps prepare your brain and body for sleep. ***What should you do if you cannot sleep?***

If you cannot sleep, or if you wake up in the middle of the night and are unable to get back to sleep, get out of bed and do something relaxing. Feeling anxious about not sleeping makes it even harder to get to sleep. Read a book or listen to soft music until you feel tired. Avoid watching television or checking your phone or computer. These activities will keep your mind active.

Create a Comfortable Sleep Environment

An uncomfortable sleep environment can contribute to insomnia. It is easier to get to sleep in an environment that you find comfortable. Even if you share a bedroom with a sibling, you can take certain actions to improve the sleep environment. The following techniques will help you create a comfortable sleep environment:

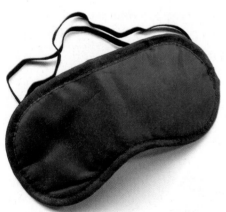

pedrolieb/Shutterstock.com

Figure 3.21
Wearing a sleep mask can help you sleep when it is not dark enough in your environment.

- **Reduce the room's temperature.** Most people sleep best in a slightly cool room, with a temperature around 65°F.
- **Keep the bedroom dark.** If light comes in through a window, install an inexpensive room-darkening shade. If you share a bedroom with a sibling, consider wearing an eye mask to create a feeling of darkness, or decide on a lights-out time (**Figure 3.21**).
- **Maintain quiet.** If you cannot eliminate noise, consider wearing earplugs or sleeping with a fan or a white noise machine to mask other sounds.
- **Make your bed as comfortable as possible.** Try to have enough room in your bed to stretch and turn comfortably. Wash your bedding, or sheets and pillowcases, at least once a week. If your mattress is uncomfortable, you might need a new one. Speak with your parent or caregiver about it. Adding a less expensive foam mattress cover may solve the problem. An inexpensive new pillow can also help.

Ways to Get a Good Night's Sleep

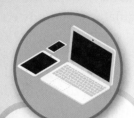

Do not bring electronics into bed with you, and stop staring at screens an hour before bedtime

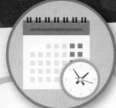

Create a sleep schedule and stick to it, even on weekends

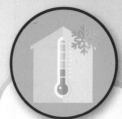

Lower the temperature; studies show it is easier to sleep in a cooler room

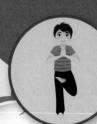

Do some light stretching before climbing into bed

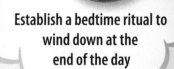

Establish a bedtime ritual to wind down at the end of the day

Control Exposure to Light

As you learned earlier in this chapter, melatonin is a naturally occurring hormone that helps regulate the sleep-wake cycle. Light affects the body's production of melatonin. When it is dark, your body produces more melatonin, which makes you feel sleepy. When it is light, your body produces less melatonin, which leads you to feel more awake and alert. Exposure to sunlight in the morning and throughout the day regulates your body's biological clock and helps you feel more active.

Many aspects of modern life can disrupt your body's natural production of melatonin and your sleep-wake cycle. For example, spending time in a school or home that does not let in natural light can make you feel sleepier during the day. If you spend the evening exposed to bright lights from a television or computer screen, your body may produce less melatonin, which makes it harder to feel sleepy.

Try natural methods of regulating your sleep schedule. The following are strategies you can use:

- Spend time outside during the day whenever possible. Eat lunch outside or go for a walk in the late afternoon.
- Keep curtains and blinds open during the day to increase the amount of natural light in your room. Move your desk or chair near a window.
- Minimize the time you spend in front of a television or computer screen at the end of the day.
- Avoid reading from an electronic device that exposes you to extra light just before you go to bed. Reading a physical book with a bedside lamp exposes your body to less light, which makes falling asleep easier.
- Use a **night-light** in the bathroom to avoid turning on a bright light in the middle of the night.
- When you wake up, open the blinds or curtains and turn on bright lights to jump-start your body's clock and help you feel more awake and alert.

Lesson 3.3 Review

1. **True or false.** Exercising for 20–30 minutes late in the evening can help you fall asleep and stay asleep.
2. People should avoid drinks and foods with _____ near bedtime.
3. Give two examples of strategies you can use to relax before bedtime.
4. When does the body produce more melatonin?
5. **Critical thinking.** How can you change your body's sleep-wake schedule in a healthy way (for example, over school breaks)?

Hands-On Activity

Create an artistic representation of an ideal sleeping situation for you. Include factors such as environment, before bed behaviors, and sleep schedule. Then, make a list of five things you can do each day or evening to achieve ideal sleep at night. Discuss your list with a partner.

Summary

Lesson 3.1 — Understanding Sleep

- People who get insufficient sleep are sleep deprived, which prevents their bodies from rejuvenating, healing, and resting. Those who do not get enough sleep experience a sleep deficit.
- Naturally occurring physical, behavioral, and mental changes in the body that follow the 24-hour cycle of the sun are called *circadian rhythms*. The body monitors light in the environment and releases melatonin at night. Disruptions to the circadian rhythm, such as using electric lights late at night, can take a while to overcome.
- Throughout one evening, you cycle through five distinct stages of sleep multiple times.
- People who get insufficient sleep are more likely to develop serious health conditions such as diabetes, heart disease, and obesity. They also have an increased risk of getting sick more often. Sleep deprivation can negatively impact young people's growth.
- People who are sleep deprived are less likely to do well in school or in sports than people who get plenty of sleep. Lack of sleep affects concentration, problem-solving skills, and memory.

Lesson 3.2 — Common Sleeping Problems

- Delayed sleep phase syndrome (DSPS) or "night owl" syndrome is a disorder that results in a person being unable to fall asleep until very late at night and naturally not waking up until much later in the morning. DSPS is common during the teenage years.
- Trouble falling or staying asleep is called *insomnia*. This affects a person's ability to get enough sleep.
- The most common forms of parasomnia are bed-wetting, nightmares, sleepwalking, restless legs syndrome (RLS), and teeth grinding.
- Sleep apnea is a potentially serious disorder in which a person stops breathing for short periods of time during sleep. This can be due to an obstruction in the person's airway (obstructive sleep apnea), or the brain failing to send the right signals to the muscles that control breathing (central sleep apnea).
- Narcolepsy affects the brain's ability to control the sleep-wake cycle, which can cause people to suddenly fall asleep for seconds or minutes at a time.

Lesson 3.3 — Developing Strategies for Getting Enough Sleep

- Setting and following a sleep-wake schedule every day of the week is one of the best ways to avoid an irregular sleeping pattern. Naps can be helpful for getting some extra sleep throughout the day as long as they are no longer than 30 minutes or are not too close to bedtime.
- Exercising at least 20–30 minutes every day can help people fall asleep and stay asleep.
- Even if they do not struggle with sleep disorders, people should avoid drinks and foods with caffeine near bedtime.
- Practicing relaxation techniques before bed can help prepare the body for sleep. A comfortable sleep environment is also important for getting the best sleep possible. Most people sleep best in a cool, dark, and quiet room.

Check Your Knowledge ⤴

Record your answers to each of the following questions on a separate sheet of paper.

1. Which of the following refers to getting enough sleep?
   A. Insufficient.
   C. Inadequate.
   B. Rejuvenated.
   D. Sleep deprived.
2. The fatigue people feel after traveling across time zones, called _____ _____, is a disruption to the body's natural circadian rhythm.
3. During which stage of sleep do most dreams occur?
4. **True or false.** Lack of sleep can impact metabolism, immune system function, concentration, and reflexes.
5. What is the most common cause of insomnia?
6. Nightmares, teeth grinding, bed-wetting, and sleepwalking are all examples of _____.
7. **True or false.** Waking a sleepwalking person could be harmful to him or her.
8. List three types of parasomnia.
9. One of the best ways to make sure you get enough sleep is to set and follow a(n) _____ _____.
10. Which of the following nap strategies can disrupt your sleep-wake schedule?
    A. Set an alarm for no more than 30 minutes.
    C. Nap in the early afternoon.
    B. Nap in your bed.
    D. Nap after dinner.
11. Why does exposure to bright light from a digital screen make it difficult to fall asleep?
12. **True or false.** Spending time outside during the day can help you fall asleep better at night.

Use Your Vocabulary ⤴

caffeine	melatonin	sleep apnea
circadian rhythms	narcolepsy	sleep deficit
delayed sleep phase syndrome (DSPS)	night-light	sleep deprived
	parasomnia	sleep-wake cycle
insomnia	REM sleep	sleep-wake schedule
jet lag	short sleepers	tryptophan

13. For each of the terms above, identify a word or group of words describing a quality of the term—an *attribute*. Team together with a classmate and discuss your list of attributes. Then, discuss your list with the whole class to increase understanding.
14. Before reading, work with a partner to write the definitions of each term above based on your current understanding. After reading the chapter, discuss any discrepancies between you and your partner's definitions and those in the chapter with another pair of partners. Finally, discuss the definitions as a class and ask your instructor for any necessary correction or clarification.

Think Critically

15. **Determine.** Why do people, especially teenagers, need sufficient sleep? What is a good bedtime for teenagers in your community?

16. **Cause and effect.** Explain the sleep cycle and how someone might feel if he or she wakes up before the end of the sleep cycle. How do naps fit into this cycle?

17. **Analyze.** What is the connection between sleep and digital screen time in the hours before bedtime?

18. **Draw conclusions.** Using reliable sources (print, online, and in person), find information, tips, and suggestions about getting better sleep. Draw conclusions from the information and share your thoughts with the class. Be sure to cite your sources.

19. **Evaluate.** Is it healthy to sleep less on weekdays and "catch up" on weekends by sleeping more? Explain.

DEVELOP Your Skills

20. **Technology and advocacy skills.** Middle school and high school students struggle to get enough sleep on a regular basis. Research the health information in this chapter on sleep, including how much sleep your age group needs and strategies for getting enough sleep. Plan an app that helps students get the sleep they need. Consider appearance as well as function. This app should represent at least one way to utilize technology to benefit the health of you and your peers.

21. **Communication skills.** Imagine you have a friend who has been having trouble sleeping. He tosses and turns almost every night for a few hours. You know this is probably because after dinner he drinks a caffeinated soda and plays video games until bedtime. Write a dialogue between you and your friend about his sleeping habits. Have him explain the health impacts he experiences from his lack of sleep. What warnings should you give about his health? What tips would you give for getting better sleep?

22. **Refusal and decision-making skills.** Imagine you have a friend who frequently invites you to come over to her house to watch movies on weeknights. You enjoy watching movies with your friend, but you stay up so late. Then, you always feel exhausted and sluggish the next day. How would you respond to your friend's next offer? Write a few possible responses.

23. **Conflict resolution skills.** Imagine you are having a disagreement with your parents about your bedtime. What are likely details of this disagreement? Consider the thoughts and feelings of you and your parents. Also, consider the information you learned in this chapter. How would you resolve the conflict so everyone agrees?

24. **Advocacy skills.** As a class, write a letter to a member of the school or district administration to share your knowledge about the sleep needs of teenagers. Provide ideas that the school or district could implement to better mesh with the sleep needs of teenagers. Prepare questions to ask administrators, too.

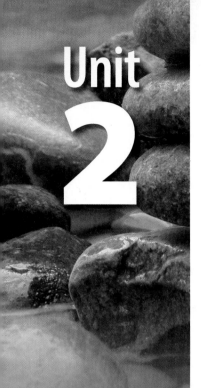

Unit 2

Promoting Mental and Emotional Well-Being

Chapter 4   Being Mentally and Emotionally Healthy

Chapter 5   Getting Help for Mental Health Conditions

Warm-Up Activity

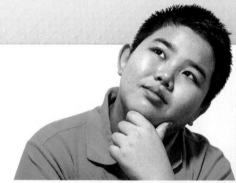

Pair Srinrat/Shutterstock.com

Prove or Disprove

Recreate the chart shown at the right on a separate sheet of paper. Before reading the chapters in this unit, fill in your thoughts for each quadrant of the chart.

When you finish reading the chapters, look at what you wrote in your chart. If what you wrote corresponds with information from the chapter, indicate that by noting the page number next to your statement. If what you wrote is disproved by your readings, cross out the statement and indicate on which page your thought was disproved.

In a different color, add additional information that you learned from the chapter. Be sure to indicate the page number on which you found the information. Then, think about the way your thoughts have been validated and changed as a result of your learning.

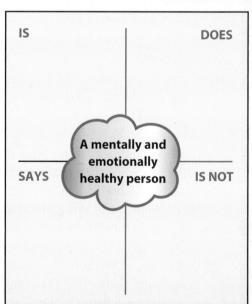

IS   DOES

A mentally and emotionally healthy person

SAYS   IS NOT

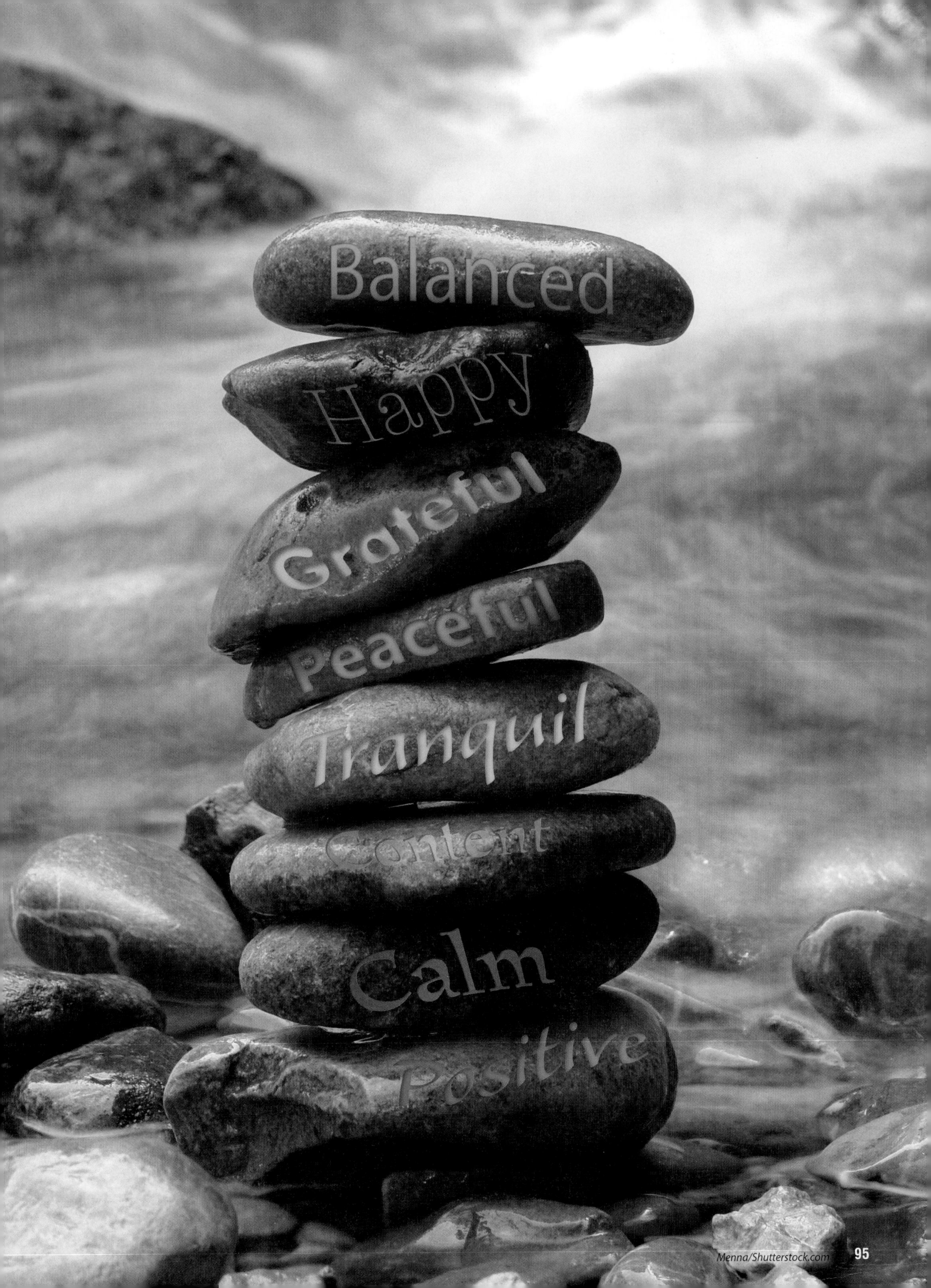

Menna/Shutterstock.com

Being Mentally and Emotionally Healthy

Essential Question ❓

Can you make sense of your own emotions?

Video ↗

Access the Chapter 4 video to start thinking about chapter topics.

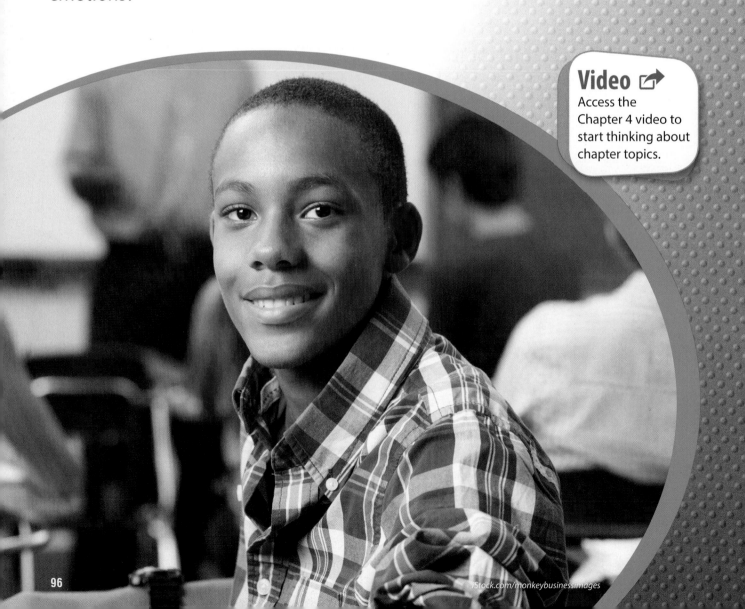

iStock.com/monkeybusinessimages

Reading Activity

Consider what each concept in this chapter might teach you about your mental health. Keep a list, placing a star beside any concepts that especially interest you. After reading this chapter, pick three of the concepts and write a few paragraphs on how these concepts can help you understand yourself.

How Healthy Are You?

In this chapter, you will be learning about mental and emotional health. Before you begin reading, take the following quiz to assess your current mental and emotional health habits.

Healthy Choices	Yes	No
Can you keep a positive outlook in stressful situations and focus on the good aspects of these situations?		
Are you tolerant and accepting of other people's beliefs, values, and feelings?		
Do you accept your strengths and weaknesses as different parts of who you are?		
Are you honest and fair in your interactions with others?		
Can you recognize your emotions and feelings and understand why you experience them?		
Can you enjoy spending time with other people, as well as spending time alone?		
Instead of bottling up your emotions, do you express them clearly to others?		
Do you help people in need and thank those who help you?		
Do you trust your own judgment and feel confident that you can make the right decision, even in difficult situations?		
Can you understand others' wants, needs, and points of view?		
Do you practice relaxation techniques, like deep breathing or meditation, to manage how your body responds to stress?		

Count your "Yes" and "No" responses. The more "Yes" responses you have, the more healthy mental and emotional health habits you exhibit. Now, take a closer look at the questions with which you responded "No." How can you make these healthy habits part of your daily life? Think about how implementing these ideas can help improve your overall health.

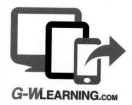

G-WLEARNING.com

While studying this chapter, look for the activity icon to

- **practice** key terms with e-flash cards and matching activities.
- **reinforce** what you learn by completing graphic organizers, self-assessment quizzes, and review questions.
- **expand** knowledge with interactive activities and activities that extend learning.

Key Terms

identity who you are, which includes your physical traits, activities, social connections, and internal thoughts and feelings

beliefs ideas or thoughts a person knows to be true, based on real experiences, scientific facts, or what a person has learned from others

attitudes set ways a person thinks or feels about someone or something

self-image your mental picture of yourself, which includes how you look, how you act, your skills and abilities, and your weaknesses; also called *self-concept*

self-esteem how you feel about yourself

Learning Outcomes

After studying this lesson, you will be able to

- **describe** the different parts of a person's identity.
- **identify** one personal value, one personal belief, and one personal attitude.
- **distinguish between** self-image and self-esteem.
- **explain** why self-esteem matters.
- **identify** factors that can affect a person's self-esteem.
- **give examples** of strategies you can use to help improve your self-image and self-esteem.

Graphic Organizer

Who Am I?

As you read this lesson, complete a chart like the one shown below for the physical, active, social, and psychological parts of your identity. For each box, identify specific examples of traits that would fall under each main topic.

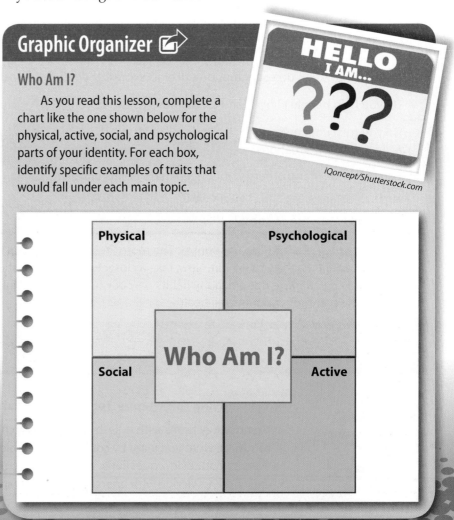

iQoncept/Shutterstock.com

Physical	Psychological

Who Am I?

| Social | Active |

In this chapter, you will learn about mental and emotional health. Your *mental and emotional health* has to do with your internal life—your thoughts and feelings. This encompasses who you believe you are and how you feel about yourself and your abilities. It includes how well you can understand and control your feelings and emotions. It also involves how well you can manage stress to promote wellness.

People with good mental and emotional health share similar traits and characteristics, such as those in **Figure 4.1**. Charlotte, who is 13 years old, has good mental and emotional health and a good sense of *self-worth*. She knows who she is, and she knows that she is a good person who deserves the respect of others. She also knows that she is valuable to others.

Charlotte feels good about herself and her life. She admits that she cannot play the trumpet very well, but she does not let that make her sad or stressed. Instead, she practices to improve. She also recognizes that she has other talents, like playing basketball.

Her friends and family say that Charlotte is usually able to laugh and have fun, even in stressful situations. She was smiling when she was nervous about giving a presentation in class. She made jokes before her first day of a new school year.

Part of Charlotte's mental and emotional health is due to her ability to understand herself and get to know herself through self-discovery. You can do this, too. By asking yourself important questions, you can get to know yourself a little better. You will figure out how you feel about this person you are becoming. If you discover that you are not happy with what you find, you can follow strategies to improve the way you feel about yourself. As you discover yourself, consider the questions in this lesson.

Characteristics of People with Positive Mental and Emotional Health

- **Having a thirst for life.** People who have a thirst for life enjoy living and are able to laugh and have fun. They strive to live life to the fullest and see the positive side of situations.
- **Being responsible.** Responsible people plan ahead and think before they act. They follow through on what they say they will do and accept the consequences of their decisions.
- **Maintaining a sense of balance.** People who maintain a sense of balance in their lives enjoy spending time with other people, but also feel comfortable spending time alone.
- **Being trustworthy.** People who are trustworthy are honest and fair in their interactions with other people. They do not lie, cheat, steal, or take advantage of others. They are loyal to their friends and family members.
- **Being respectful.** People who are respectful treat others with the same courtesy they want to be treated with themselves. They are tolerant and accepting of other people's beliefs and values, are considerate of other people's feelings, and use good manners. They listen carefully and with an open mind when other people are talking. They manage conflicts with others in constructive ways.
- **Being compassionate and kind.** People who are compassionate and kind help people who are in need and thank people who help them.
- **Being a good citizen.** People who are good citizens participate in school and community activities. They work with others to improve their schools and communities. They also stay informed about relevant issues, obey laws and rules, and respect authority.

Figure 4.1 The characteristics shown here are good indicators of someone who has positive mental and emotional health. *Which characteristics on this list do you possess?*

Who Are You?

How would you answer the question "Who are you?" Your answer will probably depend on which part of your **identity** (who you are) is your current focus. Your focus may be on your physical, active, social, or psychological identities (**Figure 4.2**).

People often focus on different parts of their identities at different ages. During early childhood, children typically define themselves by their physical and active identities. For example, a four- or five-year-old boy may describe himself as a tall boy with black hair and green eyes who runs fast.

As children enter middle childhood, around six years of age, their focus often shifts to their social identities. Friendships and relationships with peers become very important as children spend a lot of time together. Children also begin to judge one another and themselves based on their acceptance within the social group. Oftentimes, children will compete to gain *status* (social standing) within the "popular" social group. As children age, their interests expand and they get involved in new activities. Children want to join other social groups with people who share similar interests.

During the teenage years, teens tend to focus on their unique personal qualities and psychological identities. They define themselves in terms of their personal values, beliefs, and attitudes. *Values* are the things a person considers to be the most important in life. Personal **beliefs** are ideas or thoughts a person knows to be true, based on real experiences, scientific facts, or what a person has learned from others. **Attitudes** are set ways a person thinks or feels about someone or something. A person's psychological identity can be a combination of many values, beliefs, and attitudes, which often change throughout life.

How Do You See Yourself?

Now that you have identified who you are, consider how you see yourself. Do you generally like the way you look? Do you think of yourself as a good person? Are you happy with the personality traits you possess (**Figure 4.3**)?

Figure 4.2
All four different aspects of your identity combine to make up who you are. *Which part of your identity is your current focus?*

Aspects of Your Identity

Physical	Gender (being male or female), race, age, and physical characteristics, such as height, weight, and hair color
Active	Engagement in particular activities and interests, such as sports, music, and community service
Social	Connection to other people, including family members, friends, and group members
Psychological	Internal thoughts and feelings

Personality Traits

Adaptable	Dependable	Insecure	Planner
Adventurous	Detailed	Kind	Pleasant
Ambitious	Diplomatic	Leader	Productive
Analytical	Efficient	Listener	Reserved
Assertive	Emotional	Logical	Resourceful
Athletic	Empathetic	Loyal	Respectful
Bashful	Enthusiastic	Mediator	Self-reliant
Bold	Expressive	Musical	Sensitive
Calm	Faithful	Optimistic	Shy
Careful	Flexible	Orderly	Sociable
Cheerful	Forgiving	Outspoken	Spontaneous
Competitive	Friendly	Patient	Stubborn
Confident	Funny	Peaceful	Sympathetic
Considerate	Helpful	Perfectionist	Talkative
Consistent	Imaginative	Persistent	Thoughtful
Cooperative	Impulsive	Persuasive	Tolerant
Creative	Independent	Pessimistic	Understanding

Figure 4.3
This table offers some examples of the many personality traits that can describe who you are. These traits can also help you reflect on whether you are happy with yourself as a person. *Which five personality traits best describe you?*

Do you accept your strengths and weaknesses? Answering questions such as these can give you a sense of your self-image.

Your **self-image**, also called *self-concept*, is your mental picture of yourself. Your self-image is how you view your appearance, personality, skills and abilities, and weaknesses. People with good mental and emotional health accept themselves for who they are. They accept the way they look—even though they may not like all of their physical features. They have confidence in their skills and abilities and work toward improving their weaknesses.

You are not born with a self-image. It forms gradually over time, starting in childhood. Your life experiences and interactions with others influence your self-image. As you experience different events and interact with different people, your self-image may change.

The view you have of yourself is likely different from how others see you. This is because your unique personal values, beliefs, and attitudes shape your opinion of yourself. The way you see yourself affects how you relate to others. If you view yourself in a positive way, people will probably respond positively to you. If the view you have of yourself is negative, others may view you in this way, too.

How Do You Feel About Yourself?

How you feel about yourself, or your **self-esteem**, closely relates to how you see yourself. How you feel about yourself has a major impact on many different aspects of your life (**Figure 4.4**). Self-esteem varies from person to person, and many factors can affect how you feel about yourself. Some people have high self-esteem, while other people have low self-esteem. Self-esteem also changes with life experiences and new understanding.

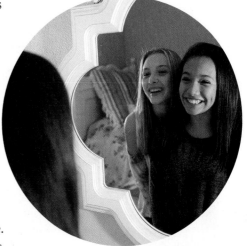

Mat Hayward/Shutterstock.com

Figure 4.4
How you feel about yourself affects how easily you make friends, how well you do in school, and how you manage disappointments and frustrations. *What is the term for how you feel about yourself?*

Factors That Affect Self-Esteem

Other people are one of the biggest factors that can affect how you see yourself. For example, healthy relationships with family and friends who accept and treat you with respect can help you develop a sense of pride in who you are. On the other hand, if you receive constant criticism and rejection from others, you may develop low self-esteem. Your personal relationships with others, whether positive or negative, can have a lasting effect on how you feel about yourself.

Other factors that can affect self-esteem include the following:

- self-image
- social interactions with family members, friends, and others
- home, school, community, and cultural environments
- life events and personal experiences
- media, such as television, movies, and social networking sites

High Self-Esteem

People who like themselves have *high self-esteem*. If you have high self-esteem, you feel good about yourself—including your skills and abilities—and you have a positive self-image. If you have high self-esteem, you also feel good about your relationships with other people. You feel loved, appreciated, and accepted by your friends and family members.

BUILDING Your Skills

How You Can Build Your Self-Esteem

Building self-esteem is not easy, but it can happen as you learn to work through issues and accept who you are. As you gain experience, you will see how you can take charge and have a positive outcome.

If you do not see yourself in a positive way, try the following strategies to help build your self-esteem:

- Take good care of yourself. Eat healthy foods, get plenty of sleep, and be physically active.
- Make a list of activities you really enjoy doing. Then, pick something from the list to do every day. Keep adding to your list as you discover new activities you enjoy.
- Spend time with people who make you feel good about yourself. Also, be someone who makes others feel good, too. Do something nice for someone else. Say a few kind words to someone. Hold the door open for someone the next time you are at a public place, such as a restaurant or store.

- Make a list of your skills and abilities. If you cannot think of anything on your own, ask friends or relatives what they think your skills and abilities are. The next time you feel down about yourself, look at the list and remember your strengths.
- Focus on your strengths and not on your weaknesses. Look at your positive qualities and concentrate on those. Rather than focusing on your weaknesses, figure out what you can do to try to improve them.

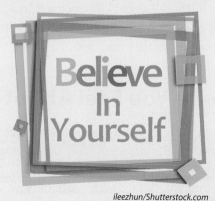

ileezhun/Shutterstock.com

Self-Esteem Stats

Nearly HALF of girls aged **11–14** refuse to take part in activities that will show off their bodies in any way

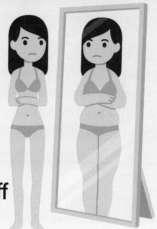

3 out of 4 girls

with low self-esteem will engage in negative activities like smoking, drinking, self-harming, bullying, or disordered eating

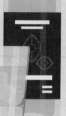

40% of boys in middle school exercise with the goal of improving their appearance by increasing their **muscle size**

Studies have shown that

social media has a negative impact on youth self-esteem due to the constant pressure to appear **perfect** online

Participation in team sports

13 **7** **12** **9**

is shown to produce **higher** self-esteem in adolescents

Having high self-esteem does not mean that you only experience good situations and never face problems or have days when you feel a little down. It just means that you cope well with unpleasant situations and disappointments.

People with high self-esteem view negative events and failures as learning experiences, not as proof of their weaknesses. Moreover, when they run into obstacles, people with high self-esteem can accept reality and make a new plan. They are also more comfortable asking other people for help and support in times of need.

People who have high self-esteem have great decision-making skills. They trust their own judgment and follow their own values. They are confident that they can make the right decision, even in difficult situations. When they feel pressure to go along with the crowd, people with high self-esteem have the courage to make the choice they believe is right or take responsibility for a poor choice.

Low Self-Esteem

People who have *low self-esteem* doubt their own self-worth and may feel negatively about their traits, skills, and abilities. If you have low self-esteem, you may wish you could change your looks, intelligence, or athletic skills. You may feel left out of social groups and disconnected from other people. You may also question whether other people like or respect you, in part, because you do not really like or respect yourself.

People with low self-esteem often worry about what other people think of them. They may try to show off because they want to convince other people of their worth. Being concerned about the opinions of others makes people with low self-esteem vulnerable to pressure. People with low self-esteem may feel unable to resist pressure to engage in unhealthy behaviors. Unfortunately, these behaviors can have long-term health consequences.

Lesson 4.1 Review

1. Name the four different parts of a person's identity.
2. **True or false.** A person's values, beliefs, and attitudes are a part of his or her identity, and do not change throughout the person's life.
3. What is the difference between self-image and self-esteem?
4. **Critical thinking.** Name four strategies you can follow to build your self-esteem.

Hands-On Activity

Create a visual representation of yourself. Using images you draw or find, create a collage that showcases who you are. About which aspects of identity do you think most positively? Which aspects of your identity do you think about most? What are most important to you? Does your collage indicate high self-esteem? Why or why not?

Making Sense of Your Emotions

Learning Outcomes

After studying this lesson, you will be able to

- **identify** pleasant and unpleasant emotions.
- **explain** what it means to have emotional awareness.
- **describe** how identifying and accepting your feelings can help you control your emotions.
- **demonstrate** how to express your emotions in a healthy way.
- **identify** characteristics of people with high emotional intelligence.

Key Terms 🔗

emotions moods or feelings you experience

emotional awareness skill of knowing which emotions you feel, and why

emotional intelligence (EI) skill of understanding, controlling, and expressing your emotions and sensing the emotions of others

optimism ability to keep a positive outlook and focus on the good aspects of stressful situations

empathy ability to put yourself in someone else's shoes, and to understand someone else's wants, needs, and viewpoints

gratitude emotion that means being thankful or grateful

resilience ability to bounce back from traumatic or stressful events

Graphic Organizer 🔗

My Emotions

Write "Making Sense of My Emotions" in the middle of a graphic organizer like the one shown below. As you read this lesson, fill in topics related to understanding your emotions in each bubble. Continue to identify and explain related topics to complete the organizer as you read this lesson.

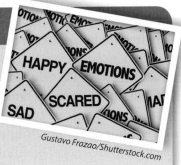

Gustavo Frazao/Shutterstock.com

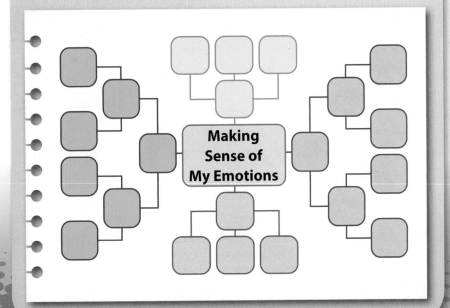

Making Sense of My Emotions

I n the previous lesson, you explored who you are and how you feel about yourself. In this lesson, you will explore how you feel about and react to people and situations around you.

Making sense of your feelings can be challenging at times, especially when you feel like you are on an emotional rollercoaster. Charlotte, from the previous lesson, experienced this today. She was upset and angry because she got a bad grade on her math test. After math, she told her friends at lunch how she was feeling. Her friends laughed and joked together to cheer her up, and she felt happy. Many people go through these emotional ups and downs, which are a normal part of experiencing life.

How you react to your feelings—what you think, say, and do—can have positive or negative effects on your mental and emotional health. People who are mentally and emotionally healthy, like Charlotte, understand their moods and feelings. They know how to control and express those feelings to others in positive ways.

Understanding Your Emotions

People experience many different emotions. Your **emotions** are the moods or feelings you experience. Emotions, which are a normal part of life, can be pleasant or unpleasant (**Figure 4.5**). Pleasant emotions represent positive feelings that make you feel good. Unpleasant emotions represent negative feelings that often make you feel bad.

As you experience life, you may feel pleasant and unpleasant emotions at the same time. For example, when the school year ends, you may feel happy because you will not have to do homework. You might also feel sad because you will not see some of your friends every day.

Sometimes, understanding your emotions can be challenging because one emotion masks or hides another emotion. If you try out for and do not make the sports team, you might feel angry with the coach for not selecting you.

Figure 4.5
Everyone experiences many different pleasant and unpleasant emotions throughout life, often at the same time. *How does emotional awareness help you control your emotions?*

How Are You Feeling Today?

Alhovik/Shutterstock.com

Alhovik/Shutterstock.com

Pleasant Emotions			Unpleasant Emotions		
Happy	Grateful	Proud	Angry	Jealous	Guilty
Loved	Excited	Hopeful	Scared	Helpless	Rejected
Kind	Cheerful	Joyful	Disgusted	Lonely	Sad

This feeling of anger may only be a result of sadness, however, because you really wanted to be part of the team.

Understanding your emotions involves knowing which emotions you feel and why. When you are aware of your emotions, you have **emotional awareness**. You are not just reacting to your emotions. Instead, you use emotional awareness to control them.

Controlling Your Emotions

Controlling your emotions is not easy. As a young child, you probably reacted to what you felt without thinking. As you grow up, however, you can learn to control your emotions by following the steps in **Figure 4.6**.

In the following sections, you will learn about the process for controlling your emotions. You will read about the feelings Jennifer is experiencing and how she responds to the situation. As you are reading, think about how you would react if you were in Jennifer's shoes. What would you do? Reflect on how identifying and accepting your feelings and expressing your feelings in healthy, positive ways can help you control your emotions.

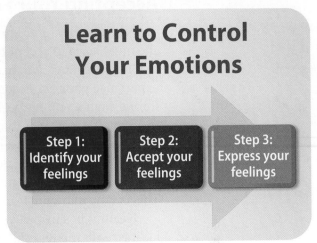

Learn to Control Your Emotions

| Step 1: Identify your feelings | Step 2: Accept your feelings | Step 3: Express your feelings |

Figure 4.6 Learning how to control your emotions can have a positive effect on your mind and body.

Identifying What You Are Feeling

The first step in controlling your emotions is to identify what emotion or emotions you are feeling. This is not always an easy task. Sometimes, identifying feelings of sadness and fear or other emotions can be confusing. To help you determine the actual emotion you are experiencing, and why, think about events or factors that might have triggered the emotion (**Figure 4.7**).

Consider Jennifer's situation. Jennifer started the day in a bad mood. She argued with her sister when her sister said it was Jennifer's turn to take the dog for a walk. On the way to school, she yelled at her brother for not keeping up with her. At lunch, Jennifer snapped at her best friend, Alia, for no reason. Alia asked Jennifer why she was in such a bad mood.

As it turns out, Jennifer was reacting negatively to a conversation she had with her mother the night before. Jennifer's mother had mentioned that she was applying for a new job in another city. If her mother gets the job, Jennifer will probably have to move, which she does not want to do. Rather than telling her mother that she did not want to move, Jennifer took out her frustrations on those around her, which is unhealthy.

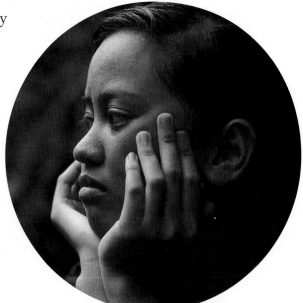

Francis Wong Chee Yen/Shutterstock.com

Figure 4.7
Spending time thinking about how you feel, and why, can help you identify your emotions.

Jennifer apologized to Alia for snapping at her and then they talked about Jennifer's situation. Jennifer identified that she was angry, but as they talked about it, Jennifer also identified that she was anxious and afraid. She was anxious about the thought of leaving her friends. She was afraid that others would not accept her at a new school. By identifying and sorting out her feelings, Jennifer took the first step toward accepting her feelings.

Accepting Your Feelings

Now that Jennifer knows her anger is a result of being anxious and afraid, she must learn to accept her feelings. Accepting your feelings does not mean that those feelings will just go away. It simply means that you allow yourself to experience your emotions. When you experience your emotions, you can work through what you are feeling so you can let it go.

Sometimes, rather than accepting your feelings, you may try to cover up or deny your emotions and hope those feelings will just go away. Denying your feelings, however, does not make what you feel go away. Burying emotions deep inside can have a negative effect on you both physically and emotionally. This is why allowing yourself to experience your emotions is so important.

Healthy, positive ways to experience your emotions may include sharing your feelings with friends and family members (**Figure 4.8**). Writing about what you are feeling in a journal is another positive way to work through your feelings. You can also work through your emotions by crying if you feel sad or running if you feel angry. These are all healthy ways to experience your feelings.

Jennifer began to accept her emotions when she admitted that her anger was a result of being anxious and afraid about moving. Talking with Alia was a healthy, positive way for Jennifer to begin to work through her emotions. Once Jennifer acknowledged her feelings and calmed down, she felt that she was ready to express her feelings to her mother.

Figure 4.8
Finding someone safe to talk with who can provide much-needed love and support can help you work through your emotions. *Why should you not deny or bury your emotions?*

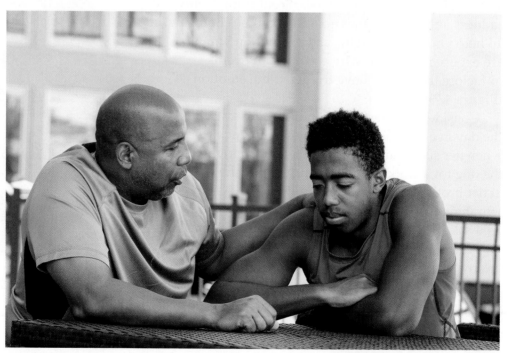

pixelheadphoto digitalskillet/Shutterstock.com

What to Do If You Feel...

Happy

Write down what made you happy that day so you can reflect on it the next time you feel down.

Express gratitude to those who helped you feel that way.

Spread the good mood to friends and family through kind words and actions.

Sad

Confide in a friend or loved one about how you are feeling.

Exercise or do something else that is physically active.

Do activities that you enjoy.

Stressed

Close your eyes and focus on your breathing for a few minutes.

Visualize a place that makes you feel happy and relaxed.

Distract yourself. Go for a walk or focus on something else for a while.

Nervous

Close your eyes and take a few deep breaths. Focus on your breathing until you feel calm.

Talk to a friend or family member about what you are feeling.

Think of five things that make you feel happy and focus on those positive thoughts.

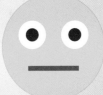

Angry

Take a mental step back before you react. Do not take action until you no longer feel angry.

Take some time alone. Get some space to clear your mind and calm down. Try taking a walk.

Once you calm down, work toward solutions. Discuss what angered you once you can keep your cool.

Lonely

Make plans to do something with friends.

Join a team, club, or activity with others who share your interests.

Spend time with family.

Play with a pet.

Faces: flower travelin' man/Shutterstock.com

Expressing Your Feelings to Others

Being able to control your emotions involves expressing your feelings clearly to others. When you are telling others how you feel, it is important to stay calm and keep your emotions under control. If you are negative and lash out at others or try to hurt someone, then you are expressing your emotions in an unhealthy way. You may cause serious harm to the relationship. Instead, be positive and think about the effect your words may have on the other person. Explain how you feel without being hurtful or negative (**Figure 4.9**).

Sometimes, you can make a situation worse if you try to confront the person who caused you to feel a certain way while you are still angry. Instead, wait until you cool off before talking about your feelings. By waiting, you can control your emotions and express them in a more positive, healthy way. You are allowing yourself time to work through and get relief from your feelings of anger. This will help you keep your emotions under control.

When Jennifer talked with her mother, she had already worked through her anger and was able to remain calm and explain her feelings about the potential move. By talking with her mom, Jennifer began to have a more positive outlook about the situation.

Developing Emotional Intelligence

Do you know people who always seem to remain positive, calm, and in control of their emotions in stressful situations? Do you know people who sense that you are feeling down, even before you say anything to them?

People who are skilled at understanding, controlling, and expressing their emotions and sensing the emotions of others have high **emotional intelligence (EI)**. Having EI is necessary to develop close personal relationships with others.

Figure 4.9
When expressing your feelings to others, be careful to avoid aggressive messages that lay blame on someone else. Instead, focus on your own actions, feelings, and needs. *Why might it be a good idea to wait a bit before talking to someone who made you angry?*

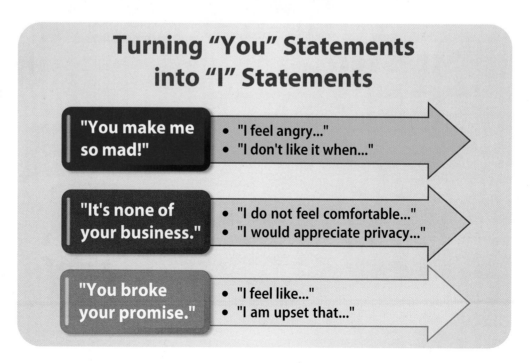

Turning "You" Statements into "I" Statements

"You make me so mad!"
- "I feel angry..."
- "I don't like it when..."

"It's none of your business."
- "I do not feel comfortable..."
- "I would appreciate privacy..."

"You broke your promise."
- "I feel like..."
- "I am upset that..."

People with high EI share similar abilities and characteristics (**Figure 4.10**). In the following sections, you will learn more about these abilities and characteristics. In the process, you will discover ways to develop your emotional intelligence and enhance personal relationships.

Control Negative Emotions

People with high EI are able to control or reduce their negative emotions. The negative emotions you experience, such as anger, jealousy, or fear, can easily become overwhelming and cloud your judgment. Controlling or reducing these emotions can help you live a happier, more fulfilling life.

One way to control your negative emotions is to change the way you think about a situation. Instead of thinking negatively about the problem, try to view the issue in different, more positive ways. For example, if your friend does not respond to your text messages, try not to think that your friend is ignoring or rejecting you. Look at other possible explanations. Perhaps your friend is very busy. Maybe your friend's cell phone is off or has a low battery.

Your friend's actions are probably more because of him or her than because of you. Try not to take your friend's lack of response personally and avoid jumping to conclusions. Instead, have optimism. **Optimism** is the ability to keep a positive outlook and focus on the good aspects of situations (**Figure 4.11**).

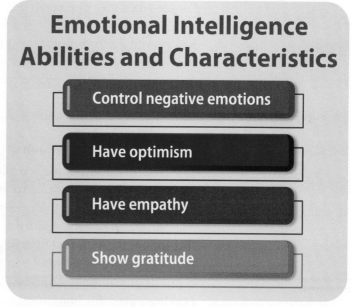

Emotional Intelligence Abilities and Characteristics

- Control negative emotions
- Have optimism
- Have empathy
- Show gratitude

Figure 4.10 You probably have high EI if you have the ability to control your negative emotions, be optimistic, have empathy, and show gratitude. *What skills do people with high emotional intelligence have?*

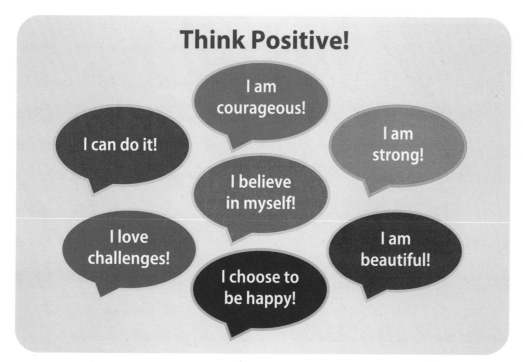

Think Positive!

I am courageous!
I can do it!
I am strong!
I believe in myself!
I love challenges!
I am beautiful!
I choose to be happy!

Figure 4.11 Responding to positive or negative situations with optimism can help you control negative emotions. *How would you rate yourself on being optimistic? Can you be more positive?*

People who have optimism are better able to cope with stressful situations because they realize situations are temporary. They know that circumstances will eventually improve. If you respond with optimism, you understand that your friend will eventually text you back.

Have Empathy

Having high emotional intelligence involves having empathy. People who have **empathy** are able to put themselves in someone else's shoes. They understand other people's wants, needs, and viewpoints. They treat others as they would expect to be treated. As a result, people who have empathy are better able to support their friends who are in need.

Can you remember a time when someone showed you empathy? How did this make you feel? Perhaps you felt valued and respected, which means you are more likely to feel good about yourself. In turn, you are more likely to make someone else feel good about himself or herself. Having empathy helps you sense the emotions of others and respond in open, positive ways.

Developing empathy involves keeping an open mind and listening carefully to what others have to say (**Figure 4.12**). People have differing opinions, and you must be able to listen to understand what people are feeling and what they need. You do not necessarily have to agree with someone else's opinion, but you can see why they feel the way they do.

Show Gratitude

The ability to have an attitude of gratitude has many benefits on your personal health and wellness. **Gratitude** is an emotion that means being thankful or grateful. People with high emotional intelligence have the ability to appreciate what is good and meaningful in their lives.

Figure 4.12
If you can recognize and understand someone else's feelings, you can better respond to their emotional needs. *What is the term for the ability to understand other people's perspectives?*

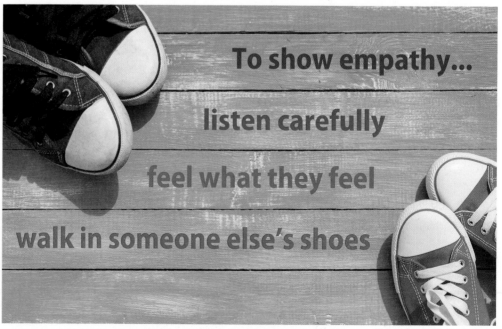

To show empathy...

listen carefully

feel what they feel

walk in someone else's shoes

Natalya Danko/Shutterstock.com

This enables people to be happier, which, in turn, often results in the ability to be nicer to others and show them gratitude.

People who can openly show gratitude to others demonstrate that they appreciate others and recognize what these people have done for them. As a result, their relationships with others improve and grow stronger.

BUILDING Your Skills

Being Thankful Makes You Healthier

> Gratitude: the quality of being thankful; readiness to show appreciation for and to return kindness.

Perhaps *gratitude* is not a new word to you. Do you realize the power of affirming the good things and people in your life? Expressing gratitude can have an immense and positive impact on your mental health, which can then translate into positive outcomes for your social and physical health. All of this from the simple act of purposefully being thankful.

Most obviously, expressing gratitude is one of the most reliable methods for improving happiness. Expressing gratitude can also reduce symptoms of depression and anxiety and help people be more resilient. There's more, too! Affirming the good in your life helps your body to work and feel better and encourages you to take better care of yourself. Social lives also improve with expressions of gratitude. People who regularly express gratitude have stronger relationships, are better able to forgive, are more connected with their communities, and are more helpful and compassionate.

Expressing Thanks

With all those reasons understood, it is time to put thankfulness into practice. Think of a person for whom you are thankful. It could be a family member, a teacher, a friend, a coach…anyone!

Now write a letter and tell the person WHY you are thankful for him or her. What has this person done for and with you? How has he or she made you feel? What is so wonderful about this person?

When you are done, choose one of the following options:

- **Option 1.** Do nothing with the letter. Just by writing the letter, you expressed gratitude and improved your health.
- **Option 2.** Give the letter to the person you wrote it to. This will boost your mental health and the other person's mental health a bit more than the first choice.
- **Option 3.** Read the letter aloud to the person you wrote it to. This will boost your mental health the most and the person you wrote it to will love hearing those words in your voice.

Regardless of which option you choose, you expressed gratitude and boosted your mental health. If you continue to be thankful for someone or something each day, you will notice the biggest impact on your health.

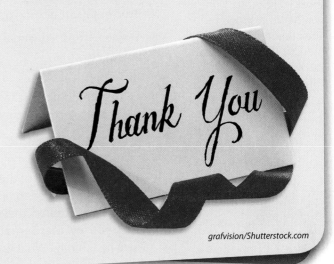

grafvision/Shutterstock.com

Show Resilience

People respond to challenges differently, and many demonstrate resilience. People who show **resilience** are able to bounce back from traumatic and stressful events, such as an act of violence, a serious health problem, or a parents' divorce. They are flexible and adapt, change, and grow as they encounter difficult experiences. When facing a life-changing situation, they think about the best way to respond to the situation and figure out what they can learn from the experience.

Having resilience requires strength, which means you need to engage in a healthy lifestyle. When you take care of yourself, you have more energy to handle challenges and respond to problems.

The care and support of others often helps people show resilience. Relationships that are positive, loving, and trusting help build a person's resilience. When experiencing emotional pain and sadness, it helps to have a strong support system of people who can offer encouragement.

Because people react to traumatic and stressful events differently, they tend to use various strategies for building resilience. The strategies that work for one person may not work for another. These strategies may include the following:

- Strengthen relationships with others and accept support when needed.
- Take action to solve problems instead of avoiding them.
- Develop a healthy self-image.
- Acknowledge your strengths and abilities, and work toward improving your weaknesses.
- Focus on what you want to accomplish and set SMART goals that enable you to succeed.
- Have optimism and remain hopeful that things will eventually get better.
- Get plenty of physical activity, eat nutritious meals, and sleep regularly.
- Learn to manage your stress (see Lesson 4.3).

Lesson 4.2 Review

1. Knowing which emotions you feel and why is called _____ _____.
2. **True or false.** Covering up or denying your feelings will make what you feel go away.
3. Which of the following is a characteristic of having high emotional intelligence?
   A. Empathy.
   B. Gratitude.
   C. Optimism.
   D. All of the above.
4. **Critical thinking.** List two positive emotions and two negative emotions. Explain how you can express these emotions in a healthy way.

Hands-On Activity

Make a list of all of the emotions you felt today. Include strong emotions that may have lasted for a while, as well as those that came and went fairly quickly. What caused these emotions? How did you react to these emotions? When you feel these emotions again, what will you do differently to respond to them healthfully? What will you do the same?

Managing Stress

Learning Outcomes

After studying this lesson, you will be able to

- **differentiate between** acute stressors and chronic stressors.

- **describe** different types of stress.

- **explain** how the body responds to stress.

- **give examples** of strategies you can use to manage the stress in your life.

- **recognize** when you should seek professional help for stress.

Graphic Organizer

What to Do About Stress

Use a graphic organizer like the one below to identify the top stressors that you are experiencing right now. For each stressor you identify, list ways that can help you manage each stressor. A sample has been done for you.

Olivier Le Moal/Shutterstock.com

Stressor 1   *I am struggling in math class.*

- *Increase the time I spend studying.*
- *Find a tutor to help me better understand the concepts.*

Stressor 2

Stressor 3

Stressor 4

Stressor 5

Key Terms

stress physical, mental, and emotional reactions of your body to the challenges you face

stressor any factor that causes stress

eustress positive stress

fight-or-flight response body's impulse to either fight off or flee from threatening situations

visualization strategy of imagining a pleasant environment when faced with stress

progressive muscle relaxation strategy of tensing and then relaxing each part of your body and breathing deeply to relieve stress

meditation strategy of clearing negative thoughts from your mind and relaxing your body to relieve stress

mindfulness strategy that involves being present in the moment and paying attention to thoughts and feelings in a nonjudgmental way

n the previous lesson, you explored how you feel about and react to people and situations around you. You also learned about the importance of developing emotional intelligence. One of the abilities of people who have high emotional intelligence is the ability to manage stress.

Many events that you experience in your life can cause stress. Remember Charlotte, from the previous lessons. She felt nervous before the first day of a new school year. She felt sick to her stomach before giving a big presentation in front of the class. She felt anxious about a bad grade on her math test. All of these are examples of Charlotte experiencing stress.

Stress is unavoidable—everyone experiences it at times. You may even feel stressed right now because of something going on in your life (**Figure 4.13**). Experiencing too much stress at once, or being unable to manage stress, can have a negative effect on your health and wellness.

In this lesson, you will learn about different types of stressors and how stress can impact your health. You will also learn some effective strategies that can help you manage the stressors in your life to promote good mental and emotional health.

Figure 4.13
Using a scale from 1–10 (10 being very stressed), determine your current level of stress in the different areas of your life.

Stress Test

1	2	3	4	5	6	7	8	9	10

Family

Do you fight with your siblings or parents? Are you adjusting to a family change? Are your parents frequently stressed? Is there a lack of communication between family members? Do you wish you had more privacy at home?

Friends and Peers

Are there any conflicts with your friends? Do some of your peers tease or bully you? Do you or your loved ones get cyberbullied on social media? Are you afraid of not being found attractive or not fitting in?

Illness

Are you (or is a loved one) suffering from disease, illness, or a loss of a loved one? Are you finding it difficult to concentrate or complete day-to-day tasks due to an illness? Are you getting the medical care and attention you need?

School

Have you just started at a new school? Do you have a big test coming up? Are you doing poorly in any of your classes? Do you complete your assignments late? Do you cram for tests at the last minute?

Activities

Do you have very little time outside of schoolwork to participate in activities you enjoy? Do you overwhelm yourself with too many activities? Do you have free time to just relax?

Types of Stressors

The physical, mental, and emotional reactions of your body to the challenges you face is **stress**. A **stressor** is a factor that causes stress. People may experience many different types of stressors, such as the following:

- **Acute (short-term) stressors.** Acute stressors include experiences that do not last very long (typically only a few hours), such as taking a final exam or giving a presentation in class.
- **Chronic (long-term) stressors.** These are occurrences that keep happening over a long period of time, such as feeling unsafe in your neighborhood or worrying about a loved one who is ill.
- **Routine stressors.** Routine stressors are small, but annoying, daily life experiences and pressures, such as getting to school on time or doing homework.
- **Major life event stressors.** Significant life experiences, such as the death of a loved one or the loss of a job are major life event stressors. **Figure 4.14** shows some examples of major life event stressors for teens.
- **Traumatic stressors.** These are experiences that could seriously threaten a person's life, such as natural disasters, wars, or major accidents.

Major Life Event Stressors for Teens
• Death of a parent
• Experience parents' divorce
• Experience parents' separation
• Moving for a parent's job
• Death of a close family member
• Experience an illness or injury
• Experience a parent's remarriage
• Parent loses his or her job
• Parents reunite after separation
• Mother goes back to work
• Family member's health changes
• Mother becomes pregnant
• Experience difficulty in school
• New brother or sister in the family
• New teacher or class
• The family finances change
• Break up with boyfriend or girlfriend
• Close friend experiences illness or injury
• Fighting more or less with brothers or sisters
• Fear of violence at school

Figure 4.14 All young people experience some of these major life events. These events can be major factors in causing stress. *What is the term for a factor that causes stress?*

Although stressors are often associated with negative events, positive events can also cause stress. If you win a big race or your sister gets married, these events can be stressful, even though they are happy occasions.

Remember, stress refers to the *reactions* of your body to the challenges you face. This means that not all stress is bad. Positive stress, or **eustress**, is good for you because it creates feelings of excitement, can be motivating, and can help you improve your performance.

The Body's Response to Stress

Sometimes stress feels unpleasant—a knot in the stomach before a big test, for example. Stress can also produce excitement, such as the surge of energy before a championship game. Your body reacts in specific ways when you encounter situations that seem threatening (for example, standing up to someone who is picking on you). All types of stressors can trigger the same bodily responses.

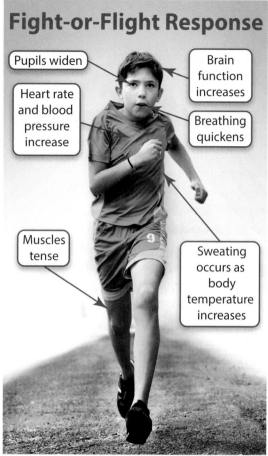

Fight-or-Flight Response

- Pupils widen
- Heart rate and blood pressure increase
- Brain function increases
- Breathing quickens
- Muscles tense
- Sweating occurs as body temperature increases

Lapina/Shutterstock.com

Figure 4.15 In the alarm stage of your body's response to stress, your body mobilizes to either attack or get away from a threat. *What is the second stage of your body's response to stress?*

If you experience a relatively brief threat, your body has plenty of resources stored up to respond. The body's response changes over time, depending on how long the stressor continues. Generally, your body's response to stress occurs in the following three stages:

1. **Alarm stage.** Your body mobilizes all of its resources to fight off a threat, either by attacking or by escaping from the threat. This reaction to a threat is the **fight-or-flight response**. To prepare for either fighting off or escaping from a predator, your body undergoes several changes (**Figure 4.15**).

2. **Resistance stage.** Your body continues to devote energy to maintaining its bodily response to the threat. Heart rate, blood pressure, and breathing are still rapid, which helps deliver oxygen and energy quickly to various parts of your body.

3. **Exhaustion stage.** If the threat persists, the body may stay in a state of high alert for a long time. In this case, the body will use up its resources and exhaustion will occur.

During times of stress, the body devotes large amounts of energy to reacting to the immediate threat. Over time, this energy can run out and the body can become open to infection or disease development. This is why people who experience chronic stress are at a greater risk of developing illnesses and diseases, such as colds, asthma, headaches, hives, or stomach disorders. Stress may also make the physical conditions a person already has, such as heart disease or high blood pressure, worse.

Strategies for Managing Stress

Learning how to manage stress is an important part of staying healthy. People who effectively manage the challenges they face and minimize the negative consequences of stress are resilient. They are able to cope with stressful situations and return to relatively normal functioning. You can use many strategies to better cope with stress and become more resilient (**Figure 4.16**). Some strategies work better in certain situations than in others.

Express Your Feelings

Talking with people you trust about your problems is a good way to manage or reduce your stress. The people you confide in may have useful advice for how to handle your problem. They might have been in a similar situation before and can provide helpful insight and suggestions. They might also help you think about the problem in a new way. Even if you do not find a solution, simply talking about your problems can be effective for reducing stress.

If you do not feel like talking with someone, you can always express your feelings by writing them down in a journal. Sharing your thoughts and feelings—instead of keeping them bottled up inside you—can reduce the amount of stress you feel.

Stress Management Strategies

Express Your Feelings	Maintain a Positive Attitude	Take Care of Yourself
• Talk through a problem with a person you trust • Ask for advice from someone who was in a similar situation • Write about your stress in a journal	• Shift your focus to something positive that has happened • See mistakes as opportunities to learn and grow • Look for the positive aspect of a negative situation	• Get enough nutrients and energy • Get enough sleep • Get regular physical activity • Spend time with your friends or family
Manage Your Time	**Distract Yourself**	**Use Relaxation Techniques**
• Break down your big tasks into smaller, more manageable ones • Create a reasonable schedule and stick to it • Say "no" to new commitments when you are already too busy	• Go for a walk • Read a good book • Find something to laugh at—a movie, TV show, videos, etc. • Work on a jigsaw or crossword puzzle	• Take slow, deep breaths • Visualize your "happy place" • Engage in muscle relaxation, meditation, or yoga • Be present in the moment and pay attention to your feelings

Figure 4.16 There are many healthy ways to manage stress to minimize its negative consequences. Some ideas are shown above.

CASE STUDY

Sameera Is in a Slump

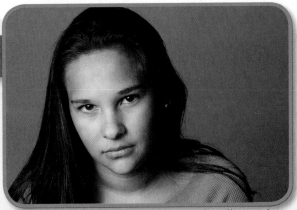

Kyle Lee/Shutterstock.com

Sameera, an eighth grader, has always enjoyed school. She likes the challenge of learning new things and the constant social interaction that comes with being in school with her friends. Math and science come pretty easily for her and she enjoys them, which makes her willing to work hard to understand the concepts. Social studies is not as interesting, but this year Sameera has a really dynamic teacher who is more like a storyteller than a teacher. This year has been great so far, until recently.

For the past few weeks, Sameera is not as excited to go to school as she used to be. Even knowing that she will see her friends in school does not motivate her to get going in the morning. She dreads waking up in the morning more than she did just a few months ago. She does not really feel like trying in any of her classes, not even math and science.

Overall, Sameera does not really feel like herself. Her friends and parents have mentioned similar thoughts to her. She is trying really hard to get back to her normal self, but she just can't.

Thinking Critically

1. What may be going on with Sameera's mental health?

2. If you were Sameera's friend and noticed these changes in her, what would you do? Explain the importance of friends advocating for friends' health during the school years.

3. Who could Sameera reach out to for help dealing with her situation? What could she say to start a conversation with these trusted people?

4. If you found yourself experiencing a dramatic change from your "normal," what would you do? Who would you reach out to for help?

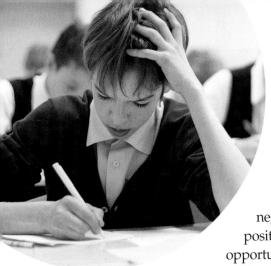

Figure 4.17
Even if you are well prepared, tests can be stressful if you have a negative attitude about them. If, however, you think of them as opportunities for learning and growth, they can be positive experiences. *What are some ways to avoid stress based on negative thoughts?*

Maintain a Positive Attitude

Some people spend lots of time each day focusing on what is not going well in their lives. They worry about upcoming exams and tryouts and become absorbed by memories of events that did not go well in the past. They may also obsess about factors they cannot change. This type of negative thinking can trigger anxiety.

It is much healthier to focus on the good events in your life. When negative thoughts enter your mind, shift your focus to something positive that has happened. Try to see mistakes or disappointments as opportunities to learn and grow, and not as major crises.

You can reduce stress by thinking about certain situations in a new and positive way. For example, if a parent picks you up late after school you may feel frustrated and anxious. Instead of focusing on your parent being late, you could come up with productive ways of using the time. You could read a book or start a homework assignment while you wait.

You can also look for positive aspects of stress-causing events—even negative events (**Figure 4.17**). Suppose you tried out for a role in a play or for a spot on the basketball team and you were not chosen. Not being chosen means you will have more time for homework, which should improve your grades.

Take Care of Yourself

During times of stress, many people neglect their physical needs. Failing to take care of yourself increases your risk for illness, which can further contribute to stress. During these times, it is important to eat well to provide your body with the energy and nutrients it needs. You also need to get plenty of sleep and physical activity.

People who engage in regular physical activity experience fewer negative physical effects of stress. Physical activity reduces the effect of stress on heart rate and blood pressure. Exercising also helps to relax the muscles.

Manage Your Time

One of the best ways to decrease or avoid stress is to manage your time well. You can avoid many stressors—such as the feeling of having too much to do at once—with careful planning, or *time management*. Planning can be very important when trying to reduce or eliminate stress.

To create a time management plan, first make a list of everything you need to do. Then break down the big tasks on your list into smaller ones (**Figure 4.18**). Create a schedule that describes when you need to accomplish each task and stick to that schedule. This technique is a simple way to keep track of what you have to do and to make sure you get everything done.

Sometimes, people take on commitments they do not have time or energy for because they have a hard time saying *no*. Being helpful to others is good, but committing to many events can create stress when your calendar is already full. Learning to set limits by saying *no* when you know you are too busy can help you avoid or reduce stress.

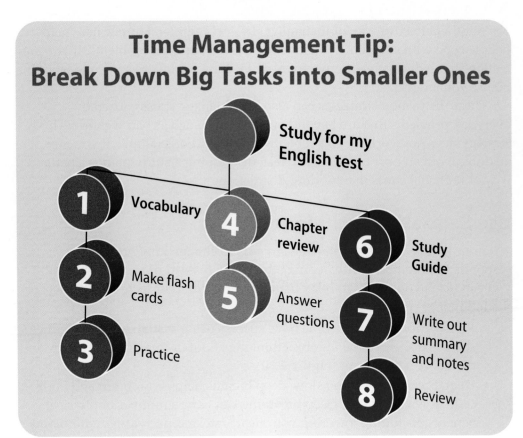

Time Management Tip: Break Down Big Tasks into Smaller Ones

Study for my English test

1 Vocabulary
2 Make flash cards
3 Practice
4 Chapter review
5 Answer questions
6 Study Guide
7 Write out summary and notes
8 Review

Figure 4.18 A big task like studying for your English test next week can seem overwhelming. Breaking it down into smaller parts can help you manage your time. *Why do people sometimes take on commitments they do not have time or energy for?*

Distract Yourself

Many situations that cause stress are either overwhelming or beyond a person's control. These situations may include family financial problems or a family member's serious illness. Intense focus on these types of problems can increase stress. Finding distractions can be a good way of managing stress that is consuming your thoughts (**Figure 4.19**). Some distraction strategies include going for a walk, volunteering in the community, or reading a good book.

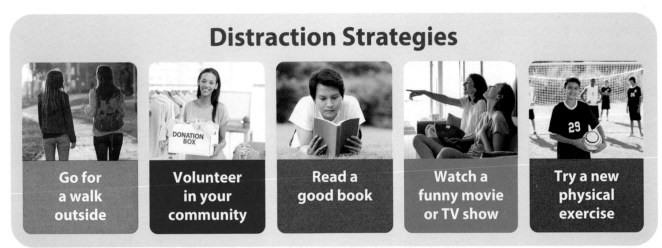

Distraction Strategies

Go for a walk outside

Volunteer in your community

Read a good book

Watch a funny movie or TV show

Try a new physical exercise

Left to right: Antonio Guillem/Shutterstock.com; wavebreakmedia/Shutterstock.com; Naypong/Shutterstock.com; Ollyy/Shutterstock.com; Monkey Business Images/Shutterstock.com

Figure 4.19 People respond differently to stress distractions, so it is important to find the method of distraction that works best for you.

Another effective way of managing stress is laughter. Humor may help people cope with stressors by distracting them from their problems. If you are feeling stressed, watch a funny movie or TV show, or talk to someone who makes you laugh.

These distraction strategies can also help manage stress caused by everyday problems that are beyond your control, such as bad weather. This strategy does not work for all problems, however. For example, if you are anxious about an upcoming science test, developing a study plan is a better way of reducing stress than finding distractions.

Use Relaxation Techniques

Another useful way to manage stress is to change how your body responds to potentially threatening situations. Instead of becoming tense, you can teach your body to relax using several different techniques, such as the following:

- **Visualization.** Some people have success using **visualization** to reduce stress. This technique involves thinking about or imagining being in a pleasant environment (**Figure 4.20**).
- **Deep breathing.** Taking slow, deep breaths helps your brain and body calm down and relax. Deep breathing can have a number of physical benefits, including lowering your heart rate and decreasing your blood pressure.
- **Progressive muscle relaxation. Progressive muscle relaxation** is a technique in which you tense and then relax each part of your body until your entire body is relaxed. Practicing deep breathing as you relax each part of your body increases the effectiveness of this technique.
- **Yoga.** Yoga involves performing a series of postures and breathing exercises. Performing yoga poses involves balance, flexibility, and intense concentration, which requires both physical and mental discipline.

Figure 4.20
If you find the beach relaxing, you might imagine the sound of waves crashing and the warmth of the sun on your skin. *What is the name of this relaxation technique?*

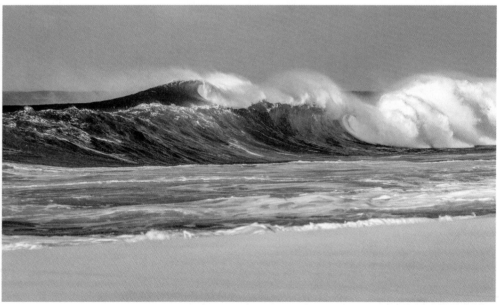

Kelly Headrick/Shutterstock.com

Basic Yoga for Beginners

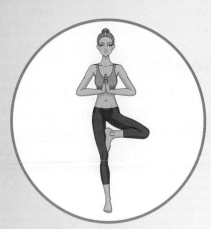

Tree Pose

From standing, shift all weight onto one leg. Place the opposite foot on the inner thigh or calf of the standing leg (never on the knee). Clasp hands at chest and balance.

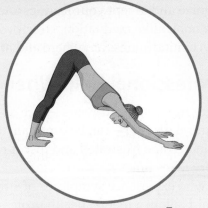

Downward-Facing Dog

Start on your hands and knees. Using straight arms, press the hips up and back reaching the chest toward the thighs. Press the heels into the floor feeling a stretch in the back of the legs. The legs are straight, or you can have a small bend at the knees to keep the back flat.

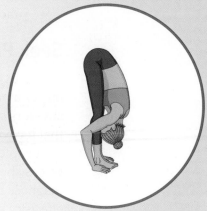

Forward Fold

Stand up straight and tall. Bend at the hips and try to touch chest to front of legs. Try to keep legs straight as you reach for the floor. Bend knees if needed.

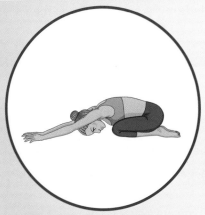

Child's Pose

Start on your hands and knees. Push hips back until buttocks rests on top of feet and forehead touches the ground. Let arms remain stretched in front of you.

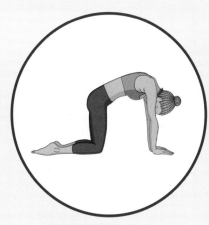

Cat Pose

Start on your hands and knees. Gently round your spine toward the ceiling as you breathe out. Inhale and lower your spine.

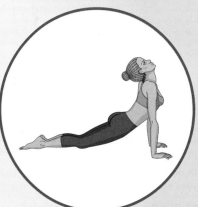

Cobra Pose

Lay face down on the floor with tops of feet touching the ground, arms against side, elbows facing feet, and palms pressed into the floor. Lift chest off floor by pushing through palms to straighten arms. Only straighten arms as much as feels comfortable for your lower back.

Baleika Tamara/Shutterstock.com

- **Meditation.** The goal of **meditation** is to reduce negative or stressful thoughts that can lead your body to become tense. During meditation, you intentionally set aside time to clear your mind of all negative and stressful thoughts and concentrate on relaxing your body.
- **Mindfulness. Mindfulness** involves being present in the moment and paying attention to thoughts and feelings in a nonjudgmental way. You recognize and accept your feelings and where you are, and then you move on. Unlike meditation, which you set aside time to do, you can practice mindfulness anywhere and at any time.

Seek Professional Help When Needed

Recovery from major stressors—such as experiencing the death of a loved one or a natural disaster—can be especially difficult. People experiencing such stressors can become frustrated and discouraged. It is helpful to remember that recovery takes time.

People who experience symptoms of stress for more than a couple of weeks should talk to a mental health professional. These trained professionals diagnose mental health conditions and help people cope with the emotional effects of stress. Professionals who can help include psychologists, social workers, therapists, and guidance counselors.

If you feel you might benefit from this type of professional help, talk to an adult you trust, such as a parent or guardian, teacher, guidance counselor, or doctor. This adult can put you in touch with a professional who can help you. If the adult you consult does not follow through, then confide in another responsible adult. Remember, asking for help is not a sign of weakness, but rather a sign of strength and courage. You do not need to struggle with mental and emotional health problems alone. Acknowledging your problem is the first step toward feeling better about your life.

Lesson 4.3 Review

1. What is the difference between an acute stressor and a chronic stressor?
2. **True or false.** Stress is always associated with negative events or experiences.
3. Your body mobilizes to fight off a threat by either attacking or escaping, which is called a(n) _____ response.
4. Meditation, yoga, visualization, and deep breathing are examples of _____ techniques to help manage stress.
5. **Critical thinking.** Name two strategies for managing stress. Why is it important that you manage the stress in your life?

Hands-On Activity

Think about a time when you felt very stressed. What was going on in your life? Was the stress caused by acute or chronic stressors or perhaps by a combination of both? Describe this time in your life in detail. What happened to your body during this time? What did you do to deal with this stress? Would you use these strategies again? What stress management techniques would you like to try out? Why?

Summary

Lesson 4.1 Getting to Know Yourself

- *Mental and emotional health* includes your self-esteem and how well you can understand and control your feelings and emotions, including stress.
- The different parts of your *identity* are physical, active, social, and psychological. Something a person accepts as true based on experiences, scientific facts, or what a person has learned is a *belief. Attitudes* are set ways of thinking or feeling.
- Your *self-image* is your mental picture of yourself, including how you look, how you act, your skills and abilities, and your weaknesses. Self-image is closely related to *self-esteem*, how you feel about yourself.
- People with positive mental and emotional health have a thirst for life and a sense of balance. They are good citizens who are responsible, trustworthy, respectful, compassionate, and kind.
- People with high self-esteem view failures as learning experiences and can adjust when faced with obstacles. They trust their judgment and stay true to their values.

Lesson 4.2 Making Sense of Your Emotions

- *Emotions* are the moods or feelings you experience. These emotions can be pleasant like joy or pride, or they can be unpleasant like anxiety or stress.
- Knowing which emotions you feel, and why, is *emotional awareness*. As you grow up, you can learn to control your emotions by identifying and accepting what you feel, and expressing those emotions in healthy ways.
- People with high emotional intelligence (EI) are skilled at understanding, controlling, and expressing their emotions. Having emotional intelligence is necessary to develop close relationships with others.
- People with high EI share similar abilities and characteristics. They are able to control negative emotions, have optimism, have empathy, and show gratitude and resilience.

Lesson 4.3 Managing Stress

- *Stress* is the physical, mental, and emotional reactions of your body to the challenges you face. The factors that cause stress, called *stressors*, can be acute (short-term), chronic (long-term), routine, major life event, or traumatic. Eustress can create excitement, add motivation, and help improve performance.
- Generally, your body responds to stress in three stages. In the alarm stage, your body mobilizes to combat a threat via the fight-or-flight response. In the resistance stage, your body devotes energy to maintaining this response. In the exhaustion stage, your body uses its resources by staying in high alert. At this stage, a body is at greater risk for illness.
- Learning how to manage stress is an important part of staying healthy. People who effectively manage the challenges they face and minimize the negative consequences of stress are resilient. They are able to cope with stressful situations and return to relatively normal functioning.

Check Your Knowledge 🡒

Record your answers to each of the following questions on a separate sheet of paper.

1. Someone who never wants to spend time alone has ____ mental and emotional health.

2. Your gender, height, weight, and age are the different attributes that make up your ____ identity.

3. What are three factors that can affect a person's self-esteem?

4. **True or false.** People with high self-esteem never encounter problems or experience bad situations.

5. **True or false.** It is possible to feel pleasant and unpleasant emotions at the same time.

6. What are three steps you can take to control your emotions?

7. People who are skilled at understanding, controlling, and expressing their emotions and sensing the emotions of others have high ____ ____.

8. The ability to keep a positive outlook and focus on the good aspects of situations is ____.

9. What is the term for a person's ability to bounce back from stressful or traumatic events?

10. Experiences that could seriously threaten a person's life, such as a major accident or war, are called ____ stressors.

11. Which of the following statements relates to *eustress*?
    A. It is a negative stress.   C. It is a positive stress.
    B. It can make you lose motivation.   D. All of the above.

12. **True or false.** Taking care of yourself by eating well, getting enough sleep, and regularly exercising can help reduce stress.

Use Your Vocabulary 🡒

attitudes	fight-or-flight response	resilience
beliefs	gratitude	self-esteem
emotion	identity	self-image
emotional awareness	meditation	stress
emotional intelligence (EI)	mindfulness	stressor
	optimism	visualization
empathy	progressive muscle relaxation	
eustress		

13. Draw a cartoon for one of the terms above. Use the cartoon to express the meaning of the term. After you finish your drawing, find a partner and exchange cartoons. Take turns explaining to each other how your cartoons show the meaning of the term you chose.

14. On a separate sheet of paper, list each of the terms above. Next to each vocabulary term, list a few words that relate to the meaning of the term. Then, work with a partner to explain how these words are related. As you discuss the terms, add any new words to your list.

Think Critically

15. **Predict.** How do gratitude, resilience, and empathy improve a person's health? Choose one of these character traits and imagine that it became a focus in your life. How would this trait impact your physical, social, and mental health?

16. **Cause and effect.** How does a person's level of self-esteem impact his or her health behaviors and decisions?

17. **Compare and contrast.** Compare and contrast positive and negative stress.

18. **Draw conclusions.** Find and explore a website that claims to provide information about adolescent mental and emotional health. After exploring the site, would you recommend this website to other middle school students? Why or why not?

DEVELOP Your Skills

19. **Stress management and accessing information.** Identify a stressor common to teenagers. Using reliable sources of information, research healthy strategies to manage this stressor. Create a presentation that explains why these strategies work for this stressor. Then, demonstrate the strategies and have your classmates give it a try, too.

20. **Community advocacy skills.** Develop and implement a campaign for your school community with a mission to increase self-esteem among adolescent students. As you plan, take into consideration the strategies for boosting self-esteem and the importance of high self-esteem discussed in the chapter. Reflect on the most common impacts on the self-image of young people. What issues most commonly harm self-esteem? What strategies most effectively build self-esteem?

21. **Stress management and technology skills.** Choose three of the relaxation techniques described in the chapter. Design and create a digital media product that exposes the reader or listener to these short relaxation techniques.

Formats for this product include a blog, website, infographic, and podcast. Present this product to your class.

22. **Stress management and communication skills.** Use a journal to record your stressors and emotions for a week. Also, record your reactions that occurred and the behaviors you chose as a result of your stressors and emotions. When the week is done, look for trends in your journal. Are the same things causing you stress and strong emotions day after day? Are your reactions under control? Are your behaviors appropriate? Use the information gained from your journal to help you better navigate your stressors and emotions next week.

23. **Communication skills.** Think about the people in your life who you tend to seek out when your emotions are strong. Make a list of these people in your life and tell them about the important role they play in your life. Even if they already know, by directly stating it, you are keeping the lines of communication open and this helps your mental health and theirs.

Chapter 5

Getting Help for Mental Health Conditions

Lesson 5.1 Recognizing Mental Health Conditions

Lesson 5.2 Treatment for Mental Health Conditions

Lesson 5.3 Preventing Suicide

Essential Question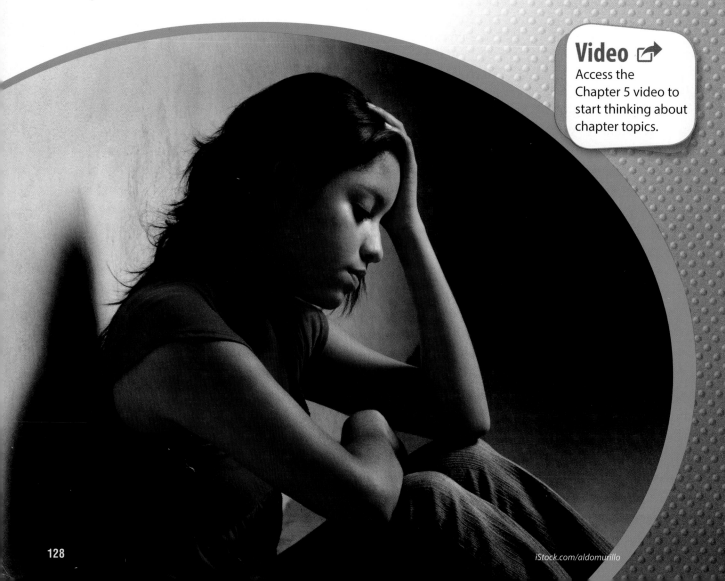

Why is getting help for mental health conditions so important?

Video

Access the Chapter 5 video to start thinking about chapter topics.

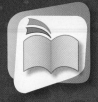

Reading Activity

Before you read the chapter, list any mental illnesses or disorders that you have heard about. As you read, look for references to the conditions you listed. After reading the chapter, review your list of mental health conditions and write two paragraphs reflecting on your list in light of what you learned in this chapter.

How Healthy Are You?

In this chapter, you will be learning about mental health conditions. Before you begin reading, take the following quiz to assess your habits in regards to preventing and treating mental health conditions.

Healthy Choices	Yes	No
Can you communicate your emotions and feelings well to other people?		
Do you regularly get at least 8 hours of sleep each night?		
If a person confides in you about having suicidal thoughts, do you take it seriously and talk to a trusted adult?		
When you are anxious, do you rarely respond with fear, dread, or panic?		
Is it uncommon for you to become panicky or upset?		
Are you able to listen to and follow instructions, focus on a task to completion, and sit still for short periods without talking or moving?		
Do you typically feel good about your skills, abilities, and relationships with other people?		
Can you usually find something that causes you to laugh and makes you happy?		
Do your family and friends support you through difficult situations?		
When you feel anxious or depressed, do you have someone to talk to about it?		
If you are suffering from a mental health condition, are you seeking the appropriate treatment options?		
If you have been diagnosed with a mental health condition, are you following the doctor's prescriptions for medication or therapy?		

Count your "Yes" and "No" responses. The more "Yes" responses you have, the more healthy mental health condition prevention and treatment habits you exhibit. Now, take a closer look at the questions with which you responded "No." How can you make these healthy habits part of your daily life? Think about how implementing these ideas can help improve your overall health.

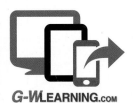

G-WLEARNING.com

While studying this chapter, look for the activity icon to

- **practice** key terms with e-flash cards and matching activities.
- **reinforce** what you learn by completing graphic organizers, self-assessment quizzes, and review questions.
- **expand** knowledge with interactive activities and activities that extend learning.

www.g-wlearning.com/health/

Recognizing Mental Health Conditions

Learning Outcomes

After studying this lesson, you will be able to

- **identify** the different types of mental health conditions.
- **describe** anxiety disorders.
- **differentiate between** mood disorders and personality disorders.
- **explain** possible causes of mental health conditions.

Graphic Organizer

Symptoms of Mental Health Conditions

As you read this lesson, use a table like the one shown below to list all the mental health conditions you learn about in this lesson. Include a list of symptoms for each condition. If multiple conditions have the same symptoms in common, highlight each repeated symptom in a different color. An example is provided.

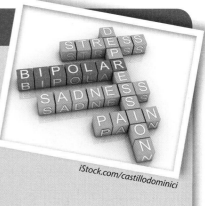

iStock.com/castillodominici

Mental Health Conditions	Symptoms
ADHD	• Difficulty paying attention • Difficulty controlling behavior • Hyperactivity

Farah, at 13 years old, has a hard time sitting still during an entire class period. She prefers to always be moving or talking to someone. She finds it difficult to listen to and follow the directions for her homework. Even if she does hear the directions, she quickly gets bored doing her homework. Because of these things, Farah's grades are suffering and she keeps getting in trouble during class.

Eleven-year-old Javier, on the other hand, has always been a good student. He loves learning, especially about history. Lately, however, he has become distracted in class because he feels deeply sad. He does not even know why he feels so sad. Sometimes, Javier will catch himself thinking about death. His teacher will scold him for zoning out, but it is not his fault! He gets irritated because he has no energy for class, even though he gets plenty of sleep.

As you learned in the previous chapter, your mental and emotional health involves how you feel about yourself, how well you can control your emotions, and how you can manage the stress in your life. In this lesson, you will learn about various mental health conditions, including those that are impacting Farah and Javier.

Types of Mental Health Conditions

Mental health conditions include mental illnesses and disorders. A **mental illness** is a mental or emotional condition so severe that it interferes with daily functioning. For example, a person might have a fear of public places. This fear may become so severe that the person avoids going to school or work. He or she might even avoid visiting with family and friends.

The terms *mental illness* and *mental disorder* both refer to serious mental health conditions. These conditions often involve thoughts, feelings, or behaviors. There are many different types of mental illnesses and disorders (**Figure 5.1**). You will learn more about these conditions in the following sections.

Types of Mental Health Illnesses and Disorders

Anxiety Disorders

- Types include: generalized anxiety disorder, social anxiety disorder, panic disorder, and phobias
- Involve inappropriate responses of fear or dread to a certain situation, experience, or object

Attention Deficit Hyperactivity Disorder (ADHD)

- Involves an inability to pay attention or control behavior
- Includes a tendency for hyperactivity

Obsessive-Compulsive Disorder (OCD)

- Involves constant and obsessive thoughts or feelings
- Usually includes rituals or repetition to make the thoughts or feelings go away

Post-Traumatic Stress Disorder (PTSD)

- Happens after an event that involves physical harm or the threat of harm
- Involves extreme stress or fear, flashbacks, angry outbursts, and nightmares

Mood Disorders

- Types include: major depression, seasonal affective disorder, bipolar disorder, and self-harm
- Involve serious changes in the way a person feels

Personality Disorders

- Types include: antisocial personality disorder and borderline personality disorder
- Involve a consistent pattern of inappropriate behavior

Schizophrenia

- Involves symptoms such as irregular thoughts, delusions, or false beliefs
- Can involve hearing voices and seeing things that are not there and paranoia

Figure 5.1 Mental illnesses and disorders come in all shapes and sizes, and can affect each person differently. *What is the name for a mental condition in which a person continually repeats an action?*

Anxiety Disorders

Almost everyone experiences anxiety in some situations. Anxiety often involves an increased heart rate, rapid breathing, sweaty palms, and an upset stomach. You may feel this way when you are nervous about something.

A person who has an **anxiety disorder** responds with extreme or unrealistic fear and dread to certain situations, experiences, or objects. These feelings and responses disrupt the person's way of life. Different types of anxiety disorders include generalized anxiety, social anxiety, panic disorder, and phobias.

People with *generalized anxiety disorder* experience anxiety about parts of their lives that they cannot control. These people may feel anxious about school or work. People with generalized anxiety disorder experience physical symptoms. These include feeling on edge, difficulty concentrating, and irritability.

People with *social anxiety disorder* feel anxious or afraid of social situations in which they might be judged. Anxious situations for these people include meeting new people, eating or drinking in public, and performing in front of others. In these situations, a person with social anxiety may worry about being embarrassed or rejected. A person with social anxiety disorder usually avoids social situations.

Panic Disorder

People with panic disorder experience *panic attacks*, or moments of intense fear. These moments of fear occur for no reason, and can happen anywhere or anytime without warning. Panic attacks include physical symptoms, such as a fast heartbeat, dizziness, trouble breathing, and chest pain.

People who have panic attacks are usually fearful of having another attack. They may avoid places where they have experienced an attack. Some become so fearful of having another attack that they will not leave their own homes.

Phobias

People with phobias have a strong fear of objects or situations that do not really pose much, if any, danger. This fear is *irrational*, meaning that it does not make sense. **Figure 5.2** describes some common phobias.

Figure 5.2
Over 30 percent of the population in the United States has arachnophobia, meaning they are deeply afraid of spiders. *If a fear is irrational, what does this mean?*

Different Types of Phobias

Phobia Name	Fear of...
Arachnophobia	spiders
Ophidiophobia	snakes
Acrophobia	heights
Agoraphobia	open or crowded spaces
Cynophobia	dogs
Astraphobia	thunder/lightning
Claustrophobia	small spaces

RiggsPhotographs/Shutterstock.com

Life with Social Anxiety

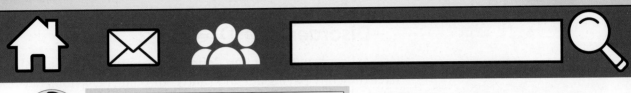

 Share your thoughts and feelings online. Will anyone care what you have to say?

Share

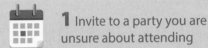 **1** Invite to a party you are unsure about attending

Your Best Friend added a new photo with **2 of your friends**

Had so much fun with these two today! All we were missing was **You**! Wish you would have come with us. 😊

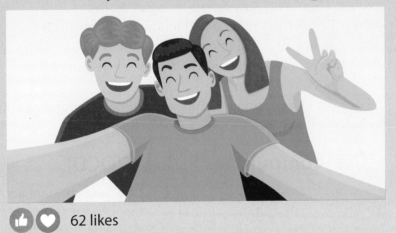

👍❤️ 62 likes

You updated your profile photo…will anyone like it?

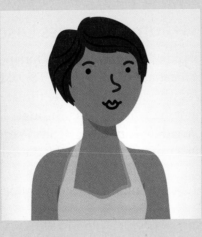

👍❤️

Chat with Your Crush

Would you maybe want to…I don't know…hang out sometime?

 Your Crush is typing…

Oh no…Did I say the wrong thing? Are you taking so long because you're going to say no? Never mind. Forget I said anything at all.

Send

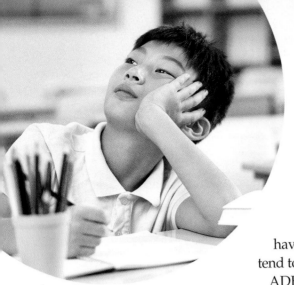

imtmphoto/Shutterstock.com

Figure 5.3
Students with ADHD are often unable to focus or sit still for the duration of the school day.
What term associated with ADHD means "overly active"?

People with phobias will try to avoid the object or situation that they fear. If they are in a situation in which they have to face their fear, they may experience physical symptoms. For example, they may experience shortness of breath, a fast heartbeat, or panic and desire to flee.

Attention Deficit Hyperactivity Disorder (ADHD)

People with **attention deficit hyperactivity disorder (ADHD)** have difficulty paying attention and controlling behavior. They also tend to be hyperactive. *Hyperactive* means overly active.

ADHD usually develops in childhood and can continue into adulthood. ADHD is the most commonly diagnosed behavioral disorder in children. A *behavioral disorder* involves serious, disruptive behaviors in children that cause problems at home, at school, or in social situations for at least six months. People who have ADHD may show the following types of symptoms:

- having difficulty focusing or sitting still
- having difficulty organizing and completing tasks
- having difficulty listening to and following instructions
- talking nonstop or being in constant motion
- being quickly bored with tasks and activities (**Figure 5.3**)
- having difficulty waiting
- blurting out inappropriate comments without awareness of the impact of this behavior on others

Obsessive-Compulsive Disorder (OCD)

People with *obsessive-compulsive disorder (OCD)* have constant and obsessive thoughts or feelings. They try to make the thoughts go away by engaging in rituals, which means they do the same thing repeatedly. For example, some people with OCD are obsessed with germs. These people may wash their hands many times a day to calm their obsessive thoughts.

Post-Traumatic Stress Disorder (PTSD)

People who live through a terrifying event may develop *post-traumatic stress disorder (PTSD)*. The event often involves physical harm or the threat of harm. For example, experiencing war or living through a natural disaster or a major accident can cause PTSD. People with PTSD experience extreme stress or fear after the danger is over. They may also experience *flashbacks* (vivid memories) of the event, angry outbursts, and nightmares or trouble sleeping (**Figure 5.4**).

Mood Disorders

People with *mood disorders* experience serious changes in the way they feel. Some mood disorders can make people feel sad all the time and lose interest in life. Other mood disorders

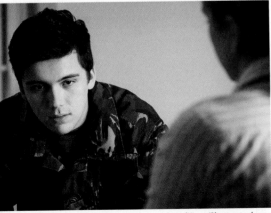

SpeedKingz/Shutterstock.com

Figure 5.4 Counseling can be an effective treatment method for people with PTSD.

can cause people to go back and forth between feelings of extreme happiness and extreme sadness. Common mood disorders include depression, seasonal affective disorder (SAD), bipolar disorder, and self-harm.

Depression

Everyone feels sad and depressed at times. These feelings are normal and usually improve and go away with time. Sometimes, however, feelings of depression are intense and do not go away. These feelings negatively affect a person's daily life.

People who experience ongoing negative feelings have **major depression**, which is also called *clinical depression*. Major depression is a serious mental disorder. Another type of depression is *seasonal affective disorder (SAD)*. People with SAD face depression in the winter months when there is less natural sunlight. SAD usually goes away in the spring and summer.

People with major depression and SAD often need professional treatment from a mental health specialist to overcome the disorder. Some people who have SAD may also benefit from light therapy.

People with depression may experience the symptoms in **Figure 5.5**. If symptoms of depression remain untreated, people who have depression are more likely to engage in harmful behaviors. They are also at greater risk of developing various health problems.

Bipolar Disorder

People who have **bipolar disorder** experience intense depression that alternates with *manic* (extremely happy and "up") moods. During the periods of depression, any of the symptoms of major depression may occur. Symptoms of the manic mood include poor judgment, little need for sleep, and hyperactive behavior. A manic mood may also include a lack of self-control. This can lead to binge drinking, binge eating, or out-of-control spending.

Self-Harm

Self-harm occurs when people hurt themselves on purpose. Cutting is the most common form of self-harm. Cutting involves a person making small cuts on his or her body with a razor blade, knife, or other sharp object. Other forms of self-harm may include burning oneself with lighters or matches, pulling out hair, punching or bruising oneself, and breaking bones.

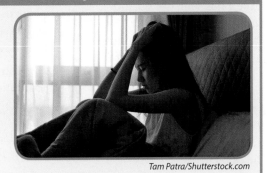

Possible Symptoms of Depression

- Loss of interest in favorite activities
- Feeling worthless
- Extreme tiredness and loss of energy
- Weight loss or gain
- Difficulty sleeping
- Trouble concentrating
- Irritability, anger, and hostility
- Recurrent thoughts of death

Tam Patra/Shutterstock.com

Figure 5.5
Depression is a serious mental disorder that has more symptoms than simply feeling sad. *What is another term for major depression?*

People typically self-harm because they cannot cope with a problem or control their emotions. They may hurt themselves because they are trying to stop feeling hopeless, angry, or lonely. Self-harm is possible to overcome by finding other ways to cope with emotions. Professional counseling may help people who self-harm learn how to control their emotions in healthier ways.

Personality Disorders

People with personality disorders show consistent patterns of inappropriate behavior. **Antisocial personality disorder** is one example of a personality disorder. People with this disorder ignore social rules and engage in impulsive and often aggressive and hostile behavior toward others.

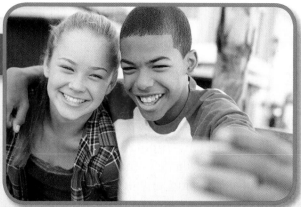

Monkey Business Images/Shutterstock.com

CASE STUDY

Best Friends: Conor and Julia

For the last few years, Conor has felt pretty lucky to have the best group of friends in the world. Together, they rode their bikes to the park, listened to music and danced, and always stuck together. He loved that he felt like he could tell them anything. His best friend is Julia. They became best friends because they both love softball and watching scary movies.

This year, however, Conor noticed that Julia is different. She does not come out for batting practice with him anymore, and she does not want to watch scary movies on the weekends. When she does hang out with their friends, she looks upset. When Conor tries to ask her if something is bothering her, she gives him an annoyed or angry look and huffs, "I'm fine." It is obvious to Conor that she is not fine, but he does not want to push her or call her a liar.

Julia fidgets all the time by rubbing her hands over her arms or legs. Conor has seen her pulling at her skin, and sometimes almost pinching it. She will do this under the table in the cafeteria or under her desk in class. He has even seen her pulling at her skin when she is at home and thinks no one is looking. Conor can tell she pinches a lot harder when she is particularly nervous or upset. A few weeks ago, he pointed out big bruises on Julia's upper arms. Since then, Julia has started wearing only pants and long-sleeved shirts, even though it is hot outside.

Conor is afraid that he will lose Julia as a best friend if he confronts her about this change in behavior. She seems so on edge about it. He is really worried about her though, and is afraid that she could be hurting herself. Conor does not know what to do.

Thinking Critically

1. What are the signs and symptoms that show Julia may have a mental health condition? Which mental health condition might she have?

2. Do you think Julia will get help to deal with her condition on her own? Why or why not?

3. If you were Conor, what would you do? How could you help her?

Sometimes, this may mean that they break the law. People with antisocial personality disorder do not show guilt or remorse if they hurt another person's feelings or cause physical harm.

People who have **borderline personality disorder (BPD)** have unstable identities and relationships. Their attitudes toward people may shift frequently. For example, people with BPD may like someone one day and then hate that same person the next day. They may get very angry with a person for canceling plans because they fear people will leave them.

Schizophrenia

People who have **schizophrenia** typically experience symptoms such as irregular thoughts, delusions, or false beliefs. Schizophrenia can also involve hearing voices and seeing things that are not there. People diagnosed with schizophrenia may experience paranoia. *Paranoia* is the belief that people are threatening or plotting against you. They may also show inappropriate emotional reactions, such as laughing when they hear someone has died.

What Causes Mental Health Conditions?

The cause or causes of most mental health conditions are unknown. Research suggests, however, that a combination of factors contribute to these conditions. These factors, as shown in **Figure 5.6** below, include the following:

- **Family history.** People who have family members with mental health conditions are at a greater risk of developing these conditions themselves.

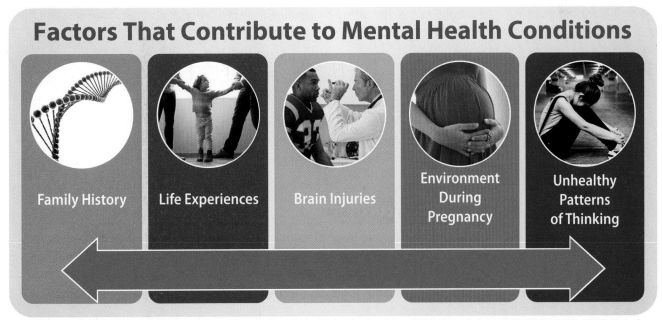

Factors That Contribute to Mental Health Conditions

Family History   Life Experiences   Brain Injuries   Environment During Pregnancy   Unhealthy Patterns of Thinking

Left to right: Jezper/Shutterstock.com; Monkey Business Images/Shutterstock.com; Rocketclips, Inc./Shutterstock.com; 10 FACE/Shutterstock.com; NARONGRIT LOKOOLPRAKIT/Shutterstock.com

Figure 5.6 Any one of these factors, or a combination of factors, can contribute to the development of mental health conditions.

- **Life experiences.** Most experts believe that a person's life experiences play a major role in whether a mental health condition actually develops. For example, a stable and loving home environment may prevent the development of a mental health condition. On the other hand, traumatic events and stressors, such as the death of a loved one, financial loss, or divorce, can increase the risk of developing a mental health condition.

- **Brain injuries.** People who experience a serious brain injury are at greater risk of developing some mental health conditions. A *traumatic brain injury (TBI)* is any blow or jolt to the head that damages the brain. Brain injuries may cause temporary or permanent changes to brain function. Permanent changes can result in depression, anxiety, personality changes, and aggression.

- **Environment during pregnancy.** A pregnant woman's environment affects the health of her baby. Certain events and behaviors in a pregnant woman's environment increase her baby's risk of developing a mental health condition. These include substance use, poor nutrition, stress, trauma, or exposure to viruses or certain chemicals.

- **Unhealthy patterns of thinking.** Having feelings of inadequacy, low self-esteem, anxiety, and anger can contribute to the development of a mental health condition. People who have unhealthy patterns of thinking may believe the negative feelings they experience will never go away. Fortunately, people can learn to change unhealthy patterns of thinking and improve their mental health.

Lesson 5.1 Review ✍

1. A person who has a(n) _____ disorder responds inappropriately with fear and dread to certain situations, experiences, or objects.

2. What does the acronym *ADHD* mean?

3. **True or false.** All mood disorders make people feel sad all the time and lose interest in life.

4. List the five factors that can contribute to a mental health condition.

5. **Critical thinking.** Describe four different possible symptoms of ADHD and explain why these symptoms might be disruptive at school, at home, or in social situations.

Hands-On Activity

Research current mental health apps to better understand the information and features provided by these types of apps. Choose one mental health condition to be the focus of your app and design a proposal including the following:

- Page 1: name, logo, description, summary of benefits and uses, target audience
- Pages 2–4: three in-app features (drawn or digital) that would be beneficial to your users

Treatment for Mental Health Conditions

Learning Outcomes

After studying this lesson, you will be able to

- **describe** treatment options for mental health conditions.
- **compare** different types of therapy.
- **summarize** barriers to seeking help for mental health conditions.
- **recognize** how to help a loved one who has a mental health condition.

Graphic Organizer

Identifying Resources

Using a graphic organizer like the one below, identify resources for people suffering from mental health conditions. Write *Resources for People with Mental Health Conditions* in the middle oval, and list any resources you can think of in the surrounding circles.

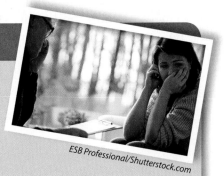

ESB Professional/Shutterstock.com

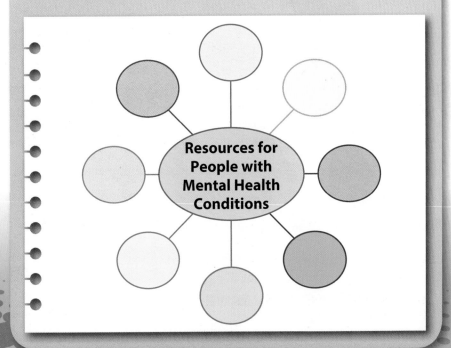

Resources for People with Mental Health Conditions

Key Terms

therapist professional who diagnoses and treats people with mental health conditions

individual therapy type of therapy that involves a one-on-one meeting with a therapist to discuss feelings and behaviors

family therapy type of therapy in which all family members meet together with a therapist to build positive, healthy relationships

support groups gatherings in which a therapist meets with a group of people who share a common problem

antidepressants medications that treat depression by making certain chemicals in the brain more available

antipsychotics medications that manage the symptoms of schizophrenia

inpatient treatment type of treatment that involves staying in a healthcare facility for a period of time

stigma mark of shame or embarrassment that is usually unfair

When mental health conditions interfere with a person's ability to control his or her emotions or cope with daily life, professional treatment from a mental health professional becomes necessary. The mental health professional can then determine which type of treatment will best meet the person's needs depending on his or her mental health condition. Different mental health conditions, and the severity of symptoms, often require different types of treatment.

Consider the examples from the previous lesson. Farah struggles with ADHD, and Javier has started to suffer from depression. These mental health conditions are causing them problems both in class and in their lives. Luckily, both of these mental health conditions are treatable.

In this lesson, you will learn about different types of treatment options that are available to treat mental health conditions. You will learn about barriers that may prevent some people with mental health conditions from getting the help they need. You will also learn how you can help a loved one who has a mental health condition.

Treatment Options

Researchers are trying to find ways of identifying people who are vulnerable to mental health conditions. These researchers work to better understand how the human brain works (**Figure 5.7**). As they learn more, researchers also create new treatments for mental health conditions. The purpose of these treatments is to help people live healthy and productive lives. Treatment may involve receiving therapy, taking medication, or staying in a healthcare facility for a period of time.

Figure 5.7
The more researchers study the brain, the more they learn about what treatment options work best for mental health conditions.

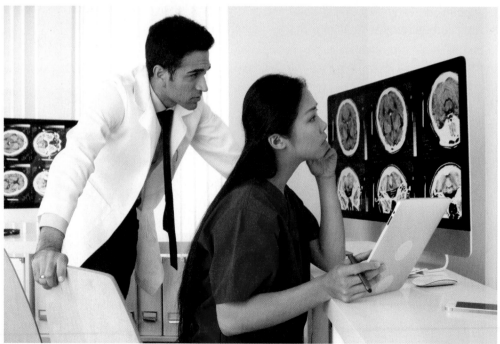

Rocketclips, Inc./Shutterstock.com

Therapy

A **therapist** is a professional who diagnoses and treats people with mental health conditions. Therapists include professionals such as psychologists, psychiatrists, social workers, and counselors.

Therapists can help people understand their feelings and behaviors in an accepting and nonjudgmental way. Therapists may also have specific suggestions for how people can understand their thought processes and help themselves feel better. Therapists can help people learn to cope with their problems in healthy, positive ways. Therapists may recommend several different types of therapy, which include the following:

- **Individual therapy** involves a one-on-one meeting with a therapist to discuss feelings and behaviors (**Figure 5.8**). The information a patient shares with his or her therapist is completely confidential in most cases. One exception is if a therapist believes a patient may hurt himself or herself, or someone else. The therapist may share that information with a parent or guardian.
- In **family therapy**, all members of a family meet together with a therapist. This type of therapy helps families build positive, healthy relationships. Family therapy can also help members of a family support one member with a mental health condition.
- In **support groups**, a therapist meets with a group of people who share a common problem. The therapist shares and discusses strategies for managing this common issue with all group members at the same time. Members of support groups also gain information about what strategies were helpful for others. Support groups can be helpful because people feel the other members truly understand their problems.

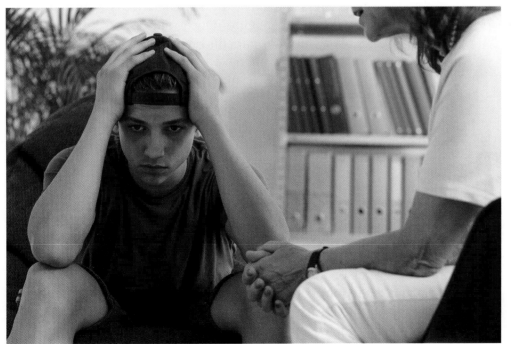

Photographee.eu/Shutterstock.com

Figure 5.8
In a one-on-one conversation, a patient can express his or her emotions and experiences. A therapist can then help create a treatment plan for any mental health conditions. *In addition to therapists, name two other types of professionals who diagnose or treat people with mental health conditions.*

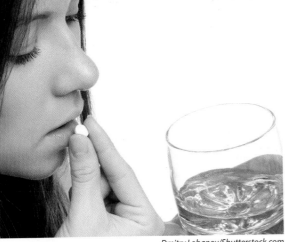
Dmitry Lobanov/Shutterstock.com

Figure 5.9 Medications often work by changing body chemistry. For example, antidepressants are believed to affect how neurotransmitters pass signals from one nerve cell to another in the brain. *Antidepressants are prescribed to treat which mental health condition?*

Medication

Doctors, usually psychiatrists, prescribe medications as a treatment option, along with therapy, for people with mental health conditions. The following are examples of medications for specific mental health conditions:

- **Depression. Antidepressants** make certain chemicals in the brain more available, which can reduce or eliminate symptoms of depression (**Figure 5.9**).
- **ADHD.** Stimulants increase the levels of certain chemicals in the brain. This helps improve memory and attention span.
- **Anxiety disorders.** Medications used to treat people with anxiety disorders often slow down the central nervous system. This makes people feel calmer and more relaxed.
- **Schizophrenia. Antipsychotics** manage the symptoms of schizophrenia, which may include hallucinations.
- **Bipolar disorder.** *Lithium* helps control the extreme highs and lows that are common with bipolar disorder.

Managing Medication Side Effects

Most medications have some side effects (**Figure 5.10**). Side effects can include tiredness and weight gain or loss. In some cases, medications can have very serious side effects. Some types of medication can cause damage to major organs. People who take certain types of antidepressants may experience *increases* in suicidal thoughts and behaviors. Due to side effects, doctors regularly monitor patients on medications.

Using Medication with Therapy

Many researchers believe that medications are most effective when used along with some type of therapy. People with depression may take medication and also benefit from therapy. Medication can effectively manage symptoms of a condition. Therapy can help people correct their negative, unhealthy thought patterns.

Possible Side Effects of Mental Health Medications

- Drowsiness
- Dizziness
- Restlessness
- Weight gain
- Nausea and vomiting
- Increases in suicidal thoughts
- Hallucinations
- Heart attack or stroke
- New or worsening mental health condition

Figure 5.10 Alert your doctor to any side effects you may experience from a medication.

Inpatient Treatment

In some cases, a person's mental health condition causes serious problems. These problems often require care in a clinic or hospital, or *inpatient treatment*. **Inpatient treatment** is necessary when people are at serious risk of harming themselves or others. People who are depressed and suicidal may need to be hospitalized for a period of time to make sure they do not attempt suicide. In the hospital, people receive around-the-clock supervision, medication, and therapy.

Barriers to Seeking Help

Unfortunately, people with mental health conditions do not always get the help they need. Only 44 percent of adults and less than 20 percent of children with mental health conditions get the help they need. Some people may assume their negative feelings will go away on their own.

BUILDING Your Skills

Talking About Mental Health

Onset of many mental health disorders occurs before 24 years of age. Getting early mental health support for children and young adults can help them before conditions interfere with their developmental needs and ability to cope with daily life. Recognizing mental health conditions in yourself and others, and knowing how to seek help, is essential to early treatment of these conditions.

It is essential to create a support system when you are young that encourages your mental health and well-being. This support system will help to guide your decisions and care for you during difficult times. The following activity will help you initiate conversations about decision-making and mental health conditions with a parent or trusted adult.

Conversations That Make a Difference

Complete this activity with a parent or trusted adult. To begin, choose one of the scenarios below. Then, discuss with your parent or trusted adult what you would do if you ever faced this situation. Together, create a plan of action. Identify what help you could provide for yourself or your loved one. What treatments may be available for this mental health condition? Summarize your conversation and include your plan of action.

Scenarios

- **Scenario 1.** Your friend cannot sit still in class. He is always getting in trouble for being off-topic during class discussions. He also has a hard time paying attention to the teacher's instructions or focusing on an assignment for more than a few minutes at a time.
- **Scenario 2.** You have your highs and lows as a middle school student. At times, you are happy and confident. At other times, you are stressed, insecure, and feel lost. Lately, the negative feelings are coming out more. You hide your emotions well, but sometimes you wish you had someone to whom you could talk.
- **Scenario 3.** Your sister is always on a roller coaster of emotions. One minute she is so happy it is almost annoying—laughing and talking loudly, running around with endless energy. Then, the next minute, she is withdrawn and tired.

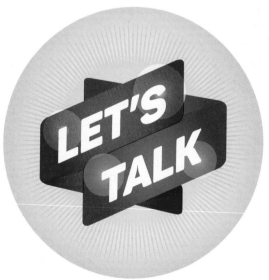

dnd_project/Shutterstock.com

Most mental health conditions, however, do not improve without treatment. Untreated mental health conditions may even get worse and lead to more severe conditions. Some people may face external barriers that prevent them from getting help for their condition. Friends and loved ones can make a big difference to help someone get the treatment he or she needs to improve his or her quality of life.

Social Stigma

Mental health conditions often carry a social stigma. **Stigma** is a mark of shame or embarrassment that is usually unfair. For example, attaching stigma to mental health conditions is unfair to the people affected by these conditions. They have done nothing to deserve shame or embarrassment. An unfair stigma may result from a lack of understanding about a mental health condition.

Social stigma may cause people with mental health conditions not to seek help. Social stigma may also cause people to deny they have a problem. Due to stigma, people may fear they will lose an opportunity because of their condition. For example, they may fear losing a job, a scholarship, or a leadership position.

People who experience a mental health condition may mistakenly believe they should be able to fix their condition on their own. In fact, a mental health condition requires a doctor's treatment just like a physical condition.

Cost of Treatment

People may be reluctant to seek help because of a cost they may be unable to afford. Although mental health professionals do charge for their services, a person's health insurance may cover a portion of the expenses. Some mental health clinics may also provide therapy services at no cost or a reduced rate.

Helping a Loved One

You may be concerned that someone you care about has a mental health condition. Share your concerns with that person in an open and honest way (**Figure 5.11**). Simply saying that you are worried and would like to help lets that person know you are available. You could also offer to find a mental health professional. You may even go with your loved one to talk to the professional.

Sometimes a person with a mental health condition is not interested in seeking help. You must intervene when you suspect someone may harm himself or herself. In other situations, you need to accept that it is not your responsibility to solve that person's problem. You should not try to protect people from the consequences of their conditions. This type of protection simply enables people to continue having the condition without treatment. For example, suppose your friend is too depressed to complete his homework. Doing the assignment for your friend just helps him hide the seriousness of his or her condition from people who could offer help.

Remember that sometimes people need more time before they are ready to get help. Take immediate action, however, if you suspect someone is suicidal. Call 911 or take the person to the hospital right away.

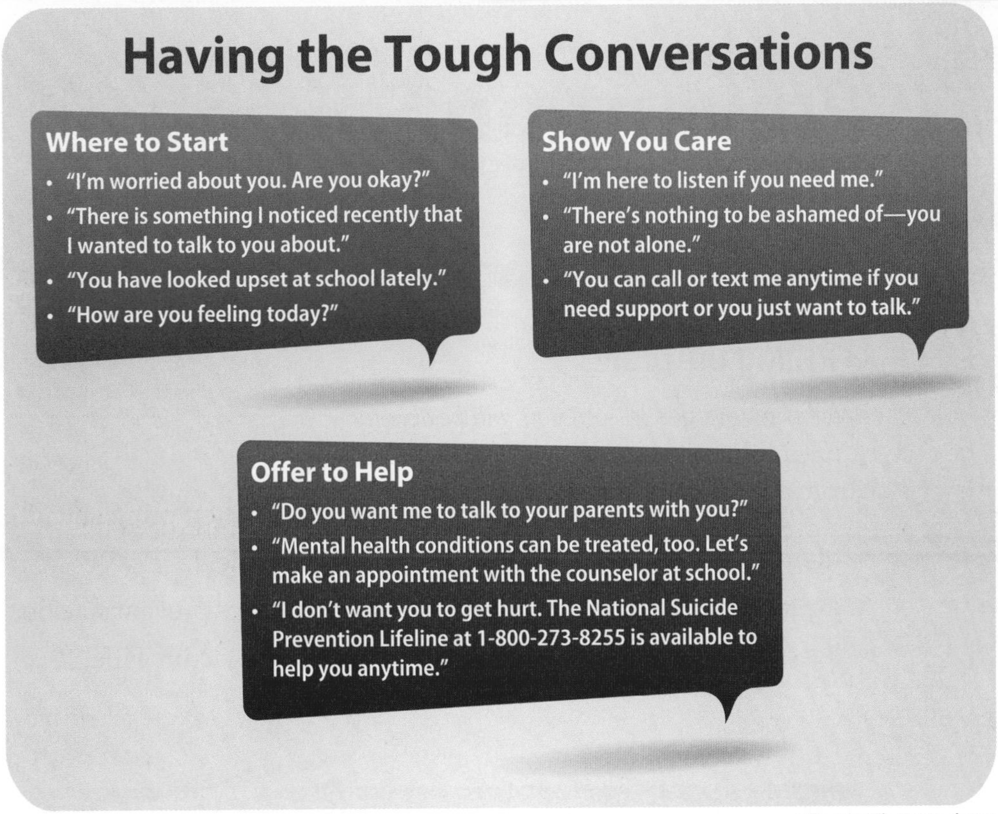

Having the Tough Conversations

Where to Start
- "I'm worried about you. Are you okay?"
- "There is something I noticed recently that I wanted to talk to you about."
- "You have looked upset at school lately."
- "How are you feeling today?"

Show You Care
- "I'm here to listen if you need me."
- "There's nothing to be ashamed of—you are not alone."
- "You can call or text me anytime if you need support or you just want to talk."

Offer to Help
- "Do you want me to talk to your parents with you?"
- "Mental health conditions can be treated, too. Let's make an appointment with the counselor at school."
- "I don't want you to get hurt. The National Suicide Prevention Lifeline at 1-800-273-8255 is available to help you anytime."

Figure 5.11

If a friend opens up to you about his or her mental health, do not promise to keep secrets. If your friend becomes a danger to himself or herself or to others, you may need to contact a trusted adult without your friend's permission.

RFvectors/Shutterstock.com

Lesson 5.2 Review

1. A professional who diagnoses and treats people with mental health conditions is called a(n) _____.

2. **True or false.** Antidepressants manage the symptoms of schizophrenia, which may include hallucinations.

3. Which form of treatment is recommended when people are at serious risk of harming themselves or others?

4. List two barriers for seeking help for a mental health condition.

5. **Critical thinking.** List the three types of therapy and explain why each could be helpful for treating a mental health condition.

Hands-On Activity

In small groups, create a real-life middle school scenario involving a mental health condition from Lesson 5.1. Have one group member be the person with the mental health condition. Other group members will be the person's friends. In your scenario, focus on ways to help the person. Create a script for each group member. Include the following information: the mental health condition involved, symptoms associated with the condition, trusted adults who can provide support, healthcare services available, and other treatment options (if applicable). Perform your scenario for the class.

Lesson 5.3

Preventing Suicide

Key Terms 📖

suicide act of taking one's own life

suicide contagion term that describes the copying of suicide attempts after exposure to another person's suicide

suicide clusters series of suicides in a particular community that occur in a relatively short period of time

survivors people who lose a loved one to suicide

Learning Outcomes

After studying this lesson, you will be able to

- **identify** risk factors of suicide.
- **recognize** signs that someone may be at risk of attempting suicide.
- **identify** ways to respond to warning signs of suicide.
- **explain** how treating mental health conditions helps prevent suicide.
- **describe** how suicide affects other people in the victim's life.

Graphic Organizer 📖

Myths and Facts About Suicide

List everything you think or have heard about suicide. Then categorize each item as a myth or a fact as shown in the table below. Compare your table with a partner's table. Add notes and corrections to your table as you read the lesson.

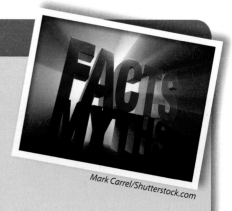

Mark Carrel/Shutterstock.com

Myths About Suicide	Facts About Suicide
Talking about suicide or asking someone if he or she feels suicidal will encourage suicide attempts.	*Talking about suicide provides an opportunity for communication for a person in need.*

People who consider death by suicide feel a sense of hopelessness and despair about their lives. They feel like things will never get better. Their emotions become too much to handle. In some cases, mental health conditions may contribute to these feelings. Remember Javier's depression from the previous lessons. Those extreme feelings of sadness could overwhelm Javier so much that he considers suicide.

The good news is that suicide is preventable. Lives and feelings can, and do, get better. Emotions often occur in cycles. There will be times of sadness, but times of happiness may be right around the corner. Treatments are available to help people with mental health conditions, like Javier, feel better. People can learn to recognize the warning signs of suicide to prevent it from happening. By getting the necessary help, people who are thinking about suicide can learn healthy ways to cope with their feelings and eventually lead fulfilling lives.

Recognize Risk Factors of Suicide

The term **suicide** describes when a person takes his or her own life. In the United States, suicide is the second leading cause of death for people ages 10 to 24. In the past 12 months, more than 9 million people had serious thoughts of suicide.

Being able to recognize risk factors of suicide can help people get the treatment they need to prevent a suicide attempt. One major risk factor is a previous suicide attempt. If a person attempted suicide before, he or she is more likely to make another attempt. **Figure 5.12** shows other factors that may contribute to suicidal behavior.

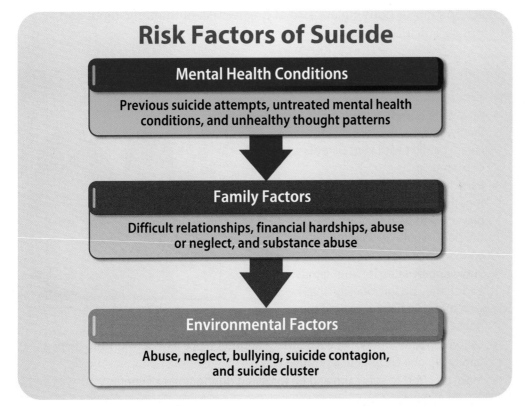

Risk Factors of Suicide

Mental Health Conditions

Previous suicide attempts, untreated mental health conditions, and unhealthy thought patterns

Family Factors

Difficult relationships, financial hardships, abuse or neglect, and substance abuse

Environmental Factors

Abuse, neglect, bullying, suicide contagion, and suicide cluster

Figure 5.12
Untreated mental health conditions, domestic abuse, and bullying are all risk factors that could lead to someone having suicidal thoughts. *Why is it so important to be able to recognize risk factors of suicide?*

Mental Health Conditions

People who consider suicide often do so because of overwhelming sadness and negative thoughts. Sometimes, a mental health condition causes these symptoms. Anxiety, depression, and other mental disorders can cause unhealthy thought patterns. These thought patterns could cause people to consider suicide. It is important to remember, however, that many people with mental health conditions never attempt suicide. Instead, they seek treatment to eliminate or reduce symptoms of their condition and change unhealthy thought patterns to lead fulfilling lives.

Family Factors

People from certain family backgrounds may be at greater risk of attempting suicide. People whose biological parents experience depression may be at greater risk of developing depression themselves. This means they may also be at greater risk of attempting suicide.

Difficult relationships among family members may also increase the risk for suicide attempts. Crises may further strain family relationships and increase risk factors. Examples of crises include financial hardships, issues of abuse or neglect, and substance abuse problems. Again, it is important to remember that many people who experience family problems never attempt suicide. They focus on improving and strengthening family relationships (**Figure 5.13**).

Environmental Factors

Serious stressors can lead someone who is depressed to consider suicide. People who experience long-term environmental stress are at greater risk of attempting suicide. Examples of environmental stress include abuse and neglect. Victims of bullying are also at greater risk of thinking about and attempting suicide.

Figure 5.13
Conflicts within your family can negatively affect your mental and emotional health. Following strategies such as those listed to the right can help you to encourage healthy relationships within your family.

Tips for Strengthening Family Relationships

- Always be honest with your family. Lying is a quick way to create conflict with your parents or siblings.
- Participate in new, fun activities together. Watch a new movie, play a board game, or go to the pool. Whatever your family enjoys, do it together.
- Show appreciation for your family and all they do for you. Say "thank you" often. Be helpful around the house in return.
- Laugh together, but not at each other. Laughter helps ease tension and helps a family see one another in a positive way.
- Make an effort to stay calm and be forgiving during times of conflict.

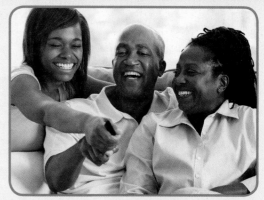
Monkey Business Images/Shutterstock.com

Hearing about someone else's suicide may increase the risk for *suicide contagion*. **Suicide contagion** is the term that describes how exposure to a suicide or suicide attempt may influence others to attempt suicide. Even hearing about a stranger's suicide can cause certain people to attempt suicide themselves.

Acts of suicide contagion may cause some communities or groups to experience *suicide clusters*. A **suicide cluster** is a series of suicides or suicide attempts in a relatively short time.

Respond to Warning Signs of Suicide

To help prevent suicide, people need to respond to warning signs of suicide. Most people who attempt suicide show some warning signs about their intentions. They often hint at or tell someone about their plans beforehand. Some people may say they feel like they have no reason to live. Others may seem obsessed with death. It is very important to take any mention of suicide seriously, even if the person seems to be joking.

The following are warning signs that may mean a person is considering suicide:

- changes in eating and sleeping habits
- withdrawal from friends, family, and regular activities
- disregard for personal appearance
- changes in personality
- giving away valued possessions
- loss of interest in activities previously enjoyed

Always take any thoughts or mention of suicide and any other warning signs very seriously (**Figure 5.14**). If you think about hurting yourself, talk to an adult you trust right away. This person can put you in touch with a trained mental health professional.

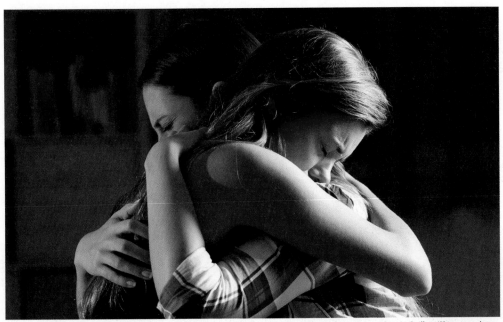

Figure 5.14
Getting help for someone who is having suicidal thoughts does not mean betraying his or her trust.

Antonio Guillem/Shutterstock.com

Watch Out for Warning Signs

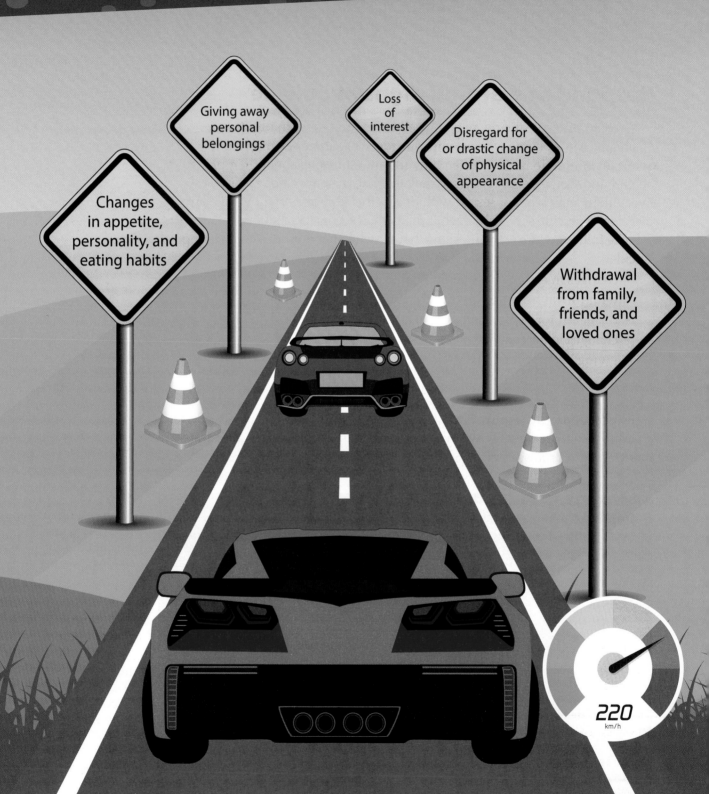

Background: Kong Vector/Shutterstock.com; Cars: HedgehogVector/Shutterstock.com; Road: pingebat/Shutterstock.com; Signs: Francois Poirer/Shutterstock.com; Speedometer: vladwel/Shutterstock.com; Construction cone: Yulia Glam/Shutterstock.com

If a person confides in you about having suicidal thoughts, you cannot keep this secret. Talk to someone who can help immediately. You can also call 911 or a suicide hotline number to reach a trained mental health professional (**Figure 5.15**).

Treat Underlying Health Conditions

The most common cause of suicide is untreated depression. Sometimes people consider suicide because of emotions resulting from a mental health condition. Anxiety, depression, and other disorders can cause sadness and negative thoughts. Treatment for these disorders seeks to reduce these symptoms. Reducing these symptoms usually means people no longer consider suicide. Getting treatment for mental health conditions helps people lead more fulfilling lives. This treatment can also help prevent suicide.

Provide Help for Survivors

The term **survivors** describes people who lose a loved one to suicide. Survivors often feel anger, guilt, and sadness. They may suffer with guilt because they were unable to prevent the death. They may feel rejected and abandoned by the victim. Suicide deaths are sudden. This means survivors are unable to prepare themselves for a loss.

Survivors may even feel embarrassed or ashamed by the suicide. Many people are uncomfortable with the topic of suicide. Unfortunately, this means survivors may not get the support they need after their loss.

The good news is that there are ways to help survivors. Some survivors may find support groups or therapy helpful. It is important to let survivors grieve. If you know someone who lost a loved one to suicide, learn about the stages of grief (**Figure 5.16** on the next page). Knowing what your friend is going through can help you be more compassionate.

Survivors may not want to talk about their loss right away. When they are ready to talk, however, just listen. Some people feel better when they talk about difficult topics. Listening is a simple way to help survivors overcome their loss.

Suicide Prevention Hotlines		
National Emergency Number	Call (and text in certain areas)	911
National Suicide Prevention Hotline	Call or chat online	1-800-273-8255
Crisis Text Line	Text	741741
Hope Line	Chat online or e-mail	www.thehopeline.com

Figure 5.15
Mental health professionals can provide effective treatment for people with mental health conditions so they can get the help they need to recover.

Stages of Grief

Stage	Description
Denial	It is normal for some people to deny sad news. People may ignore the facts and try to carry on as though nothing has changed. Not all people experience denial, but those who do are protecting themselves from emotional pain.
Anger	Some people become angry with the person who died. Although this stage is temporary, it may last a long time, and a person's anger may push family and friends away.
Bargaining	People often feel out of control and helpless in the face of death. Some people may try to bargain with a higher power that they feel has control over the situation.
Depression	Deep sadness comes with the reality of the loss. This depression is normal and can last several months.
Acceptance	As with other stages, not all people experience this stage. When they do, they accept the loss as real and begin to move on knowing that life continues.

Lesson 5.3 Review

1. **True or false.** If a person attempted suicide before, he or she is less likely to make another attempt.

2. Which of the following is *not* an example of a family factor that can increase the risk of a suicide attempt?

   A. Financial hardships.

   B. Good relationships among family members.

   C. Abuse or neglect.

   D. Substance abuse.

3. A(n) _____ _____ is a series of suicides or suicide attempts in a relatively short time.

4. What is the term for a person who has lost a loved one to suicide?

5. **Critical thinking.** List three warning signs that a person may be considering suicide. Explain how you should respond if someone you know is considering suicide.

Hands-On Activity

Write six social media posts that represent the emotional struggles of middle school students. Two of the posts should represent general feelings of sadness. Another two should indicate depression. The final two should include warning signs of suicidal thoughts. Under each post, explain whether it points toward sadness, depression, or suicidal thoughts. Describe how you would respond to the post showing empathy and compassion. Include any actions you would take to help those experiencing emotional struggles.

Review and Assessment

Summary

Lesson 5.1 Recognizing Mental Health Conditions

- A *mental illness* is a mental or emotional condition that interferes with daily functioning.
- Anxiety disorders cause inappropriate fear or dread in response to situations, experiences, or objects.
- Attention deficit hyperactivity disorder (ADHD) makes it difficult to pay attention or control behavior. Those with obsessive compulsive disorder (OCD) experience constant and obsessive thoughts or feelings.
- People with mood disorders such as depression, seasonal affective disorder (SAD), bipolar disorder, and self-harm experience extreme changes in the way they feel.
- People with personality disorders like antisocial personality disorder or borderline personality disorder (BPD) show patterns of inappropriate behavior.
- Family history, life experiences, brain injuries, environment during pregnancy, and unhealthy patterns of thinking contribute to mental health conditions.

Lesson 5.2 Treatment for Mental Health Conditions

- Treatment for mental health conditions include therapy, medication, or inpatient treatment. Therapists treat people with mental health conditions through individual therapy, family therapy, or support groups.
- Medications, in addition to therapy, can help treat specific mental health conditions. For example, antidepressants can help eliminate symptoms of depression and lithium can help control the extreme highs and lows of bipolar disorder. Some medications have side effects, so doctors regularly monitor patients on medications.
- People may choose not to seek help due to stigmas of the condition or cost of treatment.
- If you are concerned that someone you care about has a mental health condition, share your honest concerns with that person and offer to help him or her find treatment.

Lesson 5.3 Preventing Suicide

- *Suicide* describes when a person takes his or her own life. Sometimes, a mental health condition can lead to suicidal thoughts. Family and environmental factors such as financial hardship, abuse, or bullying may also lead a person to consider suicide.
- *Suicide contagion* describes how exposure to a suicide or suicide attempt may influence others to attempt suicide. A *suicide cluster* describes a series of suicides or suicide attempts that occur in a community in a relatively short time.
- Most people who attempt suicide show warning signs about their intentions. If you or someone you know experiences thoughts about suicide, talk to a trusted adult immediately. He or she can put you in touch with a trained mental health professional.
- Support groups can be helpful for survivors who often feel anger, guilt, or sadness over the loss of a loved one from suicide. It is important to let survivors grieve.

Check Your Knowledge ⤴

Record your answers to each of the following questions on a separate sheet of paper.

1. A mental or emotional condition so severe it interferes with daily functioning is called a(n) _____ _____.
2. List four common mood disorders.
3. **True or false.** People with seasonal affective disorder (SAD) face depression in the spring and summer when there is more natural sunlight.
4. How can a person overcome self-harm?
5. What are the three types of therapy available to help treat mental health conditions?
6. What is the difference between antidepressants and antipsychotics?
7. **True or false.** Inpatient treatment is necessary when people are at serious risk of harming themselves or others.
8. What could happen if a mental health condition remains untreated?
9. Are people whose biological parents have experienced depression at greater or lesser risk of developing depression themselves?
10. Suicide _____ is the term that describes how exposure to a suicide or suicide attempt may influence others to attempt suicide.
    - **A.** cluster
    - **B.** survivor
    - **C.** contagion
    - **D.** risk
11. **True or false.** Most people who attempt suicide rarely show warning signs about their intentions.
12. Give an example of a way someone could provide help for a survivor who loses a loved one to suicide.

Use Your Vocabulary ⤴

antidepressants	bipolar disorder	schizophrenia
antipsychotics	borderline personality	stigma
antisocial personality	disorder (BPD)	suicide
disorder	family therapy	suicide clusters
anxiety disorder	individual therapy	suicide contagion
attention deficit	inpatient treatment	support groups
hyperactivity disorder	major depression	survivors
(ADHD)	mental illness	therapist

13. In teams, create categories for the terms above. Then, classify as many of the terms as possible within the categories your team selected. Share your ideas with another team and discuss your categories.
14. Write each of the terms above on a separate sheet of paper. For each term, quickly write a word you think relates to the term. In small groups, exchange papers. Have each person in the group explain a term on the list. Take turns until all terms have complete explanations.

Think Critically

15. **Identify.** What are some reasons a middle school student may not seek help for a mental health condition? What can be a consequence of not receiving treatment?

16. **Draw conclusions.** How could having a mental health condition affect your physical and social health? Give a detailed answer and provide examples.

17. **Determine.** What would you do if you began experiencing depression, thoughts of self-harm, or suicidal thoughts? Identify someone you would talk to and what treatment you would seek.

18. **Compare and contrast.** Compare and contrast the following sets: experiencing mood swings and having a bipolar disorder; feeling anxious and having a generalized anxiety disorder; feeling scared and having a phobia; and being organized and having obsessive compulsive disorder. Why is it important that only a mental health professional diagnose someone with a mental health condition?

DEVELOP Your Skills

19. **Access information and technology skills.** Use reliable health-related Internet sources to research the potential symptoms of one of the mental health conditions discussed in this chapter. How might these symptoms interfere with a person's daily living? What local resources and treatment options are available in your community to support people with this condition? Create a brochure of your findings to share with the class.

20. **Analyze influences.** Analyze your favorite show or movie to determine how the media displays differences in mental health among fictional characters. Consider the following questions: Is everyone portrayed as happy? If a character has a mental health condition, is there a social stigma associated with this condition? Does your show or movie portray it as socially acceptable to have a mental health condition? How is the character with a mental health condition treated by others? Based on your analysis,

reflect on how the media shapes your view on mental health conditions. Present your findings to the class.

21. **Advocacy and teamwork skills.** With a partner or in a small group, create a poster to hang in the school to raise awareness of suicide. Consider providing information on the following: potential risk factors, warning signs, how to respond to someone who has thoughts of self-harm or suicide, different treatment options, available community resources, and other pertinent information. Do additional research as needed. With permission, hang the poster in a visible place in the school.

22. **Decision-making and communication skills.** Imagine your friend confides in you that he has considered self-harm and suicide, even though he has yet to do anything. Later, he laughs it off as a joke. Write a hypothetical dialogue explaining what you would do in this situation. What would you say to your friend? What would you do to help?

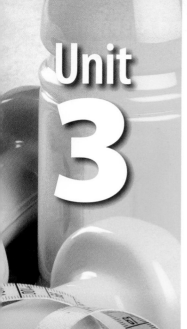

Unit 3

Nutrition and Physical Fitness

Chapter 6   Nutrition

Chapter 7   Physical Fitness

Warm-Up Activity

Setting Yourself Up for a Healthy Lifestyle

Often, the behaviors you begin today will carry into high school and adulthood. Gaining knowledge on healthy eating and personal fitness is the first step to setting yourself up for a healthy lifestyle.

Read the scenario below and decide if Caleb is setting himself up for a healthy life by making good nutritional choices and engaging in regular physical activity. Then, as a class, answer the discussion questions. When you finish reading the chapters in this unit, review the scenario and determine whether you would change any of your responses to the discussion questions.

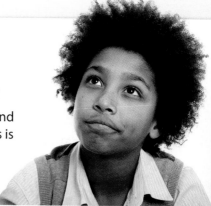

Djomas/Shutterstock.com

Scenario

Ever since Caleb was a baby, he was always a picky eater. As a 13-year-old, Caleb is still hesitant to try new foods. Breakfast is not an issue since Caleb is too busy and rushed in the morning to eat. By lunch, he is starving. School food is okay as long as it is pizza, a corn dog, or chicken nuggets. He will often order potatoes or corn as a side and chocolate milk. After school, he goes on a junk food or snacking frenzy. Caleb's parents work long hours, so dinner can be tough on the family. Luckily, they live three blocks from a burger joint. A cheeseburger, fries, and soda is Caleb's favorite meal there. He loves their milkshakes, but his parents rarely let him get them. To get their daily exercise, Caleb's family will walk to the restaurant and back. After dinner, it is often time for homework and bed.

Discussion Questions

1. Based on the information provided in the scenario about his current nutritional choices and exercise, is Caleb setting himself up for a healthy lifestyle?

2. What changes could Caleb make related to his nutritional choices in order to consume a well-balanced diet?

3. Is Caleb getting enough physical activity daily? If he is not, what changes would you recommend?

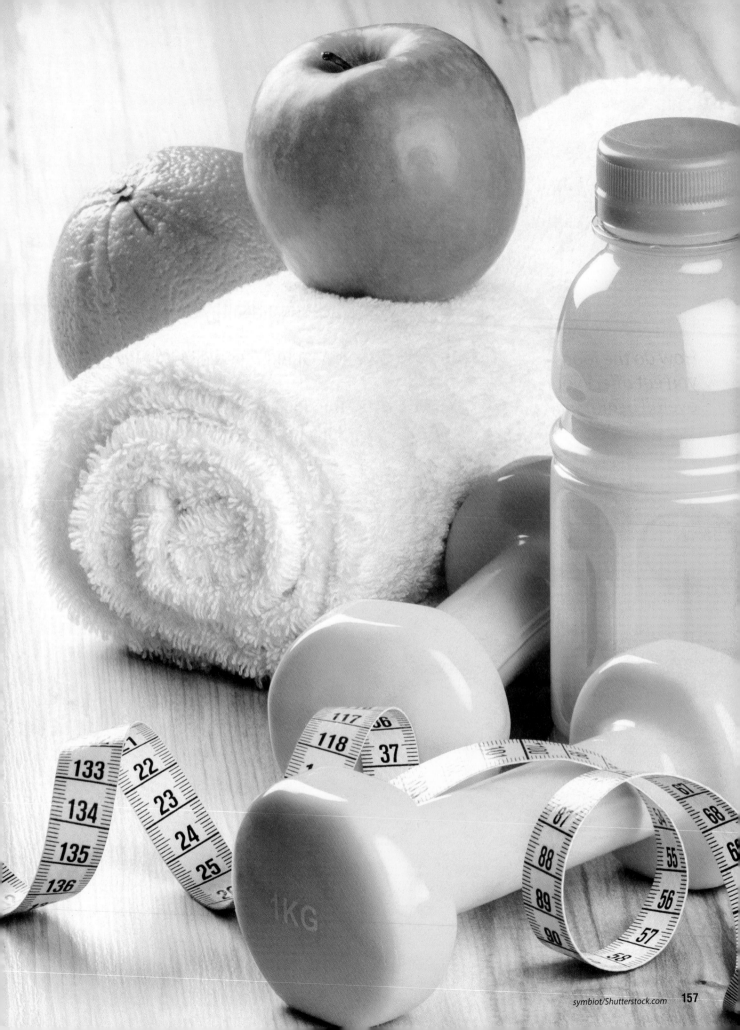

Chapter 6

Nutrition

Essential Question ?

How do the foods you eat affect your overall health?

Video ⤤
Access the Chapter 6 video to start thinking about chapter topics.

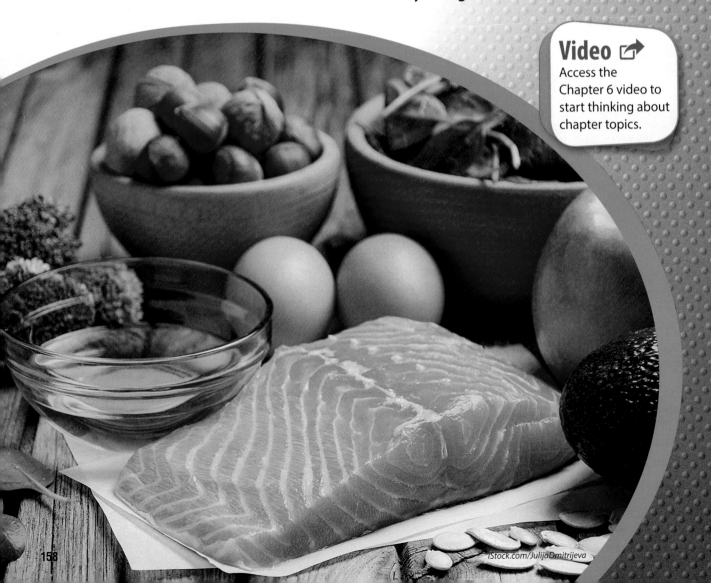

iStock.com/JulijaDmitrijeva

158

Reading Activity

Imagine you are a nutritionist and your client is using a crash diet to lose weight fast. Write a two-paragraph speech explaining your client's nutritional needs and advice for weight management and then deliver your speech to a partner. After reading this chapter, team up with your partner again to discuss what you would change about your speech based on any new information you have learned about nutrition.

How Healthy Are You?

In this chapter, you will be learning about nutrition. Before you begin reading the chapter, take the following quiz to assess your current nutrition habits.

Healthy Choices	Yes	No
Do you eat a nutritious breakfast every morning?		
Do you rarely drink soda or sugar-sweetened drinks?		
Do you eat multiple servings of fruits and vegetables every day?		
Do you rarely, if ever, have feelings of guilt or anxiety when you think about eating certain foods or certain amounts of foods?		
Do you get enough protein in your diet?		
Do you try to limit added sugars, saturated fats, and sodium in your diet?		
Do you drink 8½ to 11½ cups of water per day?		
Do you practice healthy, lifelong eating and physical activity habits?		
Do you stay away from fad diets as quick-fix weight-loss strategies?		
Are you able to identify distorted body image ideals portrayed in the media?		
Do you know about eating disorders and how to prevent them?		

Count your "Yes" and "No" responses. The more "Yes" responses you have, the more healthy nutrition habits you exhibit. Now, take a closer look at the questions with which you responded "No." How can you make these healthy habits part of your daily life? Think about how implementing these ideas can help improve your overall health.

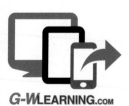

While studying this chapter, look for the activity icon to

- **practice** key terms with e-flash cards and matching activities.
- **reinforce** what you learn by completing graphic organizers, self-assessment quizzes, and review questions.
- **expand** knowledge with interactive activities and activities that extend learning.

Getting Enough Nutrients

Key Terms ☞

nutrients chemical substances that give your body what it needs to grow and function properly

carbohydrates major source of energy for the body; found in fruits, vegetables, grains, and milk products

dietary fiber tough complex carbohydrate that the body is unable to digest

protein nutrient the body uses to build and maintain all of its cells and tissues

fats type of nutrient largely made up of fatty acids, which provide a valuable source of energy

saturated fats type of fat found mainly in animal-based foods, such as meat and dairy products

unsaturated fats type of fat found in plant-based foods, such as vegetable oils, some peanut butters and margarines, olives, salad dressing, nuts, and seeds

trans fats type of fat found in foods from animals, such as cows and goats; used to be found in many processed foods, such as packaged cookies and chips

vitamins substances that come from plants or animals that are necessary for normal growth and development

minerals inorganic elements found in soil and water that the body needs in small quantities

Learning Outcomes

After studying this lesson, you will be able to

- **identify** the six types of nutrients.
- **explain** the role of each nutrient in the body.
- **identify** sources of each nutrient.
- **describe** the importance of water to good health.

Graphic Organizer ☞

Overlapping Nutrients

Most healthy foods are good sources of more than one nutrient. In the diagram below, list your favorite foods that are good sources of protein, carbohydrates, fats, minerals, or vitamins. Highlight the foods if they contain more than one nutrient. For example, a turkey sandwich on whole-grain bread is a good source of healthy protein and carbohydrates.

Hannamariah/Shutterstock.com

Protein	Carbs	Fats	Minerals	Vitamins

Rei is taller than most of the other girls and even some of the boys in seventh grade. During softball practice, her coach tells her that she throws as far as high school players. She also has not struggled yet with acne. Rei's dad says this is because of the healthy foods they eat as a family. Is Rei's dad correct? Do the foods and beverages they eat and drink affect these aspects of Rei's wellness? The answer to both questions is "yes."

Although you may not think much about the food choices you make, what you eat has a major impact on your overall health. This lesson examines *nutrition* (the processes by which you take in and use food). You will learn about different types of nutrients your body needs and how these nutrients help your body stay healthy.

Types of Nutrients

While it is enjoyable to eat a good meal or a tasty snack, food has a more fundamental role in people's lives. Food is the fuel that powers people's bodies. Food contains **nutrients**, which are chemical substances that give your body what it needs to grow and function properly. There are six general types of nutrients (**Figure 6.1**).

Some of these nutrients provide the energy your body needs to perform daily physical activities, such as playing sports and riding a bicycle. Your body also uses this energy to perform many important functions that go on within your body.

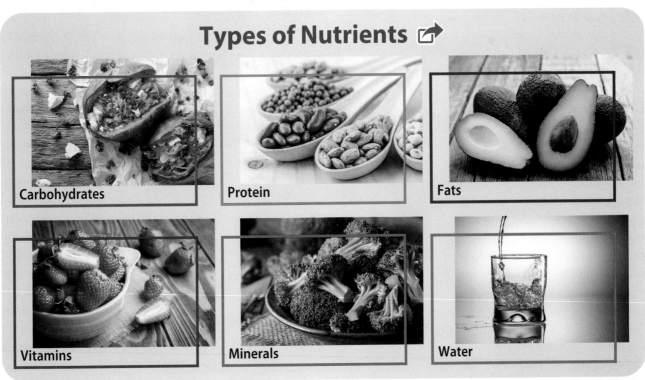

Types of Nutrients

Carbohydrates

Protein

Fats

Vitamins

Minerals

Water

Figure 6.1 You need to eat a variety of healthy foods to obtain all the nutrients your body needs.

For instance, your body has to maintain a stable body temperature. It needs to provide energy to the brain and nervous system. It also needs energy to build body tissues.

Other nutrients make it possible for your body to perform certain important functions. For example, your body needs vitamins and minerals to build new cells, strengthen bones, and carry oxygen through your blood. Nutrients also regulate basic processes in your body, such as breathing.

Carbohydrates

Carbohydrates, a major source of energy for the body, are found in fruits, vegetables, grains, and milk products. Carbohydrates are sugars and starches, and are either simple or complex (**Figure 6.2**).

Sugars are *simple carbohydrates*. These simple sugars occur naturally in some foods, including fruits and dairy products. Starches are *complex carbohydrates*. Products made from grains, such as bread, cereal, rice, and pasta, are rich sources of starch. Starch is also found in beans and in some types of vegetables, including potatoes, peas, and corn.

Figure 6.2
Simple carbohydrates are sugars, such as those found in fruit and milk. Complex carbohydrates are starches, such as those found in bread and potatoes. *What is the main function of carbohydrates in the body?*

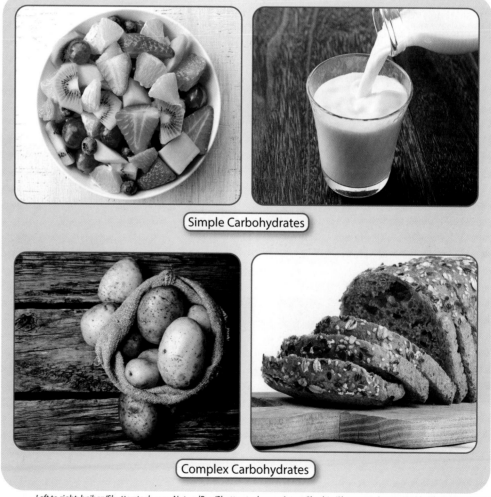

Simple Carbohydrates

Complex Carbohydrates

Dietary fiber is a tough complex carbohydrate that the body is unable to digest. This type of carbohydrate is found only in plant-based foods. Rich sources of dietary fiber include fruits, most vegetables, whole grains (such as whole-wheat bread or brown rice), and nuts.

Dietary fiber does not provide the body with energy. Still, it does have important health benefits, such as the following:

- **Lowers cholesterol.** Fiber attaches to cholesterol and carries it out of the body during digestion. *Cholesterol* is a type of fat made by the body that is also present in some foods. Having elevated levels of cholesterol in the body increases a person's risk of developing heart disease, high blood pressure, and stroke. A diet that includes enough dietary fiber can reduce the risk of these problems (**Figure 6.3**).

- **Balances level of glucose.** *Glucose* is the preferred source of energy for your brain and central nervous system. Glucose powers your brain, enabling you to concentrate and pay attention in class. By balancing the level of glucose in the blood, fiber can help control some types of diabetes.

- **Adds bulk to stools.** Fiber helps the digestive system work properly by adding bulk to stools. This can help prevent problems such as constipation (hard stools) and hemorrhoids. *Hemorrhoids* are swollen veins in the rectum that are caused by straining the muscles to pass hard stools. The condition can be painful.

- **Can prevent overeating.** High-fiber foods take longer to chew than many other types of foods. As a result, people eating a high-fiber meal are inclined to eat less than they would otherwise. Fiber also slows the movement of food out of your stomach and into your intestines. This prevents you from becoming hungry soon after eating.

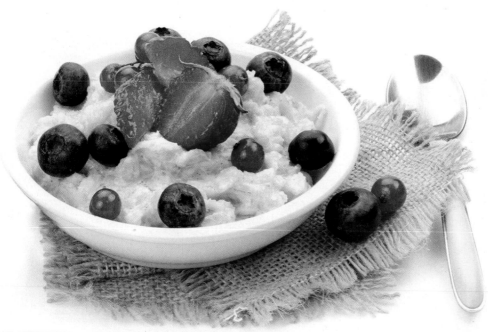

Figure 6.3
Oatmeal is an excellent source of fiber, and it is good for your heart health. You can boost the fiber content even more by adding berries or another fruit.

Vitalina Rybakova/Shutterstock.com

Protein

Protein is a nutrient the body uses to build and maintain all of its cells and tissues. Protein plays a very important role in the body (**Figure 6.4**).

Your body uses up and loses protein every day through many regular activities. For example, when you shower and brush your hair, you are actually losing protein. The shower washes some skin cells off your body. Some hair remains in the brush. Those skin cells and that hair contain protein.

Since you lose protein every day, you need to take in protein to replace it every day. Fortunately, in the United States, many foods that people eat on a regular basis contain protein. In fact, most Americans eat more protein than they need.

People who do not consume enough protein risk serious consequences. For example, the cells that help the body fight disease are made of protein. People who do not get enough protein are more likely to have weakened immune systems. This means they have an increased risk of developing infections and diseases.

Types of Protein

All proteins are made up of smaller chemical units called *amino acids*. Twenty different amino acids join in various combinations to make all types of protein. The body produces some of these amino acids, which are called *nonessential amino acids*. Other amino acids, however, are not produced in the body. You can only get them by eating particular foods. This type of amino acid is called an *essential amino acid* because it is essential that your diet includes it. Protein sources are divided into two types, depending on whether they include all of the essential amino acids (**Figure 6.5**).

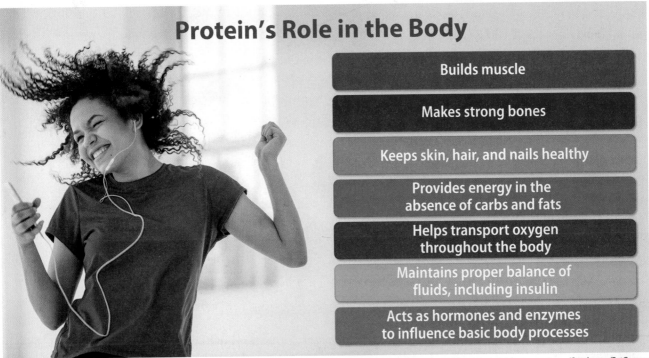

Protein's Role in the Body

- Builds muscle
- Makes strong bones
- Keeps skin, hair, and nails healthy
- Provides energy in the absence of carbs and fats
- Helps transport oxygen throughout the body
- Maintains proper balance of fluids, including insulin
- Acts as hormones and enzymes to influence basic body processes

iStock.com/FatCamera

Figure 6.4 Without protein, your body would not function properly.

Types of Protein Sources	
Complete Protein	**Incomplete Protein**
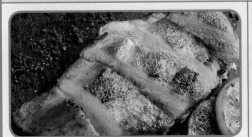 *koss13/Shutterstock.com*	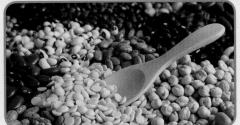 *Piyaset/Shutterstock.com*
Found in animal-based foods, such as meat, poultry, eggs, fish, and dairy products (milk and cheese).	Found in legumes (dry beans and peas), tofu, nuts and seeds, grains, some vegetables, and some fruits.

Figure 6.5
A complete protein contains all nine essential amino acids, while an incomplete protein lacks one or more of the essential amino acids. *Which type of amino acids does the body produce?*

Protein and Vegetarians

Some vegetarians avoid eating all (or most) foods from animal sources. This means they must rely on plant-based sources of protein to meet their need for protein. With knowledge and planning, a vegetarian diet can easily meet the recommended protein needs of adults and children. People who eat a vegetarian diet simply have to combine different types of foods that can work together to provide all of the essential amino acids.

For example, rice contains certain essential amino acids, though only low amounts. These same essential amino acids are found in greater amounts in dried beans. Similarly, dried beans contain less of other essential amino acids that are found in larger amounts in rice. By eating rice and beans together, a vegetarian can have adequate amounts of all the essential amino acids (**Figure 6.6**).

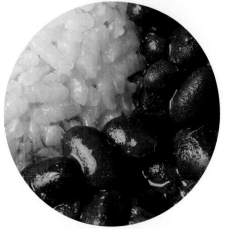
iStock.com/TiktaAlik

Figure 6.6
Eating two or more incomplete protein sources together will provide your body with all nine essential amino acids in a day. *What are some meals you eat that might combine two or more incomplete protein sources together?*

Fats

Fats are a type of nutrient largely made up of fatty acids, which provide a valuable source of energy. Fatty acids are a particularly important source of energy for muscles. Common fats in the diet include saturated fats, unsaturated fats, trans fats, and cholesterol.

Types of Fats

Saturated fats are found primarily in animal-based foods, such as meat and dairy products. Saturated fats are typically solid at room temperature.

Unsaturated fats are found in plant-based foods, such as vegetable oils, some peanut butters and margarines, olives, salad dressing, nuts, and seeds. Unsaturated fats are liquid at room temperature.

Trans fats used to be found in many processed foods, such as packaged cookies, chips, doughnuts, and crackers. Some trans fats occur naturally and are found in foods from animals, such as cows and goats.

Your body stores excess dietary fats present in the foods you eat as body fat. Despite the negative publicity that body fat gets, it is important to your body's health. Body fat has important functions, such as the following:

- supply energy to the body when food is unavailable
- act as a cushion to protect internal organs
- provide a layer of insulation to help maintain your body temperature so you do not get too hot or too cold

Fats in the Diet

Although fats are important for the body to function, some fats may be better for you than other fats. Saturated fats tend to be associated with higher levels of cholesterol in the blood. *Cholesterol* is a waxy, fatlike substance found in foods from animal sources. The body also produces cholesterol. Diets that are high in saturated fats may lead to long-term health problems (**Figure 6.7**). These problems may include heart disease, stroke, some types of cancer, and diabetes.

Some scientists believe trans fats pose major health risks as well. Many cities and states have passed laws that require restaurants to limit how much trans fat they use. In 2015, the United States Food and Drug Administration (FDA) declared that trans fats were not "generally recognized as safe." The FDA ordered food companies to remove artificial trans fats from their food products within three years.

Vitamins

Vitamins are substances that come from plants or animals that are necessary for normal growth and development. Different vitamins have different functions in the body.

Your body requires 13 different vitamins. Because your body cannot create these vitamins, you need to absorb them from the foods you eat. Unlike carbohydrates, protein, and fat, your body requires only very small amounts of vitamins. Eating a balanced diet that contains a variety of foods can easily provide you with the vitamins you need.

Figure 6.7
Replacing foods high in saturated fats with healthier options can help keep your heart healthy and your weight in check.

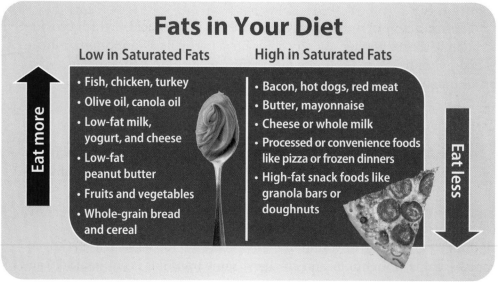

Fats in Your Diet

Low in Saturated Fats

Eat more

- Fish, chicken, turkey
- Olive oil, canola oil
- Low-fat milk, yogurt, and cheese
- Low-fat peanut butter
- Fruits and vegetables
- Whole-grain bread and cereal

High in Saturated Fats

Eat less

- Bacon, hot dogs, red meat
- Butter, mayonnaise
- Cheese or whole milk
- Processed or convenience foods like pizza or frozen dinners
- High-fat snack foods like granola bars or doughnuts

Vitamins can be divided into two distinct types—water-soluble and fat-soluble (**Figure 6.8**). *Water-soluble vitamins* dissolve in water. They pass into the bloodstream during digestion and are either used immediately by the body or are removed by the kidneys during urination. For this reason, people need these vitamins every day. The nine water-soluble vitamins are vitamin C and the B vitamins.

Fat-soluble vitamins are absorbed along with dietary fat and dissolve in the body's fats. They are stored in the body for later use. Because fat-soluble vitamins are stored for longer periods, they are not needed every day. In fact, consuming too much of them can cause serious problems. There are four fat-soluble vitamins—vitamins A, D, E, and K.

Types and Functions of Vitamins

Vitamin	Functions	Sources
Water-Soluble Vitamins		
Vitamin B$_1$ (Thiamin)	Helps change carbohydrates into energy	Pork, legumes, enriched or whole-grain products
Vitamin B$_2$ (Riboflavin)	Assists with metabolism	Milk, cheese, leafy vegetables, legumes, tomatoes, almonds
Vitamin B$_3$ (Niacin)	Promotes healthy skin and nerves; improves circulation	Eggs, lean meats, nuts, legumes, avocados, potatoes
Vitamin B$_5$ (Pantothenic acid)	Helps the body use nutrients for energy	Potatoes, sunflower seeds, cooked mushrooms, yogurt
Vitamin B$_6$ (Pyridoxine)	Helps generate energy from food; helps develop brain, nerves, and skin	Avocados, bananas, meats, nuts, poultry, whole grains
Vitamin B$_7$ (Biotin)	Assists in production of hormones and cholesterol; boosts metabolism	Milk, nuts, pork, egg yolks, chocolate
Vitamin B$_9$ (Folic acid)	Helps with cell division and growth; assists production of red blood cells	Leafy vegetables, fortified cereals, bread
Vitamin B$_{12}$ (Cyanocobalamin)	Maintains central nervous system and metabolism; helps form red blood cells	Meat, eggs, dairy products, poultry, shellfish
Vitamin C	Promotes healing within the body; helps maintain healthy teeth and gums	Citrus fruits, broccoli, cabbage, spinach, tomatoes
Fat-Soluble Vitamins		
Vitamin A	Fights infections; promotes bone health	Carrots, kale, broccoli, dairy, meats
Vitamin D	Helps absorb calcium for strong teeth and bones; regulates cell growth; reduces inflammation	Fish, egg yolks, fortified dairy products, cereals, sunlight
Vitamin E	Protects red blood cells from oxidation	Whole grains, leafy greens, nuts
Vitamin K	Assists with blood clotting	Liver, cereals, cabbage

Figure 6.8 Choose a variety of nutrient-rich foods to meet your daily requirements for vitamins. *When you spend time in the sun, which vitamin is your body absorbing?*

Minerals

Minerals are inorganic elements that are found in soil and water. Minerals are absorbed by plants from the soil and water. You then absorb minerals from the plants you eat, the water you drink, or from animal food sources that have absorbed the minerals. Your body needs minerals in small amounts to grow and develop normally.

As with vitamins, each mineral helps with different body processes (Figure 6.9). Eating a nutritious and balanced diet generally provides all of the minerals your body needs. Two very important minerals are iron and calcium.

Types and Functions of Minerals

Mineral	Functions	Sources
Major Minerals		
Calcium	Promotes muscle, heart, and digestive health; builds bone	Dairy, eggs, canned salmon or sardines, leafy vegetables, nuts, tofu
Chloride	Assists with balancing bodily fluids	Table salt
Magnesium	Contributes to bone health	Nuts, soybeans, spinach, tomatoes
Phosphorus	Assists energy processing	Red meat, dairy, fish, poultry, rice
Potassium	Assists heart function, muscle contraction, and digestive function	Legumes, potato skins, tomatoes, bananas, dry beans, whole grains
Sodium	Helps with blood pressure and bodily fluid balance	Table salt (sodium chloride), milk, spinach
Sulfur	Promotes metabolism and immune system function	Meats, fish, poultry, eggs, milk, legumes
Trace Minerals		
Chromium	Helps maintain normal glucose levels	Apples, bananas, spinach, green peppers
Copper	Assists metabolism and red blood cell formation	Shellfish, whole grains, beans, nuts, potatoes, dried fruits, cocoa
Fluoride	Prevents dental cavities; stimulates new bone formation	Fluoridated water, most seafood, tea, gelatin
Iodine	Assists thyroid hormone production	Table salt, some fish (cod, sea bass, haddock), dairy products
Iron	Carries oxygen from the lungs to the tissues	Red meat, leafy vegetables, fish, eggs, beans, whole grains
Manganese	Assists bone formation, metabolism, and wound healing	Nuts, legumes, seeds, whole grains, tea, leafy green vegetables
Molybdenum	Helps process proteins	Legumes, grains, leafy vegetables, nuts
Selenium	Protects cells from damage; regulates thyroid hormone action	Vegetables, fish, red meat, grains, eggs, chicken
Zinc	Assists immune, nervous, and reproductive system functions	Beef, pork, lamb, nuts, whole grains

Figure 6.9 Minerals are considered either major minerals or trace minerals. Your body needs major minerals in larger quantities than trace minerals. *Which minerals help build strong teeth and bones?*

The body needs *iron* so that blood cells can carry oxygen throughout the body. It needs *calcium* to build bones and teeth.

Water

Water is necessary for the body to work properly and be healthy. People can live for several weeks, and even months, without taking in any other type of nutrients. They can survive only a few days without water, however.

Your body loses water every day through urination, sweat, and even exhaling breath. For this reason, you need to take in water to replace what your body loses. Doing so prevents dehydration. *Dehydration* is a dangerous condition in which the body's tissues lose too much water. Without enough water, the body cannot cool itself.

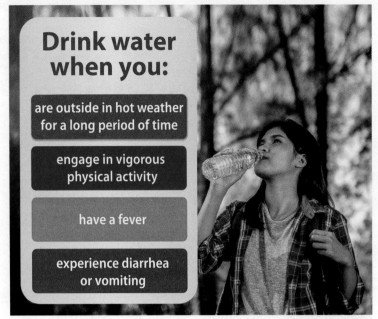

Sunti/Shutterstock.com

Figure 6.10 In certain situations, the normal amount of water may not be enough for the body to function properly. Being aware of these situations can help you maintain your health. *What is the name of the condition in which the body's tissues lose too much water?*

Individuals should drink 8½ to 11½ cups of fluids per day to have enough water in the body. Feeling thirsty is a signal that your body needs more water. Normally, most people can be sure to have enough water in their body simply by drinking when they are thirsty and when they are eating a meal. Some conditions, however, may require drinking more than normal amounts of water (**Figure 6.10**).

Lesson 6.1 Review

1. Sugars are _____ carbohydrates and starches are _____ carbohydrates.
2. **True or false.** Most Americans eat less protein than they should.
3. What are the four common fats found in the diet?
4. Individuals should drink _____ to _____ cups of fluids each day to have enough water in the body.
5. **Critical thinking.** What health benefits does dietary fiber provide your body?

Hands-On Activity

Create a poster (digitally or hand created) showing what each of the six main groups of nutrients do for the human body. For each nutrient, include an image of a healthy food that provides that nutrient.

Creating a Healthy Eating Plan

Key Terms 🔗

Dietary Guidelines United States government recommendations for forming patterns of eating that will promote health

nutrient-dense foods foods that are rich in needed nutrients and have little or no solid fats, added sugars, refined starches, and sodium

MyPlate food guidance system United States government system that helps people put the *Dietary Guidelines* into practice

undernutrition condition that results from people not receiving all the nutrients they need from the foods they eat

overnutrition condition that results from people eating too many foods that contain high amounts of added sugar, solid fat, sodium, refined carbohydrates, or too many calories

Learning Outcomes

After studying this lesson, you will be able to

- **explain** the key concepts from the *Dietary Guidelines for Americans*.
- **describe** what is meant by nutrient-dense foods.
- **demonstrate** how to use the MyPlate food guidance system to plan a healthy diet.
- **determine** steps to take to make healthy food choices.

Graphic Organizer 🔗

Food Benefits

Think about what you will be eating for lunch today. Fill in a MyPlate graphic organizer like the one below based on the ingredients of that meal. Do you have foods in every category? Are all your choices nutrient-dense foods? If not, use a different color pen to cross out any foods that are not nutrient dense. Note any foods you could add to or remove from the meal to ensure that it fulfills the nutrition guidelines.

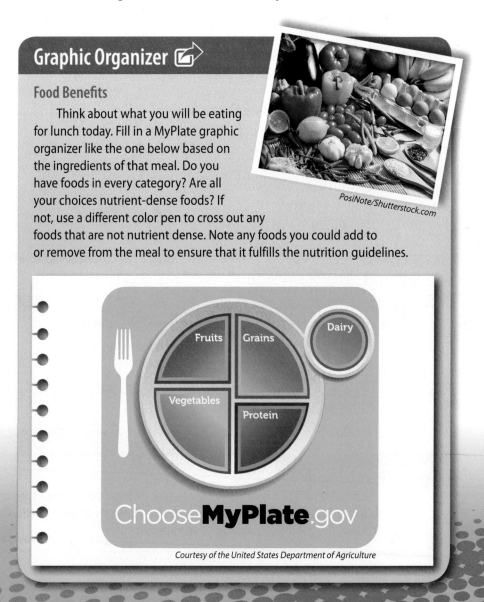

PosiNote/Shutterstock.com

Courtesy of the United States Department of Agriculture

When you eat nutritious foods today, you lower your risk of developing diseases later in life. People who follow a healthy eating plan, like Rei from the first lesson, and maintain a healthy body weight are less likely to develop serious illnesses. These may include heart disease, high blood pressure, diabetes, stroke, and cancer.

Eating a varied diet full of nutritious foods is important for maintaining good health. Rei helps her dad cook in the kitchen after school almost every day. She is learning what healthy foods to eat and what foods to avoid.

In this lesson, you will learn how to make smart food choices and how to create a balanced diet. You will also learn about the hazards of poor nutrition.

Guidelines for Healthy Eating

Each nutrient is important to having a healthy body. How do you know how to get enough of each nutrient in your diet? How do you know how to avoid eating too much?

The United States Departments of Agriculture (USDA) and Health and Human Services (HHS) publish the *Dietary Guidelines for Americans*. The USDA and HHS revise these guidelines every five years to make sure the guidelines reflect the most recent research. The *Dietary Guidelines* provides recommendations for forming patterns of eating that will promote health (**Figure 6.11**).

A healthy diet requires that the foods you choose are nutrient dense. The *Dietary Guidelines* defines **nutrient-dense foods** as foods that are rich in needed nutrients and have little or no solid fats, added sugars, refined starches, and sodium.

Figure 6.11
The *Dietary Guidelines* are based on nutrition principles that can help make and keep people healthy.

Key Concepts Promoted by the *Dietary Guidelines*

1. Follow a healthy eating pattern throughout your life.

2. Focus on the variety, nutrient density, and the amount of the foods you eat.

3. Limit how much added sugar, saturated fats, and sodium is in your food.

4. Shift to healthier food and beverage choices.

5. Support healthy patterns of eating for others you know.

The added sugars and solid fats found in some foods are called *empty calories*. These sugars and fats are called *empty calories* because they supply few, if any, nutrients to a person's diet.

Calories are a measure of the energy in a given amount of food. It is not bad to eat calories—as long as they come in nutrient-dense foods. Of course, even these good, healthy foods can be harmful to your health if you eat too much of them at a time.

MyPlate Food Guidance System

In 2011, the USDA created the **MyPlate food guidance system** to help people put the *Dietary Guidelines* into practice. The MyPlate graphic is designed to remind people about the proportion of different foods they should eat at a meal (**Figure 6.12**).

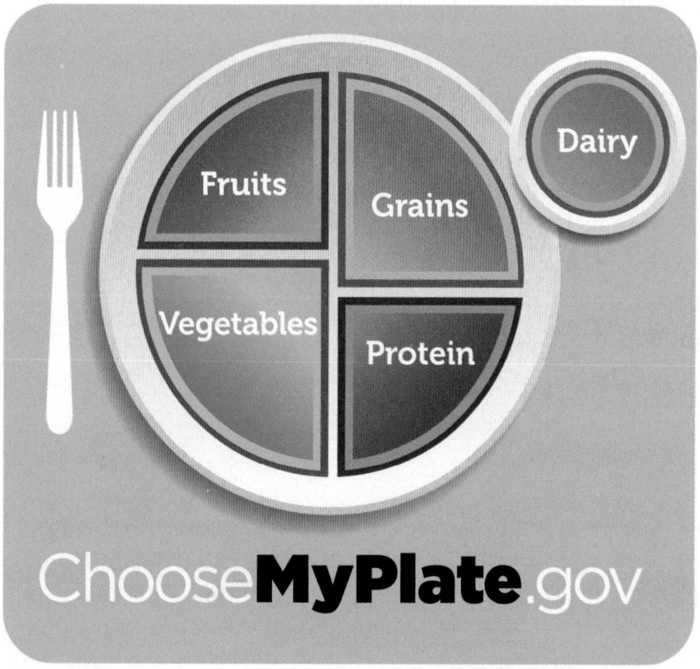

Courtesy of the United States Department of Agriculture

Figure 6.12 MyPlate illustrates the recommended proportions of the different food groups that people should eat in a day. *How does your daily diet align with these suggestions? What food groups should you eat more, or less, of?*

Food Groups

The MyPlate graphic includes the five food groups: fruits, vegetables, grains, protein foods, and dairy. Oils are not included on the MyPlate graphic because oils are not considered a food group. Oils are, however, a necessary part of a healthful diet.

Fruits

Foods in the fruits group are often good sources of fiber, vitamins, and minerals that many diets lack. These foods can be high in vitamin C and folic acid (a B vitamin). Some are rich in the mineral potassium. Fresh, frozen, canned, and dried fruits, as well as fruit juices, are included in this group.

Grains

The grains group includes foods made from wheat, rice, oats, cornmeal, barley, or other cereal grains. Grains provide carbohydrates, vitamins and minerals, and some amino acids. Foods in the grains group are either whole grains or refined grains.

Whole grains contain the entire grain kernel (**Figure 6.13**). *Refined grains* have been processed to produce a finer texture and improved shelf life, and no longer contain the whole kernel. Examples of whole grains are brown rice, oatmeal, whole-wheat bread, and wild rice. Examples of refined grains include couscous, crackers, and white bread.

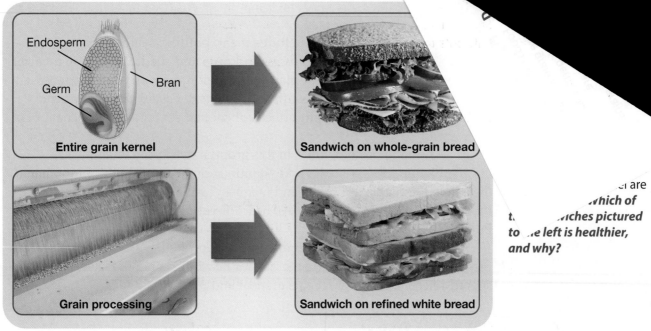

Left to right: Tefi/Shutterstock.com; Brent Hofacker/Shutterstock.com; Pavel Chagochkin/Shutterstock.com; aperturesound/Shutterstock.com

...are ...hich of t... ...ches pictured to ...e left is healthier, and why?

Vegetables

Most foods in the vegetables group are naturally low in fat and calories. They are important sources of many nutrients like potassium, fiber, folic acid, and vitamins A and C. Vegetables are often very nutrient dense. Vegetables may be fresh, frozen, canned, dried, raw, cooked, whole, cut up, or juiced.

Dairy

The dairy group includes many foods that are high in calcium. Examples of these foods are milk and milk products, such as cheese and yogurt. You should choose foods in this group that are low-fat or fat-free options (**Figure 6.14**). Dairy foods are often good sources of potassium and protein. Many are fortified with vitamin D, which helps the body use calcium.

Calcium-fortified coconut, soy, rice, almond, and cashew milks are included in the dairy group as options for people who are lactose intolerant. *Lactose* is a sugar found in cow's milk. Some people have difficulty digesting milk that has this sugar. In addition to calcium-fortified milk alternatives, people can drink lactose-free cow's milk.

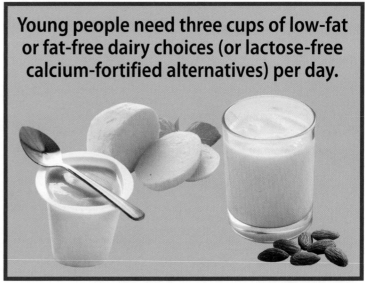

Young people need three cups of low-fat or fat-free dairy choices (or lactose-free calcium-fortified alternatives) per day.

Left to right: meaofoto/Shutterstock.com; Wichy/Shutterstock.com; Tanya Sid/Shutterstock.com

Figure 6.14 Dairy products such as fat-free yogurt, low-fat mozzarella cheese, and calcium-fortified almond milk are great choices to get the calcium you need without a high amount of saturated fats.

Protein Foods

The protein foods group includes meat, poultry, seafood, beans and peas, eggs, processed soy products, and nuts and seeds. Including a variety of protein foods in your meal plan each week improves your nutrient intake and supplies health benefits. The *Dietary Guidelines* recommend that you include at least eight ounces of cooked seafood in your meal plan each week.

In addition to protein, foods in this group may supply vitamins like niacin, thiamin, riboflavin, B_6, and vitamin E. Some foods in this group have the needed minerals iron, zinc, and magnesium. Some seafood contains fats that may work to reduce the risk of heart disease (**Figure 6.15**). Plant-based proteins are often rich in fiber.

Some animal-based proteins are high in saturated fats. As you have read, these substances may increase the risk for heart disease. For this reason, you should select lean or low-fat cuts of meat and poultry.

Oils

Oils are not considered a food group, but they do provide essential nutrients and must be included in your diet. Oils are naturally present in many plants and fish. The oil is often extracted from a food source and sold as liquid oil. These oils are then used for cooking or flavoring. For instance, olive oil is extracted from olives. Other examples are corn oil and canola oil. Avocados, nuts, and some fish are common sources of oils that are typically included in the diet.

Because they are unsaturated fats, oils are usually liquid at room temperature. Saturated fats, however, are not oils and come from animal sources. Saturated fats commonly found in the diet include butter, milk fat, beef fat, pork fat, and poultry fat. Saturated fat in the diet may contribute to such serious conditions as heart disease.

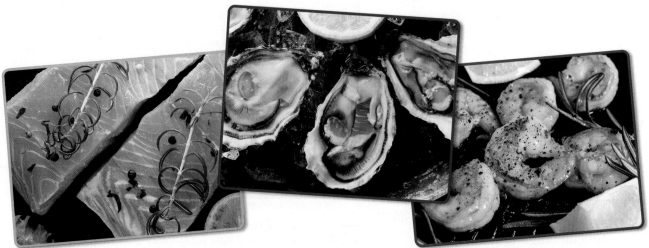

Left to right: Timolina/Shutterstock.com; Lisovskaya Natalia/Shutterstock.com; Tema_Kud/Shutterstock.com

Figure 6.15   According to the MyPlate guidelines, eating about eight ounces of seafood each week can help prevent heart disease. Some popular nutrient-dense seafood choices include salmon, oysters, and shrimp. *Do you get enough seafood in your diet each week?*

Recommended Amounts

The MyPlate food guidance system provides tools to help you develop a personalized daily checklist that shows what and how much you should be eating. This daily checklist outlines the amounts you should consume from each food group (**Figure 6.16**). It also provides information to help you choose nutrient-dense foods.

The amount of food you need from each of the food groups is affected by several factors. These factors include age, gender, height, weight, and level of physical activity.

Nutrition for Pregnant Women

Women who are pregnant have special nutritional needs. They have to meet these needs for their own health and for the health of the baby they are carrying.

Women who are pregnant or breast-feeding should avoid seafood that is high in mercury. Examples are shark, swordfish, tilefish, and King mackerel. They should also limit canned white tuna (albacore) to less than six ounces per week.

United States Department of Agriculture

ChooseMyPlate.gov

MyPlate Daily Checklist
Find Your Healthy Eating Style

Everything you eat and drink matters. Find your healthy eating style that reflect your preferences, culture, traditions, and budget—and maintain it for a lifetime! The right mix can help you be healthier now and into the future. The key is choosing a variety of foods and beverages from each food group—*and making sure that each choice is limited in saturated fat, sodium, and added sugars.* Start with small changes—**"MyWins"**—to make healthier choices you can enjoy.

Food Group Amounts for 2,200 Calories a Day

Fruits	Vegetables	Grains	Protein	Dairy
2 cups	3 cups	7 ounces	6 ounces	3 cups
Focus on whole fruits	**Vary your veggies**	**Make half your grains whole grains**	**Vary your protein routine**	**Move to low-fat or fat-free milk or yogurt**
Focus on whole fruits that are fresh, frozen, canned, or dried.	Choose a variety of colorful fresh, frozen, and canned vegetables—make sure to include dark green, red, and orange choices.	Find whole-grain foods by reading the Nutrition Facts label and ingredients list.	Mix up your protein foods to include seafood, beans and peas, unsalted nuts and seeds, soy products, eggs, and lean meats and poultry.	Choose fat-free milk, yogurt, and soy beverages (soy milk) to cut back on your saturated fat.

Limit

Drink and eat less sodium, saturated fat, and added sugars. Limit:
- Sodium to 2,200 milligrams a day.
- Saturated fat to 24 grams a day.
- Added sugars to 55 grams a day.

Be active your way: Children 6 to 17 years old should move at least 60 minutes every day.

Courtesy of the United States Department of Agriculture

Figure 6.16 Depending on your age, gender, height, and weight, the MyPlate Daily Checklist provides tips for getting the right amount of the best foods for your health.

Poor Nutrition

Healthy eating plans identify the amounts and types of food individuals should eat so they get the nutrients needed for good health. These plans help people avoid the problems that result from poor nutrition, or malnutrition. Poor nutrition can include both undernutrition and overnutrition (Figure 6.17).

Undernutrition

When people do not receive all the nutrients they need from the foods they eat, they experience **undernutrition**. This means that they take in too few nutrients for health and growth.

Healthy eating is especially important for children and teenagers. The bodies of children and teens undergo a large amount of growth and development. Children and teens need to be sure to get enough nutrients for that growth and development to be healthy. Children who do not receive enough nutrients may never reach their full height. Undernutrition can also lead to serious and even life-threatening problems. Examples are brain damage, impaired vision and blindness, and bones that do not form properly.

Overnutrition

Although many people think about poor health in terms of not getting *enough* nutrients, it can also be caused by eating *too much* of some nutrients. This type of **overnutrition** is often a result of eating too many foods that contain high amounts of added sugar, solid fat, sodium, refined carbohydrates, or simply too many calories.

Figure 6.17
Poor nutrition can involve not getting enough of the nutrients your body needs, or getting way more of certain nutrients than your body needs. *Why is good nutrition especially important for children and teenagers?*

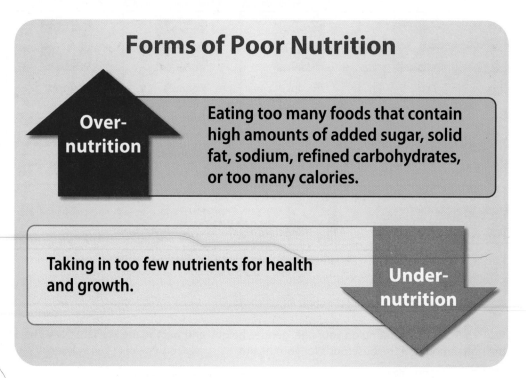

Forms of Poor Nutrition

Over-nutrition — Eating too many foods that contain high amounts of added sugar, solid fat, sodium, refined carbohydrates, or too many calories.

Taking in too few nutrients for health and growth.

Under-nutrition

Foods high in solid fats, added sugars, refined grains, and sodium are believed to be linked to a variety of health conditions. For instance, as the amount of sodium a person consumes goes down, so does his or her blood pressure. Maintaining a normal blood pressure reduces the risk of heart and kidney diseases.

Making Healthy Food Choices

There are many ways to be sure to make healthy food choices. These ways may include using the MyPlate system, choosing nutrient-dense foods, eating breakfast every day, and being aware of calories. Using nutrition information wisely and thinking about influences on food choices are also ways to make healthy food choices. Remember, you can also encourage others to make healthy food choices. Keeping food safe and preparing it in healthy ways also contribute to a healthy diet.

BUILDING Your Skills

Choosing Healthy Foods

Have you ever heard the saying, "You are what you eat?" Most of you probably have at one time or another. Do you think this statement is true? The answer is yes.

The foods you choose to eat are important and can have a great effect on your body. Foods nourish your body and help it function properly. Foods give you the energy you need to complete all of your daily activities. Foods can affect all aspects of physical and mental health. This is why the foods you choose to eat are so important to your overall health and wellness.

Many resources are available to help you learn how to make healthy food choices. The ChooseMyPlate website is one such resource. To start on the right path of making your own healthy food choices, you may want to begin by evaluating your current choices.

Evaluating Your Food Choices

For two days, keep track of all the foods, beverages, and amounts you eat. Record these foods, beverages, and amounts in a table similar to the one below. Then, answer the questions to help evaluate your food choices. Write a summary about what you learned. Explain how you can make healthier food choices.

1. Which of the foods you ate would be considered nutrient-dense foods?

2. How did your food choices compare with the MyPlate daily recommendations? Explain.

3. Did you make mostly healthy choices? In what areas do you need to improve?

Daily Food Choices Tracking Form		
Meal or Snack	**Day 1—Food/Beverage Amounts**	**Day 2—Food/Beverage Amounts**
Breakfast		
Morning snack		
Lunch		
Afternoon snack		
Dinner		
Evening snack		

Using the MyPlate System

Nutrition can seem complex and confusing to many people. Yet people need to eat several times a day to stay healthy. How can you make healthy choices given all the complexity?

The best place to start is by following the MyPlate guidance system. Follow these guidelines to eat a balanced diet of foods high in all the nutrients you need. Following these guidelines will also help you avoid eating too little or too much.

Choosing Nutrient-Dense Foods

Remember to choose nutrient-dense foods. The foods you eat should be high in carbohydrates, protein, vitamins, and minerals. While you need some fats in your diet, most people can generally get enough fat without adding it to foods. Avoid empty calories from added sugars and saturated fats (**Figure 6.18**). Following these guidelines is an easy way to make healthy food choices.

Eating Breakfast Every Day

Eating a healthy breakfast every day is very important. Children and teens need a morning meal to give them energy. Breakfast does more than provide energy for young people's bodies, however. It also helps children and teens learn and it helps their brains grow. Eating breakfast every day is especially important for youth who have difficulty getting enough nutrients.

Using Information Wisely

There is plenty of good information about the nutrients in foods that people can use to make healthy food choices. Packaged foods are required to have a Nutrition Facts label that shows the nutrients in each serving of the food.

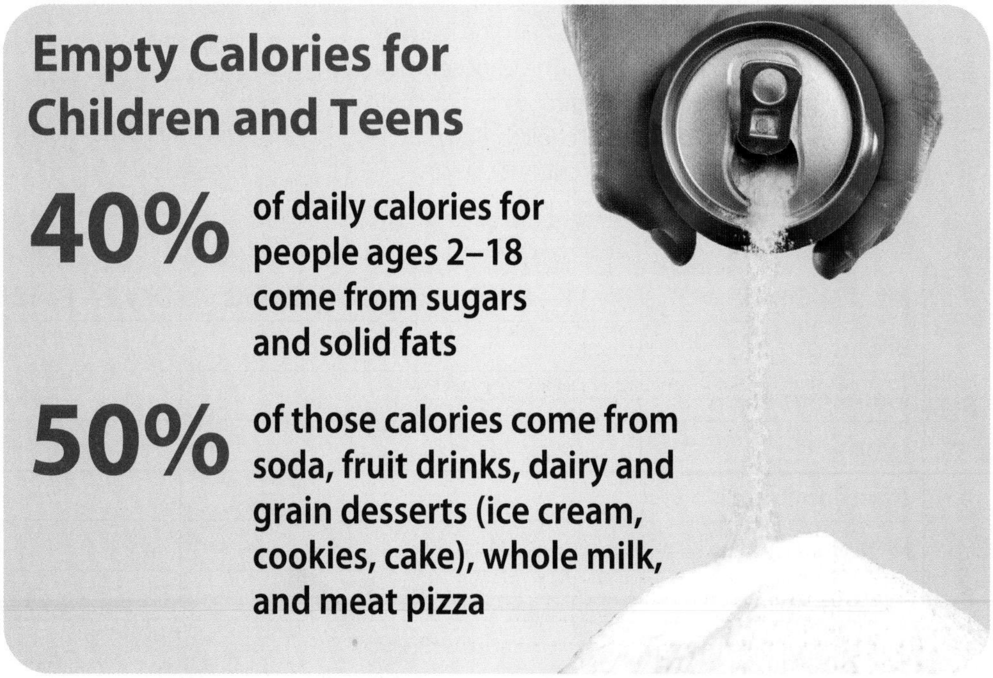

Figure 6.18
"Empty calories" come from foods that are high in added sugars and saturated fats and low in other nutrients like vitamins, minerals, protein, and carbohydrates.

Empty Calories for Children and Teens

40% of daily calories for people ages 2–18 come from sugars and solid fats

50% of those calories come from soda, fruit drinks, dairy and grain desserts (ice cream, cookies, cake), whole milk, and meat pizza

Marcos Mesa Sam Wordley/Shutterstock.com

This label also indicates how much of the recommended daily value of that nutrient is in the serving. People can use these labels to help choose nutrient-dense foods. The information on these labels is scientifically tested and proven. You can rely on it. **Figure 6.19** shows an example of a Nutrition Facts label.

Some of the information about nutrients in food is not reliable, however. You need to be sure that the nutrition information you use is valid or true. Some companies make false claims about popular diets or pills that provide vitamins and minerals. How can you tell if the claims are false? Use online sources to try to learn about the claim. Remember that websites from the domains *.gov* are very reliable. Websites from the domains *.org* and *.edu* are usually reliable as well, but some may have false information. Visit the website to see what its claims are based on. Look for other websites that comment on the claims to see what they have to say.

Thinking About Calories

Along with nutrients, health experts also look at the calories in food. Remember that calories show the food energy in a food. The number of calories a person should eat each day depends on three factors. These factors include gender, age, and level of physical activity. Generally, males need more calories than females and physically active people need more calories than those who are not active.

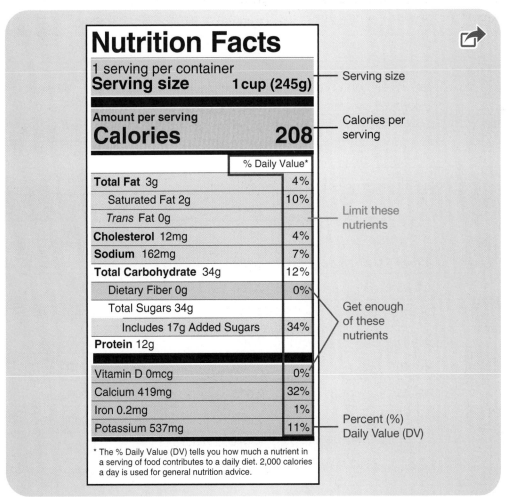

Figure 6.19
A Nutrition Facts label provides information about serving size, calories, nutrients, and how this food can fit into a person's daily eating plan.

Courtesy of the Food and Drug Administration

Adults between the ages of 19 and 30 typically need more calories than middle-aged and older adults need. In fact, adults ages 51 and over need the least number of calories. **Figure 6.20** shows the recommended daily calorie intake for males and females ages 10 through 65.

Healthy Eating Away from Home

You can also make healthy food choices when eating away from home. Start by getting information about the nutrients in restaurant food. Many popular chain restaurants publish information about the nutrients in their foods. People going out to eat can look up this information online. Armed with the facts, they can make healthy food choices.

Some companies that provide food for school lunches also provide nutrition information. You can use this information to make healthy choices. Remember to choose nutrient-dense food options in school.

Figure 6.20
The amount of calories a person needs to eat during a day depends on many factors, including age and gender. *What is the third factor that can impact how many calories a person should eat each day?*

Recommended Daily Calorie Intake		
	Male **Moderately Active**	**Female** **Moderately Active**
Age	**Calories**	
10	1,800	1,800
11	2,000	1,800
12	2,200	2,000
13	2,200	2,000
14	2,400	2,000
15	2,600	2,000
16	2,800	2,000
17	2,800	2,000
18	2,800	2,000
19–20	2,800	2,200
21–25	2,800	2,200
26–30	2,600	2,000
31–35	2,600	2,000
36–40	2,600	2,000
41–45	2,600	2,000
46–50	2,400	2,000
51–55	2,400	1,800
56–60	2,400	1,800
61–65	2,400	1,800

Influences on Food Choices

Making healthy food choices also involves being aware of influences on food choices. These influences can be internal or external.

Family is a major influence on food choices. Parents play an important role in helping children establish healthy eating habits. This helps a person maintain a healthy weight. Children who have a normal weight are less likely to become overweight as adults (**Figure 6.21**).

Media is another important influence on food choices. Commercials for restaurants and food companies aim to persuade people to buy their foods. To do so, they try to make them look as tasty and appealing as possible. These ads often say nothing about the nutritional value of the foods. They may completely ignore how many calories are in a dish. It is important to use other sources of valid information to check on these ads.

Peers have an effect on food choices, too. The foods your friends choose can influence you. Having solid knowledge and information about healthy food can help you resist the pressure to choose foods that are not nutrient-dense options. You can also encourage healthy food choices by others. One way is to model healthy food choices. When you choose nutrient-dense foods, you can influence your friends in a positive way. Another way is to speak to others about making healthy choices. Let friends know what you know about healthy eating habits.

Figure 6.21
A young person's home environment can greatly impact his or her nutrition habits as a child, and these habits often become lifelong habits.

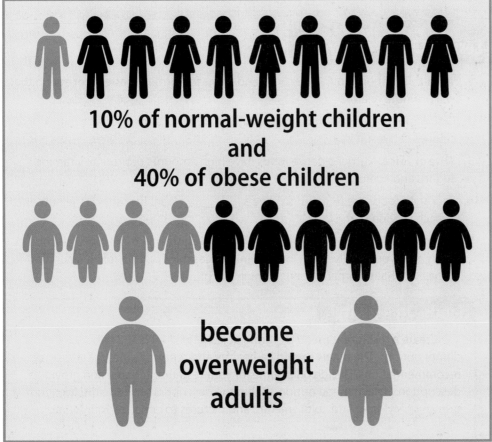

10% of normal-weight children
and
40% of obese children

become overweight adults

Sudowoodo/Shutterstock.com

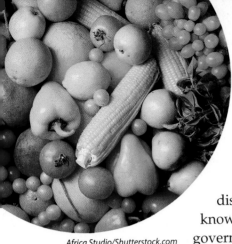

Africa Studio/Shutterstock.com

Figure 6.22
To select the best quality produce, look for brightly colored fruits and vegetables that have firm skins without bruises or cracks. *What is the term for disease-causing substances that can appear on food and make it spoil?*

Keeping Food Safe

Eating a healthy diet also calls for keeping food safe. Buying fresh fruits and vegetables rather than processed foods can give you more nutrients (**Figure 6.22**). Make sure that you eat those fresh foods before they spoil. By doing so, you will ensure that you get the full benefit of those nutrients.

Sometimes, contaminants can affect foods. *Contaminants* are disease-causing substances that can appear on food. When the government knows that a certain food product has been tainted by a contaminant, the government issues a warning. The food may be *recalled*, which means that anyone who purchased the product should return it to the seller.

Storing food properly helps keep food safe, too. Food in jars and cans can be stored in cabinets before the container is opened. Once the container is opened, however, the food needs to be refrigerated. Meat, fish, eggs, and dairy products should also be refrigerated. Frozen foods should be defrosted in the refrigerator, not left out on a table or counter. This will prevent bacteria from growing on foods as they thaw.

Preparing Healthy Food

Food needs to be prepared in healthy ways. Proteins should be cooked at high enough temperatures to kill bacteria present in the food. Avoid cooking foods in too much fat or adding too much sodium.

Lesson 6.2 Review

1. What publication provides recommendations for forming patterns of eating that will promote health?
2. Eating too many foods that contain high amounts of added sugar, sodium, or calories can result in _____.
3. **True or false.** Nutrient-dense foods have high amounts of protein, vitamins, sugars, and sodium.
4. Packaged foods are required to have a _____ _____ label that shows the nutrients in each serving of the food.
5. **Critical thinking.** Describe what healthy food choices you can make at a birthday party with your family. What internal influences might play a role in your food choices? What external influences might be present?

Hands-On Activity

Create a restaurant menu featuring at least two lunch and two dinner options. The meals should be healthy and represent the MyPlate recommendations. Decide on a name for your restaurant. Name and provide a description of each menu option. Within the description, include the five food groups of MyPlate. Add color, images, and pictures to enhance your menu.

Managing Your Weight

Learning Outcomes

After studying this lesson, you will be able to

- **describe** ways to determine healthy weight.
- **explain** the poor health results of being underweight, overweight, or obese.
- **identify** healthy weight-management strategies.
- **describe** unhealthy weight-loss strategies.
- **identify** healthy weight-gain strategies.

Graphic Organizer

Healthy Weight Management

As you read this lesson, use a table similar to the one below to list the strategies for healthy weight management. Then, write one or more summary statements that briefly describes the strategy. Put an asterisk next to the strategy or strategies you believe are most effective. Then, put a check mark next to those you would likely do. Think about other strategies you might use for healthy weight management and add them to your list. An example is provided for you.

iStock.com/Martinina

Strategies	Summary Statements
Think positively	Remember that permanent change takes time and that everyone has brief slip-ups.

Key Terms

body composition ratio of the various components—fat, bone, and muscle—that make up a person's body

body mass index (BMI) measure used to estimate whether a person is a healthy weight for his or her height

overweight having excess body weight from fat

obesity having a considerable excess of body weight from fat

underweight having less body fat than what is considered healthy

fad diets weight-loss plans that often forbid eating certain types of food groups and may require the purchase of special, and often costly, prepared meals

fasting not eating any food or drink except water for an entire day

Many Americans have difficulty controlling their weight. In recent years, rates of obesity in the United States doubled for adults and tripled for children. Approximately 17 percent of children and adolescents, from two to 19 years of age, are obese.

As you learn more about this topic, you will understand that weight management is a complex and sensitive issue. It is important to remember that all people deserve understanding, support, and respect (**Figure 6.23**).

Rei, from the previous lessons, sometimes wishes she weighed more than she actually does. She is much skinnier than her friends and other classmates. She wants to gain muscle like the professional softball players she watches on TV, but she is just too skinny. When Rei says this to her dad, he tells her that comparing her weight to her peers or to celebrities is a bad idea. He says that her ideal weight is the weight at which her body is healthy. She should not compare her weight to the weight of someone else.

Determining a Healthy Weight

Weight is discussed often and in many places. People share concerns about their own weight with family and friends. One friend may tease another friend about how much lunch he or she is eating and the impact that will have on his or her weight. Commercials promote low-calorie products and weight-loss plans. News reports warn of new studies about the health effects of being overweight. Doctors warn about the harmful effects of the latest fad diet. What is the truth? What weight is a healthy weight? How much does that vary from one person to another? What factors explain why it varies? What are the risks of being over or under that healthy weight? You will learn the answers to these questions as you read this lesson.

Figure 6.23
Remember to show respect for everyone you meet and to appreciate the differences among people.

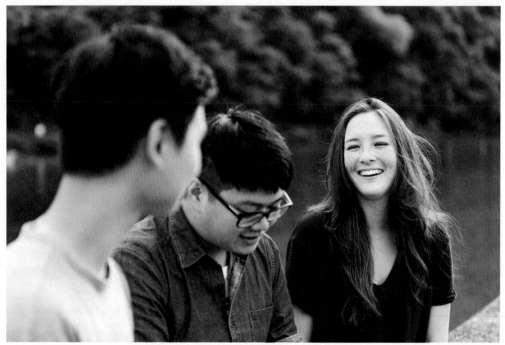

iStock.com/GCShutter

Weight and Body Composition

The factors that determine what you should weigh include your age, height, body composition, and gender. Weight is viewed differently for children and teens than it is for adults. The reason is that children and teens are still growing (**Figure 6.24**).

Body composition is the ratio of the various components—fat, bone, and muscle—that make up your body. The size and shape of two people who weigh the same, but differ in body composition, can be very different. To understand how that can be, imagine what one pound of metal looks like compared to one pound of plastic wrap. It should be easy to see that the plastic wrap will take up much more space than the metal. The same is true of people. A person who weighs 160 pounds and has a higher ratio of fat to bone and muscle will be larger than a 160-pound person with a lower ratio of fat to bone and muscle.

The reason for these differences is that muscle and bone weigh more than fat. A person may weigh more than someone else because he or she is more muscular, not because he or she is overweight. Athletes often train for long hours, which builds muscle and increases bone density. Therefore, it should not be a surprise that athletes often have considerably lower body-fat averages than nonathletes (**Figure 6.25**).

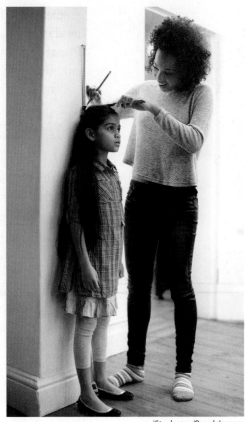

iStock.com/PeopleImages

Figure 6.24 As you grow and become taller, your healthy weight range naturally increases. ***What are the factors that determine what you should weigh?***

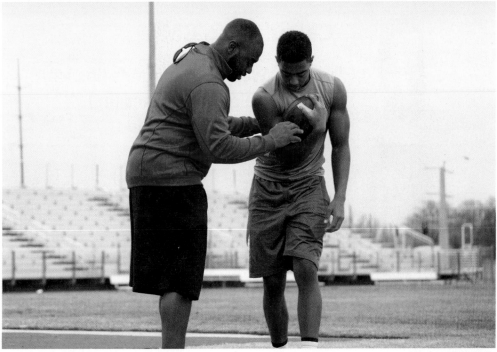

Figure 6.25 Athletes tend to have lower body-fat percentages than nonathletes due to their increased physical activity, muscle content, and bone density. ***What is the term for the ratio of fat, bone, and muscle that make up the body?***

iStock.com/digitalskillet

Gender affects body composition and body weight. Male bodies tend to have more muscle than those of females. Female bodies tend to have a greater proportion of fat. On average, adult males have a body-fat percentage of 15 percent and adult females have a body-fat percentage of 25 percent. Women have a higher percentage of body fat than men to support their role in reproduction.

BMI for Children and Teens

In recent years, experts have come to use body mass index (BMI) and other measures to assess body composition and fat distribution. **Body mass index (BMI)** is used to estimate whether or not a person is a healthy weight for his or her height. This index is calculated by dividing a person's weight in pounds by his or her height in inches squared and then multiplying the quotient by a factor of 703 (**Figure 6.26**).

BMI is calculated in the same way for children, teens, and adults. The resulting number, however, is interpreted differently for different age groups. This is true because children and teens are still growing. As a result, their BMI values are plotted on growth charts based on their age and gender. The BMI percentile for children and teens indicates the relative position of the person's BMI compared with others of the same gender and age. (See the *Appendix* in the back of this book to view the BMI charts for boys and girls.)

For children and teens, the Centers for Disease Control and Prevention (CDC) define **overweight** as having excess body weight from fat for a particular age, gender, and height. The CDC defines **obesity** as having a considerable excess of body weight from fat for a particular age, gender, and height. In simpler terms, to be overweight is to have moderately more body fat than recommended. To be obese is to have excessively more body fat than recommended. A person can also be **underweight**. This is the case if he or she has a weight that is lower than what is considered healthy.

Figure 6.26
The formula for calculating BMI can help indicate if you are within a healthy weight range for your age, gender, and height.

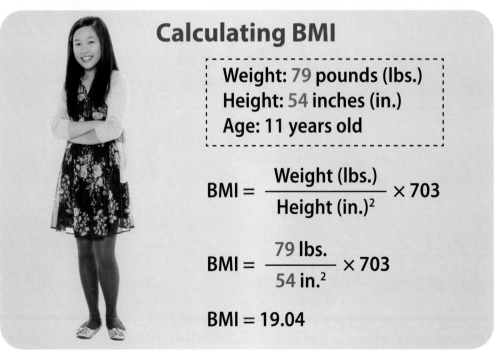

Calculating BMI

Weight: 79 pounds (lbs.)
Height: 54 inches (in.)
Age: 11 years old

$$BMI = \frac{Weight\ (lbs.)}{Height\ (in.)^2} \times 703$$

$$BMI = \frac{79\ lbs.}{54\ in.^2} \times 703$$

$$BMI = 19.04$$

iStock.com/JohnnyGreig

BMI Is a Range

Health experts do not identify one BMI measure as being the only healthy level for a person. For children, teens, and adults, healthy BMI is a range of BMIs. For children and teens, that range is based on weight, height, age, and gender (**Figure 6.27**).

The CDC compares each teen to all the teens who took part in a study that was carried out to determine healthy BMI. Teens whose weight is in the range of 5 to 85 percent of all others the same age and gender are at a healthy weight. A 12-year-old boy who is 5 feet tall can have a healthy weight ranging from 77 to 107 pounds.

A teen is underweight if his or her weight is in the lowest five percent of values for age and gender. Someone is overweight if his or her weight falls in the range of the highest 85 to 95 percent of those of the same age and gender. Someone is obese if his or her weight is in the highest five percent for the same age and gender.

Health Consequences of Underweight and Overweight

Regardless of how it is measured and assessed, a person's weight clearly has an impact on his or her health. Being underweight, overweight, or obese can cause a variety of health conditions. Weight control can affect a person both in the short term and in the long term.

Being Underweight and Your Health

Many more people in the United States are overweight than underweight. Some people, however, do struggle with being underweight.

Causes for being underweight include medical conditions such as cancer or alcohol or drug abuse. A person's genetic makeup can lead to being underweight. Psychological problems, such as depression or an eating disorder, can also be involved. The most common cause of being underweight, however, is a lack of access to food. Getting insufficient nutrients over time can result in poor health. **Figure 6.28** shows some of the health risks associated with being underweight.

Being Overweight and Your Health

Being overweight or obese raises the risk for several health issues. People who are overweight are at an increased risk of death, especially death caused by heart disease.

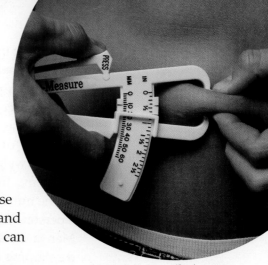

iStock.com/airet

Figure 6.27
It is important to seek the advice of a healthcare professional to provide a healthy weight range for children and teens since the interpretation of BMI depends on so many factors. A doctor may use measurement techniques such as the skinfold test shown above to determine BMI.

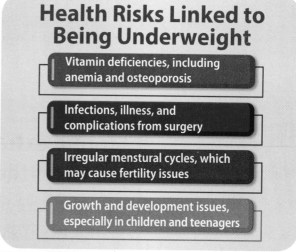

Health Risks Linked to Being Underweight

- Vitamin deficiencies, including anemia and osteoporosis
- Infections, illness, and complications from surgery
- Irregular menstural cycles, which may cause fertility issues
- Growth and development issues, especially in children and teenagers

Figure 6.28   One in five American children do not always have access to enough nutrients, which can result in becoming underweight. Being underweight can cause various health issues. *What is another potential cause of being underweight?*

One of the most common health conditions associated with obesity is type 2 diabetes. In this disorder, the body is unable to utilize blood glucose properly. About 5,000 children under age 20 develop type 2 diabetes each year. One in three children who were born in one recent year are likely to develop this disease at some time in their lives.

Being overweight is also associated with other health issues. People who are overweight and obese are more likely to have breathing, sleep, and joint problems. In addition, people who are overweight or obese may not receive all the nutrients needed for health. Interestingly, where weight is located on a person's body can help predict the physical consequences of overweight. Men and women who store extra fat around their waists are at greater risk of developing diabetes, hypertension, and heart disease than those who store extra fat in their lower bodies (**Figure 6.29**).

Strategies for Healthy Weight Management

Many people have unhealthy eating habits or are physically inactive. Healthy weight management requires a lifelong commitment to a healthy eating and physical activity plan. Several strategies can help people manage their weight. Bear in mind that making permanent changes requires patience and persistence.

Set and Reward Realistic Goals

One very good strategy for healthy weight management is to set realistic, short-term goals regarding eating and physical activity. For example, you might decide to do the following:

- stop snacking between meals
- eat an apple instead of chips as a mid-morning snack
- go for a walk with a friend instead of watching television after school

Figure 6.29
Where the body stores extra fat can be a risk factor for developing certain diseases.

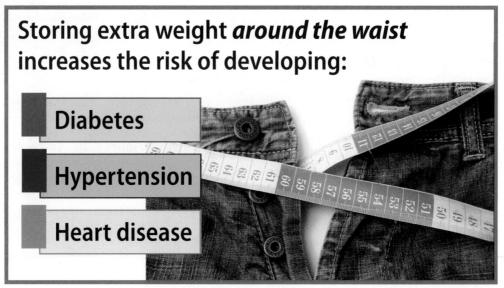

Storing extra weight *around the waist* increases the risk of developing:

Diabetes

Hypertension

Heart disease

Jorge Casais/Shutterstock.com

The Healthy Weight Journey

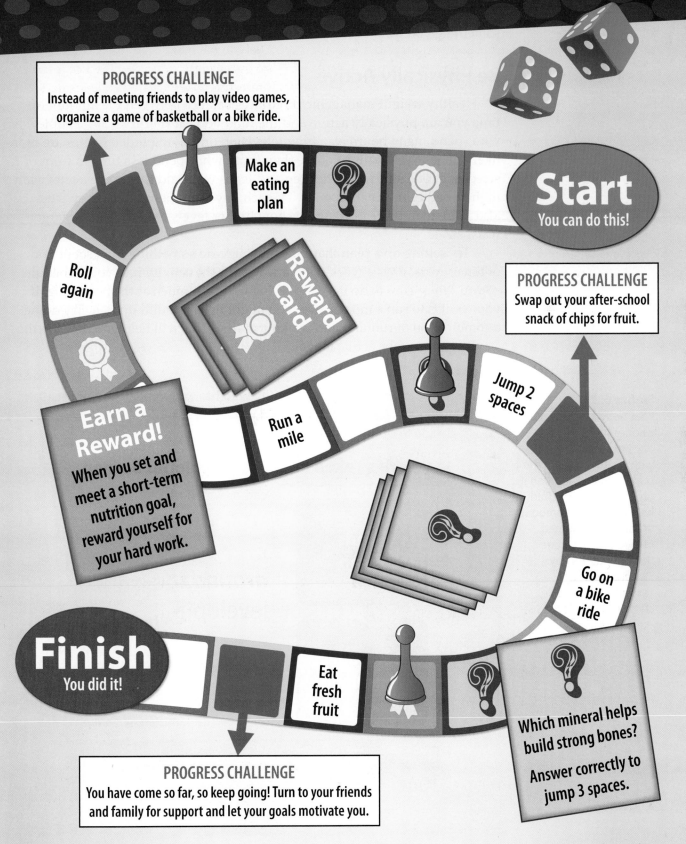

PROGRESS CHALLENGE
Instead of meeting friends to play video games, organize a game of basketball or a bike ride.

Make an eating plan

Start
You can do this!

Roll again

Reward Card

PROGRESS CHALLENGE
Swap out your after-school snack of chips for fruit.

Jump 2 spaces

Run a mile

Earn a Reward!
When you set and meet a short-term nutrition goal, reward yourself for your hard work.

Go on a bike ride

Finish
You did it!

Eat fresh fruit

Which mineral helps build strong bones?

Answer correctly to jump 3 spaces.

PROGRESS CHALLENGE
You have come so far, so keep going! Turn to your friends and family for support and let your goals motivate you.

Board game: EkaterinaP/Shutterstock.com; Pieces: JSlavy/Shutterstock.com; Dice: d-e-n-i-s/Shutterstock.com; Award: Classica2/Shutterstock.com

Setting and meeting short-term goals allows you to feel good about having some success. It inspires you to feel more confident that you can achieve your longer-term goal for overall health. Also, be sure to reward yourself for meeting your short-term goals. For example, after successfully running three miles or substituting water for soda for one month, reward yourself with something you want to do. Avoid using food as a reward.

Be Physically Active

Healthy weight management requires balance between the amount of time you are physically active and the food you eat (**Figure 6.30**). People who spend many hours watching television or playing video games are more likely to be overweight or obese than those who spend less time in front of screens. In one study, the children and teens who said they have a television in their bedroom watched more TV each day than their peers. They were also more than twice as likely to show higher levels of body fat and larger waist sizes.

Try setting up a plan that calls on you to do something for a set period of time several days a week. Find a way to fit the activity into your schedule so you can be sure to do it. Avoid trying to do too much at the beginning. If your goal is to run a mile or two, you might need to build up to it. Try doing a combination of running and walking at first. This will help you develop the staying power to be active longer.

Figure 6.30
Your body naturally burns calories throughout the day just by keeping up with the functions of the body systems. Additional physical activity should help balance the amount of calories consumed in food and beverages throughout the day.

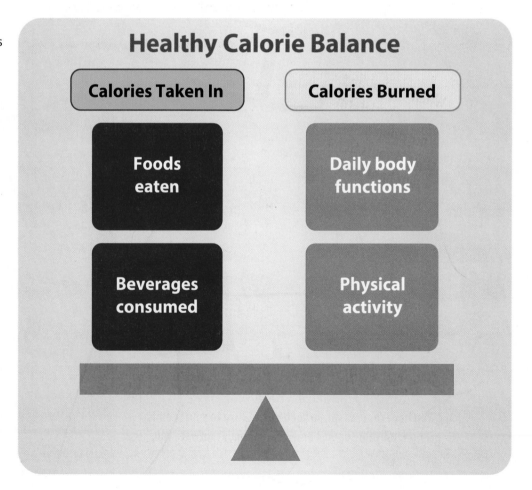

Healthy Calorie Balance

Calories Taken In — Foods eaten — Beverages consumed

Calories Burned — Daily body functions — Physical activity

What kind of physical activity is healthy? Any kind of activity is better than nothing. Simply choosing to walk or ride a bike instead of taking a bus to get somewhere will help. Choosing physical activities you enjoy is a good idea (**Figure 6.31**). Then, you are more likely to stay active.

Think Positively

Another way to reach your goal is to think positively about your healthy eating and physical activity plan. First, remember that making permanent changes takes time. Do not attempt to make too many changes all at once. Changing habits gradually is more likely to ensure the habits become permanent. Second, remember that everyone who is trying to create new eating and activity habits will have some slip-ups or lapses. The important thing is to keep these lapses brief. Return to the new habits you are trying to adopt as quickly as possible.

Enlist the Support of Friends and Family

Changing eating and physical activity behaviors can be difficult. Having support from those around you can help, though. Talk honestly with parents, other family members, and friends about your goals. Ask them for their support and encouragement. You can also ask people who have succeeded in changing their eating and physical activity patterns how they were successful. They might have some helpful suggestions for you.

Your plans are more likely to be effective if your parents are involved and supportive. The best results occur when parents change their own habits and provide healthier foods for their children (**Figure 6.32**).

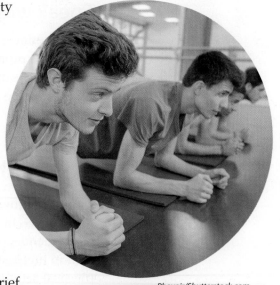

Phovoir/Shutterstock.com

Figure 6.31
Having a friend who will go to the gym or do other physical activities with you can help you stick to adding physical activity into your routine.

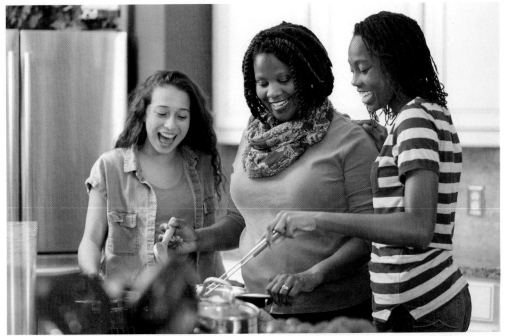

iStock.com/fstop123

Figure 6.32
To motivate changes in your family's eating habits and make sure that you are getting the nutrients you need, offer to help your parents cook.

Speak with a Healthcare Professional

Sometimes people struggle with weight management. Talking to a healthcare professional about the problem is always a good idea. These professionals can help you determine the strategy that is best for your health. They might be able to provide helpful advice on how to view your progress as time goes on.

Unhealthy Weight-Loss Strategies

Major growth spurts often occur during middle childhood. For this reason, weight-loss strategies that include calorie restriction generally are not recommended. In fact, these strategies may result in greater weight problems later in life. Instead, making healthy changes to eating patterns, increasing physical activity, and allowing your height to catch up to your weight are preferred.

Nonetheless, as many as 45 million adults in America diet each year. Americans spend a tremendous amount of money—an estimated $33 billion each year—on weight-loss programs and products. Unfortunately, these programs and products often promise more than they can deliver.

Many people try to lose weight using **fad diets**. These diets often forbid eating certain types of food groups, such as carbohydrates (**Figure 6.33**). They may also require the purchase of special, and often costly, prepared meals. Some so-called weight-loss experts even suggest fasting. **Fasting** means not eating any food or drink except water for an entire day.

The goal of most fad diets is to lose a lot of weight in a very short time. This is not a healthy approach to weight loss, however. First, these types of diets can result in the loss of muscle and gaps in meeting nutritional needs.

Figure 6.33
Restricting a food group does not enable your body to get all the nutrients it needs. Instead, make healthy choices from all food groups. *What is the term for a diet that restricts a certain food group?*

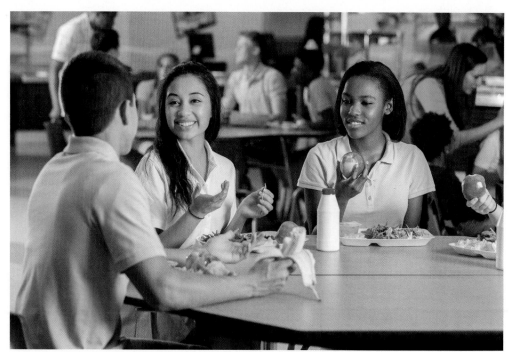

iStock.com/asiseeit

Both of those results are dangerous to a person's health. Second, any weight lost so quickly is almost always quickly regained. The reason for this is that the poor habits that led to the initial weight gain persist.

People may also try different types of drugs to help them lose weight. *Appetite suppressants* trick the body into believing that it is not hungry, or that the stomach is full. These drugs work by increasing levels of chemicals in the brain that affect mood and appetite. These quick-fix approaches are not healthy either. Dietary supplements do not require approval by the Food and Drug Administration, as do most other drugs. As a result, they can have harmful side effects.

Healthy Strategies for Gaining Weight

Some people are naturally thin, probably due to their genetic makeup and high rate of metabolism. It is possible to be very thin, but also healthy. It is also possible to be too thin, however.

Someone who a healthcare professional identifies as underweight needs to find healthy ways to gain weight. These strategies should focus not just on eating more food, but on eating more nutrient-dense food. This approach ensures that the added food can be used to help the body heal, build muscle, and strengthen bones. Foods that supply empty calories from added sugars and fats may add pounds, but will not benefit your health.

Lesson **6.3** Review

1. **True or false.** Fat weighs more than muscle and bone.
2. The healthy range of _____ for children and teens is based on height, age, and gender.
3. List three strategies for healthy weight management.
4. Strategies for healthy weight gain should include eating more _____ foods and fewer _____ calories.
5. **Critical thinking.** Describe the effectiveness of using fad diets to lose weight, especially in a short period of time. What effects do fad diets have on a person's health?

Hands-On Activity

Go to the KidsHealth website and click on the link for "Teens." Search for body mass index, and scroll through the article until you come to the *KidsHealth BMI Calculator.* Then, input the information requested to discover your BMI score. Be sure to print your results. What does this information tell you about yourself? Do you think this is an accurate indicator of your status in this area of health? Why or why not? Why does looking at BMI one time over the course of your teenage years not always provide accurate information in this area of health? What does a teen need to do in order to use BMI data appropriately?

Treating and Preventing Body Image Issues

Key Terms 📑

body image person's thoughts and feelings about how he or she looks

anabolic steroids artificial hormones used to treat certain types of muscular disorders that can have harmful side effects

eating disorder serious illness that causes major disturbances in a person's daily diet

anorexia nervosa eating disorder in which people have an intense fear of gaining weight and lose far more weight than is healthy

bulimia nervosa eating disorder in which a person has recurrent episodes of binge eating followed by purging

binge-eating disorder eating disorder characterized by people eating very large amounts of food with no control

Learning Outcomes

After studying this lesson, you will be able to

- **compare and contrast** positive and negative body image.
- **identify** several factors that can influence a person's body image.
- **describe** the symptoms of three eating disorders.
- **explain** approaches for treating eating disorders.

Graphic Organizer 📑

Self-Assessment

Everyone struggles with body image issues on some level. As you read this lesson, complete the sentences below on a separate sheet of paper.

Anna Tkach/Shutterstock.com

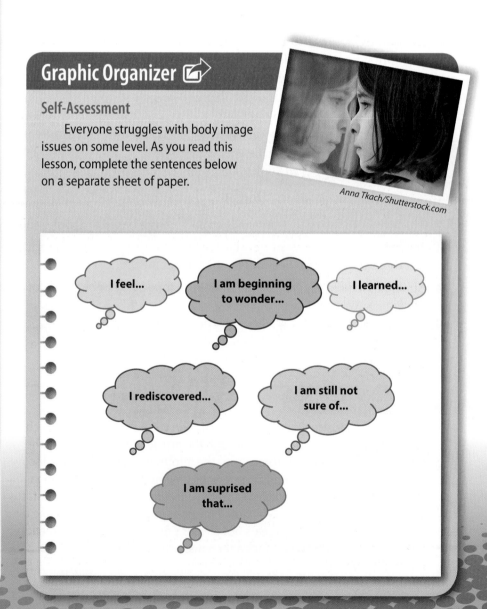

I feel...

I am beginning to wonder...

I learned...

I rediscovered...

I am still not sure of...

I am suprised that...

How do you feel about your body? Do you marvel at its strength and agility, which allow you to engage in many different types of physical activities? Do you appreciate the organs in your body that accomplish amazing feats? For example, did you know that your heart pumps about 2,000 gallons of your blood each day?

Many young people do not think about these facts when asked how they feel about their bodies. Consider Rei, from the other lessons. Instead of appreciating her body's functions, she thinks about how much weight she wants to gain. She worries about not having enough muscle. These types of feelings are common among adolescents whose bodies are changing rapidly in many ways. The thoughts and feelings people have about their bodies, however, can affect their physical and emotional health in powerful ways.

In this lesson, you will learn about body image and factors that can influence your body image. You will also learn about the prevention and treatment of eating disorders.

Body Image

Your thoughts and feelings about how you look make up your **body image**. Your body image does not describe what your body *actually* looks like. Your body image refers to how you *think* it looks (**Figure 6.34**). How your body actually looks and how you feel about it are not necessarily related. For example, someone who is fit and considered attractive by many people may dislike aspects of his or her body. If so, this person has a poor body image. On the contrary, someone whose body type is not considered ideal or attractive by many people may still feel good about his or her body. This person has a positive body image.

People who have a positive body image have an accurate perception of the shape and size of their bodies. They see the parts of their bodies as they truly are. They appreciate and value their bodies. They recognize that a person's physical appearance has no impact on his or her character, values, and worth.

iStock.com/ronstik

Figure 6.34 A person may think his or her body looks differently than it actually does. *What is the term for how you feel about your body and how you think it looks?*

Although men and boys can have poor body images, girls and women are more likely to have negative thoughts about their bodies. One reason for this is that girls and women are defined by their physical appearance more often than men and boys.

Female Body Image

Think quickly—who is the most attractive female television or film star? Whoever came to mind is almost certainly thin. Virtually all images of women in American media—including in movies, on television, in music videos, and on the covers of magazines—show very thin women.

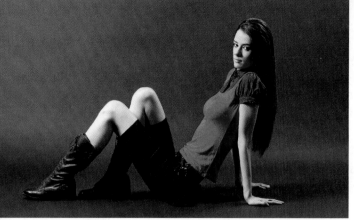

Popular media employs images of women who are consistently young and thin, promoting a standard of attractiveness against which women are measured (**Figure 6.35**). In one study, teen girls said their ideal body size was five feet seven inches tall and 100 pounds. These dimensions are both taller than the average woman (by more than 3 inches) and substantially lighter (by over 50 pounds). A person with these body dimensions would have a BMI of less than 16. People with this BMI meet the criteria for having a serious illness, as you will learn about later in this lesson.

iStock.com/adipelcz

Figure 6.35 Images such as the one shown above build an expectation of body shape and size for women that is not healthy.

Male Body Image

Like females, males are feeling increased pressure to meet an unrealistic body image. As images of women in the media have become increasingly thin, those of men have become more muscular. Many images in the media show men with muscled abdomens and chests and large biceps. Most male bodies do not look like this, but the bodies of male models, celebrities, and sports stars that appear in the media do.

The drive to achieve an unrealistically muscular figure has led some boys and men to take extreme measures, such as using *dietary supplements* and steroids to change their body shape and size (**Figure 6.36**). **Anabolic steroids** are artificial hormones used to treat certain types of muscular disorders. People also use anabolic steroids illegally to strengthen and increase the size of their muscles. (You will learn more about anabolic steroids in Chapter 10 of this text.)

Medical experts do not recommend the use of performance-enhancing or muscle-building drugs and supplements. These substances can cause both short- and long-term physical and psychological problems. In addition, some of these drugs are illegal and use of them can result in serious consequences.

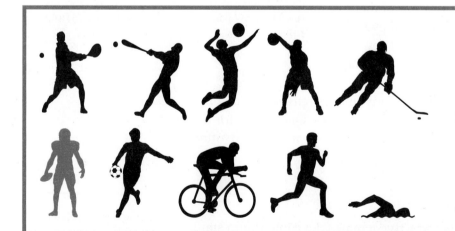

An estimated 1 in 10 male high school athletes has tried a dietary supplement. Nearly 1.6% of high school seniors have taken steroids.

Left to right: o_vishnevska/Shutterstock.com; Michal Sanca/Shutterstock.com; Miceking/Shutterstock.com

Figure 6.36 The increased pressure for boys and men to be overly muscular leads boys to use dangerous dietary supplements or steroids to change their body shape and size. *Give an example of a legal reason a person may use anabolic steroids.*

Influences on Body Image

People are not born with a body image. A person's body image develops over time and a number of factors influence it. These factors include family members, peers, the media, and ethnicity.

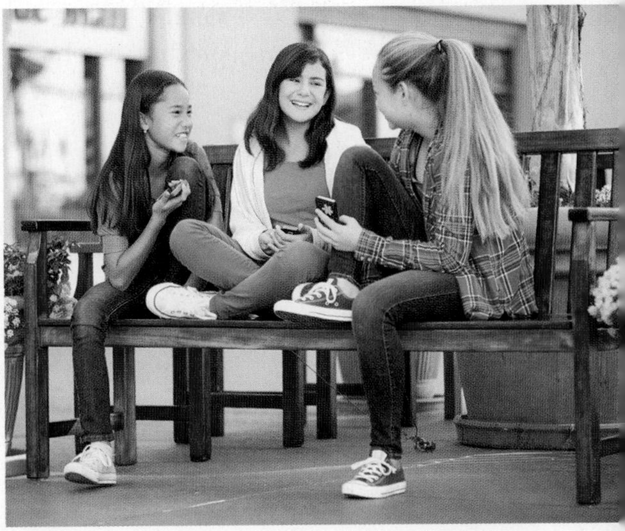

Family Members and Peers

Parents can influence a child's body image if they emphasize the importance of body weight and shape. Girls who believe their parents value being thin are more likely to be concerned about their weight. One study found that 40 percent of 9- and 10-year-old girls who were trying to lose weight by dieting were urged to do so by their mothers. These family pressures can lead to serious eating disorders.

Friends can also influence a teen's body image. To fit in with a peer group, teenagers may feel pressured to have a certain body shape or size (**Figure 6.37**). When teens worry that their bodies will not be attractive to potential dating partners, teens may feel extra pressure.

Unfortunately, teens sometimes make unhealthy choices when attempting to change their body shape or size. Girls may go on unhealthy crash diets. Likewise, boys may feel pressured to use steroids or other types of drugs to become more muscular. All teens feel self-conscious about their bodies at some time, and wish they could change some aspects of their appearance. This feeling usually goes away with time, and with age and greater self-confidence.

The Media

Every day, people are exposed to media messages communicating what is considered attractive in their culture. Ads for various products—such as shampoo, lipstick, and clothing—convey messages about what culture regards as attractive. People also regularly see images of celebrities, actors, and models. These figures and images can influence how people feel about their bodies (**Figure 6.38**).

The problem is that these standards are not appropriate. First, they are not based on what is *healthy*. Models, for instance, are often very thin. Second, the people being held up as standards base their careers on how they look. They spend a great deal of time working out—more time than many ordinary people can manage to devote to physical activity. Sometimes, advertisers will also digitally retouch photos to make a person appear more attractive. For example, wrinkles or body hair may be removed or teeth may be whitened.

iStock.com/bowdenimages

Figure 6.37 Teens who hang out with friends who have a similar body type—very thin or very muscular, for example—can feel pressured to conform to that body type.

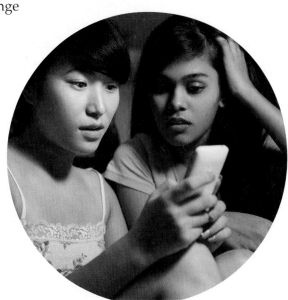

iStock.com/gawrav

Figure 6.38 Seeing highly edited, unrealistic, idealized images on social media can make young people develop negative feelings about their own bodies.

Finally, remember that ads are trying to sell something. They suggest that their product can help people look attractive. The product ad, however, may have nothing to do with attractiveness.

Ethnicity

Ethnic differences can shape body image, too. Some groups think people with larger bodies are more attractive than people who have thinner ones. As a result, a teen girl in that group may think she needs to add weight to be attractive. A girl from another group who is exactly the same size might think that she needs to lose weight to be attractive.

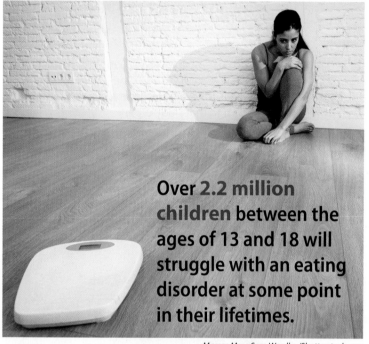

Over 2.2 million children between the ages of 13 and 18 will struggle with an eating disorder at some point in their lifetimes.

Marcos Mesa Sam Wordley/Shutterstock.com

Figure 6.39 Many people who struggle with eating disorders begin to develop these disorders during adolescence. *What are the three main types of eating disorders?*

Eating Disorders

An **eating disorder** is a serious illness that causes major disturbances in a person's daily diet. These disturbances can include eating only extremely small amounts of food, or eating huge quantities of food in a small amount of time. People with eating disorders often focus so much on their food and weight that they have difficulty paying attention to other areas of their lives.

Although eating disorders may develop during childhood or later in life, they often begin during the teen years (**Figure 6.39**). Eating disorders can result in many health problems. They can even lead to death. There are three main types of eating disorders: anorexia nervosa, bulimia nervosa, and binge-eating disorder.

Anorexia Nervosa

Anorexia nervosa is a disorder in which people have an intense fear of gaining weight, refuse to maintain a healthy weight, and practice ongoing, severe calorie restriction. People who have anorexia nervosa demonstrate symptoms such as the following:

- extreme thinness
- an unending drive to be thin
- intense fear of gaining weight
- distorted body image
- self-esteem that is heavily influenced by perceptions of body weight and shape
- denial of the seriousness of low body weight
- lack of menstruation among girls and women

The most obvious signs of anorexia nervosa are an extremely thin body and very little eating (**Figure 6.40**). A person with anorexia may also engage in eating rituals as a way to avoid eating. For example, he or she may also skip meals entirely or eat very small amounts of food, such as a single Cheerio for breakfast.

Bulimia Nervosa

Bulimia nervosa is an eating disorder in which a person has recurrent episodes of binge eating followed by purging. During binge eating, the person eats very large quantities of food in one sitting.

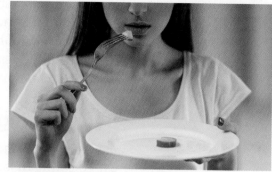

VGstockstudio/Shutterstock.com

Figure 6.40 Eating very little, cutting food into small portions, or eating slowly are signs that a person may be suffering from anorexia nervosa.

CASE STUDY

Asher's Quest—Losing to Win

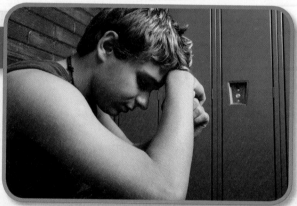

iStock.com/asiseeit

For as long as Asher could remember, he wanted to be part of the school wrestling program. His dad and grandpa had both wrestled and *won* at the local and state levels. His grandpa even participated on an Olympic wrestling team. Asher was glad to have finally made the middle school team this year.

Asher wanted to continue the tradition of "winning" for his family—but there was a problem. He weighed 117 pounds at the beginning of the school year. Asher knew he would have a better chance of winning in the 106-pound weight class (one of the official weight classes for his state). Ignoring the coach's instruction on good nutrition and drinking plenty of water for good hydration, Asher set out to lose weight.

He made up his mind to get to 106 pounds by the first meet in three weeks. Asher was eating fewer than 800 calories per day, and was drinking a lot less water than was good for him. He ran morning and night, and worked out in the weight room every day after school. Asher felt like he was always starving, but at the same time was feeling good and strong. He made his weight goal for the first meet and won.

Throughout the season, Asher kept up his weight-loss routine—he was afraid of gaining weight and not winning. When he looked at himself in the mirror, all he saw was excess fat and knew it had to go if he was to keep winning. It was such a fight to keep his weight down. In addition to eating less, Asher started using laxatives to lose weight, too.

About halfway through the season, Asher was tired all the time and his grades began to suffer—and he lost several matches. Others were noticing how thin he was, but it did not matter to him. Asher believed he needed to keep his weight down at all costs to be a winning wrestler. So, he kept up his routine of eating less and working out more, and spending even less time with his friends.

Thinking Critically

1. Analyze Asher's goal to lose weight for wrestling. Was this a realistic goal? Why or why not?

2. How did Asher's attitude toward weight loss change throughout the wrestling season? How did striving for his goal affect his life—physically, mentally, and socially?

3. Do you think it is possible that Asher is working himself into an eating disorder? Why or why not?

4. If you were Asher's friend, what would you do if you noticed these changes in him?

Purging refers to efforts people make to get rid of that food afterward. These efforts typically include forcing themselves to vomit or excessive exercise.

People with bulimia nervosa often have negative emotions. These feelings both lead to and result from their unhealthy behaviors. Often, a negative emotion, such as anxiety, tension, or sadness, will trigger a binge-purge episode.

Binge-Eating Disorder

The most common eating disorder is binge-eating disorder. **Binge-eating disorder** is characterized by people eating very large amounts of food with no control. The bingeing period typically lasts over a period of about two hours.

Binge-eating disorder has two key features. One key feature involves frequent periods of uncontrollable binge eating. The second key feature relates to feelings of extreme distress during or after bingeing. Unlike people with bulimia nervosa, people who have binge-eating disorder do not regularly try to get rid of the calories they ate. They do often feel guilt, disgust, and depression, however. They worry about what their destructive eating behavior is doing to their bodies. They feel terrible that they do not have the self-control to stop binge eating.

Prevention of Eating Disorders

Eating disorders are serious illnesses that have a negative effect on people's health. Fortunately, there are ways to help prevent eating disorders (**Figure 6.41**). Many communities and schools have programs to help prevent eating disorders.

Ways to Prevent Eating Disorders

Learn More

- Learn all you can about eating disorders to avoid mistaken attitudes about food, weight, or body shape.
- Avoid categorizing foods as "good" and "bad" or "safe" and "dangerous."
- Recognize that everyone needs to eat a balanced variety of foods for good nutrition.

Challenge the Ideal

- Question the false belief that only being thin or muscular is desirable.
- Remember that body fat and weight gain do not indicate worthlessness or laziness.
- Discourage the idea that a particular body shape or size will lead to happiness.
- Avoid judging others and yourself based on body shape or weight.

Assess Your Values

- Value yourself based on your accomplishments, talents, and character.
- Do not let the way you feel about your body determine the course of your day.
- If you think someone has an eating disorder, express your concerns and gently encourage the person to seek professional help.

Figure 6.41 Addressing different mindsets that help contribute to the development of eating disorders is a primary goal of preventing eating disorders.

Eating Disorders by the Numbers

30 million
Americans of all ages suffer from an eating disorder

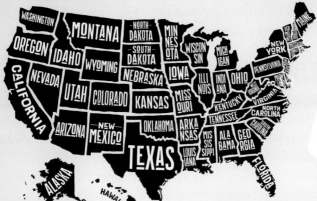

35–57%
of adolescent girls have engaged in unhealthy eating behaviors in an attempt to modify their weight

Only **4** out of **20** adolescents suffering from eating disorders seek treatment

80%
of 10-year-olds are afraid of being fat

Every **62** minutes,
at least one person dies as a direct result of an eating disorder

Top to bottom: MJgraphics/Shutterstock.com; Forest Foxy/Shutterstock.com; Okuneva/Shutterstock.com; estudio Maia/Shutterstock.com; h0lyland/Shutterstock.com

These programs arm people with the knowledge about the dangers of eating disorders. Many programs teach strategies for engaging in healthy eating and physical activity behaviors. People also learn about various factors that influence eating, such as their moods, other people around them, and portion sizes. Through these programs, people learn how to make healthy food and physical activity choices.

Another effective approach for preventing eating disorders is learning to critique media images of women. As described earlier in this lesson, thin images of women in the media can contribute to the development of eating disorders. In turn, programs which help people learn that this thin ideal is unhealthy and may be falsely created through photo-editing techniques can help prevent disordered eating.

Treatment of Eating Disorders

Many people with eating disorders are embarrassed to admit their behavior. They may believe that their disorders will go away without treatment. Some of these people are afraid that treating their disorder will cause them to gain weight.

Eating disorders rarely go away without proper treatment, so it is important for people struggling with these disorders to get professional help. By getting help, they can feel better about themselves. They can also avoid serious, long-term health consequences of the disorder. Eating disorders are mental disorders. Therefore, mental health professionals should treat these disorders.

Lesson 6.4 Review

1. **True or false.** How your body actually looks and what you think your body looks like are always related.

2. What type of disorders can result from family pressure to have a certain body weight and shape?

3. The eating disorder in which people have an intense fear of gaining weight and practice ongoing, severe calorie restriction is called _____ _____.

4. What is the most common eating disorder?

5. **Critical thinking.** Name one male and one female celebrity that are widely considered to be attractive. What influence can seeing these people in the media have on a young person's body image?

Hands-On Activity

Take and print (or draw) a selfie that you really like. Use that picture to create a "self-poster" that includes a word cloud identifying aspects you like about yourself (physically, socially, and mentally). Also, include all the factors that influence your body image. What do you notice about the words you chose? What conclusions can you draw about your body image and self-esteem? Do you need to improve? If needed, what could you say to yourself and/or choose to do to improve your self-esteem and body image?

Review and Assessment

Summary

Lesson 6.1 Getting Enough Nutrients

- Nutrients allow your body to grow and function properly. These include carbohydrates, fats, proteins, minerals, vitamins, and water.
- Carbohydrates are the body's major source of energy. Protein helps build muscles, bones, skin, hair, fingernails, and organs. Fats provide a valuable source of energy.
- Vitamins are necessary for normal growth and development. Minerals are consumed through the plants and animal products you eat and the water you drink.
- You can survive for weeks without other nutrients, but only a few days without water.

Lesson 6.2 Creating a Healthy Eating Plan

- The *Dietary Guidelines for Americans* recommend eating patterns that promote health. Using the MyPlate food guidance system helps people put the guidelines into practice. This system outlines how much you should consume from each food group: fruits, vegetables, grains, protein, and dairy. Although oils are not a food group, they are an important part of a nutritious diet.
- *Undernutrition* involves taking in too few nutrients for health and growth. *Overnutrition* often involves eating too many foods with a high content of sugar, solid fat, sodium, carbohydrates, or calories.
- Healthy food choices can include using the MyPlate system, choosing nutrient-dense foods, using nutrition information wisely, being aware of internal and external influences, keeping food safe, and preparing food in a healthy way.

Lesson 6.3 Managing Your Weight

- Your age, height, body composition, and gender all impact what you should weigh. *Body composition* is the ratio of fat, bone, and muscle in your body.
- *Body mass index (BMI)* estimates how healthy a person's weight is for his or her height. A person who has less body fat than recommended is *underweight*. A person who has moderately more body fat than recommended is *overweight*, and excessively more is *obese*.
- Healthy weight management methods include setting and rewarding realistic goals, physical activity, and enlisting the support of family and friends. Weight loss strategies including fad diets, fasting, and appetite suppressants can be dangerous to your health.

Lesson 6.4 Treating and Preventing Body Image Issues

- The media often portrays women as very thin and men as very muscular. Unrealistic standards such as these often impact a person's *body image* (thoughts and feelings about how they look). Other factors that can affect a person's body image may include family members, peers, and ethnicity.
- An eating disorder is a serious illness that causes major disturbances in a person's daily diet. This can include anorexia nervosa, bulimia nervosa, and binge-eating disorder. Eating disorders rarely go away without professional help.

Check Your Knowledge ⤇

Record your answers to each of the following questions on a separate sheet of paper.

1. Name the six general types of nutrients.
2. **True or false.** Vegetarians must get the protein they need by eating foods from animal sources.
3. How many different vitamins does the body require through diet?
4. ____ foods are rich in nutrients and have little added sugars, starches, and sodium.
5. **True or false.** The five food groups included in the MyPlate food guidance system are protein, carbohydrates, fats, vitamins, and minerals.
6. Storing fresh foods at the appropriate temperatures can keep disease-causing substances called ____ from affecting the foods.
7. What are the three main components that make up body composition?
8. **True or false.** BMI is calculated and interpreted in the same way for each age group.
9. People who are overweight are at an increased risk for which of the following health conditions?
   A. Type 2 diabetes.
   B. Hearing loss.
   C. Liver damage.
   D. Lung cancer.
10. ____ ____ are artificial hormones sometimes used illegally to increase the strength and size of muscles.
11. **True or false.** Anorexia nervosa involves eating only extremely small amounts of food.
12. What are the two parts of a bulimia nervosa episode?

Use Your Vocabulary ⤇

anabolic steroids	eating disorder	overnutrition
anorexia nervosa	fad diets	overweight
binge-eating disorder	fasting	protein
body composition	fats	saturated fats
body image	minerals	trans fats
body mass index (BMI)	MyPlate food guidance	undernutrition
bulimia nervosa	system	underweight
carbohydrates	nutrient-dense foods	unsaturated fats
dietary fiber	nutrients	vitamins
Dietary Guidelines	obesity	

13. Working in pairs, locate a small image online that visually describes each of the terms above. Create flash cards by writing each term on a note card and pasting the image on the opposite side.
14. Write the definition for each of the terms above in your own words. Then, read the text passages in this lesson. Double-check your definitions by using the text glossary.

Think Critically

15. **Evaluate.** How do you make decisions about what to eat each day? What internal and external influences have the strongest impact on your decisions?

16. **Make inferences.** What impact does a person's food choices and nutrition status have on that person's academics, activities, social life, and mental health?

17. **Cause and effect.** Does social media usage cause issues with body image? Why or why not?

18. **Assess.** What personality characteristics and social skills do you possess? Do you need to improve to increase acceptance of all body types?

DEVELOP Your Skills

19. **Leadership and advocacy skills.** Examine the lunch offerings in your school cafeteria and look at what young people typically choose to eat. Compare the food options presented and those that young people choose with the *Dietary Guidelines*. Create a new menu that meets the Guidelines and that young people will actually eat. Use the resources on www.choosemyplate.gov to help create your menu plan, such as the "Healthy Eating on a Budget" resources for planning weekly meals and making a grocery list.

20. **Communication, teamwork, conflict resolution skills.** With your family's grocery shopper, discuss what you have learned about nutrition and your family's meals. Then, help plan your family's meals for a week (you can use the meal-planning resources on www.choosemyplate.gov). Create a grocery list that includes healthier foods that you and your family will actually eat for a week. Share this list with your family's grocery shopper and discuss any issues with purchasing these foods. If there are barriers to getting everything on your list, communicate with the shopper to figure out low-cost, healthy solutions that work for everyone. Once you have a grocery list that you are both happy with, help with the shopping and enjoy the food all week.

21. **Advocacy and literacy skills.** Write a children's book to promote healthy eating and healthy body image. Include accurate information. Make it interesting with a kid-friendly story line and illustrations. Submit your book to your teacher for review. Make any changes needed for accuracy. Then, with their parent's permission, share your story with children you may know.

22. **Goal-setting skills.** Write a personal plan to improve your nutrition and/or body image. Be sure to include your overall goal and the small steps you will take to achieve it. Also, consider obstacles that may hinder your progress or success, and develop a plan to overcome them.

Chapter 7

Physical Fitness

Essential Question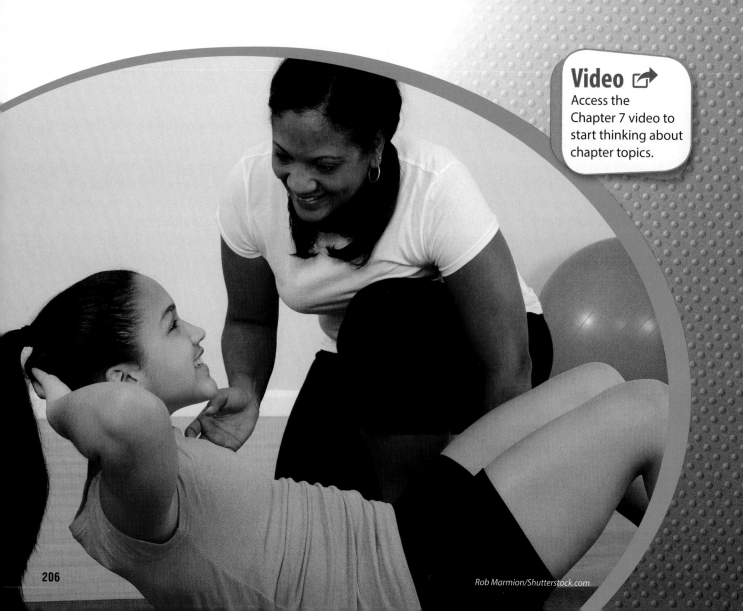

How physically fit are you?

Video
Access the Chapter 7 video to start thinking about chapter topics.

Rob Marmion/Shutterstock.com

Reading Activity

Arrange a study session to read the chapter aloud with a classmate. Take turns reading each lesson. Stop at the end of each lesson and identify its main points. Take notes of your study session to share with the class.

How Healthy Are You? ↗

In this chapter, you will be learning about physical fitness. Before you begin reading, take the following quiz to assess your current physical fitness habits.

Healthy Choices	Yes	No
Do you follow the rules of any physical activity, especially sports, in which you participate?		
Are you physically active for a total of 60 minutes or more each day?		
Do you do cardio activities like playing sports, riding your bike, or taking a dance class?		
Can you balance on one foot, do a handstand, or ride a skateboard?		
Do you drink lots of water before, during, and after physical activity?		
Do you do anaerobic workouts like push-ups, sit-ups, or squats for 20 to 30 minutes, two or three days a week?		
Do you regularly do yoga, Pilates, or some type of stretching?		
Do you tend to walk up the stairs instead of taking an elevator or escalator?		
Do you make personal fitness plans to identify which parts of your fitness need the most improvement?		
Do you have the energy to perform life's daily activities?		
Do you warm up your muscles before any type of physical activity?		
Do you do a cooldown after physical activity to stretch and help your heart rate return to a normal, lower level?		

Count your "Yes" and "No" responses. The more "Yes" responses you have, the more healthy physical fitness habits you exhibit. Now, take a closer look at the questions with which you responded "No." How can you make these healthy habits part of your daily life? Think about how implementing these ideas can help improve your overall health and wellness.

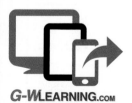

G-WLEARNING.com

While studying this chapter, look for the activity icon ↗ to

- **practice** key terms with e-flash cards and matching activities.
- **reinforce** what you learn by completing graphic organizers, self-assessment quizzes, and review questions.
- **expand** knowledge with interactive activities and activities that extend learning.

What It Means to Be Physically Fit

Learning Outcomes

After studying this lesson, you will be able to

- **define** the terms *fitness*, *exercise*, and *physical activity*.
- **describe** the benefits of physical activity.
- **summarize** the key guidelines for children and teens, adults, and older adults as outlined in the *Physical Activity Guidelines for Americans*.
- **evaluate** how you can improve your health by doing activities you enjoy.

Graphic Organizer 👉

Have Fun Getting Fit

In a table like the one shown below, list five physical activities you enjoy doing and include a list of health benefits for each activity. If multiple physical activities have the same benefits in common, highlight each repeated benefit in a different color.

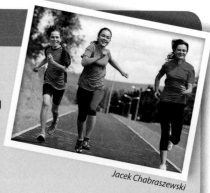

Jacek Chabraszewski

Physical Activities I Enjoy	Health Benefits of These Activities
1. Running	• Improves heart and lung function • Helps control weight
2.	
3.	
4.	
5.	

Madison is in sixth grade and loves being active. She walks to school every day. After school, she enjoys riding her bike to her friend Danny's house. Almost every weekend she goes out with her family for a hike or a bike ride.

Madison's friend Danny does not always have the energy for those types of physical activities. He does like to play baseball once a week with friends, and he will occasionally do some push-ups or pull-ups. Lately, however, Danny has noticed that he gets very tired throughout the day. He becomes out of breath quickly when walking up stairs or riding his bike. If he wants to go to the park or go to Madison's house, he asks his mom to drive him.

In this lesson, you will learn what the terms *fitness*, *exercise*, and *physical activity* mean. You will discover how leading an active lifestyle can benefit your health and wellness. You will find out how you can improve your health simply by doing physical activities you enjoy.

Fitness Defined

You often hear the terms *physical fitness*, *exercise*, and *physical activity*, but do you know what these words really mean? The term **fitness** refers to the body's ability to meet daily physical demands. People who are fit can meet the day's physical challenges without tiring out too easily. Becoming physically fit is one of the most important actions you can take to promote good health and well-being.

To become physically fit, you need to get plenty of exercise and physical activity. Many people think that the terms *exercise* and *physical activity* have the same meaning, but there is a difference. **Exercise** is a type of planned, structured, and purposeful physical activity. Exercise could be running daily to train for a marathon or doing a routine of sit-ups, push-ups, and pull-ups in PE class. The term **physical activity** is broader because it includes both structured exercise and other activities that use energy (**Figure 7.1**).

Deciding to exercise is a good lifestyle choice if you want to be physically fit. You do not need to engage in structured exercise, however, to improve your fitness level. Your health and fitness can benefit from many types of physical activities.

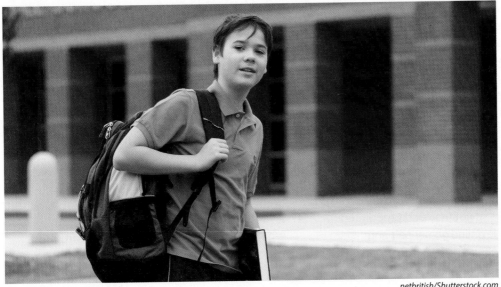

Figure 7.1
You probably would not call walking to school exercise, but it is a physical activity. *What defines a physical activity?*

netbritish/Shutterstock.com

By setting SMART goals—goals that are specific, measurable, action oriented, relevant, and timely—you can start taking steps toward improving your physical fitness.

The Benefits of Physical Activity

There are many benefits of engaging in physical activity. Regular physical activity improves heart and lung function, and builds strong bones and muscles. It lowers the risk of certain diseases, such as heart disease or diabetes. Engaging in regular physical activity also reduces your risk of developing some cancers. In fact, physical activity increases your chances of living longer.

These are not the only benefits of physical activity, however. Physical activity also helps you control your weight and improve your quality of sleep. It improves your mental health and mood. It can make you feel better about yourself or certain situations. It can provide opportunities to meet new friends and become closer with old ones. Engaging in regular physical activity can even help you improve your concentration and focus, enabling you to do better in school.

CASE STUDY

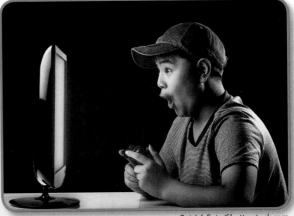

Patrick Foto/Shutterstock.com

Walk in My Shoes: Jaquan's Story

Thirteen-year-old Jaquan is a good student and does not mind going to school. His parents have high academic expectations for him. As long as he gets good grades, Jaquan can do whatever he wants after school. What he really likes to do is play video games.

For his birthday, Jaquan got a new gaming system and several games. Most days, he will play four to six hours. This often leaves him exhausted and not very motivated to do other activities.

Recently, Jaquan has gained some weight. He realizes that this is because he is spending more time being sedentary while playing his video games. The extra weight in his stomach does make him feel a little insecure at school. He usually tries to escape these insecurities by retreating to his room after school. Jaquan is not really worried about his weight gain because he figures he has plenty of time to lose weight.

Jaquan does not really enjoy sports. His parents pushed him, with little success, to try soccer, football, and even lacrosse when he was younger. Jaquan felt that he was never fast or coordinated enough to keep up with the other boys. He is not mad or disappointed about it. Jaquan has made online gamer pals and would rather play video games with them.

Thinking Critically

1. How could Jaquan benefit from being physically active at his age? Consider how being physically active could positively affect his current physical, mental, social, and emotional health.

2. How could Jaquan enjoy playing video games and achieve health-related fitness?

3. If you were Jaquan's friend, what activities would you recommend to help him stay physically fit, aside from playing sports?

4. If Jaquan's sedentary lifestyle continues, what are the possible long-term health outcomes?

Benefits of Physical Activity

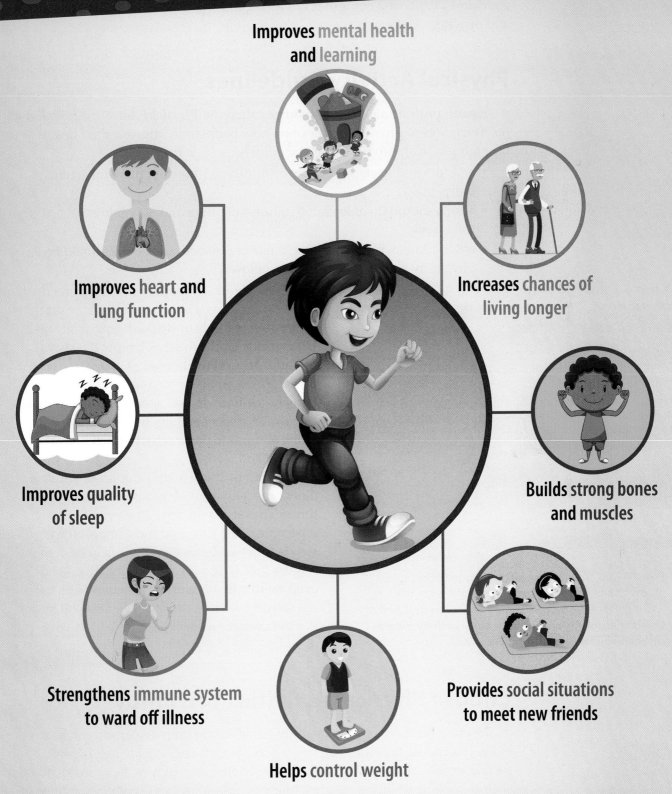

Improves mental health and learning

Improves heart and lung function

Increases chances of living longer

Improves quality of sleep

Builds strong bones and muscles

Strengthens immune system to ward off illness

Provides social situations to meet new friends

Helps control weight

Center: GraphicsRF/Shutterstock.com; Clockwise from top: Lorelyn Medina/Shutterstock.com; Iconic Bestiary/Shutterstock.com; Victor Brave/Shutterstock.com; wet nose/Shutterstock.com; Lorelyn Medina/Shutterstock.com; teamplay/Shutterstock.com; Victor Brave/Shutterstock.com; chombosan/Shutterstock.com

Although the benefits of regular physical activity are clear, most people do not get enough activity each day. Many people spend much of their days doing activities that involve sitting and using very little energy. These people are being **sedentary** (inactive). Living a sedentary lifestyle can result in developing a chronic health condition, such as diabetes. Sedentary behaviors can include watching TV, playing computer or video games, going to the movies, reading, and driving.

Physical Activity Guidelines

Health professionals use a resource called the *Physical Activity Guidelines for Americans* to provide guidance on how people can improve their health through physical activities. The key guidelines state the following:

- children and teens should get 60 minutes (1 hour) of physical activity daily
- adults should do at least 150 minutes (2 hours and 30 minutes) of activity each week
- older adults who cannot do 150 minutes of activity a week should be as physically active as their abilities allow

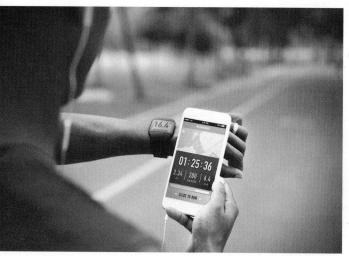

Rawpixel.com/Shutterstock.com

Figure 7.2 You can use technology to improve your fitness habits. Apps can record workouts, set reminders, and track fitness goals. *According to the* Physical Activity Guidelines for Americans, *how much activity should children and teens engage in each day?*

Think about the types of activities you do on a regular basis. Do you jog, swim, or skate? Do you lift weights or do push-ups or sit-ups? Do you ride a bike to school, mow the lawn, or dance around the house? Do you stretch or do yoga? Do you play on a school sports team? How much time do you spend doing activities? Does your current activity level measure up to the 60-minute daily activity guideline for children and teens?

Making physical activity a part of your daily or weekly routine can be challenging at times. The more you do it, however, the easier it becomes. The first, and most important, step is to set aside time each week to be active (**Figure 7.2**). If you are usually inactive, then even as little as 10 minutes of activity at a time is a step in the right direction. Before you know it, physical activity will become part of your daily life.

Choose Physical Activities You Enjoy

Meeting the daily physical activity guideline for your age group can be easy when you choose activities you enjoy. Some people really enjoy team sports, such as basketball or field hockey. Other people like activities they can do alone, such as walking or lifting weights. Many people enjoy both types of activities. Think about what you like the most. Do you prefer outdoor or indoor activities?

Do you like to exercise alone or with other people? Also, consider which physical activities are appropriate for your levels of fitness and development.

If you like to exercise with other people, try to find someone who will be active with you. Do you have a friend who would take a brisk walk with you after school? What about going on a bike ride? You could even make new friends by joining a sports team or fitness group. An exercise class might be a good place to meet new people. A pick-up baseball game at a local park could help you meet new people, too.

Many schools and communities provide free or low-cost ways to enjoy physical activities. Community centers often offer dance lessons and sports and exercise programs. Many communities also have places you can use for free or at a reduced cost, such as the following:

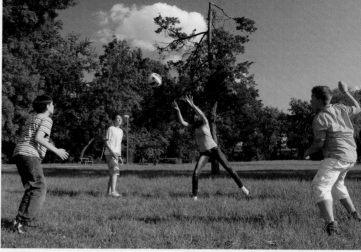

Sasa Prudkov/Shutterstock.com

Figure 7.3 Going to a community park is a great, free way to stay active with your friends without spending money on a gym membership.

- parks and green spaces for playing Frisbee, throwing a baseball, or playing soccer (**Figure 7.3**)
- outdoor sports areas, such as baseball or softball fields and tennis and basketball courts
- indoor sports areas, such as swimming pools, basketball courts, and running tracks
- walking and biking trails and skate parks
- public pools

Lesson 7.1 Review

1. What is the term for planned, structured, and purposeful physical activity?
2. Which of the following is *not* a benefit of physical activity?
   A. Improves quality of sleep.   **C.** Increases risk of disease.
   B. Helps concentration and focus.   **D.** None of the above.
3. What is the name of the resource that health professionals use to provide guidance on how people can improve their health through physical activities?
4. **Critical thinking.** Identify two activities that would be categorized as physical activity and two that would be considered exercise. Explain the difference.

Hands-On Activity

Choose one of the activities you identified in question number four above and do this activity at least three times on three different days. After doing this activity, reflect on how it made you feel. Did you enjoy the activity? How likely are you to keep doing this activity? Write a summary of your findings.

Fitness Types

Key Terms

health-related fitness type of fitness a person needs to perform daily activities with ease and energy

aerobic exercise activity involving the use of oxygen to fuel processes in the body

resistance opposition

anaerobic exercise activity involving the use of energy stored in the muscles to supply the body with the fuel it needs

endurance ability to continue an activity over a period of time without tiring

skill-related fitness type of fitness that improves a person's performance in a particular sport

Learning Outcomes

After studying this lesson, you will be able to

- **describe** five parts of health-related fitness.
- **compare** and **contrast** aerobic activities and anaerobic activities.
- **explain** the two types of endurance.
- **differentiate between** health-related fitness and skill-related fitness.
- **identify** the six aspects of skill-related fitness.

Graphic Organizer

Many Ways to Be Fit

In an organizer like the one below, identify the five aspects of health-related fitness and the six aspects of skill-related fitness. After each aspect of fitness, offer an example of a physical activity that uses this aspect.

Africa Studio/Shutterstock.com

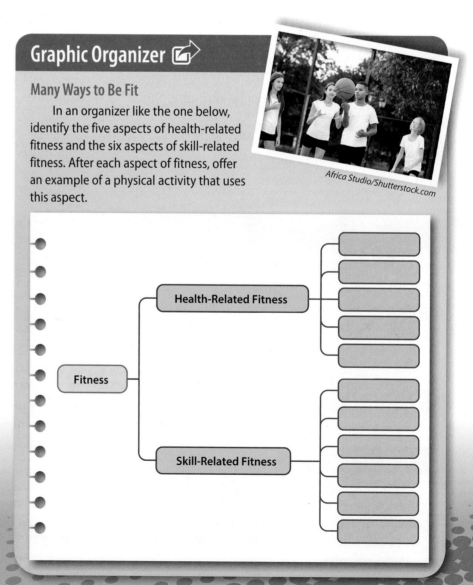

Fitness

Health-Related Fitness

Skill-Related Fitness

As people engage in physical activities, they develop some parts of their fitness more than other parts. For example, how fast, and how long, can you run? Are you able to touch your toes? How many push-ups and pull-ups can you do?

Recall from the previous lesson, Madison and Danny's different physical activities. Madison's hiking and biking develop different parts of her fitness than Danny's push-ups and pull-ups. Hiking and biking improve balance or heart and lung strength, while push-ups improve muscle strength and power. These activities represent different types of fitness. In this lesson, you will learn about health-related fitness and skill-related fitness.

Health-Related Fitness

Health-related fitness is the type of fitness you need to perform daily activities with ease and energy. There are different parts of health-related fitness. These parts include heart and lung strength, muscle strength, endurance, flexibility, and body composition.

Heart and Lung Strength

Your heart and lung strength affects how well you can do physical activities. In **aerobic exercise**, the heart and lungs work together to deliver oxygen to the muscles. As you exercise, your heart beats faster and your breathing quickens. Your lungs must work harder to provide your muscles with oxygen so you can keep moving. Examples of aerobic (also called *cardio*) exercises include running, dancing, swimming, walking briskly, and riding a bike (**Figure 7.4**).

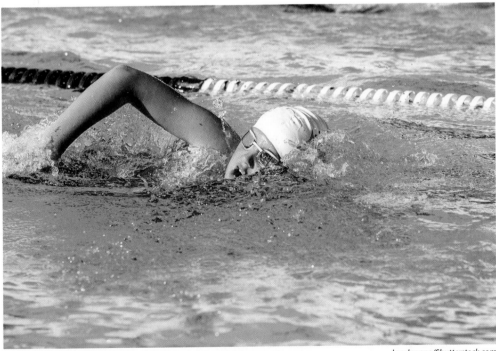

Figure 7.4
Aerobic exercises like swimming help improve heart and lung function and build strong muscles and bones. *What is another name for aerobic exercise?*

karelnoppe/Shutterstock.com

Most of your 60 minutes of activity each day should be spent doing aerobic activities. Engaging in regular aerobic activity strengthens the heart and lungs. The stronger your heart and lungs become, the more physically fit you become.

Muscle Strength

Muscle strength is the ability of a muscle to exert force against **resistance** (opposition). Imagine you are arm wrestling with a friend. Assume that you have stronger arm muscles than your friend. As you push against your friend's weaker arm muscles, your force will overcome your friend's resistance. This will result in you winning the match.

You can measure your muscle strength in many ways. For example, you can measure how much weight (resistance) you can lift. You can also measure how much weight you can push, and how much weight you can pull.

When you lift weights or do push-ups and pull-ups, you are engaging in anaerobic exercise. In **anaerobic exercise**, the energy stored in your muscles supplies your body with the fuel it needs. Anaerobic activities differ from aerobic activities. Anaerobic activities occur in short bursts, while aerobic activities occur over a longer stretch of time (**Figure 7.5**). Children and teens can improve their muscle strength by doing anaerobic exercises at least three days each week.

Endurance

Another important part of health-related fitness is a person's endurance. **Endurance** refers to the ability to continue an activity over a period of time without tiring. There are two types of endurance—aerobic and muscle. *Aerobic endurance* describes a person's ability to engage in cardio exercises over a period of time.

Figure 7.5
Examples of anaerobic exercises include sit-ups, push-ups, sprinting, and weight lifting. *How often should children and teens do anaerobic exercises?*

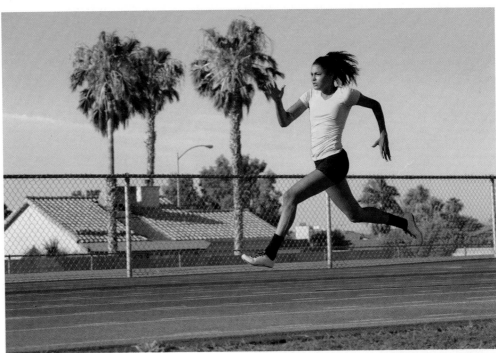

LifetimeStock/Shutterstock.com

Muscle endurance refers to the length of time for which a group of muscles can continue to exert force. Muscle endurance is different from muscle strength. Muscle endurance has to do with the duration of performance. Muscle strength has to do with the amount of force used to move or lift an object.

Some types of physical activity require high levels of both aerobic and muscle endurance. For example, consider marathon runners who run long distances for hours at a time. These runners must have great aerobic endurance for their hearts to continue pumping at higher-than-normal levels throughout the run. They must also have great muscle endurance for their leg muscles to continue exerting force for such a long time.

Flexibility

You probably know what it means to be flexible. People who are flexible are able to fully and easily move their muscles and joints. One measure of flexibility is *range of motion*, which tells how far a joint can move in a certain direction (**Figure 7.6**).

Some people are very flexible. They are easily able to move their muscles and joints into difficult positions. Ballet dancers and gymnasts are good examples. They have great flexibility, enabling them to perform moves such as backbends and the splits. Other people are not so flexible, and will often have tight or stiff muscles. Their range of motion is limited. This can make normal daily activities, such as tying their shoes, difficult to do.

Everyone benefits from having some flexibility. Flexibility helps improve performance in many physical activities. It also lowers the risk of getting an injury. Regularly (and safely) stretching your muscles can increase your flexibility. Fitness guidelines suggest that everyone engage in some type of stretching activity at least two or three days each week.

Body Composition

Body composition is an important part of health-related fitness. As you may recall, *body composition* is the ratio of fat, bone, and muscle that naturally make up a person's body. Two people may be the same weight, but their body composition can be very different. Some people have much more muscle than fat, while others have more fat than muscle. If a person has too much body fat, he or she has a higher risk of developing a chronic health condition. These conditions may include heart disease, diabetes, or high blood pressure.

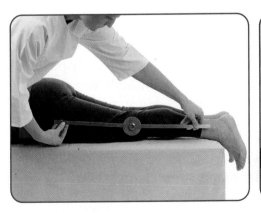 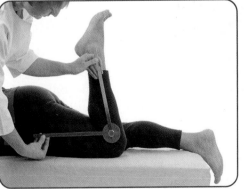

Figure 7.6
Having good range of motion is important for your health and wellness, and can be improved over time with stretching exercises.

pryzmat/Shutterstock.com

Engaging in regular physical activity can improve a person's body composition. People who engage in strength training, which includes push-ups, sit-ups, or lifting weights, can increase their muscle mass. Increasing muscle mass, and reducing a high percentage of body fat, is important to prevent chronic health conditions.

Skill-Related Fitness

Skill-related fitness refers to the kind of fitness a person needs to successfully perform a sport or leisure activity. The different aspects of skill-related fitness include speed, agility, balance, power, coordination, and reaction time.

Speed

If you participate in or watch sporting events, then you know what *speed* is. Many sports require people to be fast. Runners and swimmers must be fast, especially if they are racing short distances. Sprinting requires more speed than long-distance running or swimming. Soccer players must be fast to get to the ball first. Speed is an important aspect of skill-related fitness that is needed to be successful in many sports.

Agility

Another type of skill-related fitness is agility. *Agility* is the ability to rapidly change the body's momentum and direction. This skill involves accelerating in a particular direction from a position of standing still. It can also involve rapidly changing from movement in one direction to movement in another direction. Agility describes a person's ability to go under, over, or around obstacles that he or she may encounter (Figure 7.7).

Balance

Balance means holding a certain body posture and position on a stable or unstable surface. Balance is very much a part of some sports, such as diving and gymnastics, as well as many leisure activities. Can you do a handstand or ride a skateboard? What about hopping on one foot? These are all examples of activities that involve the ability to balance.

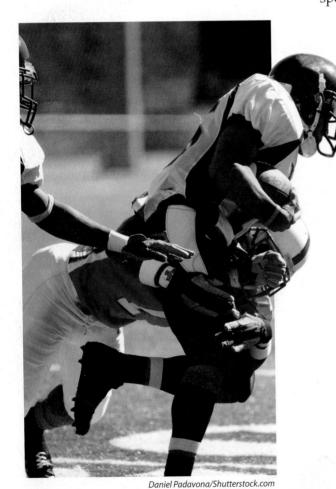

Daniel Padavona/Shutterstock.com

Figure 7.7 A running back on a football team must have agility to move around and away from players on the other team to avoid getting tackled.

Types of Fitness

Start ▶

Choose Your Abilities ▲

Health-Related Fitness

Heart and Lung Strength
Provides oxygen to the muscles to keep you going longer

Muscle Strength
Allows you to lift objects and push against resistance

Endurance
Allows you to be physically active for long periods of time without tiring

Flexibility
Allows you to fully and easily move your muscles and joints

Body Composition
The amount of muscle and fat in your body

Choose Your Skills ▲

Skill-Related Fitness

Speed
How fast you can move

Power
A mix of strength and speed

Balance
Holding a certain body posture on a stable or unstable surface

Coordination
Allows you to perform various movements easily and smoothly

Agility
The ability to rapidly change the body's momentum and direction

Reaction Time
The quickness of a response

Power

Power is a mix of strength and speed. Some athletes are strong, but not fast. Other athletes are fast, but not strong. The athlete who combines strength and speed can be powerful. Power is an important skill in many sports, such as football and baseball. An outstanding volleyball hitter is usually one of the more powerful players on the team.

Coordination

Having good *coordination* enables you to perform various movements easily and gracefully (**Figure 7.8**). Soccer players, hockey players, and other athletes who must have agility also have high levels of coordination. Some people are naturally more coordinated than others. Many athletes who perform complex movements do so smoothly, however, as a result of practice. Natural ability and practice lead to better coordination.

sirtravelalot/Shutterstock.com

Figure 7.8 Coordination relates closely to balance. Gymnastics, for example, requires both balance and coordination to perform complex movements. *What is another physical activity that requires good coordination and balance?*

Reaction Time

Reaction time refers to the quickness of a response. How quickly do you react to someone else's movement? A person's reaction time is important in many sports. You must be able to react quickly to hit a tennis ball, hit a baseball, or block a soccer ball.

Lesson 7.2 Review

1. **True or false.** Health-related fitness helps you perform daily activities with ease and energy.
2. Name the two types of endurance.
3. Heart and lung strength, muscle strength, endurance, flexibility, and body composition are all parts of _____ fitness.
4. What are the six aspects of skill-related fitness?
5. **Critical thinking.** How does aerobic exercise differ from anaerobic exercise?

Hands-On Activity

Write down each physical activity you perform this week. Make sure to record how long you do each activity. Next to each item, identify whether it is an aerobic activity or an anaerobic activity. Which types of activities do you want to improve? Do you need to improve your aerobic endurance? Do you get enough anaerobic activity? Write a summary describing which types of activities you want to improve.

Fitness Safety

Learning Outcomes

After studying this lesson, you will be able to

- **give examples** of rules you have learned in sports.
- **identify** common safety equipment for physical activities.
- **explain** why it is important to start slowly and not overdo it when starting a fitness program.
- **describe** why drinking water is important before, during, and after physical activity.
- **list** steps you can take to ensure your safety when exercising in hot or cold weather.
- **compare** and **contrast** a sprain, dislocation, and fracture.

Graphic Organizer

Staying Safe

This lesson is about preventing fitness-related injuries. Before reading this lesson, make five predictions of safety strategies you think might be included in the lesson. For each prediction, explain why you think this is an important guideline for avoiding injuries. Use your previous personal experience, as well as information you may have learned elsewhere, to fill in a table like the one below.

kazoka/Shutterstock.com

Safety Strategy	Why Is This Important?
1.	
2.	
3.	
4.	
5.	

Key Terms

hyperthermia serious condition that results when the heat-regulating mechanisms of the body are unable to deal with the heat from the environment, which results in a very high body temperature

hypothermia serious condition that results when a person's body loses heat faster than it can produce it

frostbite injury caused by the freezing of skin and body tissues

sprain common sports injury involving the stretching or tearing of ligaments (tissues that hold joints together)

dislocation serious injury in which bones move out of their normal position

fracture broken bone

concussion type of brain injury that results from a blow or jolt to the head or upper body

As you know, engaging in regular physical activity is an important part of staying healthy. You probably also know that you cannot engage in regular physical activity if you are injured. This means that following accepted guidelines and taking the necessary precautions when exercising are critical to your health.

Remember Madison from the previous lessons. When she goes for a bike ride, she always wears her helmet. When she goes for a hike with her family, they always make sure to bring a first-aid kit and plenty of water. When Danny plays baseball, he wears a batting helmet to protect himself from injury.

This lesson will examine actions you can take to be safe, avoid common injuries, and treat injuries that might occur.

Follow the Rules

Many physical activities, especially sports, have certain rules you must learn. These rules exist, at least in part, to help people stay safe. Knowing and following the rules of your chosen activity can keep you and your teammates safe and free from injury.

Rules can vary based on the activity. For example, a rule in football or soccer states that all activity on the field must stop when the referee blows the whistle. A rule to obey traffic laws is important for activities such as biking, running, or rollerblading. Because rules can vary for activities, make sure you practice safety by learning the rules of an activity before you participate.

Use Proper Equipment

When you exercise or play sports, you will need to have the necessary safety equipment to prevent injuries (**Figure 7.9**). The equipment you use needs to fit well. Do not use hand-me-downs or used equipment that is overly worn or the wrong size for you. Common safety equipment for popular activities includes the following:

- **Helmets.** Helmets protect your head from injury and are necessary for sports such as baseball, softball, and football. Also, wear a helmet when biking, skiing, and rollerblading.
- **Mouth guards.** Mouth guards protect your teeth and tongue. They are needed in sports such as lacrosse, ice hockey, and football.
- **Goggles and face masks.** Goggles and face masks provide protection for the eyes. Swimmers often use goggles to protect their eyes. Ice hockey goalies and baseball catchers are examples of athletes who wear face masks.
- **Padding for wrists, knees, hips, shoulders, and elbows.** Padding prevents injuries common in sports such as ice hockey, football, soccer, and lacrosse. Padding may also be needed while ice-skating, rollerblading, and snowboarding.
- **Reflective gear.** Reflective gear makes you more visible when you are riding your bike or running along the side of a road.

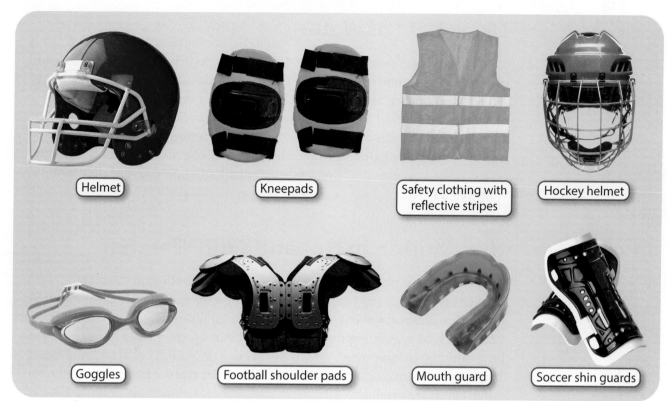

Helmet | Kneepads | Safety clothing with reflective stripes | Hockey helmet

Goggles | Football shoulder pads | Mouth guard | Soccer shin guards

Left to right: pbombaert/Shutterstock.com; TerraceStudio/Shutterstock.com; krolya25/Shutterstock.com; Supertrooper/Shutterstock.com; Martina_L/Shutterstock.com; wacpan/Shutterstock.com; Mega Pixel/Shutterstock.com; MaZiKab/Shutterstock.com

Figure 7.9 Safety equipment prevents injuries, which can stop you from getting to play sports or do other physical activities. *What are two kinds of safety equipment that help protect your head?*

Start Slowly and Do Not Overdo It

If you are just starting a fitness program, take care to start slowly (**Figure 7.10**). It can be tempting to exercise too much or too strenuously when you first start. You should resist this temptation because over-exercising can be harmful. If you overdo any type of physical activity during the first couple of days, you increase your chances of an injury. Then, you will have to wait until you heal before you can get back on track.

Once you feel more comfortable with physical activity, you can increase the time, frequency, and intensity of your exercise. For example, you could walk, roller skate, or bike for 30 minutes instead of just 10 to 20 minutes. You could jog instead of walk. Gradually increase the demands on your body. Be patient rather than trying to do too much too soon.

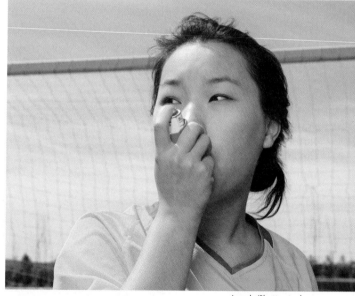

Lopolo/Shutterstock.com

Figure 7.10 People with preexisting conditions, such as asthma or diabetes, should see a doctor before starting any new physical activity. *Why should someone with asthma see a doctor before trying a new physical activity?*

Drink Lots of Water

Your body sweats during physical activity, which decreases the amount of fluids in your body. The loss of too much fluid causes dehydration. This affects your body's ability to function properly. Fluid loss also makes the heart work harder to circulate blood throughout your body. A loss of fluid can also lead to muscle cramps, dizziness, and fatigue. Therefore, drink lots of water before, during, and after physical activity. Make sure to bring water when you exercise. Remember to drink often to prevent dehydration (**Figure 7.11**).

Use Caution in Hot and Cold Weather

Exercising or playing sports outside in hot or cold weather can be dangerous if you are not careful. The term *hyperthermia* describes heat-related illnesses and *hypothermia* describes cold-related illnesses. **Hyperthermia** occurs when the heat-regulating mechanisms of the body are unable to deal with the heat from the environment, which results in a very high body temperature. **Hypothermia** is a result of a very low body temperature that occurs from too much exposure to cold weather.

If you are engaging in physical activity outside when it is hot and humid, make sure to drink plenty of water before, during, and after your exercise to avoid dehydration. Wearing light-colored and lightweight clothing can prevent you from becoming too overheated. You can use misting sprays to keep cool, too. Also, be aware of the signs and symptoms of heat-related illnesses. These symptoms may include heavy sweating and a rapid pulse, confusion, dizziness, fainting, headache, nausea, and weakness. If you have any of these symptoms, tell your coach or someone who is with you right away.

Figure 7.11
Drinking water is important before, during, and after engaging in physical activity.
Why is drinking water important for engaging in physical activity?

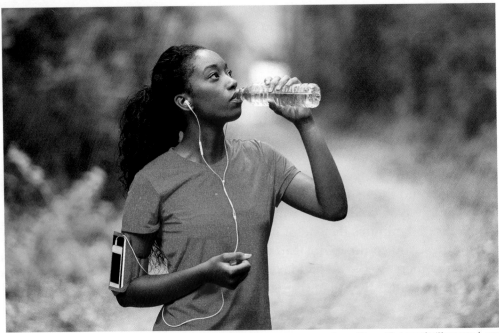

Samuel Borges Photography/Shutterstock.com

If you are engaging in physical activity outside in very cold temperatures, you need to stay safe. Steps you can take to ensure your safety include the following:

- Check the temperature—including the wind chill factor—carefully before you go outside.
- Dress warmly with several layers of clothing.
- Make sure to protect your head, ears, hands, and feet, which are especially vulnerable to frostbite (**Figure 7.12**). **Frostbite** is an injury caused by the freezing of skin and body tissues. Symptoms of frostbite may include numbness, loss of feeling or a stinging sensation, intense shivering, slurred speech, and a loss of coordination.
- Drink plenty of fluids, just as you would when exercising in hot weather.

Treat Injuries

Sports activities and falls are common causes of injuries. Some of the most common injuries related to physical activities are sprains, dislocations, fractures, and concussions.

A **sprain** is an injury to tissues called *ligaments* that hold joints together. If a joint moves suddenly beyond its normal range of motion, the ligaments stretch and tear. The ankle, knee, and wrist are the most commonly sprained parts of the body. Swelling and pain around the affected area are familiar signs of a sprain.

First aid for a sprain follows the R.I.C.E. treatment (**Figure 7.13**). If a sprain does not improve after two to three days, see a doctor. You may also need to see a doctor if swelling or pain worsens. The doctor may prescribe medication to help reduce the pain and swelling.

Several layers of loose-fitting clothing

Hat

Scarf

Water-resistant coat

Water-resistant boots

Mittens or gloves

Evgeny Bakharev/Shutterstock.com

Figure 7.12 In cold weather, protective clothing can help prevent hypothermia and frostbite. *Which parts of the body are especially vulnerable to frostbite?*

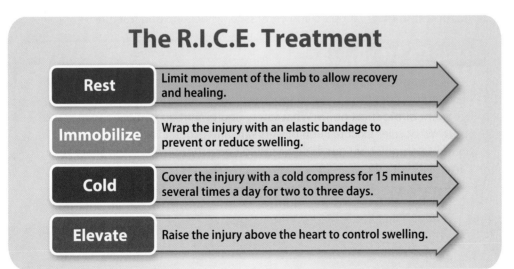

The R.I.C.E. Treatment

Rest	Limit movement of the limb to allow recovery and healing.
Immobilize	Wrap the injury with an elastic bandage to prevent or reduce swelling.
Cold	Cover the injury with a cold compress for 15 minutes several times a day for two to three days.
Elevate	Raise the injury above the heart to control swelling.

Figure 7.13 When following the R.I.C.E. treatment, do all four parts at the same time. *What are the tissues called that stretch and tear when you experience a sprain?*

If you experience a more serious injury, such as a dislocation or fracture, seek medical treatment right away. A **dislocation** is a condition in which bones move out of their normal positions. A **fracture** is a broken bone. Never try to force a bone back into place. This can seriously damage muscles, joints, and nerves.

Always seek medical treatment right away for a concussion, too. A **concussion** is a type of brain injury that results from a blow or jolt to the head or upper body. Contact sports injuries, such as those from football, soccer, wrestling, or hockey, often result in concussions. Concussions result in disorientation, confusion, nausea, weakness, memory loss, or unconsciousness. Concussions are usually temporary, but they can lead to serious permanent complications.

If you do experience an injury that requires medical treatment, be sure to follow your doctor's instructions. These instructions could include taking appropriate medications, performing recommended exercises and stretches, or receiving physical therapy. Be sure to follow the doctor's recommendations regarding amount of time to refrain from certain physical activities. Returning to the activity that led to your injury too soon after the injury increases your risk of re-injury.

Lesson 7.3 Review

1. Which of the following is *not* an example of safety equipment for physical activities?

   A. Swim goggles.

   B. Reflective gear.

   C. Baseball bat.

   D. Shin guards.

2. Why is it important to start slowly and not overdo it when starting a fitness program?

3. **True or false.** Drinking lots of water is only important after physical activity.

4. _____ refers to heat-related illnesses, while _____ refers to cold-related illnesses.

5. **Critical thinking.** Compare and contrast a dislocation and fracture.

Hands-On Activity

Pick a sport that you would like to learn more about. Talk to people who play the sport or who know the sport well. You may also choose to watch a live event of the sport on TV. What safety equipment do you need to play the sport? What rules exist to keep players safe and protect them from injury? Create a pamphlet of your findings called *Know the Rules of _____*. Share your pamphlets with the rest of the class.

A Personal Fitness Plan

Learning Outcomes

After studying this lesson, you will be able to

- **determine** your current level of fitness.
- **identify** your personal fitness goals.
- **explain** what FITT means.
- **determine** your maximum heart rate and your target heart rates for moderate- and vigorous-intensity activities.
- **create** a tracking report to help you achieve your fitness goals.

Key Terms 📲

pulse person's heart rate

intensity measure of how much energy is used during exercise

FITT acronym used to focus on the key fitness factors of frequency, intensity, time, and type

target heart rate heart rate to aim for while performing aerobic exercise to get the best results from a workout; varies by age

maximum heart rate number of beats per minute a person's heart can achieve when working its hardest; varies by age

sets anaerobic exercises done in groups of repetitions followed by rest

Graphic Organizer 📲

Make the Most of Your Fitness

In a table like the one shown below, write the main headings of this lesson. As you read this lesson, take notes and organize them by heading. Draw a star beside any words or concepts you do not yet understand.

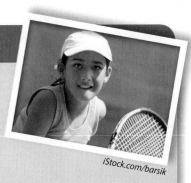

iStock.com/barsik

Checking Your Health-Related Fitness Level
Setting Your Goals
Maximizing Your Workouts

Most people, even those who appear fit, can improve some aspects of their fitness. From the previous lessons, even though he is strong, Danny can improve his heart and lung strength to prevent getting so out of breath. Madison can hike and bike, but she might still have problems with her flexibility or balance. That is why fitness plans are "personal." You can work on the parts of your fitness most in need of improvement. Madison and Danny's fitness goals may be very different from yours.

In this lesson, you will learn how to create your personal fitness plan. You are already well on your way. You know how much, and what types of, physical activity you need. You have also had a chance to choose activities you would enjoy doing. The next steps in creating your plan are to check your current level of fitness and set your goals. Then, you will be ready to get moving and experience the benefits of physical fitness.

Checking Your Health-Related Fitness Level

To check your current fitness level, you will need to measure the different parts of health-related fitness. This includes your heart and lung strength, muscle strength, endurance, flexibility, and body composition. As you check your fitness level, be sure to record your results. Ask your teacher to look at your results and help you identify the areas in which you may need to improve. Keep your results in a safe place so you can keep track of your progress as you work toward your goals.

To begin, measure the following areas of fitness:

- Check aerobic fitness by timing yourself to see how long it takes you to briskly walk one mile. Before you start, check and record your **pulse** (your heart rate). Check and record your pulse again after you finish. See **Figure 7.14** for ways to take your pulse.
- Measure your muscle strength and endurance by counting how many push-ups you can do at one time. If you are not very physically active, you may want to do modified push-ups on your knees.
- Check your flexibility by noting how far you can reach forward, toward your toes, while sitting with your legs straight in front of you.
- Measure your waist circumference and determine your body mass index (BMI) using the formula you learned in Chapter 6: *Nutrition.* (Also, see the BMI charts for boys and girls in the Appendix at the back of this text.)

Taking Your Pulse

Taking your pulse at the wrist is very easy when you use the following steps:

- Find your pulse on the artery of the wrist, in line with your thumb.
- Place the tips of your index and middle fingers over the artery and press lightly.
- Start counting on a beat, which is zero (not one).
- Count the number of heartbeats for a full 60 seconds. You can also count for six seconds and multiply by 10.

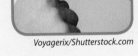
Voyagerix/Shutterstock.com

Heart rate monitors and some *fitness trackers* worn around the wrist can also measure your pulse. These devices measure your pulse by shining a light into the blood vessels in your wrist. The light measures changes in blood volume each time your heart beats and blood is pushed through your body. Less light reflected back into the sensor on your wrist means more blood volume and a faster pulse.

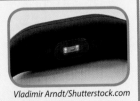
Vladimir Arndt/Shutterstock.com

Figure 7.14 You can check your pulse manually or use a device.

Setting Your Goals

If you currently do not meet the daily physical activity guideline for your age group, you might want to set goals that will help you work toward being more active every day. Perhaps you already get plenty of physical activity, but you would like to perform at a certain level of **intensity** (measure of how much energy is used during exercise). Maybe you would like to set a goal to exercise at a certain time of day, such as every morning. You might even want to set a goal to join a sports team or take dance lessons.

BUILDING Your Skills

Be SMART, Stay Motivated

Have you ever tried achieving fitness goals and given up? Perhaps you just never knew where to start. Adopting a more physically fit lifestyle is not easy, and there are often many obstacles to overcome along the way. By setting SMART goals, you are more likely to be successful and stay motivated. Following are some examples of ways to write, and not to write, SMART goals:

- **Specific**—"Ride my bike five miles after school on Monday and Thursday."
  NOT: "Ride my bike."

- **Measurable**—"Do five unassisted pull-ups."
  NOT: "Build arm muscle."

- **Achievable**—"Lose one pound a week."
  NOT: "Lose 10 pounds by the dance next Friday."

- **Relevant**—"Swim 30 minutes three days a week to increase stamina."
  NOT: "Lose 15 pounds to increase stamina."

- **Timely**—"Join an aerobics class by the end of the month."
  NOT: "Join an aerobics class."

For ideas on how to start writing your SMART goals, remember the acronym *FITT*. Also, keep in mind that you are much more likely to be successful when you choose activities you enjoy. Be sure to include both short-term goals and long-term goals. Your short-term goals should act as stepping stones to the long-term goals. For example, a long-term goal might be to run a five-mile race at the end of the summer. A short-term goal might be to run one mile three times this week.

Setting SMART Fitness Goals

Using the tips above, write your own SMART fitness goals. Once you create your fitness goals, design a one-week plan of action. You can use a chart like the one shown in Figure 7.16 to guide you through creating your plan. The next step is to get moving. Begin your daily exercise plan and fill in your chart. In the comments section of the chart, record your thoughts and feelings related to each activity. After completing your plan for a week, reflect on your progress and identify any changes you would want to make to your plan. Make any necessary changes and create a new chart for next week. Continue this activity until your behavior becomes a lifestyle.

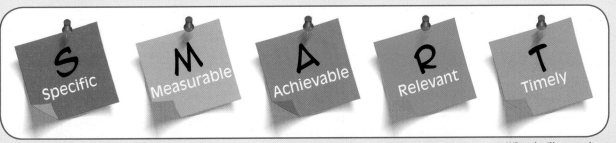

WDstocker/Shutterstock.com

As you set your goals, use the acronym *FITT* to keep your focus on key fitness factors. **FITT** stands for frequency, intensity, time, and type. When using FITT factors, consider the following:

- **Frequency.** Frequency involves how often you engage in physical activity. According to the *Physical Activity Guidelines for Americans*, children and teens need to engage in various aerobic activities every day.
- **Intensity.** Intensity is measured by the amount of energy your body uses per minute while engaging in an activity (**Figure 7.15**). You can judge the intensity of a physical activity by how it affects your heart rate and breathing.

Figure 7.15
Different physical activities performed at different intensities affect the number of calories burned. *If you weighed 100 lbs. and ran at a rate of 6 miles per hour for 30 minutes, how many calories would you burn?*

Approximate Calories Burned in 60 Minutes*

Activity	Calories Burned	Activity	Calories Burned
Running: 6 mph (10 min./mile)	480	Hiking	288
Sergey Novikov/Shutterstock.com		*Blend Images/Shutterstock.com*	
Swimming laps (vigorous)	480	Stretching (yoga)	192
Blacqbook/Shutterstock.com		*wong yu liang/Shutterstock.com*	
Jumping rope	480	Volleyball	144
Pressmaster/Shutterstock.com		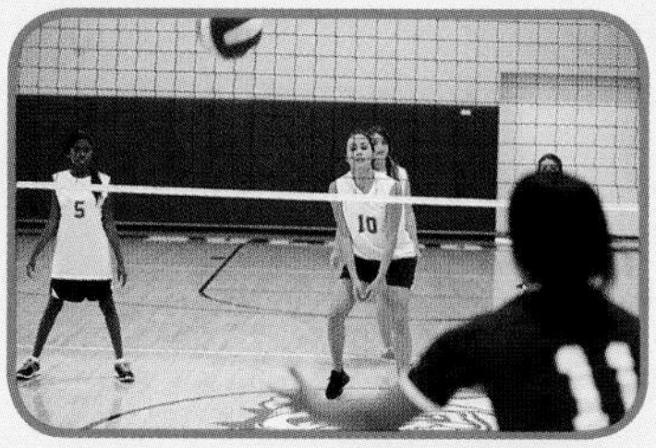 *Monkey Business Images/Shutterstock.com*	
Bicycling: 12–13.9 mph	384	Lifting weights (general)	144
Jacek Chabraszewski/Shutterstock.com		*Rob Marmion/Shutterstock.com*	

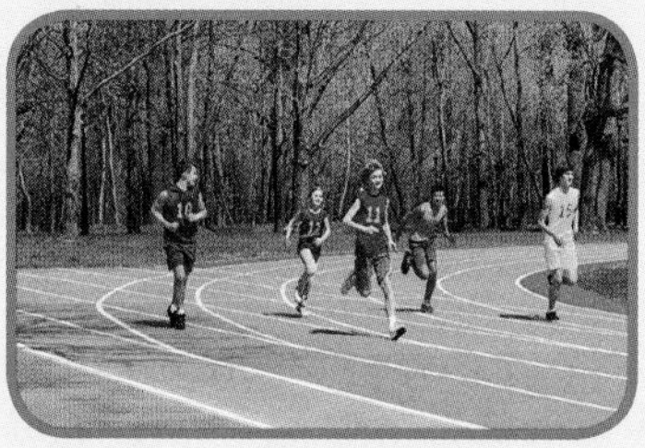

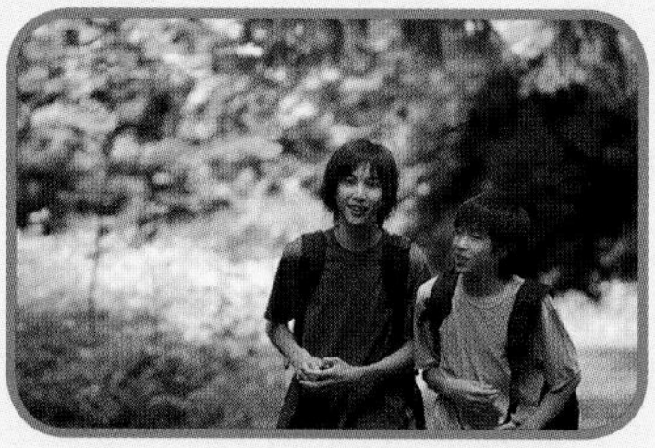

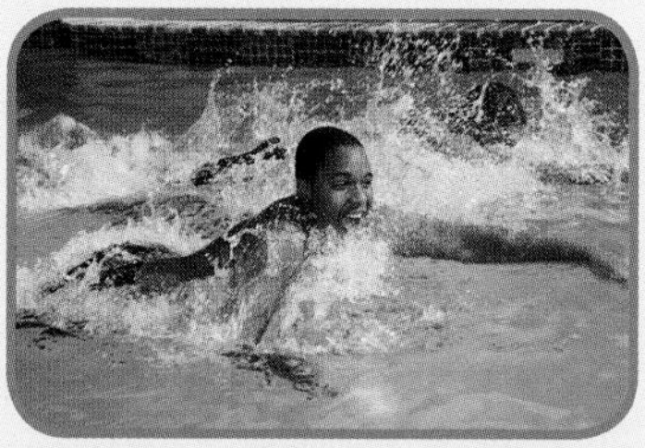

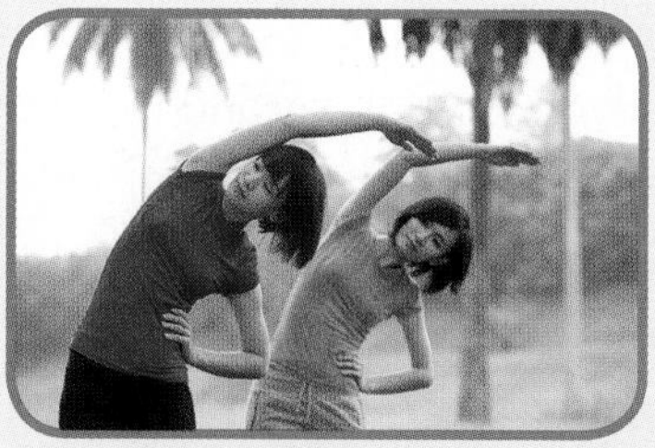

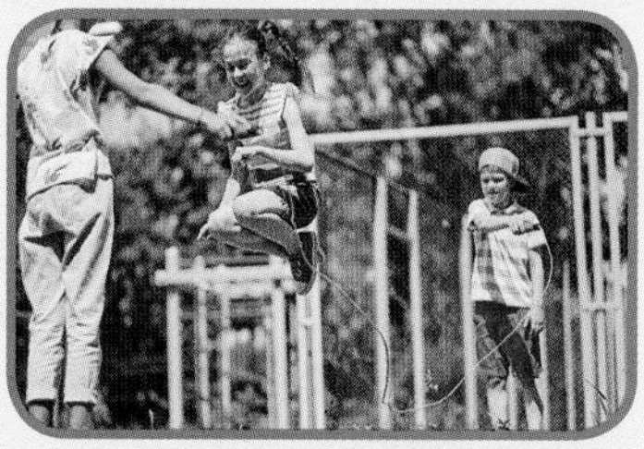

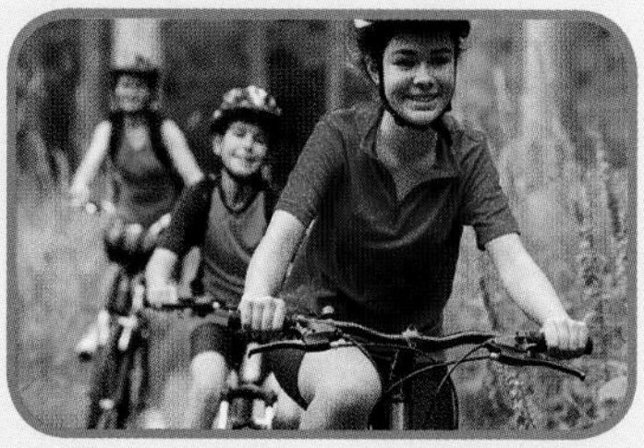

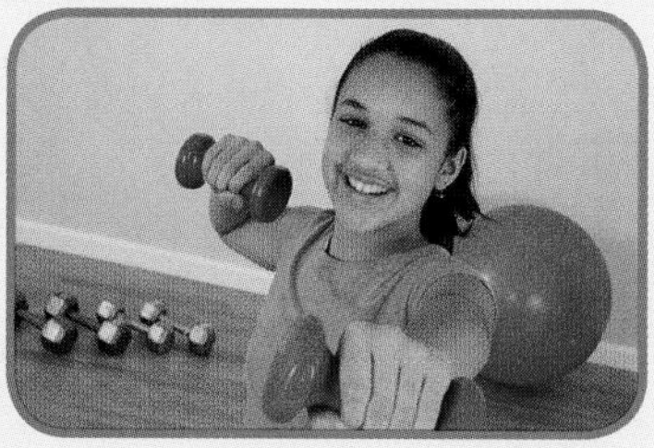

*Based on the average calories burned per hour for a 100-lb. person.

- **Time.** Time refers to the duration of your activity. Children and teens should be active for at least 60 minutes every day. How you choose to use this time depends on your schedule. You may choose to do all 60 minutes at once. Some people, however, prefer to break up their activities into smaller chunks of time. For example, you may do 30 minutes of exercises in PE class. Then, you may take a 30-minute walk after school.
- **Type.** Type refers to the different activities you do. The types of activities you choose to engage in should be ones you enjoy. Choosing activities that you enjoy helps set you up for success in achieving your goals.

Maximizing Your Workouts

Once you have identified and set your fitness goals, you are almost ready to get moving. Before you begin, however, figure out how you want to keep track of your progress. You may want to keep a fitness log or create a spreadsheet to record your progress. Use whatever tracking method works best for you. **Figure 7.16** shows a sample tracking report.

Recording your workouts will ensure that you stay on track with your goals. If a certain exercise is not working for you, or a time of day is not good, you may need to revise your fitness plan. Assess your progress regularly and adjust your goals as needed to ensure success.

Sample Tracking Report				
Day	**Physical Activity**	**Time**	**Achievement**	**Comments**
Sunday				
Monday				
Tuesday				
Wednesday				
Thursday				
Friday				
Saturday				

Figure 7.16
This example of a basic fitness log can help you track your fitness achievements over time. *If your fitness plan is not working for you, what should you do?*

Now that you are ready to start your workout, there are a few important guidelines to remember. In the following sections, you will learn how to make the most of your workouts.

Warm-Ups

No matter what type of physical activity you do, it is important to warm up your muscles before you begin. A simple 5- to 10-minute warm-up helps get much-needed blood to your muscles. This brief warm-up time helps to prevent injuries.

The warm-up should include the following two distinct parts:

- a low-intensity aerobic activity, such as light jogging, jumping jacks, or brisk walking
- at least 5 minutes of muscle stretching, starting at the top of your body and moving to your lower body

Some experts suggest doing a light version of the activity you are about to do as your warm-up. For example, just before a basketball game, you might shoot some baskets and retrieve missed shots. Before a tennis match, you might casually hit some balls back and forth with a partner.

Aerobic Workouts

To maximize your aerobic workouts, you need to perform aerobic activities at a moderate- or vigorous-intensity level. During an activity of *moderate intensity*, your heart rate and breathing are faster than normal, but you can still carry on a conversation. During an activity of *vigorous intensity*, your heart rate and breathing are much faster than normal (**Figure 7.17**). It is difficult to talk during vigorous-intensity activity.

Figure 7.17
You can play basketball at either moderate or vigorous intensity. *How do you know if your activity is of vigorous intensity?*

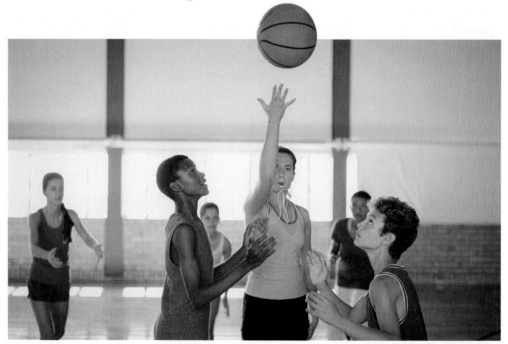

wavebreakmedia/Shutterstock.com

Reaching your **target heart rate** will help you get the best results from your workout. For moderate-intensity activity, a person's target heart rate should be 50 to 70 percent of his or her maximum heart rate. For vigorous-intensity activity, a person's target heart rate should be 70 to 85 percent of his or her maximum heart rate.

What is maximum heart rate? Your **maximum heart rate** is the number of beats per minute your heart can achieve when working its hardest. A single, standard maximum does not exist. A person's maximum heart rate depends on his or her age. There are numerous apps available to help you measure your target and maximum heart rates.

You can also calculate your maximum heart rate by subtracting your age from 220. Once you determine your maximum heart rate, you can calculate your target heart rate for different levels of physical activity. **Figure 7.18** shows how to calculate your maximum heart rate and target heart rates.

Anaerobic Workouts

During anaerobic workouts, you will be performing exercises such as sit-ups, push-ups, pull-ups, and squats. To get the most out of these workouts, do anaerobic exercises for 20 to 30 minutes, two or three times a week. Do not perform any type of anaerobic activity unless you know the proper form for each exercise. Proper form includes holding a position correctly and paying attention to your breathing. Using improper form can lead to injuries and less-than-desirable increases in strength and endurance.

Figure 7.18
Achieving your target heart rate can help you optimize your aerobic workouts.

Calculating Your Maximum and Target Heart Rates

Use the following formula to calculate your maximum heart rate:

220 – age in years = maximum heart rate in beats per minute (bpm)

Example: If you are 13 years of age, you would calculate your maximum heart rate as follows:

220 – 13 = 207 bpm

Multiply your maximum heart rate in bpm by the minimum and maximum levels for moderate- and vigorous-intensity activities to find your target heart rates. Following are the calculations for the example of the 13-year-old:

207 (bpm) x 50% (min. moderate-intensity level) = 103.5

207 (bpm) x 70% (max. moderate-intensity level/ min. vigorous-intensity level) = 144.9

207 (bpm) x 85% (max. vigorous-intensity level) = 175.95

As you can see, a 13-year-old should try to engage in physical activities that cause a heart rate between 104 and 176 bpm. If the goal is moderate-intensity physical activity, this person should maintain a heart rate between 104 and 145 bpm. If the goal is vigorous-intensity physical activity, this person's heart rate should be between 145 and 176 bpm.

The following are some guidelines for achieving anaerobic fitness:

- Start with a 5- to 10-minute warm-up. This includes a low- or moderate-intensity aerobic activity to get blood flowing to your muscles.
- Do two or three **sets** (groups of repetitions followed by rest) of an exercise. For example, you could choose to do three sets of 10 squats.
- As you become stronger, you may choose to do more sets to build muscle endurance.
- Rest your muscles for at least one full day after doing muscle-strengthening exercises. This gives the muscles time to recover.
- Stop right away if you feel sharp pain or experience swollen joints. These are signs that you have done too much. Some muscle soreness is a normal part of exercising. Intense pain, however, indicates a problem.

Cooldowns

A simple 5- to 10-minute cooldown is important after engaging in physical activity. The cooldown helps your heart rate return to a normal, lower level. A cooldown should include some gentle stretching. Stretches help prevent your muscles from feeling stiff and sore the next day. Any light activity can serve as your cooldown. Many people just slow down to low levels of their current activity for a cooldown.

Lesson 7.4 Review

1. Which of the following is a good way to determine your current level of fitness?
   - **A.** Weigh yourself.
   - **B.** Run a marathon.
   - **C.** Test your flexibility.
   - **D.** Take your blood pressure.
2. What does the acronym *FITT* stand for?
3. The maximum _____ _____ is the number of beats per minute a person's heart can achieve when working its hardest.
4. What two parts should be included in a warm-up before physical activity?
5. **Critical thinking.** Why are *FITT* factors important when considering fitness goals?

Hands-On Activity

Using the formulas in Figure 7.18, calculate your maximum heart rate and target heart rate range. Write these numbers on a piece of paper. Then, engage in aerobic activity for 30 minutes, checking your pulse as soon as you finish exercising. Answer the following questions:
- Was your heart rate within your target heart rate range for moderate- or vigorous-intensity exercise?
- Do you need to adjust the intensity level of your exercise to maximize your workout? Why or why not?

Review and Assessment

Summary

Lesson 7.1 — What It Means to Be Physically Fit

- Becoming physically fit is one of the most important actions you can take to promote good health and well-being.
- To become physically fit, you need to get plenty of exercise and physical activity.
- Regular physical activity has many benefits, one of which is increasing your chances of living longer.
- According to the *Physical Activity Guidelines for Americans*, children and teens should get 60 minutes of physical activity every day.

Lesson 7.2 — Fitness Types

- There are two types of fitness: health-related fitness and skill-related fitness.
- The different parts of health-related fitness include heart and lung strength, muscle strength, endurance, flexibility, and body composition.
- *Aerobic exercises* use the heart and lungs together to deliver oxygen to the body's muscles, as in running, dancing, or riding a bike. *Anaerobic exercises* use the energy stored in your muscles for the fuel your body needs, like when you lift weights or do push-ups.
- Skill-related fitness is what you need to play sports or other leisure activities. Aspects of skill-related fitness include speed, agility, balance, power, coordination, and reaction time.

Lesson 7.3 — Fitness Safety

- Knowing and following the rules of activities can help keep you and the people you are playing with safe and free from injury.
- When engaging in physical activities, wear safety equipment to avoid injury. To avoid dehydration, drink lots of water before, during, and after physical activity.
- Exercising or playing sports outside in hot or cold weather can be dangerous if you are not careful. *Hyperthermia* describes heat-related illnesses, and *hypothermia* describes cold-related illnesses, including frostbite.
- First aid for a sprain follows the R.I.C.E. (rest, immobilize, cold, elevate) treatment. For dislocations, fractures, and concussions, seek medical treatment right away.

Lesson 7.4 — A Personal Fitness Plan

- Checking your health-related fitness level will help you identify areas in which you may need to improve.
- The *FITT* factors of frequency, intensity, time, and type are important to remember when setting fitness goals.
- Recording your workouts will ensure that you stay on track with your goals. Assess your progress regularly and adjust your goals as needed to ensure success.
- Doing warm-ups and cooldowns are important to help prevent injuries.

Check Your Knowledge ↗

Record your answers to each of the following questions on a separate sheet of paper.

1. Is walking to school an example of exercise or physical activity?
2. People who spend much of their days doing activities that involve sitting and using very little energy are being _____.
3. **True or false.** Adults should get one hour of physical activity daily.
4. Most of a teen's activity each day should be spent doing _____ (anaerobic/aerobic) activities.
5. **True or false.** Anaerobic activities occur in short bursts, while aerobic activities occur over a longer stretch of time.
6. Which type of fitness refers to the kind of fitness a person needs to successfully perform a sport or leisure activity?
7. What safety equipment is necessary when playing football?
8. The loss of too much fluid from the body causes a condition called _____.
9. A condition in which bones move out of their normal position is called a _____.
   A. dislocation   C. sprain
   B. fracture   D. concussion
10. Which of the following is *not* one of the FITT factors?
    A. Time.   C. Frequency.
    B. Temperature.   D. Intensity.
11. Shooting some baskets and retrieving missed shots before you play a game of basketball is an example of a(n) _____ activity.
12. **True or false.** Reaching your maximum heart rate will help you get the best results from your workout.

Use Your Vocabulary ↗

aerobic exercise	frostbite	pulse
anaerobic exercise	health-related fitness	resistance
concussion	hyperthermia	sedentary
dislocation	hypothermia	sets
endurance	intensity	skill-related fitness
exercise	maximum heart rate	sprain
fitness	physical activity	target heart rate
FITT	*Physical Activity Guidelines*	
fracture	*for Americans*	

13. Write each of the terms above on a separate sheet of paper. For each term, quickly write a word that you think relates to the term. In small groups, exchange papers. Have each person in the group explain a term on the list. Take turns until all terms have complete explanations.
14. Choose four words from the list above. On a separate sheet of paper, write a paragraph correctly using all four of these words. Read your paragraphs in class.

Think Critically

15. **Evaluate.** What could you do to make sedentary activities more active? Give a detailed response providing several examples.

16. **Determine.** Does a person need to be thin or lean to be physically fit? Provide a detailed answer.

17. **Identify.** Identify reasons some teens are fit and physically active while others are not.

18. **Draw conclusions.** Why are teens less likely to follow safety rules such as wearing a helmet while skateboarding or wearing reflective gear at night while biking?

DEVELOP Your Skills

19. **Advocacy and leadership skills.** For years, school districts across the United States have discussed eliminating PE in elementary schools to reduce the school district budget and allow more time for core subjects, such as reading and math. Imagine your former elementary school is considering this change. As a former student, you want to advocate and be the voice for the younger students who will be impacted. Write a letter to your state senator to voice your concerns. Include the following information in your letter: five or more benefits of exercise (include ones that are personal to you), the physical activity guidelines for children based on the *Physical Activity Guidelines for Americans*, how you were personally impacted by your PE experience in elementary school, and other relevant information.

20. **Access information and technology skills.** Investigate current fitness-based apps. Begin by searching best fitness apps for kids. In small groups, choose one app that you feel is the best one for teens. The app should be fun, increase motivation to exercise, and include a variety of exercises. Create a presentation about your app highlighting three appealing features and three benefits to using the app. Present it to the class.

21. **Communication and goal-setting skills.** Talk with your family about their daily exercise habits and health-related fitness. Discuss current obstacles and ways to overcome them. As a family, create a plan to improve family health. This plan may include opportunities to exercise alone, with one family member, or as an entire family. Display your plan in a visible place in your house.

22. **Decision-making skills.** In the last couple of years, many parents are questioning whether to allow their children to play football due to the short- and long-term effects of concussions. Some professional football players have dropped out of the NFL claiming that the benefit of playing football does not outweigh the risks associated with the game. Imagine you are a parent and your son is begging you to play football. Would you allow him to play? Do additional research on the impact of repetitive concussions and decide if you would let him play. Write an essay reflecting on the following questions: Would you let him play tackle football? Does the benefit of playing football outweigh the risk of concussions? What is the benefit of playing? What are the short- and long-term effects of concussions?

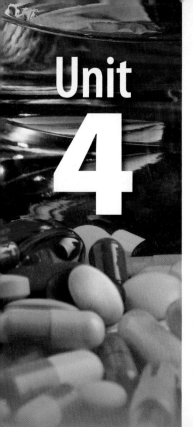

Unit 4

Understanding and Avoiding Hazardous Substances

Warm-Up Activity

Pros and Cons

While in middle school, you may encounter a situation in which you are asked to try tobacco, alcohol, or other drugs. Read each of the scenarios below. Then, on a separate sheet of paper, list all of the possible pros and cons to each of the scenarios from the person's perspective in the scenario. Consider short-term and long-term pros and cons if this behavior continues. Share your answers with a partner. Add to your pros and cons list based on your partner's responses.

During this unit, you will learn more about tobacco, alcohol, and other drugs. After you finish reading the chapters, revisit these scenarios and add to or change your answers.

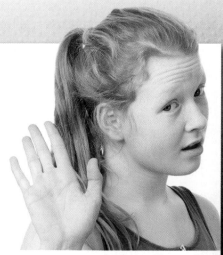

Pete Pahham/Shutterstock.com

Scenario 1
While at overnight camp, one of Maria's roommates pulls out a pack of cigarettes from her suitcase. Maria has never tried a cigarette before and wonders what it would be like to smoke one.

Scenario 2
Mason's parents trusted him and his friend, James, to stay home while they went to dinner. While Mason plays video games, James explores the house until he finds the liquor cabinet. James breaks the lock and takes two big gulps of liquor, then offers it to Mason. Mason does not want James to tease him for not drinking.

Scenario 3
While at the school dance, several of Kristina's friends invite her to meet in the bathroom to smoke marijuana. Not wanting to be left out, Kristina walks with her friends to the bathroom.

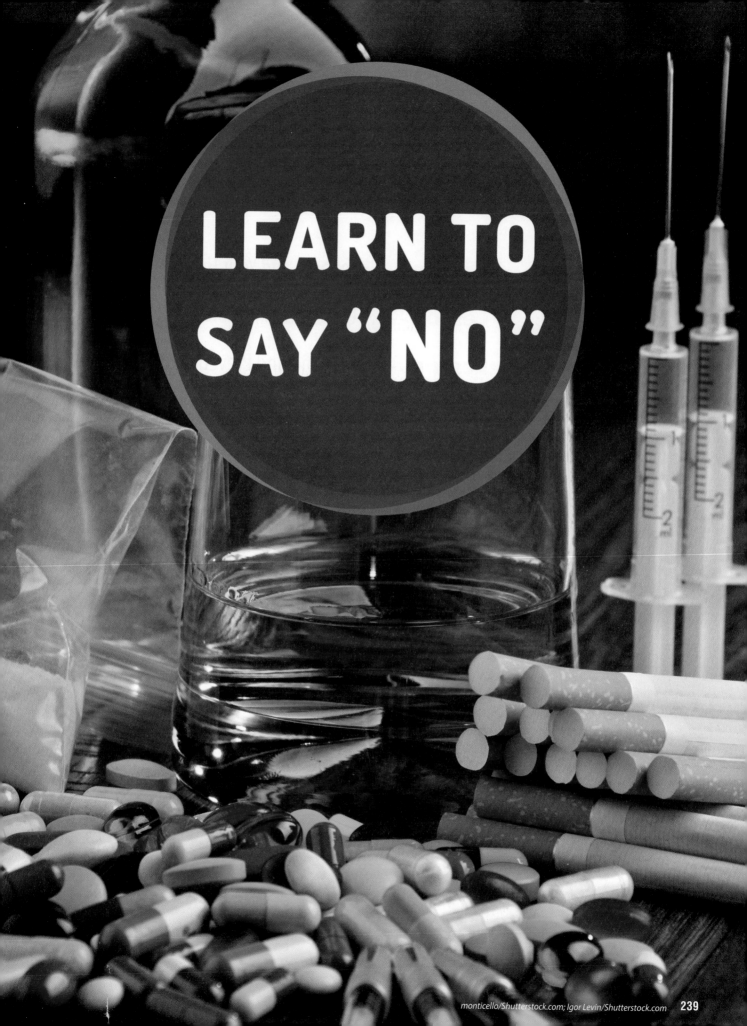

LEARN TO SAY "NO"

Chapter 8

Tobacco

Essential Question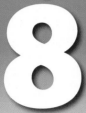

How is tobacco hazardous to the human body?

Video ↗
Access the Chapter 8 video to start thinking about chapter topics.

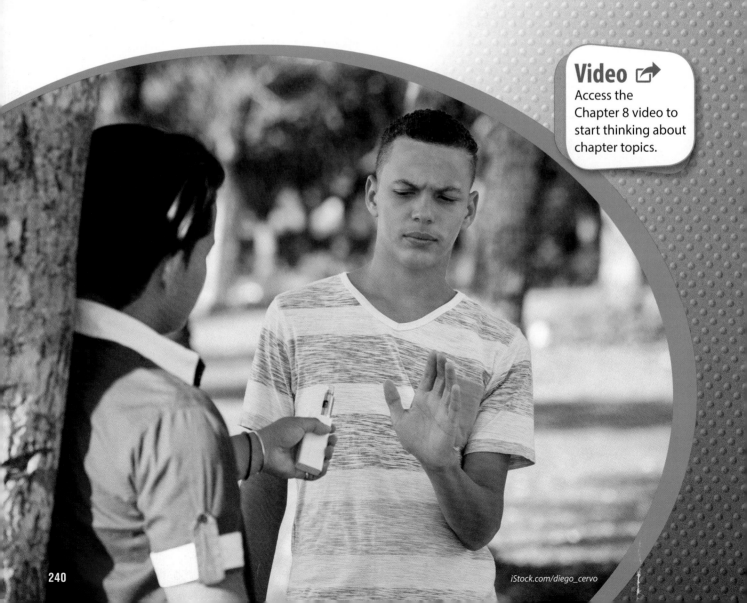

iStock.com/diego_cervo

Reading Activity

In what ways do you think tobacco is harmful to your health? Before reading the chapter, write a two-paragraph essay explaining some of the health effects of tobacco. After you finish reading the chapter, consider what information you might add to your essay. Share your essay and any additions with a partner.

How Healthy Are You? ⬏

In this chapter, you will be learning about tobacco. Before you begin reading, take the following quiz to assess your current tobacco habits.

Healthy Choices	Yes	No
Do you refuse to use tobacco products, such as cigarettes, electronic nicotine delivery systems (ENDS) or e-cigarettes, cigars, pipes, or chewing tobacco?		
Do you avoid exposure to secondhand smoke whenever possible?		
Can you identify the many, severe health hazards of using tobacco products?		
Do you understand the financial, social, and physical costs of smoking?		
Are you confident in your ability to say "no" to friends or peers who ask if you want to smoke?		
Can you recognize the signs and symptoms of nicotine addiction?		
Do you understand the danger of beginning to "experiment" with tobacco product use?		
Can you identify the symptoms of withdrawal from nicotine?		
Do you know the best techniques for quitting tobacco use?		
Can you evaluate the messages you see in tobacco advertisements and the products sold by tobacco companies to avoid manipulation?		

Count your "Yes" and "No" responses. The more "Yes" responses you have, the more healthy tobacco habits you exhibit. Now, take a closer look at the questions with which you responded "No." How can you make these healthy habits part of your daily life? Think about how implementing these ideas can help improve your overall health.

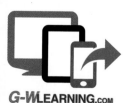

G-WLEARNING.com

While studying this chapter, look for the activity icon ⬏ to

- **practice** key terms with e-flash cards and matching activities.
- **reinforce** what you learn by completing graphic organizers, self-assessment quizzes, and review questions.
- **expand** knowledge with interactive activities and activities that extend learning.

Tobacco and Your Health

Learning Outcomes

After studying this lesson, you will be able to

- **identify** various forms of tobacco and the addictive substance in tobacco products.
- **assess** the hazardous effects of tobacco use on heart and lungs.
- **describe** how tobacco use can affect a person's appearance.
- **explain** the impact of secondhand smoke on individuals.

Graphic Organizer 🡒

Tobacco Cause and Effect

Create a graphic organizer like the one below to connect information about tobacco products to the effects they can have on your health. Add as much information as you can, and make your columns as long as you need them to be.

Stuart Miles/Shutterstock.com

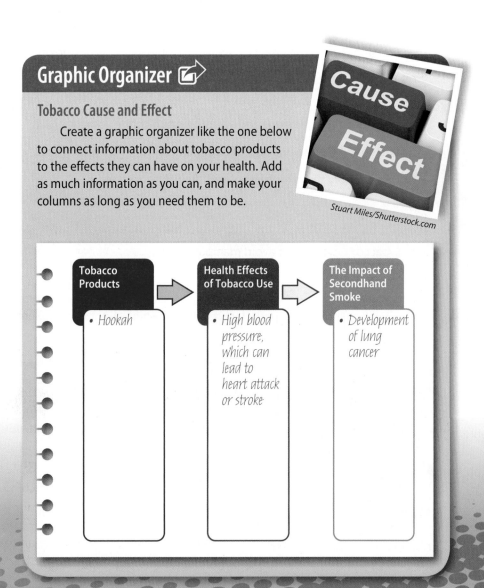

Tobacco Products	Health Effects of Tobacco Use	The Impact of Secondhand Smoke
• Hookah	• High blood pressure, which can lead to heart attack or stroke	• Development of lung cancer

Olivia is 13 years old and is around people who smoke all the time. Her parents smoke cigarettes, even inside the house and car. Someone is always smoking near her during family parties so she has gotten used to the smell. Even though her parents tell her not to smoke, she wonders how bad it can be if they do it.

Catalina is 11 years old and is grateful that her family does not smoke tobacco. She thinks it smells terrible and knows how bad it can be for your health. One of her peers has recently started vaping, however. Catalina thought that might not be bad for her health since there is not any tobacco.

Are Olivia and Catalina's assumptions about smoking correct? What mistakes are they making that may impact their health and wellness?

Smoking is the leading cause of preventable death in the United States. Smokers and the people around them experience many health issues (**Figure 8.1**). This lesson examines different types of tobacco products, the physical effects of tobacco use on the body, and the health impact of being around others who smoke.

Tobacco Products

Tobacco is a plant used to create tobacco-related products, such as cigarettes and chewing tobacco. Tobacco leaves contain the chemical **nicotine**. This toxic substance makes tobacco products **addictive** (habit-forming).

Smoking cigarettes is the most common method of using tobacco. Other methods include cigars, pipes, and smokeless tobacco. Newer methods of tobacco use include electronic nicotine delivery systems (ENDS) such as vaporizers and electronic cigarettes (e-cigarettes). Some people believe that these other methods of tobacco use are safer, healthier, or less addictive than regular cigarettes. The reality is that all forms of tobacco use may cause addiction and serious health issues.

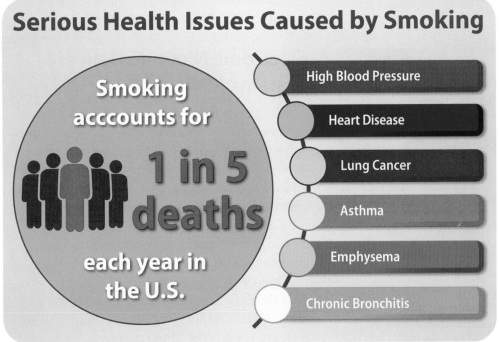

Serious Health Issues Caused by Smoking

Smoking acccounts for

1 in 5 deaths

each year in the U.S.

High Blood Pressure

Heart Disease

Lung Cancer

Asthma

Emphysema

Chronic Bronchitis

Andy Dune/Shutterstock.com

Figure 8.1
Smoking can cause many health issues, which can help explain why so many deaths in the United States are a result of smoking.

Chemicals Found in Cigarettes

Chemical	Other Locations
Acetic acid	Ingredient in hair dye
Acetone	Found in nail polish remover
Ammonia	Common household cleaner
Arsenic	Used in rat poison
Benzene	Found in rubber cement
Butane	Used in lighter fluid
Cadmium	Active component in battery acid
Carbon monoxide	Released in car exhaust fumes
Formaldehyde	Embalming fluid
Hexamine	Found in barbecue lighter fluid
Lead	Used in batteries
Methanol	Main component in rocket fuel
Naphthalene	Ingredient in mothballs
Nicotine	Used as insecticide
Tar	Material for paving roads
Toluene	Used to manufacture paint

Figure 8.2 Cigarettes are made of deadly chemicals that can all cause harm to the body.

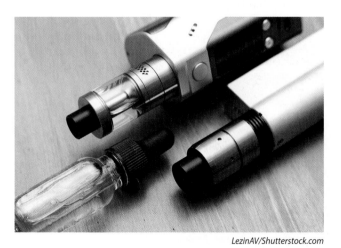

LezinAV/Shutterstock.com

Figure 8.3 While cigarette use has declined in recent years, the use of ENDS has nearly doubled. ***What substance in ENDS causes addiction?***

Cigarettes

A *cigarette* consists of finely cut tobacco, chemical additives, a filter, and a paper wrapping. Cigarettes are the most common method of tobacco use. When a person smokes a cigarette, he or she inhales 7,000 chemicals and **toxic** (poisonous) substances that harm the body (**Figure 8.2**).

The purpose of the filter on a cigarette is to minimize the smoke a person inhales. Modern filters, however, only hold back a small portion of smoke. These filters do not make cigarettes healthier or safer.

Smokeless Tobacco

Smokeless tobacco is a type of tobacco a person chews, inhales, or dissolves rather than smokes. People absorb the nicotine in smokeless tobacco through their mouth tissues. Like cigarettes, smokeless tobacco contains many chemicals, toxic substances, and carcinogens that can harm the body. Forms of smokeless tobacco include the following:

- Chewing tobacco involves placing wads, or *plugs*, of tobacco leaves between the cheeks and gums.
- Snuff is a finely cut or powdered tobacco that a person inhales or places between the cheek and gums.
- Dissolvable tobacco consists of flavored liquid drops, strips, or sticks that a person places in his or her mouth.

Electronic Nicotine Delivery Systems (ENDS)

Electronic nicotine delivery systems (ENDS) are devices that convert nicotine and flavored liquids into a vapor. Types of ENDS include vaporizers, vape pens, electronic cigarettes, hookah pens, e-pipes, and others (**Figure 8.3**). ENDS are the most commonly used tobacco product among youth.

Electronic cigarettes, or *e-cigarettes*, use cartridges of liquid that contain nicotine, flavorings, and other chemicals. The battery-powered e-cigarette contains a heating device. This device warms the liquid in the cartridge and converts it into a vapor. This is why using e-cigarettes is often called *vaping*.

Unlike regular cigarettes, ENDS do not use any actual tobacco. This means that ENDS users inhale fewer toxic chemicals than regular cigarette smokers. ENDS, however, still provide nicotine and contain an unhealthy dose of chemicals that can harm the body.

Health Effects of Tobacco Use

On average, long-term tobacco users die 13 to 15 years earlier than people who do not use tobacco products. Tobacco use increases a person's risk for developing a number of major health conditions like cancer, heart disease, and breathing problems. In the following sections, you will learn how tobacco use affects a person's heart and blood vessels, lungs, and even appearance.

Heart and Blood Vessels

The *circulatory system* includes the heart and blood vessels in the body (**Figure 8.4**). (You will learn more about the circulatory system in Chapter 17.) Health issues such as heart disease and high blood pressure affect the circulatory system. People who use tobacco products have a higher risk of developing these health issues than people who do not use tobacco products. Tobacco users are also twice as likely as non-tobacco users to die from a heart attack.

When people use any form of tobacco, nicotine enters their bloodstream. Nicotine triggers the release of the hormone *adrenaline*, which increases nervous activity in the body. Adrenaline causes an increase in heart rate, breathing rate, and blood pressure. As a result, the heart works harder to pump blood faster around the body. This puts stress on the heart, making heart disease more likely.

Nicotine also causes the blood vessels to *constrict*, or narrow. The heart must work harder to pump blood through narrowed vessels. Gradually, nicotine causes changes in the blood vessels. These changes make it easier for fatty substances to build up in the arteries. Fatty deposits restrict the movement of blood. Buildup of fatty substances can disrupt the overall flow of blood through the body.

Over time, more nicotine in the body leads to more buildup of fatty substances. This buildup increases the risk of a heart attack or stroke. These health emergencies occur when an artery becomes completely blocked.

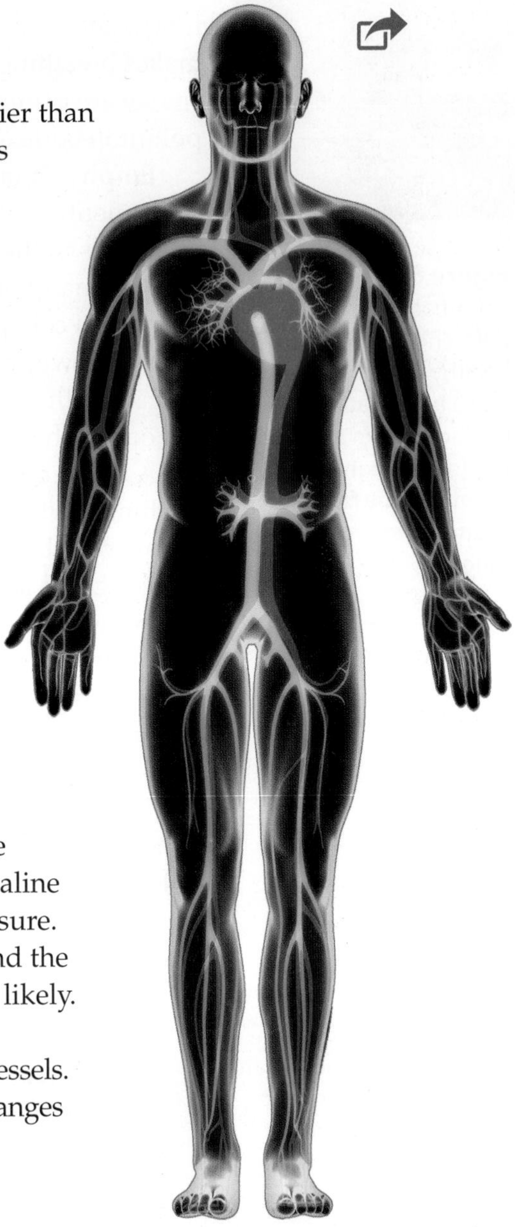

CLIPAREA | Custom media/Shutterstock.com

Figure 8.4 As tobacco enters the bloodstream, blood vessels carry the carcinogens throughout the entire body. *How does nicotine affect blood vessels and increase heart problems?*

Lungs

The *respiratory system* includes the lungs, as well as other structures that you will learn more about in Chapter 17. Smoking damages the respiratory system and makes breathing more difficult.

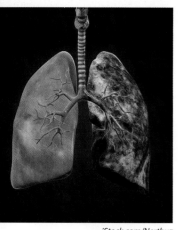

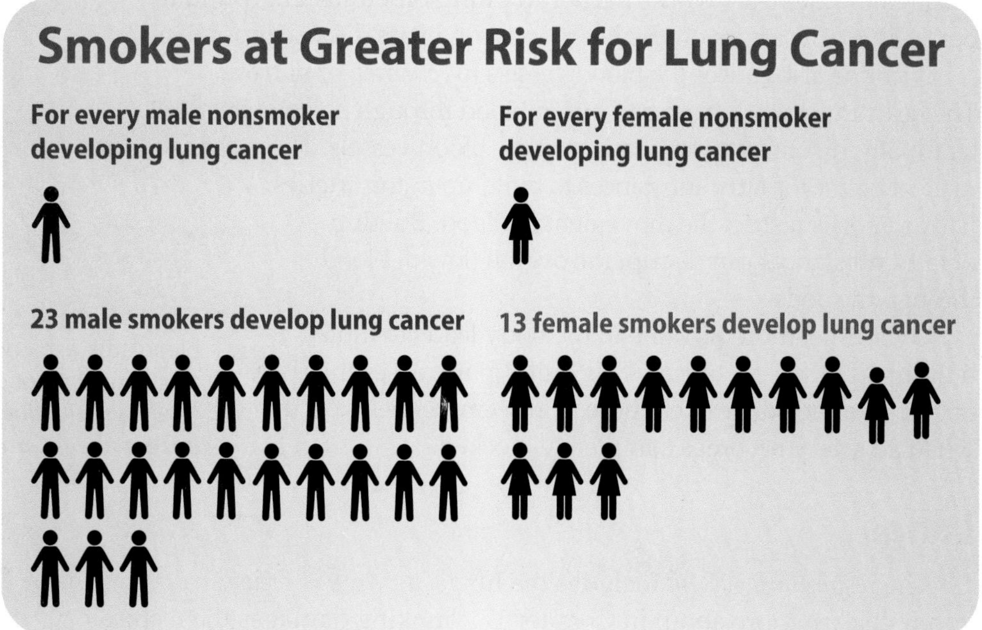

AlexHliv/Shutterstock.com

iStock.com/Nerthuz

Figure 8.5
This image shows the difference between a healthy lung (on the left) and a lung that has been damaged from tobacco use (on the right).
What residue from tobacco damages the lungs?

Burning tobacco produces a residue known as **tar**. This substance consists of small, thick, sticky particles. As smoke repeatedly passes through the respiratory system, tar builds up in the lungs (**Figure 8.5**). Smoking-related damage to the lungs contributes to the development of chronic respiratory diseases and can trigger asthma attacks. It can also lead to lung cancer.

Chronic bronchitis is an ongoing condition in which small tubes in the lungs, known as *bronchioles*, become swollen and irritated. This condition makes breathing more and more difficult. Smoking and inhaling secondhand smoke are primary causes of chronic bronchitis. Regularly inhaling air pollution adds to the condition as well.

Emphysema is a disease that causes the airways in the lungs to become permanently enlarged. This enlargement results from damage to the *alveoli*, or air sacs in the lungs. Typically, the lungs contain many small alveoli, which provide many places for air to enter the lungs. In a person with emphysema, the alveoli collapse and create large air spaces, meaning that air enters the lungs in fewer places. This reduces the amount of oxygen that can enter the lungs and the bloodstream. As a result, people with emphysema are frequently out of breath. Smoking is the most common cause of this condition.

Asthma is a chronic disease caused by blockages of the airflow to and from the lungs. When a person with asthma inhales tobacco smoke, the lining of the airways becomes irritated. This irritation can then cause an asthma attack. Smoking and secondhand smoke can cause this type of irritation.

Lung cancer occurs when abnormal cells in one or both lungs grow rapidly and form a mass of cells, which is called a *tumor*. This growth usually happens in the cells that line the air passages. As the tumors grow, they interfere with the lungs' ability to transport oxygen to the bloodstream. Tumors can also spread from the lungs to other parts of the body.

Tobacco smoke contains over 70 **carcinogens**, or cancer-causing agents, that can lead to the abnormal growth of cells in the mouth, throat, and lungs. This is why smokers have higher rates of cancer than nonsmokers (**Figure 8.6**).

Figure 8.6
Men who smoke are 23 times more likely to develop lung cancer than men who do not smoke. Women are 13 times more likely, compared to nonsmokers.

Smokers at Greater Risk for Lung Cancer

For every male nonsmoker developing lung cancer

For every female nonsmoker developing lung cancer

23 male smokers develop lung cancer

13 female smokers develop lung cancer

Cancers Caused by Smoking

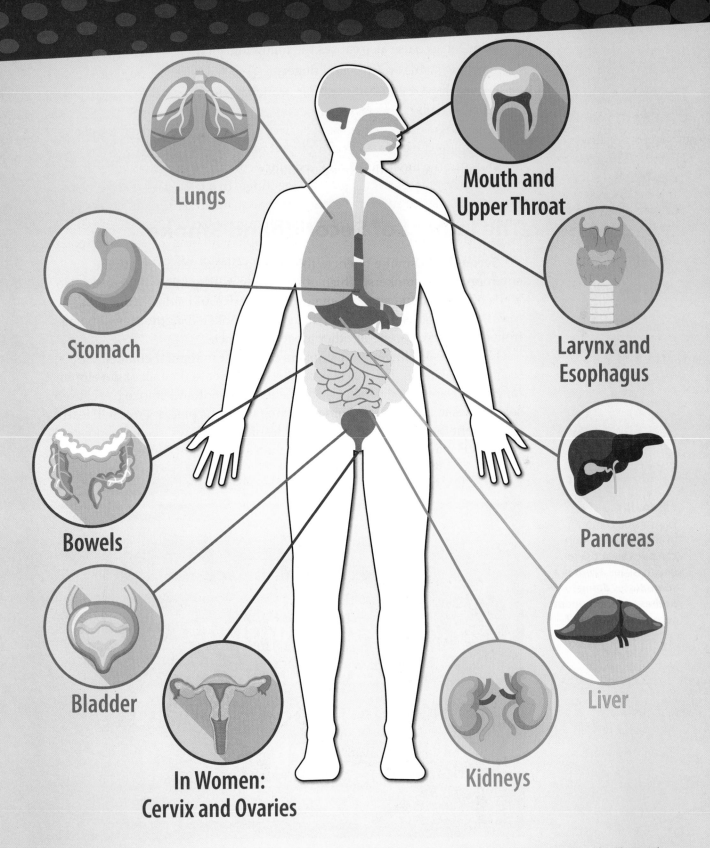

Lungs

Mouth and Upper Throat

Stomach

Larynx and Esophagus

Bowels

Pancreas

Bladder

Liver

In Women: Cervix and Ovaries

Kidneys

Larynx and esophagus icon: AlexHliv/Shutterstock.com; Pancreas and stomach icons: Rvector/Shutterstock.com; Cervix and ovaries: Nadia Buravleva/Shutterstock.com; Other body part icons: Macrovector/Shutterstock.com; Body: elenabsl/Shutterstock.com

Appearance

Tobacco use not only causes many problems inside the body, but it also affects a person's outward appearance. People who smoke for at least 10 years show more wrinkles in their skin. This is because of the effect nicotine has on blood vessels. As blood vessels get smaller, oxygen and nutrients cannot reach the skin. Tobacco use also causes the following:

- yellow stains on teeth and fingers
- gum disease and bad breath
- brittle nails
- hair loss
- sagging skin
- clothes and hair that smell of smoke

The Impact of Secondhand Smoke

Secondhand smoke refers to the tobacco smoke released into the environment by smokers, which other people nearby inhale. There are two kinds of secondhand smoke—mainstream smoke and sidestream smoke. *Mainstream smoke* is the smoke exhaled by a smoker. *Sidestream smoke* comes from a burning cigarette or other tobacco product.

Living or socializing with smokers can result in regular contact with secondhand smoke. This regular contact can increase the risk of developing lung cancer or heart disease. Concern about secondhand smoke has caused some states to pass laws banning smoking in public places. (You will learn more about these laws in Lesson 8.3.) Despite these laws, secondhand smoke still affects many people in the United States each year (**Figure 8.7**).

Figure 8.7
Even a small amount of secondhand smoke can put you at risk for health issues. *What are some states doing to address concern about secondhand smoke?*

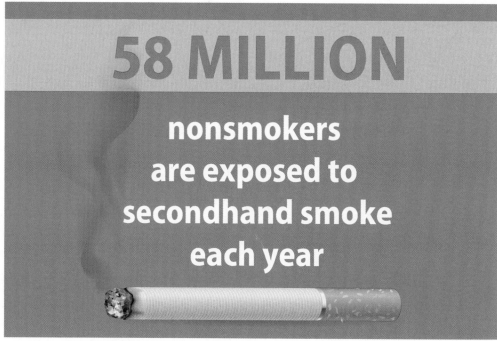

58 MILLION

nonsmokers are exposed to secondhand smoke each year

The health concerns related to secondhand smoke are serious. In children, exposure to secondhand smoke can cause ear infections, asthma attacks, bronchitis, and pneumonia. More than 300,000 children suffer each year from these conditions due to secondhand smoke exposure. In adults, health risks include heart disease, lung cancer, and stroke.

Exposure to nicotine is particularly dangerous for a *fetus*, or unborn baby. When a pregnant woman smokes, nicotine and carbon monoxide pass to the fetus. Women who smoke while pregnant increase their risk of *miscarriage* (loss of pregnancy). In addition, their babies may be born too early or with low birthweight.

The risk of *sudden infant death syndrome (SIDS)* is also higher among babies born to mothers who smoked or breathed secondhand smoke during pregnancy. SIDS is the unexpected and sudden death of a baby less than one year after birth.

To maintain good health, avoid exposure to secondhand smoke whenever possible. Choose restaurants and other public places that do not allow smoking. If someone is smoking near you, leave the area or ask the person to stop smoking. If your parents or friends smoke, consider explaining the health risks to them and ask them to stop. You might just convince them to quit!

Lesson 8.1 Review

1. What is the name of the toxic and addictive chemical contained in tobacco?

2. **True or false.** On average, long-term tobacco users die 13 to 15 years earlier than people who do not use tobacco products.

3. Smokers have higher rates of cancer than nonsmokers due to the _____ in tobacco smoke.

4. Name two examples of effects tobacco use can have on your outward appearance.

5. **Critical thinking.** Consider the different kinds of secondhand smoke and the health effects it can have on your body even if you do not smoke. How often are you exposed to secondhand smoke? How can you set boundaries about smoking with your family or friends?

Hands-On Activity

Create a new design for the front and back of a pack of cigarettes aimed to prevent smoking. You may sketch this design on paper or use a computer to create a digital design. Include the following on your cigarette pack:

- brand
- chemicals and poisons contained in a cigarette
- health problems caused by smoking
- graphic anti-tobacco pictures
- other information you feel would discourage someone from buying a pack of cigarettes

Key Terms ☞

peer pressure influence that people your age have on your actions

addiction physical and psychological need for a substance or behavior

tolerance effect that occurs when the body needs more and more of a substance to experience the desired effects

dependence effect that occurs when the body needs an addictive substance in its system to function "normally" or feel "normal"

triggers reminders that cause people to feel a strong desire for a substance

withdrawal unpleasant symptoms that occur when someone addicted to a substance tries to stop using that substance

Learning Outcomes

After studying this lesson, you will be able to

- **summarize** the factors that cause teens to try smoking.
- **analyze** the stages of addiction in relation to tobacco use.
- **describe** two types of dependence.
- **give examples** of withdrawal symptoms people with a nicotine addiction may experience.

Graphic Organizer ☞

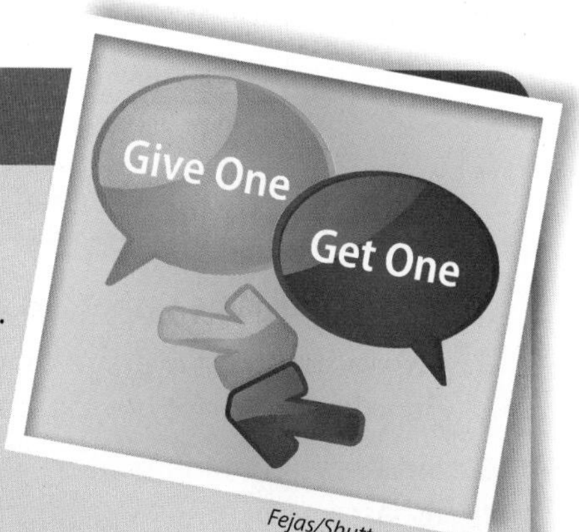

Give One, Get One

Create a table like the one shown below. Include as many rows as you need. Before reading the lesson, list facts you already know about people's tobacco use in the *Give One* column. In the *Get One* column, list facts you learn as you read the lesson. After you finish reading the lesson, team up with a classmate and discuss each other's lists. Are there items you would add to your list?

Fejas/Shutterstock.com

Give One (facts I already know)	Get One (new information)
Peer pressure can lead to experimenting with tobacco use.	Good friends can use positive peer pressure instead to encourage healthy behaviors.

In the previous lesson, you learned about health issues associated with tobacco use. You also learned that secondhand smoke puts family members and friends of smokers at risk for health issues. Given these facts, you may wonder why anyone would start smoking or using other tobacco products. Unfortunately, more than 30 million people in the United States smoke cigarettes (**Figure 8.8**).

Consider Catalina and Olivia from the previous lesson. Catalina sees her peers and people on social media vaping. She thinks it looks cool and is considering experimenting with it. Olivia is more likely to try smoking since her family environment encourages that behavior. Olivia's parents, however, would tell her that they would like to quit smoking, and have tried to quit before, but find it too difficult.

In this lesson, you will learn about several factors that may cause someone to try smoking. These factors include the influence of parents, friends, and the media. This lesson also discusses the difficulties a person faces when trying to quit smoking.

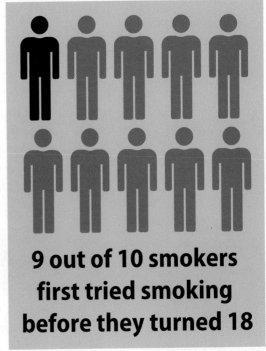

9 out of 10 smokers first tried smoking before they turned 18

Visual Generations/Shutterstock.com

Figure 8.8 The majority of people who smoke tried their first cigarette before age 18.

Why Young People Try Smoking

Unfortunately, more young people start to smoke each day. Most young people who begin to smoke do plan to quit. They believe that quitting will be easy. They soon find out, however, that smoking is a very hard habit to break. The majority of young people who smoke become adults who regularly smoke.

Various factors may cause a young person to try smoking (**Figure 8.9**). These factors include identity exploration, parents and environment, peer pressure, and the media.

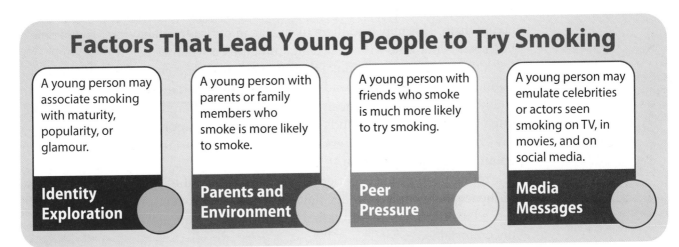

Figure 8.9 Many influences can cause a young person to consider smoking, despite the health risks.

Identity Exploration

Some young people start to smoke as a way of trying out a new identity. Young people may associate smoking with maturity, popularity, or glamour. They may believe that smoking will make them seem older or cooler. Young people may also begin smoking because they want others to view them as rebellious and tough. They buy cigarettes even though doing so is illegal for middle school students and most high school students.

Most young people do not view smokers as popular or cool, however. Surveys have found that young people see smokers as unhealthy and foolish. In fact, avoiding smoking rather than trying it may make you seem more mature.

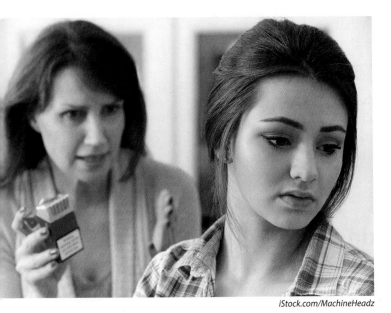

iStock.com/MachineHeadz

Figure 8.10 Parents who set clear rules and consequences to smoking are less likely to have children experiment with smoking.

Parents and Environment

Parents' attitudes and behaviors about smoking strongly influence whether or not young people smoke. Young people are much less likely to start smoking if their parents set clear expectations. This means parents must discuss and follow through on consequences for smoking (**Figure 8.10**).

Parents' attitudes toward smoking create an environment that influences young people's behavior. Some parents are strongly against smoking. These parents are not smokers, and they may prohibit guests from smoking in the house. In this environment, young people are less likely to smoke. Other parents are more open-minded toward smoking, and may even smoke in the home environment. Young people in this environment are more likely to try smoking.

Peer Pressure

During the school-age years, the influence of friends can be much stronger than the influence of family members. Most young people want their friends to accept them. This may lead them to engage in unhealthy behaviors. The people you spend your time with have a big influence on whether you try smoking.

Many young people smoke their first cigarette or e-cigarette with a friend. Young people who have friends who smoke are much more likely to try smoking. Young people whose friends smoke are offered cigarettes much more often than those whose friends do not smoke. It is important to learn how to say "no" when someone offers you tobacco products. (You will learn more about this in the next lesson.)

Young people may experience peer pressure to smoke. **Peer pressure** is the influence that people your age have on your actions. Peer pressure is negative if used to encourage an individual to do something unsafe, unhealthy, or uncomfortable.

Young people may worry that not smoking means others will not like or accept them. If someone forces you to try smoking, he or she is not really your friend. Real friends do not want their friends to engage in unhealthy behaviors.

Sometimes peer pressure is positive (**Figure 8.11**). You can use the influence you have over your friends to encourage them to practice healthy behaviors.

Media Messages

You are constantly receiving messages from the media. These messages may be commercials you see on TV or ads that you see on the Internet. Companies are always trying to get you to buy their products. This includes companies that sell tobacco products. Young people are more likely to want to try new products after seeing ads about them.

Think about your favorite celebrity or athlete and the image he or she presents to others (**Figure 8.12**). If your role model engages in healthy behaviors, copying what he or she does can have a positive effect on your health and wellness.

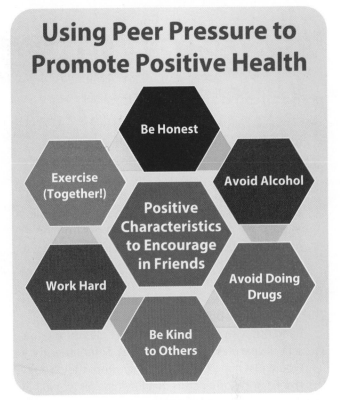

Figure 8.11 There are many ways peer pressure can be used to inspire healthy behaviors. Encouraging your friends not to smoke is one example. *Give an example of a time when you influenced someone, or were influenced by someone else, with positive peer pressure.*

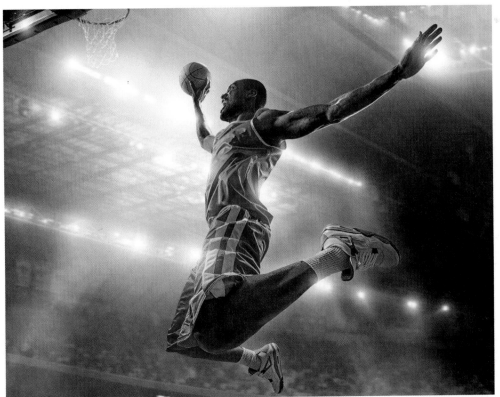

iStock.com/peepo

Figure 8.12
Young people often want to copy what their favorite celebrity wears, eats, or drinks. If a celebrity publicly smokes, this may cause his or her fans to want to try this action, too. *Who is your favorite celebrity role model? Is this person a positive influence? Why or why not?*

Kevin's First Cigarette

Kevin did not think it was that big of a deal when he tried his first cigarette. It was at the beginning of last school year. He was waiting after school for his mom to pick him up and an older group of boys dared him to smoke. His friend Max was standing next to Kevin, and he chose to walk away. Kevin recognized two of the boys from his neighborhood so he did not think it was a big deal. Secretly, he hoped that he would fit in with the older boys and maybe they would think he was cool.

The older boys did ask Kevin if he wanted to hang out with them several more times during the school year. Kevin always said yes. Sometimes they would just hang out, while other times they would smoke or do other stuff that Kevin never would have done with his old friends like Max.

Today, Kevin is grounded and his parents are so disappointed. Kevin and the older boys were caught vandalizing an old abandoned building. Kevin did not think this was a good idea, but he went along with the other boys anyway. The police checked their pockets and one of his friends had cigarettes. The police turned them over to their parents and Kevin confessed everything. He was tired of keeping secrets.

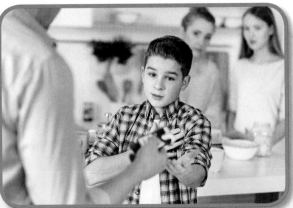

iStock.com/yacobchuk

He wishes he could go back in time. He would not have smoked that cigarette. Instead, he would have just walked away with Max.

Thinking Critically

1. Why does experimenting with one risky behavior, such as tobacco use, often lead to other risky behaviors?

2. Kevin wanted to fit in and be accepted by older boys. What are positive ways to fit in and feel accepted within a group?

3. If you were Max, what could you have said to Kevin before he accepted his first cigarette?

4. What are two ways that Kevin could have respectfully and assertively refused the cigarette?

Does your role model smoke or engage in other unhealthy behaviors? Imitating the smoking habit or other unhealthy behaviors of a celebrity you admire can negatively impact your overall health. This is why it is so important to choose your role models carefully.

Why Quitting Smoking Is Difficult

Most people cannot use tobacco in a casual way. It is much more likely that a person will become addicted to tobacco. As mentioned earlier, the nicotine found in tobacco is an addictive substance. Nicotine makes cigarettes, e-cigarettes, chewing tobacco, and other tobacco products addictive. Tobacco users develop a physical and psychological need for nicotine. This means that the body and mind both crave the feeling that nicotine creates. Addiction makes it very difficult to quit smoking.

Stages of Addiction

Addiction is the physical and psychological need for a given substance or behavior. Recall that the term *psychological* refers to a person's mental and emotional state. Addiction to a substance usually develops in four stages—experimentation, regular use, tolerance, and dependency (Figure 8.13).

Experimentation

People often choose to use a substance such as cigarettes or chewing tobacco "just to try it." This is the stage of experimentation. In this stage, a person is trying a substance. He or she may begin to use the substance more regularly. Experimentation with a substance often leads to the regular use of a substance. "Just trying" a tobacco product can easily lead to regular use.

Regular Use

After experimentation, people usually increase their substance use. Over time, people may slowly increase the amount of times they smoke per week. Users are then likely to develop a regular pattern of smoking cigarettes. For example, people may smoke at a certain time of day or while performing a certain activity.

Tolerance

People who regularly use a substance develop a tolerance for that substance. A **tolerance** develops when the body gets used to a substance. This means the body needs more of a substance than was previously needed to experience the same effects. The body can quickly develop a tolerance to nicotine and require more cigarettes to achieve the original effect.

Stages of Addiction to a Substance	
Stage one: experimentation	Experimentation with a substance begins. Substance use may stop at this stage, or may rapidly develop into other stages.
Stage two: regular use	The user develops a habit of regularly using a substance.
Stage three: tolerance	The user's body develops a tolerance to the substance. Gradually, the user feels the need for more and more of a substance to achieve the same effects as before.
Stage four: dependence and addiction	The user becomes reliant on having the substance present in the body to function "normally" or feel "normal." Substance use also interferes with personal responsibilities and relationships. The user is physically and psychologically addicted to the substance.

Figure 8.13
People can move through the four stages of addiction more quickly than they might think. *What are the two types of need in addiction?*

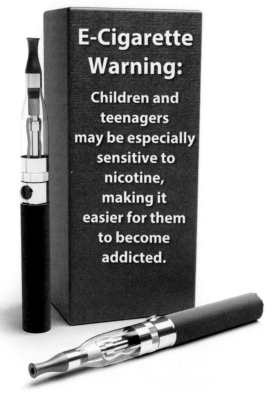

Franck Boston/Shutterstock.com

Figure 8.14 Young people are extra vulnerable to developing many unhealthy habits, including nicotine addiction.

During experimentation, a person may smoke one cigarette a week. This may increase to one cigarette each day with regular use. Once a tolerance develops, a person may need to smoke three cigarettes each day to feel the effects of nicotine (**Figure 8.14**).

A tolerance to nicotine is dangerous because it causes people to smoke more cigarettes. This increases the damage done to the body. Even if someone is not feeling the effect of the nicotine, the substance is still entering the body. The more a person smokes, the more damage he or she causes.

Dependency

After repeated use, the body becomes dependent on the way nicotine makes it feel. This means the body adjusts to the feelings that nicotine causes. **Dependence** occurs when the body needs an addictive substance in its system to function "normally" or to feel "normal." There are two types of dependence—physical and psychological.

A *physical dependence* occurs when the body needs a certain amount of a substance to function "normally." Without the substance in the body, the dependent person feels uncomfortable and even sick. If a dependent person is unable to smoke a cigarette for a whole day, he or she may feel sick.

People who smoke also develop a *psychological dependence*. This causes people to believe that they need a certain substance to feel "normal." Psychological dependence relates to mental and emotional factors. If a dependent person is unable to smoke, he or she may feel irritable.

People may develop patterns for using a substance, such as smoking a cigarette after dinner every day. Patterns such as this can connect a substance with certain triggers (**Figure 8.15**). **Triggers** are like reminders that cause people to feel a strong desire for a substance. In this case, the end of the meal becomes the trigger to have a cigarette. When smokers encounter triggers that they connect with smoking, they feel a strong psychological need to smoke.

Withdrawal Symptoms

Withdrawal occurs when someone addicted to a substance tries to stop using that substance. The term *withdrawal* describes unpleasant symptoms. These symptoms vary based on the addictive substance. People addicted to nicotine may experience irritability, difficulty concentrating, fatigue, nausea, and weight gain during withdrawal. They also experience intense cravings for nicotine. This occurs because their body is addicted to having this chemical.

Withdrawal is one of the reasons tobacco users have such difficulty quitting. The withdrawal symptoms for tobacco last several weeks or even months. Some former smokers have occasional tobacco cravings for years after quitting.

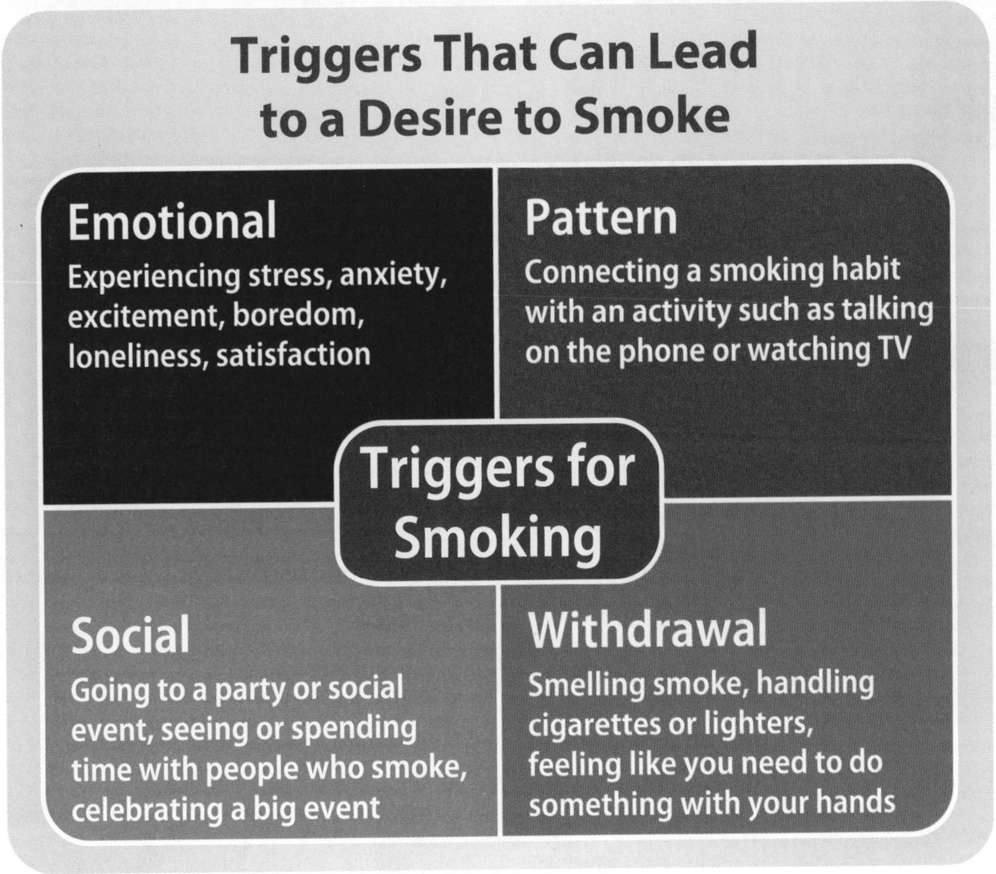

Triggers That Can Lead to a Desire to Smoke

Emotional
Experiencing stress, anxiety, excitement, boredom, loneliness, satisfaction

Pattern
Connecting a smoking habit with an activity such as talking on the phone or watching TV

Triggers for Smoking

Social
Going to a party or social event, seeing or spending time with people who smoke, celebrating a big event

Withdrawal
Smelling smoke, handling cigarettes or lighters, feeling like you need to do something with your hands

Figure 8.15
People can connect smoking mentally with a certain feeling, habit, person, or situation that can increase their desire to smoke. *Which type of dependence is related to mental and emotional factors such as stress?*

Lesson 8.2 Review

1. **True or false.** Most young people view smokers as popular, cool, and mature.

2. Young people are much _____ (more/less) likely to start smoking if their parents discuss and follow through on consequences for smoking.

3. What are the four stages of substance addiction?

4. Which of the following is *not* a common symptom of withdrawal from nicotine?

   A. Hunger.

   B. Fatigue.

   C. Irritability.

   D. Difficulty concentrating.

5. **Critical thinking.** Compare and contrast a physical dependence and a psychological dependence in the final stage of nicotine addiction.

Hands-On Activity

In small groups, create an anti-tobacco message to encourage students at your school to say "no" to tobacco products. Possible formats include a message for the morning announcements, a poster or flyer, an article for a newspaper, a brochure, or a social media post. Include some of the following in your message: factors that make kids want to try tobacco, consequences of tobacco use, anti-tobacco pictures, and statistics related to tobacco use.

Quitting and Preventing Tobacco Use

Learning Outcomes

After studying this lesson, you will be able to

- **identify** steps someone can follow when trying to quit tobacco.
- **describe** treatment methods for nicotine addiction.
- **outline** effective strategies to prevent and discourage tobacco use.
- **demonstrate** skills for resisting tobacco.

Graphic Organizer 📑

KWL Chart: Treating Addiction

Create a table like the one shown below. Before you read the lesson, outline what you know and what you want to know about treating and preventing nicotine addiction. After you have read the lesson, outline what you learned.

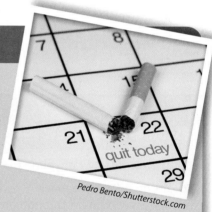

Pedro Bento/Shutterstock.com

K	W	L
What I <u>K</u>now	**What I <u>W</u>ant to Know**	**What I Have <u>L</u>earned**
Nicotine gum or the nicotine patch can help curb withdrawal symptoms for tobacco users.	What does the government do to help prevent tobacco use?	More than half of people who have had a heart attack or surgery resulting from lung cancer continue to smoke.

n Lesson 8.1, you learned how tobacco products harm the body and negatively affect a person's health. In Lesson 8.2, you learned that smoking is a very addictive activity, and it can be difficult to quit. Quitting is possible, however.

From the previous lessons, Olivia has encouraged her parents to quit smoking. They know how harmful it is for their own health and for Olivia to be near all of that secondhand smoke. In this lesson, you will explore some strategies for breaking the tobacco habit. Olivia's parents, for example, will buy the nicotine patch since they know they will have withdrawal symptoms.

Of course, the best option to prevent smoking is never to begin using tobacco products. Catalina, for example, found out that vaping can still be harmful to her health and that there is still nicotine in ENDS. Because of this, she has decided not to smoke at all. Therefore, this lesson also discusses ways to prevent tobacco use.

Breaking the Tobacco Habit

Tobacco use is a hard habit to break. Often, the threat of serious health problems is not enough to make someone quit. More than half of the people who have had a heart attack or surgery resulting from lung cancer continue to smoke. There is still time for these people. It is never too late for someone to stop using tobacco.

Tobacco users who quit successfully experience a number of health benefits (**Figure 8.16**). Within just a few days of quitting, people see a decrease in blood pressure, heart rate, and coughing. Within a year after quitting, people see a decreased risk of heart attack and cancer. These benefits increase over time. The longer someone avoids using tobacco, the lower the risk of developing major health issues.

Health Benefits from Quitting Tobacco Use

Within a Few Days
- Lower blood pressure
- Slower heart rate
- Less coughing

Within a Year
- Decreased risk of heart attack
- Decreased risk of cancer

After a Year
- Health benefits continue to increase
- Decreased risk of developing major health issues

Figure 8.16 The body experiences long-term health benefits when a person quits smoking, but it also shows benefits within a few days.

Quitting tobacco use is a difficult task to undertake. If you or someone you know is trying to quit tobacco use, the following steps may help:

- attend individual or group counseling
- talk to a school guidance counselor, doctor, teacher, or other trusted adult
- call a helpline that provides free counseling to people trying to quit using tobacco
- research online resources that have information on quitting

Although quitting tobacco can be difficult, nicotine addiction is treatable. Treatment methods include nicotine replacement and self-management techniques.

Nicotine Replacement

Some approaches to quitting smoking, or **smoking cessation**, rely on nicotine replacement. A smoker's body is used to nicotine and its effects. Stopping nicotine intake completely can cause withdrawal symptoms. These symptoms may be so severe that people give up on quitting.

In **nicotine replacement**, tobacco users continue to put nicotine into their bodies. They do not do this, however, through the use of tobacco products. Instead, tobacco users typically use *nicotine gum* or the *nicotine patch* as replacements (**Figure 8.17**). These replacements lessen withdrawal symptoms. In this way, nicotine replacement makes smoking easier to quit.

Nicotine replacement treatment enables tobacco users to gradually treat their addiction to nicotine by using smaller and smaller amounts of the substance. Eventually, people find they are no longer dependent on nicotine.

Self-Management Strategies

Self-management strategies often involve developing ways to resist temptation. First, tobacco users must identify situations that trigger their desire for tobacco. Once they have that information, tobacco users can respond with two techniques—stimulus control and response substitution.

Figure 8.17
Nicotine gum and nicotine patches can help tobacco addicts quit smoking. *What treatment method involves nicotine gum and patches?*

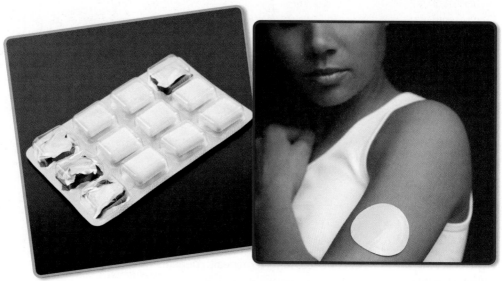

Left to right: jcjgphotography/Shutterstock.com; bikeriderlondon/Shutterstock.com

Stimulus control involves trying to avoid tempting situations and managing feelings that lead to nicotine use. Through stimulus control, people learn to avoid or manage each stimulus that causes them to smoke. A *stimulus* is a thing or event that causes a specific reaction in the body. In this case, the reaction is a craving for tobacco. The stimulus can be anything from a stressful day to seeing someone else smoke.

With stimulus control, the goal is to avoid triggers that cause a desire for smoking. People may not always be able to avoid their triggers, however. If someone feels triggered to smoke, he or she can use response substitution.

Through **response substitution**, people learn to respond to difficult feelings and situations with behaviors other than smoking. They may use stress management, relaxation, and coping skills. For response substitution to work, the first step is to recognize the stimulus that triggers the desire to smoke. Then, a person can respond with an appropriate substitution for the behavior.

BUILDING Your Skills

Addiction Prevention

Many factors determine the likelihood that a young person will use tobacco products. Most people form their smoking habits as young people, and one of the most important ways to prevent tobacco addiction is never to use it in the first place.

There will be many negative influences in a young person's life that may influence him or her to try smoking, including peer pressure and representations of smoking in the media. There are also positive influences that may convince young people *not* to smoke. The power of positive peer pressure can weigh heavily on someone's decision. You have the power to be a positive influence on your friends' (and classmates') decisions to be tobacco-free.

Tobacco-Free Pledge and Personal Promise

Design a *Tobacco-Free Pledge* and encourage your friends and classmates to sign one, too. See the basic example below to better understand the wording in a pledge. Do additional research to get ideas for what a pledge could look like. In addition to the pledge statement, add the following extra information to make your pledge special:

- an inspirational quote
- at least one image
- at least three harmful effects of tobacco use
- at least two benefits of being tobacco-free
- other relevant information or images (if applicable)

If you are choosing to be tobacco-free, sign the pledge. With teacher permission, hang the pledges at your school to advocate for tobacco-free youth.

Tobacco-Free Pledge

I Am Saying NO to Tobacco!

I, _____, pledge to be tobacco-free.
        (person's name)

Preventing Tobacco Use

Most adult smokers picked up the habit as young people. Therefore, experts believe the best way to reduce the smoking rate is to prevent smoking. Prevention strategies include government-based regulations, antismoking campaigns, and personal skills for refusing tobacco.

What the Government Is Doing

Governments recognize the serious threat to public health associated with the use of tobacco products. They focus on preventing nicotine use and helping tobacco users quit to lessen that threat. Governmental strategies may involve passing state and federal laws. Sometimes, government organizations such as the Food and Drug Administration (FDA) create regulations for tobacco products. Typical laws and regulations cover the sale, advertisement, labeling, and cost of tobacco products.

Sales Restrictions

Perhaps the best way to prevent tobacco use among young people is to make it difficult for them to get the products. Several laws exist to restrict the sale of tobacco products to young people.

In 1996, the United States government passed a law banning the sale of tobacco products to anyone younger than 18 years of age. In 2009, the government passed the *Family Smoking Prevention and Tobacco Control Act*. This law prohibits the sale of tobacco products containing flavorings. Tobacco companies often add flavorings to appeal to young people. Banning these flavorings makes it harder for tobacco companies to reach young people.

In 2010, the *Prevent All Cigarette Trafficking (PACT) Act* was passed. *PACT* requires Internet and mail order retailers to include age verification in their sale processes. This ensures that these retailers cannot sell tobacco products to young people.

Recently, some states and government organizations passed legislation to address electronic cigarettes. In 2016, the FDA finalized a *Tobacco Rule* that bans the sale of e-cigarettes to anyone younger than 18 years of age (**Figure 8.18**). The rule also requires that retailers verify the age of anyone trying to buy these products.

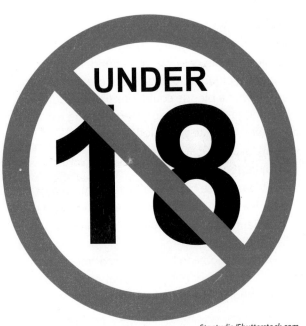

Ste studio/Shutterstock.com

Figure 8.18 Cigarettes and e-cigarettes are illegal to purchase for those under 18 years of age in the United States, including online. *How do retailers help enforce this rule?*

Advertising and Labeling

Several laws focus on the messaging surrounding tobacco products. These laws include requirements and restrictions on tobacco advertising and labeling. The *Family Smoking Prevention and Tobacco Control Act*, or *Tobacco Control Act*, is one of those laws. This law requires prominent, graphic warning labels on cigarette packaging. It also requires large text warnings on smokeless tobacco products. Beginning in 2018, an FDA rule requires ENDS packaging to include a warning stating that these products contain nicotine.

The *Tobacco Control Act* also restricts the language that tobacco companies can use. This law prohibits the use of terms such as *light*, *low*, or *mild* to describe tobacco products. These terms can suggest that tobacco products are less harmful. This law also limits the coloring and design elements companies can use on tobacco product packaging and advertisements. Companies often use bright colors to appeal to young people.

Laws that require warning labels on tobacco products increase awareness about health risks associated with those products (**Figure 8.19**). More people know about these health risks now than before. Awareness, however, can always increase. The more people hear about the potential health risks, the more likely they may be to stop smoking, or to never start smoking.

State Smoking Bans

In recent years, several states passed laws to ban smoking in certain public places. These laws typically cover three locations—workplaces, bars, and restaurants. Each state's law covers these locations in different ways. Only 27 states ensure a smoke-free environment in all three locations. Five states cover two of these locations, and five other states only cover one location. Currently, thirteen states have no smoke-free laws. You can find out your state's smoke-free laws by visiting the Centers for Disease Control and Prevention website.

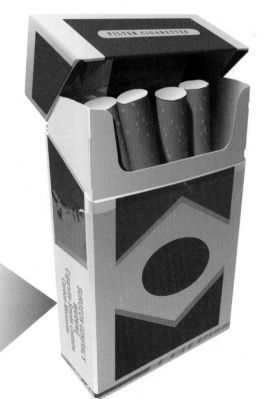

Figure 8.19 All tobacco product labels are required to include prominent, graphic warnings for potential health effects that accompany the use of that product.

SURGEON GENERAL'S WARNING: Smoking Causes Lung Cancer, Heart Disease, Emphysema, and May Complicate Pregnancy

Bill Fehr/Shutterstock.com

There is currently no federal law banning smoking in public places. This means that each state can decide where to ban smoking. Until there is a federal law, smoking bans will vary from state to state.

Increasing Taxes on Cigarettes

Cigarettes are expensive. When people continue to smoke, they have less money to buy other items they need and want. Raising federal, state, and local taxes on tobacco products can cause people to quit smoking. When tobacco products are so expensive, quitting helps save money. Increased taxes may even discourage people from starting to smoke.

Antismoking Campaigns

Antismoking campaigns are a commonly used method to help prevent smoking. Successful antismoking campaigns often use someone's personal experience to emphasize the long-term negative health effects of smoking (Figure 8.20). For example, an antismoking campaign may show a former smoker telling how he now has to use an oxygen tank at all times to breathe.

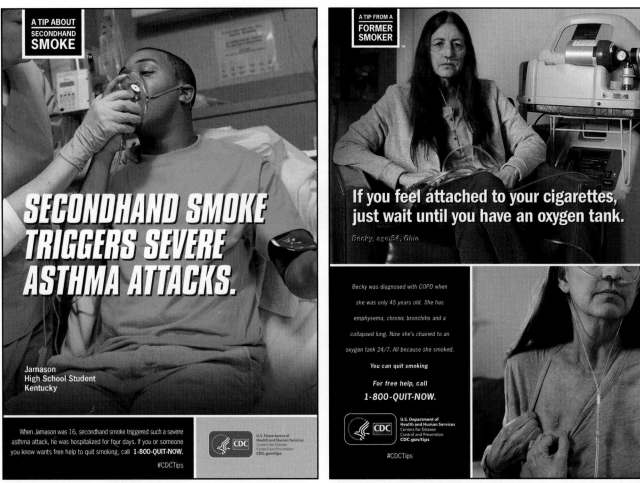

Courtesy of the Centers for Disease Control and Prevention

Figure 8.20 Most antismoking advertisements depict one of the serious health effects that can occur as a result of tobacco use. *Why are these ads so effective?*

When people actually see the harmful effects of smoking, they are less likely to smoke.

Youth-oriented antismoking campaigns often include strategies for refusing tobacco offers. Campaigns such as these are successful because they help young people develop refusal skills. These campaigns also spread the fact that many young people do not smoke. Young people who regularly see these advertisements and campaigns are less likely to smoke. Antismoking campaigns show young people they are not alone in their decision not to smoke.

Skills for Resisting Tobacco

Resisting pressure to begin smoking can be challenging. You may feel this pressure from your peers and from the media. Luckily, specific skills can help you prepare for and respond to situations that may involve tobacco use.

The best way to avoid smoking is to spend time with friends or peers who do not smoke. If your friends do smoke, however, be clear with them about your own feelings toward smoking. Make sure that they know you do not want to use tobacco or be around their secondhand smoke. Firmly explain the reasons behind your decision (**Figure 8.21**). Stick to your decision and refuse to give in. Your true friends will support your decision not to smoke.

Refusal skills are strategies you can use to stand up to pressures and influences that want you to engage in unhealthy behaviors. Strong refusal skills help you stick to your own beliefs and values in the face of peer pressure. These skills can help you in situations when you feel pressured to try tobacco.

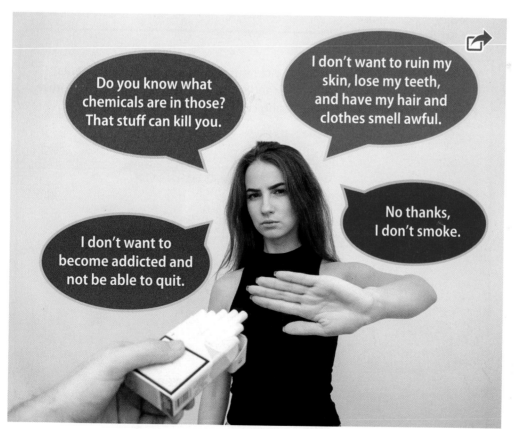

Do you know what chemicals are in those? That stuff can kill you.

I don't want to ruin my skin, lose my teeth, and have my hair and clothes smell awful.

No thanks, I don't smoke.

I don't want to become addicted and not be able to quit.

Simikov/Shutterstock.com

Figure 8.21
Saying no to your friends can be extremely difficult, but having a few practiced responses in mind can help when faced with peer pressure. *What skills help a person stand up to peer influences and pressures?*

For example, suppose that when you hang out with a certain group of friends, several of them offer you cigarettes. Your response may be, "No thanks, I want to keep my lungs healthy for track and field." You may also say, "I don't want my hair, clothes, and breath to smell like cigarettes," or "I like my lungs. I don't want to damage them."

Remember that practice makes perfect. Imagine situations in which someone offers you tobacco, and then practice your responses. Play out each situation in your mind so you are ready to respond firmly. With time, your refusal skills will become stronger. Eventually, you will feel confident when you tell people that you choose to stay tobacco-free.

Lesson 8.3 Review

1. Nicotine replacement and self-management techniques are two approaches to smoking _____.
2. What is the name of the method in which a smoker tries to avoid tempting situations and manages feelings that lead to nicotine use?
3. **True or false.** Most people pick up smoking habits in adulthood.
4. Making sure your friends know you are tobacco-free and sticking to that decision in the face of pressures and influences require _____ skills.
5. **Critical thinking.** Identify the health benefits of smoking cessation that occur throughout the years after you quit, as well as those you see within a few days.

Hands-On Activity

On a separate sheet of paper, write refusal responses to the statements below. Then, team up with a partner and share your responses with each other. Practice your responses out loud using clear and assertive language.

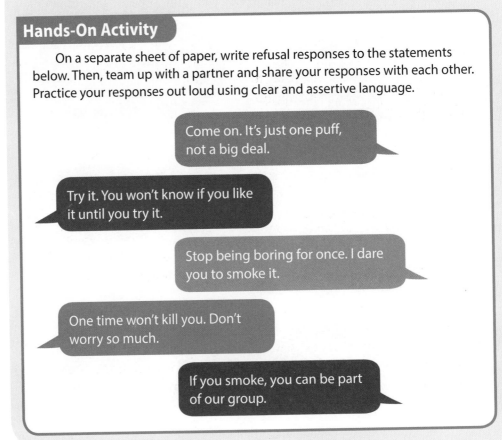

Come on. It's just one puff, not a big deal.

Try it. You won't know if you like it until you try it.

Stop being boring for once. I dare you to smoke it.

One time won't kill you. Don't worry so much.

If you smoke, you can be part of our group.

Summary

Lesson 8.1 Tobacco and Your Health

- *Tobacco* is a plant used to create products such as cigarettes and chewing tobacco. Tobacco leaves contain the chemical *nicotine*, which makes tobacco products addictive. Cigarettes are made of 7,000 chemicals and toxic substances and over 70 carcinogens.
- Smokeless tobacco is chewed, inhaled, or dissolved rather than smoked, but still contains the same chemicals, toxic substances, and carcinogens. *ENDS*, such as vape pens, e-cigarettes, and hookah pens, convert nicotine and flavored liquids into a vapor.
- Tobacco increases the risk for cancer, heart disease, high blood pressure, bronchitis, asthma, and emphysema. Tobacco also causes yellow teeth or fingers, gum disease, bad breath, brittle nails, hair loss, sagging skin, and clothes and hair that smell like smoke.
- *Secondhand smoke* refers to tobacco released into the environment by smokers. Even brief exposure to the toxins in tobacco can cause health issues.

Lesson 8.2 Understanding Tobacco Use

- Common reasons young people start to smoke include: to try out a new identity or due to influences of their family or home environment, friends, peers, or celebrities in the media.
- *Addiction* is the physical and psychological need for a substance, such as nicotine. This typically develops in four stages—experimentation, regular use, tolerance, and dependency.
- People may develop patterns for using a substance, which can connect a substance with certain triggers, causing people to feel a strong desire for a substance.
- When someone addicted to a substance tries to stop using that substance, he or she goes through withdrawal.

Lesson 8.3 Quitting and Preventing Tobacco Use

- Within a few days of quitting smoking, blood pressure, heart rate, and coughing decrease. Within a year, risk of heart attack and cancer decreases. Health benefits increase over time.
- Some approaches to quitting smoking rely on nicotine replacement through products such as nicotine gum or a nicotine patch, which help lessen withdrawal symptoms. *Stimulus control* and *response substitution* rely on the user developing a way to resist the temptation to smoke. The most effective method to reduce the smoking rate, however, is to prevent people from smoking in the first place.
- To prevent and discourage nicotine use, the government passes laws and regulations over the sale, advertisement, labeling, and cost of tobacco products.
- Tips for refusing to smoke include: being clear with your friends about your attitude toward smoking, standing by your values and decisions, and practicing situations and preparing potential refusal responses.

Check Your Knowledge ➦

Record your answers to each of the following questions on a separate sheet of paper.

1. **True or false.** Vaporizers or electronic cigarettes are less addictive than regular cigarettes.
2. What do the toxic chemicals used in paving roads, rocket fuel, and rat poison have in common?
3. Chewing tobacco and snuff are forms of _____ _____.
4. List four health conditions that can develop as a result of smoking-related damage to the lungs.
5. Some young people start to smoke as a way of exploring a new _____.
6. **True or false.** Peer pressure can be negative or positive.
7. Even people who use tobacco casually can form an _____ and have a difficult time quitting.
8. When a person's body gets used to a substance, this is called a(n) _____.
9. What are two products a former smoker can use to ease the withdrawal symptoms of smoking cessation?
10. What is the goal of stimulus control?
11. _____ involves the use of stress management, relaxation, and coping skills as an appropriate substitution for smoking.
    A. Stimulus control
    B. Response substitution
    C. Nicotine replacement
    D. Withdrawal
12. Youth-oriented antismoking campaigns are successful because they help young people develop _____ skills.

Use Your Vocabulary ➦

addiction	nicotine	tar
addictive	nicotine replacement	tobacco
asthma	peer pressure	tolerance
carcinogens	response substitution	toxic
chronic bronchitis	secondhand smoke	triggers
dependence	smoking cessation	withdrawal
emphysema	stimulus control	

13. Work with a partner to write the definitions of the terms above based on your current understanding before reading the chapter. Then, pair up with another pair of students to discuss your definitions and any discrepancies. Finally, discuss the definitions with the class and ask your instructor for any necessary correction or clarification of terms.
14. Choose two of the terms above. Use the Internet to locate photos or graphics that show the meaning of these two terms. Create a digital presentation of these photos or graphics and show them to the class. Explain how they show the meaning of the terms.

Think Critically

15. **Predict.** If an adolescent chooses to try vape pens with his or her peers and this behavior continues, predict the impact of this decision on his or her body, family, and future generations.

16. **Identify.** List some reasons a young person might try an ENDS for the first time. Why is it difficult for a young person to just say "no" to risky behaviors like smoking?

17. **Compare and contrast.** Compare and contrast a cigarette or smokeless tobacco product to a vaporizer or e-cigarette in terms of health consequences and addiction.

18. **Assess.** Calculate the financial cost of a tobacco addiction. How much would it cost to buy two packs of cigarettes every week for one year? What else could you purchase with this amount of money?

DEVELOP Your Skills

19. **Analyze influences and technology skills.** Think about an example of where you see tobacco being glamorized on television, in social media, in magazines, or in music. What message about tobacco is being portrayed? Reflect on the influence of this message and write a summary describing the post, picture, show, movie, or song. How might this message negatively affect young people?

20. **Communication skills.** Imagine you have a friend or family member who is a current smoker. Consider his or her potential reasons for having started smoking and why he or she may continue to smoke. Write a letter to this person about the use of tobacco, the harmful effects it has on the body, reasons for quitting, strategies used to quit, and the immediate as well as long-term benefits of quitting. As you write, keep in mind your conflict resolution skills and empathy.

21. **Access information and advocacy skills.** Create a brochure that can act as a guide to quitting tobacco use. In your guide, include motivation such as financial and health benefits, behaviors that will help, and local resources that can assist. Consider the difficulty of overcoming nicotine addiction and include strategies for doing so. Present your guide to the class.

22. **Teamwork and advocacy skills.** In small groups, create a life-size representation of the long-term effects of tobacco on the body. To begin, have a group member lie down on bulletin board paper to allow the others to trace his or her body. Once the body is traced, research the long-term effects on the body from the top of the head to the tip of the toes. This should include visible body parts as well as internal organs affected by tobacco use. View pictures of the long-term effects to assist in drawing. On the inside of the traced body, draw and label the effects of tobacco use. Obtain permission to hang your life-size representation in the hallway of your school to teach others about the harmful effects of tobacco.

Chapter 9

Alcohol

Essential Question ?

What are some health risks of underage drinking?

Video ↗
Access the Chapter 9 video to start thinking about chapter topics.

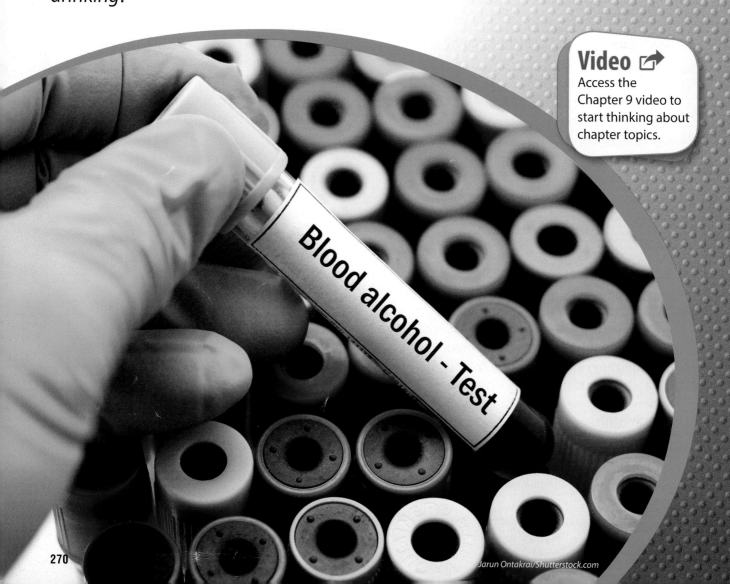

Reading Activity

Review the key terms for this chapter and write them on a separate piece of paper. Look up these terms in the dictionary. Then, write definitions for each term using your own words. Underneath each definition, write an example of the term's meaning in action. After reading this chapter, update your examples and review them with a partner.

How Healthy Are You?

In this chapter, you will be learning about alcohol. Before you begin reading, take the following quiz to assess your current alcohol habits.

Healthy Choices	Yes	No
Do you understand the health hazards of alcohol use on the muscles, nervous system, and brain?		
Do you understand that alcohol is an addictive substance?		
Do you understand the consequences of underage drinking?		
Do you understand the consequences of consuming excessive amounts of alcohol?		
Do you surround yourself with friends who choose not to drink?		
Do you try to limit your exposure to people drinking in movies and TV shows?		
In social situations where you feel nervous or awkward, would you give in to peer pressure to drink alcohol?		
Do you stay away from experimenting with drinking alcohol?		
Have you prepared refusal skills to help when you are offered alcohol?		
If you or someone you care about has a problem with alcohol, do you know what help is available?		

Count your "Yes" and "No" responses. The more "Yes" responses you have, the more healthy alcohol habits you exhibit. Now, take a closer look at the questions with which you responded "No." How can you make these healthy habits part of your daily life? Think about how implementing these ideas can help improve your overall health.

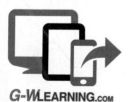

While studying this chapter, look for the activity icon to

- **practice** key terms with e-flash cards and matching activities.
- **reinforce** what you learn by completing graphic organizers, self-assessment quizzes, and review questions.
- **expand** knowledge with interactive activities and activities that extend learning.

G-WLEARNING.com

Key Terms ↱

alcohol type of drug (known as a *depressant*) found in drinks—such as beer, wine, and liquor—that can cause a person to act and feel differently

moderate drinking consuming no more than one drink per day for women and no more than two drinks per day for men; also called *social drinking*

binge drinking consuming four drinks for women and five drinks for men on the same occasion

heavy drinking consuming eight or more drinks for women and 15 or more drinks for men in one week; can lead to alcohol dependence

blood alcohol concentration (BAC) percentage of alcohol that is in a person's blood

inhibition self-control that keeps people from taking dangerous risks

zero-tolerance policy rule that results in punishment of young people caught driving with any level of alcohol in their system

alcohol-use disorders conditions that occur when the recurrent use of alcohol causes problems that interfere with a person's health and responsibilities at school, home, or work

Learning Outcomes

After studying this lesson, you will be able to

- **differentiate** moderate drinking, binge drinking, and heavy drinking.
- **analyze** the effects of alcohol on the brain.
- **relate** alcohol use to long-term health consequences.
- **explain** the consequences of underage drinking.
- **assess** the role of alcohol in accidents and violence.
- **summarize** how alcohol use can increase the risk of developing alcohol-use disorders.

Graphic Organizer ↱

Alcohol and Your Health

As you read this lesson, use a chart like the one below to organize your notes. After you finish reading the lesson, compare your notes with those of a classmate. Together, discuss similarities and differences in your notes. What items would you add to or delete from your list? Adjust your list, if necessary.

iStock.com/WellfordT

- Alcohol Use
- Health Effects
- Effects on Your Life
- Alcohol-Use Disorders

Santiago and Priya are in seventh grade together and have the same group of friends. Priya's family is very open about drinking alcohol. Her older siblings are still under 21 years old, but are allowed to moderately drink alcohol at family dinners. Priya herself has tried a small amount of alcohol before at a family party. Her parents also frequently drive home after drinking.

Santiago's family is not this accepting of alcohol. They would never let Santiago drink alcohol until he turns 21, and they would never drive drunk. Santiago's cousin ended up in the hospital last year because of alcohol poisoning from heavy drinking. It opened Santiago's eyes to just how dangerous alcohol can be.

Alcohol is the third leading preventable cause of death in the United States (**Figure 9.1**). Drinking alcohol has an immediate effect on the body, and can cause lifelong health issues. In this lesson, you will learn about alcohol use and the damaging effect alcohol can have on people's health and lives.

Alcohol Use

Alcohol is a type of drug (known as a *depressant*) found in drinks—such as beer, wine, and liquor—that can cause a person to act and feel differently. In the United States, a person must be 21 years of age to legally drink alcohol. Following are people who should not drink alcohol:

- people under 21 years of age
- women who are pregnant or may be pregnant
- people who are driving or operating equipment
- people who are taking certain medications
- people who are unable to control their alcohol use or who have a family history of alcohol-use disorders

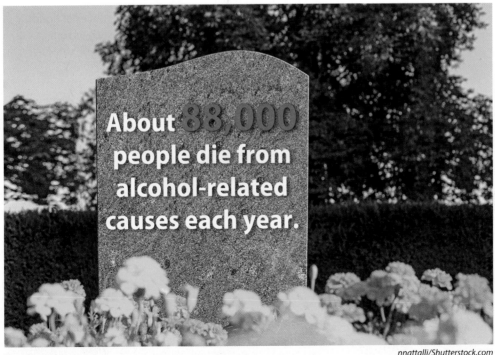

About 88,000 people die from alcohol-related causes each year.

nnattalli/Shutterstock.com

Figure 9.1
Alcohol can lead to death in many ways, including liver failure, car accidents, and alcohol poisoning. *How old does a person have to be in the United States to legally drink alcohol?*

Alcohol is an addictive substance that can have many harmful effects on the user. The best way to avoid the harmful effects of alcohol is not to drink. Some adults, however, choose to use alcohol. If someone does drink alcohol, it should be in moderation only.

Moderate drinking, also called *social drinking*, involves consuming no more than one drink on the same occasion for women and no more than two drinks on the same occasion for men. When experts talk about an alcoholic drink, they are referring to any drink that contains 0.6 ounces (14.0 grams or 1.2 tablespoons) of pure alcohol. **Figure 9.2** shows the one-drink equivalents for beer, wine, and liquor.

People who drink in moderation do not drink every day. Moderate drinking describes when legal adults *occasionally* consume alcohol. For example, an adult might have a drink at a dinner party or other special event. Moderate drinking is less likely to cause harmful effects, but it could easily lead to binge drinking or heavy drinking.

Binge drinking involves consuming four or more drinks for women and five or more drinks for men on the same occasion, and in a short amount of time. The majority of alcohol consumed by underage drinkers is in the form of binge drinking. Binge drinking can result in many harmful effects.

Heavy drinking is drinking eight or more drinks in one week for women and 15 or more drinks in one week for men. Heavy drinking can lead a person to become psychologically and physically dependent on alcohol.

When a person is *psychologically dependent* on alcohol, he or she has a strong mental need for alcohol. This person may feel that he or she needs to drink alcohol to feel "normal." When a person is *physically dependent* on alcohol, he or she needs to consume alcohol to function "normally."

Figure 9.2
Although the total liquid ounces are very different in each of the alcoholic drinks shown here, the drinks have exactly the same amount of pure alcohol. *What is the best way to avoid the harmful effects of alcohol?*

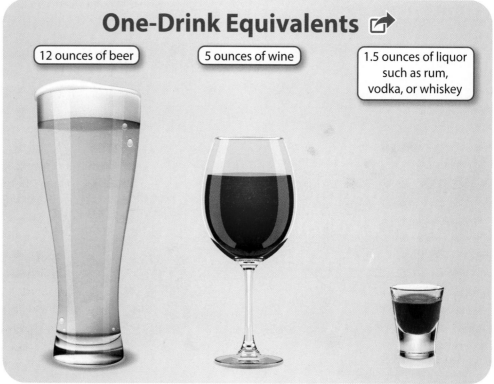

One-Drink Equivalents

12 ounces of beer

5 ounces of wine

1.5 ounces of liquor such as rum, vodka, or whiskey

Left to right: Neyro/Shutterstock.com; VikaSuh/Shutterstock.com; StudioSmart/Shutterstock.com

Health Effects of Alcohol Use

The effects of alcohol vary from person to person, depending on several factors (**Figure 9.3**). Even when people consume small amounts of alcohol, they experience minor effects. When people consume larger amounts of alcohol, they can face life-threatening health problems. The following sections describe some of the immediate and long-term health effects of using alcohol.

Immediate Health Effects

When someone drinks alcohol, the substance is quickly absorbed into the person's bloodstream. The blood carries the alcohol to different parts of the body. When someone drinks a lot of alcohol in a short period of time, the body is unable to break down the alcohol fast enough. As a result, the alcohol builds up in the bloodstream. **Blood alcohol concentration (BAC)** is the percentage of alcohol that is in a person's blood. People who have a BAC of 0.08 or above are considered legally impaired, also known as *intoxicated* or *drunk*. A person who is intoxicated shows substantial physical and mental impairments.

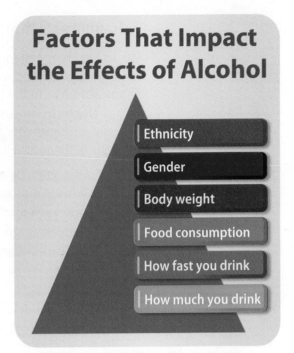

Factors That Impact the Effects of Alcohol

Ethnicity

Gender

Body weight

Food consumption

How fast you drink

How much you drink

Figure 9.3 Because these factors change from person to person or from day to day, it is hard to predict the effect alcohol will have on a person's body.

Central Nervous System

Alcohol affects every cell in the body and slows down the *central nervous system*, which consists of the brain and spinal cord. (You will learn more about the central nervous system in Chapter 17.) The central nervous system directs many functions in the body. When alcohol enters the central nervous system, it negatively affects those functions. Certain brain functions slow, chemical changes occur, and a person's inhibition is reduced (**Figure 9.4**). **Inhibition** is the self-control that keeps people from taking dangerous risks.

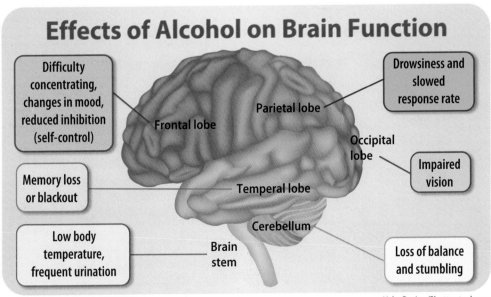

Effects of Alcohol on Brain Function

Difficulty concentrating, changes in mood, reduced inhibition (self-control)

Drowsiness and slowed response rate

Frontal lobe

Parietal lobe

Occipital lobe

Impaired vision

Memory loss or blackout

Temperal lobe

Low body temperature, frequent urination

Brain stem

Cerebellum

Loss of balance and stumbling

Figure 9.4 Alcohol has many effects on brain function that result in impaired physical and mental abilities. *Which body system consists of the brain and spinal cord?*

Yoko Design/Shutterstock.com

Hangover Symptoms and Alcohol Poisoning

Drinking too much in a short period of time can cause a hangover or even alcohol poisoning, which can be life threatening. The effects of drinking alcohol can continue in the body—even up to 24 hours—after a person stops drinking.

The term *hangover* describes the negative symptoms caused by drinking large amounts of alcohol in one occasion. Examples of hangover symptoms include the following:

- tiredness, headaches, and muscle aches
- nausea and vomiting
- dizziness and a feeling that the room is spinning
- increased sensitivity to light and sound
- difficulty sleeping
- thirst
- shakiness
- depression, anxiety, and irritability
- difficulty concentrating

Alcohol poisoning is a medical emergency that occurs when a large amount of alcohol enters the bloodstream in a short period of time. Alcohol poisoning can result in loss of consciousness, low blood pressure, low body temperature, and difficulty breathing. Extreme levels of alcohol consumption can lead to permanent brain damage and death. Given the serious consequences of alcohol poisoning, you should know the danger signs (**Figure 9.5**). Call 911 immediately if you suspect a person is experiencing alcohol poisoning.

Long-Term Health Effects

Young people who start drinking face serious lifelong health consequences. Alcohol is distributed throughout the entire body, so it affects every single organ and body system. Therefore, regularly drinking large amounts of alcohol is associated with serious and even life-threatening consequences.

Figure 9.5
People who have alcohol poisoning may experience life-threatening consequences that require immediate medical attention.

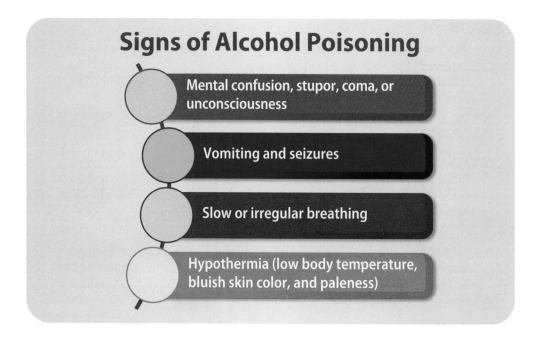

Signs of Alcohol Poisoning

- Mental confusion, stupor, coma, or unconsciousness
- Vomiting and seizures
- Slow or irregular breathing
- Hypothermia (low body temperature, bluish skin color, and paleness)

Brain Development

Alcohol use has immediate effects on brain function. It also causes long-term effects, especially for young people who start drinking. People who begin drinking early in life experience changes in their brain development. One recent study found that young people who binge drink show permanent changes in their brains, including problems with learning and memory. People who consume large amounts of alcohol on a regular basis can experience issues such as dementia, stroke, memory problems, confusion, and drowsiness.

Chronic Diseases

A *chronic disease* lasts three months or more. Over time, drinking too much alcohol can lead to the development of several types of chronic diseases. These may include high blood pressure, heart disease, and certain types of cancer. Another chronic disease associated with heavy drinking is cirrhosis.

Cirrhosis is a buildup of scar tissue in the liver. Heavy drinking often causes liver damage. High levels of alcohol cause fat to build up in the liver, which blocks blood flow. Eventually this lack of blood flow can cause cirrhosis (**Figure 9.6**).

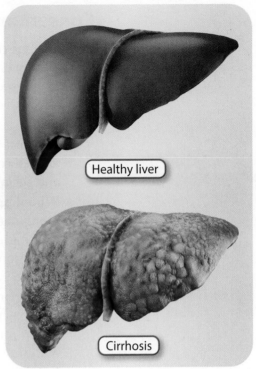

Healthy liver

Cirrhosis

iStock.com/eranicle

Figure 9.6 Cirrhosis of the liver is one of the 15 leading causes of death in the United States. *What often causes liver damage?*

Alcohol and Pregnancy

When a pregnant woman drinks, the alcohol she consumes passes from her bloodstream to the bloodstream of the fetus. Women who drink during pregnancy risk giving birth to babies with *fetal alcohol spectrum disorder (FASD)*. This condition results in lifelong physical and mental effects. For example, babies with FASD often experience poor growth (both in the womb and after birth). They may have decreased muscle tone and poor coordination, as well as heart and facial conditions. Delayed development and problems with thinking, speech, movement, and social skills may also occur.

Effects on Your Life

In the United States, you must be 21 years of age to buy alcohol. Unfortunately, even with this law, many young people have serious problems due to alcohol use. Alcohol use contributes to the deaths of more than 4,300 Americans younger than 21 years of age each year. In addition, alcohol use increases the likelihood of engaging in other risky behaviors. Young people who use alcohol are more likely to use drugs or engage in sexual activities. Alcohol use affects young people's lives in a variety of ways. It can even cause dangerous situations that lead to accidents and violence.

Consequences of Underage Drinking

Underage drinkers, or those under 21 years of age, account for 11 percent of all alcohol consumed in the United States. In fact, alcohol is the most commonly used and abused drug among youth in the United States. Young people who drink alcohol are at greater risk of experiencing the following problems:

- **Physical problems.** Hangovers, illnesses, and injuries may result from alcohol consumption. These physical problems can interfere with school and social relationships.
- **School problems.** Young people who consume alcohol may experience more school absences, difficulty focusing in class, and declining or failing grades. These consequences can have a negative impact on future educational plans, such as going to a technical school or university (**Figure 9.7**).
- **Family and social problems.** Alcohol use can cause strained relationships with family and friends. Feelings of guilt and fear may result from disappointing their loved ones. Young people may also withdraw from sports, clubs, or other extracurricular activities.
- **Legal problems.** Alcohol use is illegal for those younger than 21 years of age. Youth who use alcohol can be arrested. This arrest could appear on a young person's permanent record and affect his or her future life and career goals.

Alcohol use can also lead to unsafe behaviors with long-term effects. Young people who drink alcohol are more likely to start abusing other drugs. Even drinking small amounts can lead to long-term problems with alcohol. In fact, people who start drinking before 15 years of age are five times more likely to develop alcohol dependence than those who begin drinking as adults.

Figure 9.7
Young people who do not engage in underage drinking have a higher success rate of achieving their school and career goals than young people who do drink alcohol.

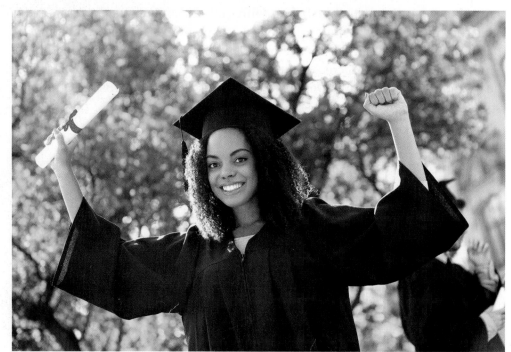

Pandora Studio/Shutterstock.com

The Consequences of Underage Drinking

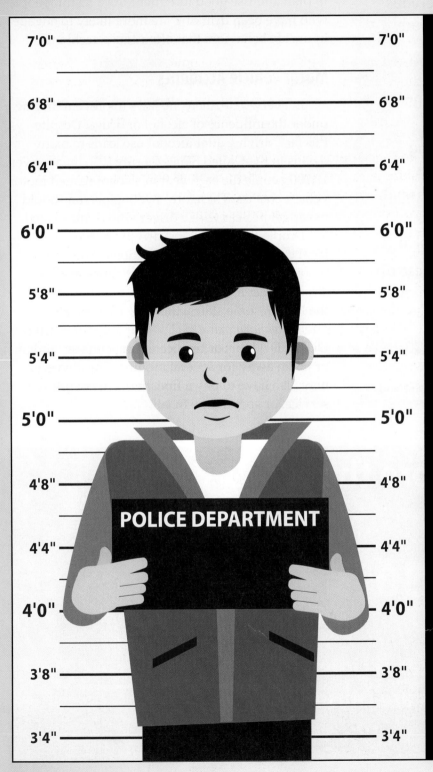

7'0"	7'0"
6'8"	6'8"
6'4"	6'4"
6'0"	6'0"
5'8"	5'8"
5'4"	5'4"
5'0"	5'0"
4'8"	4'8"
4'4"	4'4"
4'0"	4'0"
3'8"	3'8"
3'4"	3'4"

POLICE DEPARTMENT

CHARGES

HEALTH PROBLEMS
- Alcohol poisoning
- Changes in mood/behavior
- Hangover
- Increased risk of chronic illnesses

SCHOOL PROBLEMS
- Difficulty focusing
- Increased amount of absences
- Declining or failing grades

FAMILY/SOCIAL PROBLEMS
- Strained relationships
- Feelings of guilt and fear
- Withdrawal from activities, teams, and hobbies
- Feelings of isolation

LEGAL PROBLEMS
- Can be arrested
- Potential for jail time
- Fines and fees
- May have to appear in court
- Offenses can show up on permanent record

Background: Alhovik/Shutterstock.com; Boy: Busyok Creative/Shutterstock.com

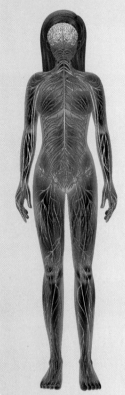

Alcohol's Effects on the Central Nervous System

When alcohol slows down the nervous system, the body experiences

- decreased reaction time
- difficulty coordinating movements
- decreased ability to plan or problem solve
- decreased use of good judgment

BlueRingMedia/Shutterstock.com

Figure 9.8 As alcohol filters into the brain and bloodstream, it affects a person's ability to think and move quickly and correctly.

Alcohol Use and Accidents

Alcohol slows down the central nervous system, which affects the body in various ways. **Figure 9.8** shows some of these effects. These include a decrease in reaction time, difficulty coordinating movements, and a decreased ability to plan and use good judgment. As a result, people who have been drinking are more likely to engage in unsafe behaviors that often cause accidents.

Motor Vehicle Accidents

In every state, there are laws to prevent driving under the influence of alcohol or drugs. Despite this fact, driving after alcohol use leads to many deaths in the United States (**Figure 9.9**). In fact, over 10,000 people die each year in alcohol-related motor vehicle crashes. Therefore, a young person should never get in a car with a driver who is intoxicated.

People who drink and drive can face legal consequences for their actions. Adults who drive with a BAC of 0.08 or above are *driving under the influence (DUI)*, which is against the law. In some states, this may also be called *driving while intoxicated (DWI)*. If a driver receives a DUI or DWI, his or her license may be suspended, or taken away for several months. This driver may also have to pay a fine, perform community service, or spend time in jail.

Figure 9.9
Because of alcohol's effects on the body's reflexes, motor skills, and alertness, driving after drinking alcohol frequently results in deadly car accidents. *What is the legal term for a person who has consumed too much alcohol before driving a vehicle?*

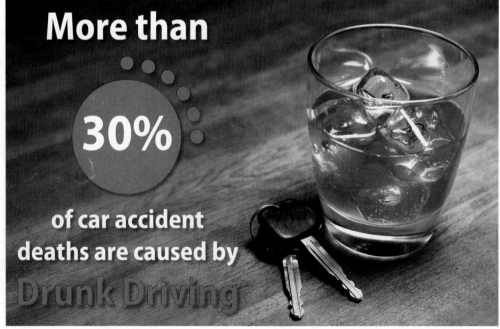

More than 30% of car accident deaths are caused by Drunk Driving

Glass and keys: iStock.com/dehooks

Many states follow a **zero-tolerance policy** for people under 21 years of age. Under this policy, young people caught driving with any level of alcohol in their system are punished. Punishment for violating a zero-tolerance policy varies from state to state.

Other Types of Accidents

Alcohol use is also associated with other types of accidents and injuries. Under the influence of alcohol, people experience high rates of the following:

- falls
- burns
- homicides
- suicides
- unintentional firearm injuries
- electrical shocks
- incidents of near drowning
- accidental death while bicycling or swimming

CASE STUDY

Keisha's Babysitting Conundrum

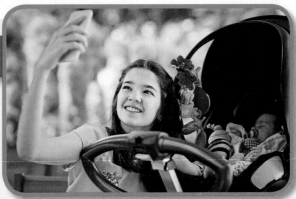
iStock.com/praetorianphoto

Keisha, who is in the eighth grade, frequently babysits for the Patel family. Vera and Toshiro Patel are fun little kids with whom Keisha enjoys spending time. Babysitting is a perfect job for Keisha.

The Patels live a half mile down the street from Keisha's family. When Keisha babysits during the day, she often rides her bike to and from the Patel's house. When Keisha babysits at night, her parents drop her off and the Patel parents bring her home.

Keisha has babysat for the Patels many times without any problems. One evening, however, the Patel parents went to a fancy party. Everything had gone as planned that evening. The kids ate dinner, played, and went to bed without any arguments. Once the kids were asleep, Keisha spent time watching TV, doing a little bit of cleaning up, and periodically checking on the kids. Mr. and Mrs. Patel returned home around midnight as Keisha expected. What she did not expect was for them both to have been drinking.

Keisha was not sure how drunk Mr. Patel was, but he stumbled when he walked into the house. He was also slow to respond to any of her questions. Mrs. Patel almost immediately fell asleep on the couch. Keisha was uncomfortable getting into a car with Mr. Patel driving, but he was so nice and she did not know how to refuse. Keisha decided that it was only a couple of blocks to her house, so she got into the car with Mr. Patel.

Thinking Critically

1. Why was Keisha uncomfortable in this situation? What could go wrong on the car ride to her house? Who could get hurt?

2. What other options does Keisha have in this situation? How do you think she would feel about these alternative solutions?

3. How might refusing a ride from Mr. Patel affect her relationship with him? Do you think it would be worth it?

4. If you were in a situation like Keisha, what would you do?

Alcohol Use and Violence

People who have been drinking are more likely to behave violently than those who have not been drinking. About 35 percent of victims of some type of violent attack report that the person who assaulted them was under the influence of alcohol. Alcohol use is also associated with many cases of violence within families, including child abuse and violence between romantic partners. (You will learn more about abuse and violence in Chapter 15.)

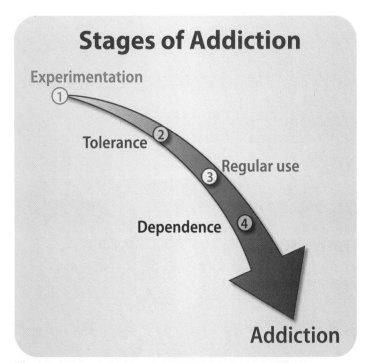

Stages of Addiction

Experimentation ①

Tolerance ②

Regular use ③

Dependence ④

Addiction

Figure 9.10 People who never drink alcohol will never develop an addiction to alcohol. *When does an alcohol-use disorder occur?*

Alcohol-Use Disorders

Like smoking, drinking alcohol can be addictive, especially for some people more than others. Alcohol use can increase the risk of developing alcohol-use disorders. **Alcohol-use disorders** occur when the recurrent use of alcohol causes problems that interfere with a person's health and responsibilities at school, home, or work. Alcohol-use disorders may range from mild to moderate to severe. They generally follow the stages of addiction (**Figure 9.10**).

The first stage of addiction is experimentation. *Experimentation* occurs when people are trying a substance. Young people may try alcohol after seeing their parents or someone in a movie try alcohol. They may also feel pressured by their friends to try alcohol.

Some people who experiment with alcohol decide they do not like it and quit drinking. For other people, experimentation with alcohol can lead to *regular use*. During this stage, people develop a habit of using a substance on a regular basis. People who engage in moderate drinking limit their alcohol intake so they do not drink too much. Regular use, however, often causes people to drink more than they should, resulting in a mild to moderate alcohol-use disorder.

Regular use of alcohol causes the body to develop a *tolerance* for alcohol. In this stage, a person's body gets used to a certain amount of alcohol (**Figure 9.11**). Gradually, a person must consume larger amounts of alcohol than were previously needed to feel the same effects. Regular use of alcohol can easily lead to heavy drinking, a severe alcohol-use disorder, and dependence on alcohol.

Dependence occurs when the user is psychologically and/or physically dependent on alcohol. Once a person is dependent on alcohol, he or she must have the substance in the body to function "normally" and feel "normal." At this stage, a person may experience withdrawal symptoms if he or she tries to stop drinking. These symptoms may include hallucinations, impaired coordination, and disruptions in brain function.

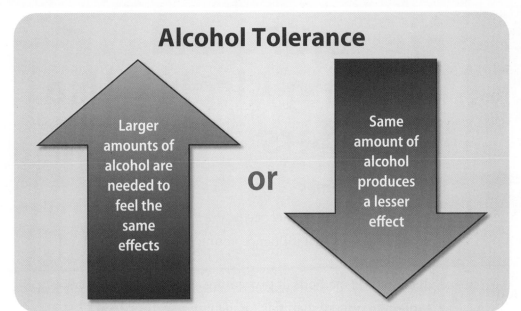

Alcohol Tolerance

Larger amounts of alcohol are needed to feel the same effects

or

Same amount of alcohol produces a lesser effect

Figure 9.11
A tolerance for alcohol means that a person's body has grown used to a certain amount of alcohol. *What stage of alcohol addiction causes a person to develop a tolerance for alcohol?*

People with an *alcohol addiction* show a number of symptoms. They may have a strong craving for alcohol. They may not be able to limit their drinking. They may also experience memory loss or a *blackout* (forget what happened while drinking). People with an alcohol addiction often continue to drink despite serious problems with their physical and mental health, as well as trouble with their family, school, or work responsibilities.

Lesson 9.1 Review

1. In the United States, a person must be _____ years of age to legally drink alcohol.
2. The majority of alcohol consumed by underage drinkers is in the form of _____ drinking.
3. **True or false.** Changes in the brain, hangovers, and alcohol poisoning are long-term health effects of drinking alcohol.
4. List four problems young people who drink alcohol are at greater risk of experiencing.
5. **Critical thinking.** How many ounces are equivalent to one drink for beer, wine, and liquor? What does this mean about consumption of these types of alcohol?

Hands-On Activity

Think of your favorite activities to do—playing a sport, going to the theater, reading, listening to music, drawing, cooking, etc. Using information from the text about the immediate health effects of alcohol use, write about how these activities would be impacted if you tried to do them after drinking alcohol. Then, consider and write about how these activities would be impacted if you experienced the long-term health effects of alcohol use.

Preventing and Treating Alcohol-Use Disorders

Key Terms

detoxification process of completely stopping all alcohol use to remove the substance from the body

Alcoholics Anonymous (AA) self-help program for people with alcohol-use disorders to help them change how they think about drinking

enabling encouraging a person's unhealthy behaviors, either intentionally or unintentionally

Alateen support group where young people who have loved ones with an alcohol-use disorder come together to share their experiences and learn ways to cope with problems

Al-Anon Family Groups support group where family members and friends who have loved ones with an alcohol-use disorder come together to share their experiences, receive encouragement, and learn ways to cope with problems

Learning Outcomes

After studying this lesson, you will be able to

- **describe** factors that influence young people's beliefs about alcohol use.
- **demonstrate** methods of preventing alcohol-use disorders.
- **explain** treatment methods for alcohol-use disorders.
- **demonstrate** how to help someone who has an alcohol-use disorder.

Graphic Organizer

Alcohol Use

Before you read this lesson, think about how you would answer the following questions:

- What influences lead young people to try alcohol the first time?
- What are some ways to prevent underage drinking?
- What treatment is available for people with alcohol-use disorders?

As you read this lesson, take notes about these topics using a graphic organizer like the one shown here.

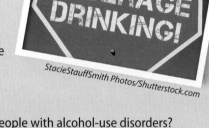

StacieStauffSmith Photos/Shutterstock.com

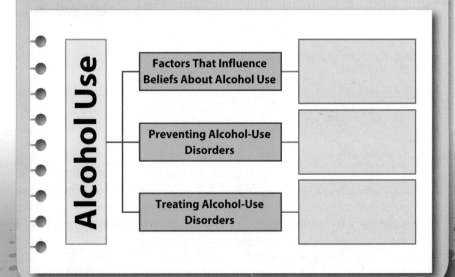

According to the most recent Youth Risk Behavior Survey conducted by the CDC, 33 percent of high school students drank some amount of alcohol during the past 30 days (**Figure 9.12**). This is an alarming percentage considering that alcohol use is illegal for people younger than 21 years of age.

Remember Priya and Santiago from the previous lesson. Because of her family's openness toward alcohol use, Priya does not see the dangers associated with alcohol as Santiago does. Last week, she even snuck a bottle of alcohol to a sleepover and shared it with her friends. Due to Priya's carefree attitude toward alcohol, Santiago may feel peer pressured into drinking by Priya and his other friends. Santiago thinks about telling his parents about Priya's alcohol use, but he does not want to get her in trouble.

This lesson will explore some of the factors that may influence young people's beliefs about alcohol use, such as Priya's family influence and Santiago's peer pressure. You will also learn about strategies for preventing alcohol use and the development of alcohol-use disorders. Luckily, treatment methods exist to help people overcome alcohol-use disorders.

Identifying Factors That Influence Beliefs About Alcohol Use

Several factors may influence young people's beliefs about alcohol use. These factors may include family influences, peer pressure, and media messages. Certain people in a person's environment can influence that person's beliefs and expectations about alcohol. These people include parents, siblings, peers, and media figures. Generally, people who have the most influence are those the person considers important, and whose opinions he or she values. If these important people model unhealthy behaviors about alcohol, young people are more likely to engage in that unhealthy behavior.

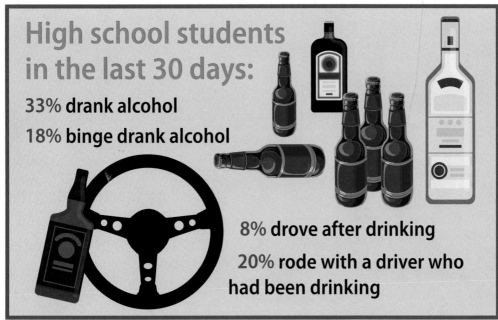

High school students in the last 30 days:

33% drank alcohol
18% binge drank alcohol

8% drove after drinking
20% rode with a driver who had been drinking

Figure 9.12
Because they fear the consequences of asking an adult for help, young people have a higher likelihood than adults of agreeing to drive under the influence and getting into a car with a drunk driver.

Alcoholic beverages: Andrii Bezvershenko/Shutterstock.com; SlipFloat/Shutterstock.com; Steering wheel: Miceking/Shutterstock.com

Influences on Drinking

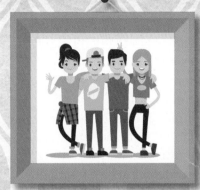

Your "cool" older classmates who you believe are drinking

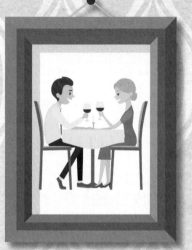

Your parents or guardians who drink more than they should

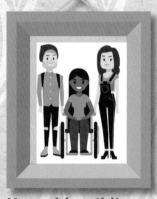

Your older siblings who drink around you and with their friends

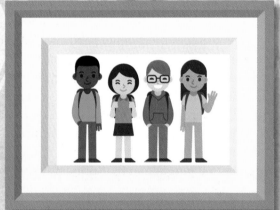

Your friends who want you to try it with them

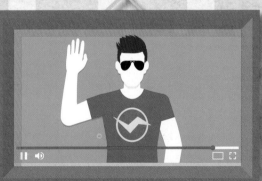

People you see drinking and having fun on social media

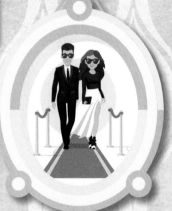

Your favorite celebrity, who makes drinking look fun or glamorous

Family Influence

Families have their own attitudes, beliefs, and rules about alcohol use, which influence their children's attitudes toward alcohol. Some parents or guardians may keep and drink alcohol in the home, but have rules about alcohol use to protect their children. Other parents or guardians may have strong beliefs about alcohol use, leading them not to allow any alcohol in the home.

Unfortunately, some young people have parents or guardians with alcohol-use disorders (**Figure 9.13**). These parents or guardians may have a dependence on alcohol, which can be very difficult for young people. This experience may influence them to try alcohol or avoid alcohol completely. Young people who have parents or guardians with an alcohol-use disorder are more likely to develop one, too. Some young people, however, decide never to try alcohol because of how it affected their parents or guardians.

Siblings can also affect how a young person feels about alcohol use. Young people often look up to older siblings as role models. If a young person's older sibling uses and abuses alcohol, the young person may consider this acceptable and "cool" behavior.

Peer Pressure

Friends can also influence a young person's alcohol use. People tend to drink more alcohol when they have friends who drink. This may be due to peer pressure. As you learned in Chapter 8, *peer pressure* is the influence that people your age have on your actions. Young people who drink may pressure their friends into trying alcohol. Aggressively pressuring someone to drink alcohol is a form of bullying. Real friends will not pressure you into engaging in unhealthy behaviors.

Peer pressure can be indirect. Young people often believe that their peers are drinking. This may lead them to try alcohol to fit in with the "cool kids" they imagine are drinking. Young people may also view using alcohol as a way to seem older, but teens and young adults do not drink as much as you might think. In fact, many young people are often uncomfortable with alcohol use (**Figure 9.14**).

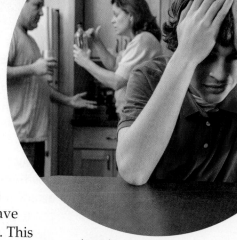
threerocksimages/Shutterstock.com

Figure 9.13
Having a parent or guardian with an alcohol-use disorder can cause stress and conflict for young people. It can also increase their risk of developing an alcohol-use disorder themselves. *Why might an older sibling influence a young person's personal beliefs about alcohol use?*

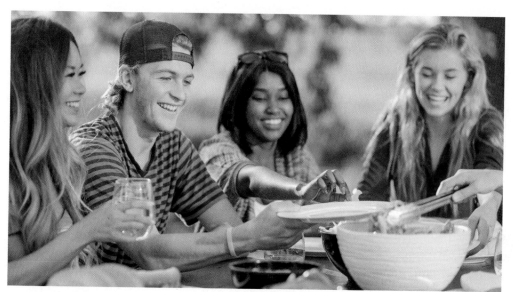
iStock.com/FatCamera

Figure 9.14
Despite common assumptions, most teens and young people do not drink alcohol even with their friends. *What is the term for the influence people your age have on others their age?*

Media Messages

Media messages may also contribute to alcohol use. Young people form attitudes about alcohol use by watching television and movies. Advertisements for alcohol products can also influence these attitudes. Films, even those marketed to young people, frequently show alcohol use. Young people who see drinking in movies tend to view alcohol use more positively. These young people are also more likely to plan to drink alcohol as adults.

In addition, young people may model behavior and attitudes about alcohol use after their favorite celebrities. Do your favorite celebrities drink large amounts of alcohol every weekend and post about it on social media? Imitating this behavior can lead to negative effects on your health and life. Always remember to choose your role models wisely.

BUILDING Your Skills

Making IDEAL Decisions

Do you know how to make healthy decisions in the best possible way for yourself? Making decisions in the adolescent years is tough. Your parents tell you one thing, while your friends may say something different. Movies, TV, and other media showcase yet another opinion. All the while, your gut may be telling you something very different. So, how should you make *healthy* decisions about alcohol and other health behaviors? Try the following IDEAL strategy:

Identify the situation or problem
Describe all the possible solutions
Evaluate all those solutions
Act on the best solution
Learn from the experience

When you are making a big decision, about alcohol or something else, it helps to write down your thoughts for each of the letters in the IDEAL strategy. If the situation is complicated, more than one problem may be involved. Remember that there are usually several possible solutions to any problem. It is okay, and even good, to get ideas for solutions from other people—your parents, friends, siblings, or teachers.

When you evaluate these solutions, brainstorm and write a list of the pros and cons. Be careful though. Just because one option has more pros than another option does not necessarily mean it is the better choice. You have to account for how important each of those pros are to you and how you value them. For example, you may realize that making your parents proud of your decisions or doing well in sports may outweigh all the other pros involved.

Once you have acted, be sure to reflect on the experience and learn from what happened. Think about what went well, and what you will do again in future situations. Also, consider the things you thought did not go well. What will you change if faced with a similar situation again?

Using the IDEAL Process

Think about a big decision you are facing. On a sheet of paper, use the steps in the IDEAL process to help you come up with the best choice.

I D E A L

Preventing Alcohol-Use Disorders

Alcohol-use disorders can cause serious short- and long-term consequences. Alcohol use in young people can lead to changes in brain development and long-term dependence on alcohol later in life. Therefore, preventing alcohol use in young people is especially important. Fortunately, certain strategies exist to help prevent alcohol-use disorders and improve health and well-being. These strategies include education and refusal skills and government approaches.

Education and Refusal Skills

Schools have developed many education programs to decrease risky drinking, especially in underage drinkers. These programs include information about the physical, social, and mental consequences of alcohol use. This information might mention the health risks and physical effects of alcohol use on the body. It might also mention the risk of strained personal relationships, which can occur when a person drinks too much. This information might also emphasize the legal consequences of young people possessing alcohol (**Figure 9.15**).

Education can disprove the beliefs some young people have about their peers' alcohol use. Young people may believe that using alcohol is the norm among their peers, but the truth is very different. Many studies show that most young people do not drink. In fact, most young people wish there was less drinking in their environment. Educating young people about this fact can encourage them not to drink. For example, some colleges give new students information showing that many of their fellow students are also uncomfortable with how much drinking occurs on campus. Students who receive such information report drinking less alcohol than students who do not receive this information.

Education is important, but you must also learn refusal skills. Even if you are aware of the many negative consequences of alcohol use and have made the decision not to drink, alcohol may still be present in your environment. Though it is not the norm, some young people do use alcohol. Developing and practicing refusal skills can help when someone offers you alcohol (**Figure 9.16**).

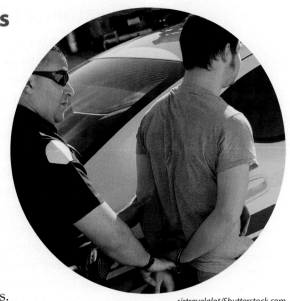

sirtravelalot/Shutterstock.com

Figure 9.15
Underage drinking is illegal and can result in an arrest.

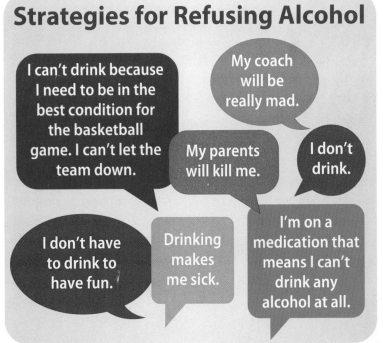

Strategies for Refusing Alcohol

I can't drink because I need to be in the best condition for the basketball game. I can't let the team down.

My coach will be really mad.

My parents will kill me.

I don't drink.

I don't have to drink to have fun.

Drinking makes me sick.

I'm on a medication that means I can't drink any alcohol at all.

FMStox/Shutterstock.com

Figure 9.16   Refusal skills can help you resist pressure to try alcohol. The more you practice your refusal skills, the better prepared you will be to resist peer pressure.

Government Approaches

The government seeks to make it difficult for young people to access alcohol. One of the most obvious and effective government approaches to preventing alcohol-use disorders is setting the minimum legal drinking age at 21. Forbidding people who are younger than 21 years of age from purchasing alcohol makes it more difficult for young people to have access to alcohol. Similarly, making it illegal to use a fake ID to purchase alcohol reduces alcohol use among young people.

Other public policy approaches also exist to limit access to alcohol. For example, in some states, people cannot buy alcohol on Sundays or in grocery and convenience stores. States may also raise the sales tax on alcohol, which makes buying alcohol more expensive.

The government does create some educational materials about alcohol use. Some drinking prevention programs focus on the negative effects of alcohol use. You have probably seen television and magazines ads that portray the negative consequences of drunk driving. Public policies may also place limits on alcohol advertisements, including the hours in which such ads can appear on television and what they can include. These policies seek to prevent young people from seeing alcohol advertisements.

Addiction Treatment Strategies

Detoxification

Support Groups

Self-Management Strategies

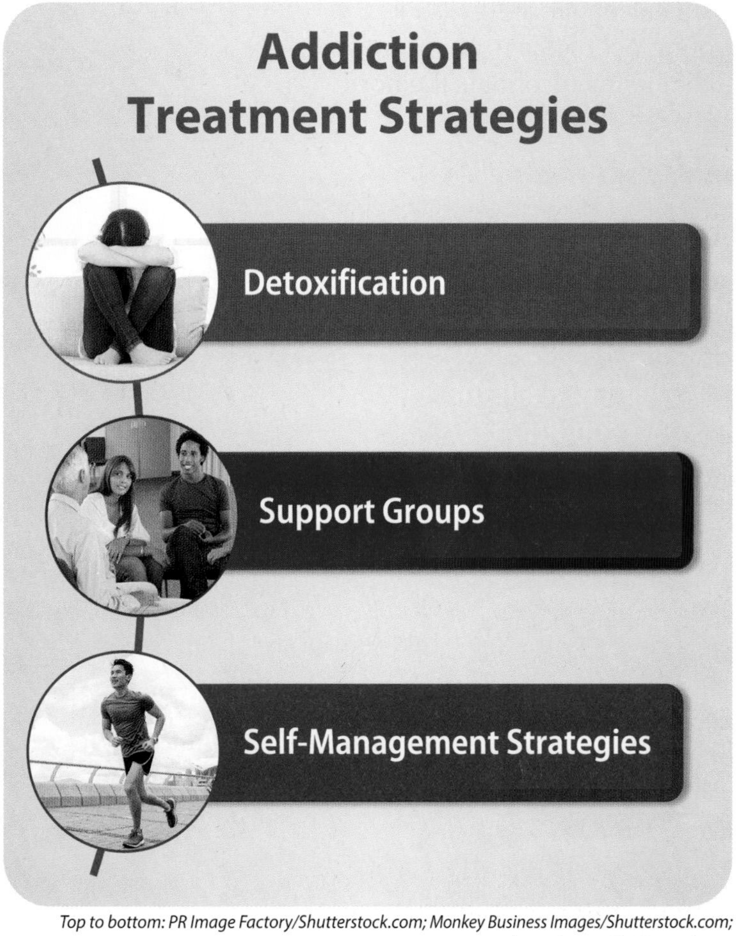

Top to bottom: PR Image Factory/Shutterstock.com; Monkey Business Images/Shutterstock.com; leungchopan/Shutterstock.com

Figure 9.17 Overcoming an addiction to alcohol is not easy, but with support recovery may seem more possible.

Treating Alcohol-Use Disorders

People with severe alcohol-use disorders are often physically and psychologically addicted to alcohol. Although breaking this addiction is difficult, there are a number of strategies that can help people quit drinking (**Figure 9.17**).

Detoxification

One of the first steps in recovery from an alcohol-use disorder is **detoxification**. This is the process of completely stopping all alcohol use to remove the substance from the body. Detoxification is a necessary step in recovering from a physical addiction to alcohol. This process, which is sometimes called *drying out*, may take up to a month. The process may or may not include time spent in the hospital. Detoxification can include severe withdrawal symptoms, such as intense anxiety, tremors, and hallucinations. A doctor may prescribe medications to lessen these symptoms.

Support Groups

Community support groups can be helpful tools for those overcoming alcohol-use disorders. *Support groups* are groups of people with a common problem who share struggles and examples of getting through that problem.

Alcoholics Anonymous (also known as *AA*) is the most well known and widely used self-help program for people with alcohol-use disorders. The program includes a support group element. The goal of AA is to help people with alcohol-use disorders change how they think about drinking. This program involves going through 12 distinct steps, which are a set of guiding principles designed to help people recover from addiction.

According to AA, when a person with a severe alcohol-use disorder consumes even a small amount of alcohol, the presence of alcohol in the bloodstream leads to an irresistible craving for more alcohol. Thus, the goal for recovery is never to drink any alcohol again.

During AA meetings, group members share with other group members any alcohol-related problems they have experienced (**Figure 9.18**). This process of sharing their experiences may help people stop drinking.

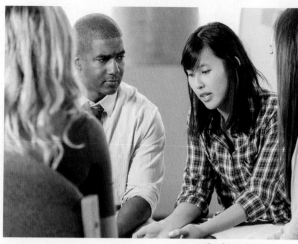

iStock.com/asiseeit

Figure 9.18 People who are trying to quit drinking may attend frequent AA meetings. *What is the goal of AA?*

Self-Management Strategies

Many programs that help people with alcohol-use disorders also teach self-management skills. First, these programs focus on helping people become aware of why they drink. Understanding the motivations that lead someone to drink is an important first step in learning how to avoid alcohol-use disorders.

Next, people develop skills for managing the situations that lead them to want to have a drink. These skills include the following:

- avoiding situations where alcohol is present
- responding in new ways to these situations
- learning new strategies for handling stress
- developing strategies for refusing alcohol

People can use these types of self-management skills in combination with other treatments for alcohol-use disorders. Other treatments may include attending AA meetings or undergoing detoxification.

Helping a Loved One with an Alcohol-Use Disorder

Loving and caring about someone with an alcohol-use disorder can be very difficult. People who have loved ones with an alcohol-use disorder may feel ashamed, angry, afraid, and guilty. Other people feel so overwhelmed by their loved one's alcohol-use disorder that they just deny the problem and pretend that nothing is wrong.

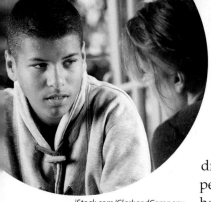

iStock.com/ClarkandCompany

Figure 9.19
Hiding a loved one's alcohol-use disorder can allow that person's behavior to continue. To help a loved one, it is best to speak to a trusted adult. *Who would you feel comfortable talking to about a serious problem?*

If you care about someone who has an alcohol-use disorder, you must first get support for yourself. Try to find an adult you can talk openly and honestly with about the problem. This trusted adult may be a family member, guidance counselor, school nurse, doctor, religious leader, or coach (**Figure 9.19**).

Some people feel they should try to solve or fix their loved one's alcohol-use disorder. They may try to punish, threaten, or bribe their loved one to stop drinking. They may beg their loved one to stop drinking and try to make the person feel guilty about his or her alcohol use. The first step to alcohol recovery, however, is for a person to recognize that he or she has a problem. He or she has to want to change. You cannot force a person to stop drinking.

People may also try to hide their loved one's alcohol use. They may cover up the problems caused by the person's drinking or hide evidence of the drinking. These actions simply help the person avoid the natural consequences of his or her behavior. Hiding a person's alcohol use is an enabling behavior. **Enabling** involves encouraging a person's unhealthy behaviors.

Many young people who have family members with alcohol-use disorders find joining support groups helpful. These groups can help young people learn how to cope with the difficulties of their loved one's alcoholism. Support groups can also be comforting because they show that other people are facing the same challenges.

Young people who have loved ones with an alcohol-use disorder may find Alateen to be helpful. **Alateen** members include young people whose lives have been affected by someone else's drinking. In Alateen meetings, young people come together to share their experiences, gain encouragement, and learn ways to cope with problems. In Alateen, young people can find other people their age who have the same problems and worries.

Alateen is part of the **Al-Anon Family Groups** organization in which family members and friends who have loved ones with an alcohol-use disorder come together to share their experiences, receive encouragement, and learn ways to cope with problems.

Lesson 9.2 Review

1. List three factors that may influence young people's beliefs about alcohol use.
2. **True or false.** Most young people experiment with drinking alcohol.
3. How does raising the sales tax on alcohol help prevent alcohol-use disorders?
4. Encouraging a person's unhealthy behaviors, such as an alcohol-use disorder, is called _____.
5. **Critical thinking.** Compare the three strategies described in this lesson for treating alcohol-use disorders.

Hands-On Activity

Conduct interviews with your parents, older siblings, and/or grandparents about any alcohol-use disorders they may know about in your family. Find a time to talk seriously, openly, and honestly with them. How was this conversation—easy, difficult? What did you learn? What questions would you still like to have answered?

Chapter 9 · Review and Assessment

Summary

Lesson 9.1 · The Effects of Alcohol

- *Alcohol* is a drug found in drinks that can cause a person to act and feel differently. Depending on the amount consumed, drinking alcohol can be considered moderate drinking, binge drinking, or heavy drinking.
- *Blood alcohol concentration (BAC)* is the percentage of alcohol in a person's blood. People with a BAC of 0.08 or above are considered intoxicated.
- As a person drinks alcohol, brain functions slow down. This may result in the following: stumbling, difficulty concentrating, memory loss, seizures, and frequent urination.
- Most people who drink too much will experience a hangover. Symptoms may include headaches, muscle aches, vomiting, dizziness, and sensitivity to light and sound.
- *Alcohol poisoning* is a medical emergency that results from too much alcohol in the bloodstream. Extreme cases can lead to permanent brain damage or death.
- Drinking alcohol long-term is associated with serious consequences, including permanent problems with learning and memory and chronic diseases like cirrhosis.
- Alcohol is the most commonly abused drug among youth in the United States. Young people who drink alcohol are at greater risk of experiencing problems with their physical health, at their school, with their family and friends, and with the law. Drinking alcohol also puts people at greater risk for accidents.
- Alcohol-use disorders occur when the use of alcohol causes problems that interfere with a person's health and responsibilities. People with an alcohol addiction continue to drink despite these problems.

Lesson 9.2 · Preventing and Treating Alcohol-Use Disorders

- The people in a young person's life can influence their decision to drink or avoid alcohol. These people may include a person's siblings, parents, peers, friends, and media figures.
- Young people are more likely to experiment with alcohol use if their parents or older siblings use or abuse alcohol. Their friends and peers may also try to pressure them into trying alcohol. The messages young people see in the media, such as TV commercials, social media, or in magazines, can also influence this decision.
- Education programs can help disprove the beliefs young people have about drinking and help them learn the physical, social, and mental consequences of alcohol use. Refusal skills can also help young people avoid drinking alcohol.
- The government has made alcohol difficult to obtain for young people with a minimum legal drinking age and sales tax.
- People with severe alcohol-use disorders can use detoxification, support groups like Alcoholics Anonymous, and self-management strategies for treatment. Enabling a person's unhealthy behaviors by covering up their problems will not treat the alcohol-use disorder.

Check Your Knowledge ⤤

Record your answers to each of the following questions on a separate sheet of paper.

1. Alcohol is a type of a drug known as a(n) _____.
2. For moderate drinking, how many alcoholic drinks can men and women consume on the same occasion?
3. **True or false.** Drinking eight or more drinks in one week for women and 15 or more drinks in one week for men can lead a person to become dependent on alcohol.
4. A person with a BAC of _____ or above is considered intoxicated or drunk.
5. **True or false.** Alcohol affects and is associated with health issues in every single organ and body system.
6. What is the name of the disorder that occurs when the use of alcohol causes problems that interfere with a person's health and responsibilities at school, home, or work?
7. **True or false.** A person's siblings, parents, peers, and celebrity idols do not have much of an influence on whether he or she decides to use alcohol.
8. Developing and practicing _____ skills can help when someone offers you alcohol.
9. What is the most obvious and effective government approach to prevent alcohol-use disorders among young people?
10. Which of the following is *not* an effective treatment method for alcohol-use disorders?
    A. Support groups.
    B. Detoxification.
    C. Enabling.
    D. Self-management.
11. The most well-known and widely used support group for people with alcohol-use disorders is _____.
12. What is the sub-group of AA that helps young people come together to share their experiences of having been affected by someone else's drinking?

Use Your Vocabulary ⤤

Al-Anon Family Groups	alcohol-use disorders	enabling
Alateen	binge drinking	heavy drinking
alcohol	blood alcohol	inhibition
Alcoholics	concentration (BAC)	moderate drinking
Anonymous (AA)	detoxification	zero-tolerance policy

13. With a partner, choose two words from the list above to compare. Create a Venn diagram to compare your words and identify differences. Write one term under the left circle and the other term under the right circle. For each term, write descriptions in each respective circle. Where the circles overlap, write three characteristics the terms have in common.
14. In small groups, create categories for the terms above and classify as many of the terms as possible. Then, share your ideas with another pair and discuss your categories.

Think Critically

15. **Assess.** Why are rules and laws about alcohol use needed? What are the intentions behind a minimum legal drinking age, laws against drinking and driving, or zero-tolerance policies?

16. **Compare and contrast.** Many factors influence a person's decision to use alcohol. Which influences do you think impact teens the most? Why?

17. **Draw conclusions.** For a person who is dependent on alcohol, draw conclusions about which level of dependency would be more difficult to overcome. Why?

18. **Identify.** What are the different options for treating alcohol-use disorders? Use valid resources to identify three treatment facilities or programs in your community.

DEVELOP Your Skills

19. **Conflict resolution and communication skills.** Imagine that a member of your family or someone you know is showing signs of an alcohol-use disorder. How would you address this problem? What if this person does not agree with your thoughts and is adamant that his or her alcohol use is safe and under control? What would you do?

20. **Decision-making and advocacy skills.** Create a public service announcement (PSA)—print, audio, or video—targeted toward students in your school. Focus your PSA on the promotion of having fun without drinking alcohol. Spotlight healthy alternatives to drinking alcohol. Mention the dangers of alcohol use as a teenager. Be sure to include information about how students can access help for alcohol-use disorders.

21. **Refusal and communication skills.** Practice makes permanent! Write at least three statements that are true for you and will clearly express your desire not to drink alcohol. Examples: "I'm not interested in drinking because I have alcoholism in my family." "No thanks, my parents would be so mad at me."

22. **Refusal and communication skills.** With a classmate, role-play a situation for the class in which one person is pressuring another to go to a party where "everyone" will be drinking alcohol. In the role-play, demonstrate your effective refusal skills.

23. **Access information.** Find a current news story (print or video) from the last six months that involves adolescent alcohol use. In writing, summarize the article and discuss the accuracy of the facts about alcohol presented. What can a teen learn from this situation, and what questions may remain? Properly cite the news story.

24. **Decision-making skills.** Many teens feel the effects of someone else's drinking, and Alateen and Al-Anon can help. Go to the Al-Anon Family Groups' website and click on the self-quiz for teens. On a sheet of paper, write your answers to the quiz questions. Use your decision-making skills to determine whether Alateen is a group that might be helpful to you.

Chapter 10

Medications and Drugs

Essential Question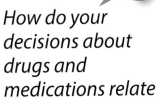

How do your decisions about drugs and medications relate to your health?

Video ↗
Access the Chapter 10 video to start thinking about chapter topics.

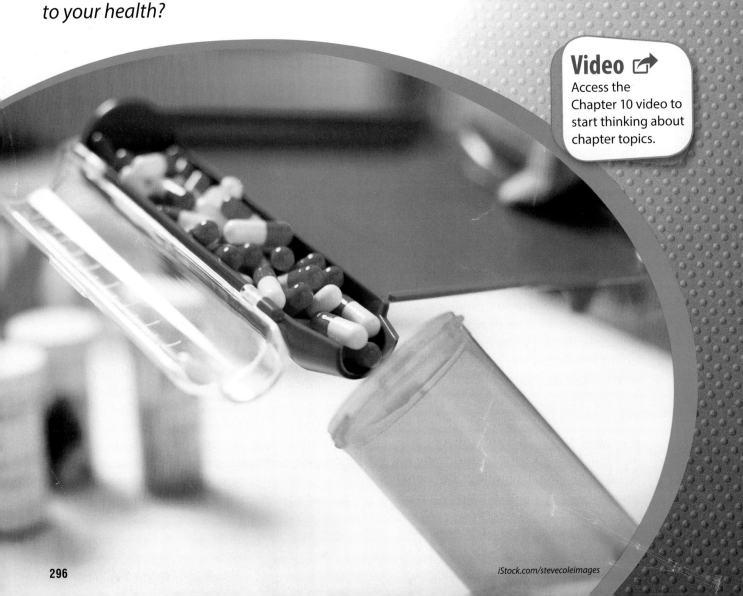

iStock.com/stevecoleimages

Reading Activity

Before reading the chapter, look at the illustrations and write a prediction about how the image illustrates a text concept. As you read the chapter, write notes about what information the text gives regarding these illustrations. After you finish reading the chapter, compare your predictions with your notes.

How Healthy Are You?

In this chapter, you will be learning about medications and drugs. Before you begin reading, take the following quiz to assess your current medication and drug habits.

Healthy Choices	Yes	No
Are you aware of the possible side effects of any medication you may take?		
Are you aware of the health risks caused by your medication interacting with other medications, dietary supplements, foods, or drinks?		
Are you aware of any allergies you have to medications?		
Do you always carefully read and follow the instructions for taking medication?		
Do you refuse to take medicine prescribed for someone else?		
Do you only use medication for the purposes and in the doses intended?		
Do you refuse to consume illegal drugs, including marijuana and club drugs?		
Do you understand the serious health risks, especially to adolescents, of using anabolic steroids?		
Do you avoid self-medicating with drugs to treat mental health conditions?		
Do you feel confident that you could refuse a friend's offer to try drugs?		
Do you avoid going to parties where drugs are present?		
Do you know about the resources at your school, in your community, and online that can help educate you about the dangers of abusing drugs?		

Count your "Yes" and "No" responses. The more "Yes" responses you have, the more healthy medication and drug habits you exhibit. Now, take a closer look at the questions with which you responded "No." How can you make these healthy habits part of your daily life? Think about how implementing these ideas can help improve your overall health.

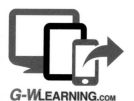

G-WLEARNING.COM

While studying this chapter, look for the activity icon ⤵ to

- **practice** key terms with e-flash cards and matching activities.
- **reinforce** what you learn by completing graphic organizers, self-assessment quizzes, and review questions.
- **expand** knowledge with interactive activities and activities that extend learning.

www.g-wlearning.com/health/

Key Terms 🔗

medications drugs and medicines used to treat symptoms of an illness or to cure, manage, or prevent a disease

drugs medications and other substances that change the way the body or brain functions

legal drugs medications that can treat health conditions to improve a person's health and enhance wellness

over-the-counter (OTC) medications medicines people can purchase without a doctor's written order or prescription to treat the symptoms of many minor health conditions

prescription medications medicines that people can only purchase with a doctor's written order for the treatment of a specific illness or condition

side effect unpleasant and unwanted symptom that occurs from taking a medication

overdose taking too much of a medication; often causes dangerous, life-threatening consequences

medication misuse taking medication in a way that does not follow the medication's instructions; often unintentional

medication abuse intentionally taking a drug in a way other than its intended use

Learning Outcomes

After studying this lesson, you will be able to

- **differentiate between** over-the-counter and prescription medications.
- **explain** three health risks of taking medications.
- **identify** strategies for using medications safely.
- **summarize** the different functions of different types of prescription medications.
- **differentiate between** medication misuse and abuse.

Graphic Organizer 🔗

Safe Medication Use

In a graphic organizer like the one shown below, write eight statements about strategies for using medications safely. As you read the lesson, note any health benefits of safe medication usage not previously known.

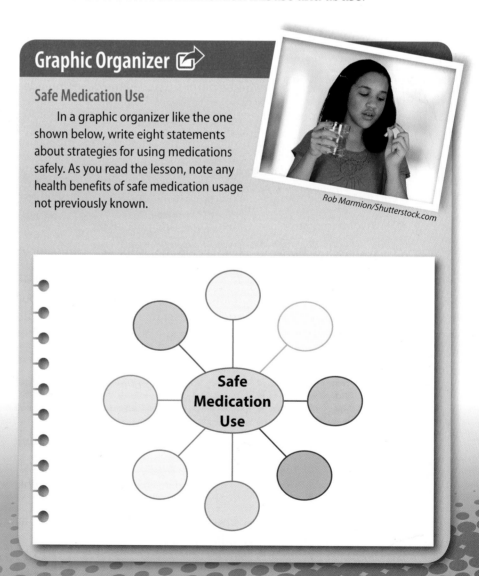

Rob Marmion/Shutterstock.com

Safe Medication Use

Jamal is 12 years old. He has to stay home from school today because he is sick. His dad gives him an ibuprofen to treat his low-grade fever and tells him to get some sleep. Jamal has a hard time resting, however, because of his cough. When it starts to become painful, Jamal's dad drives to the drugstore and buys some over-the-counter cough syrup and cough drops to help soothe his throat. Jamal takes one dose of cough syrup and another one after his two-hour nap. He did not read the label, so he does not know that he is only supposed to take one dose every four to six hours.

Ibuprofen and cough medicine are examples of medications and legal drugs that people like Jamal can take to treat symptoms of an illness or prevent a disease. These drugs and medications come with specific instructions, however, that must be followed.

Defining Medications and Drugs

When you hear the terms *medications* and *drugs*, would you define them in the same way? Sometimes, you might say they are the same. At other times, you would not. **Medications** are drugs and medicines used to treat symptoms of an illness or to cure, manage, or prevent a disease. **Drugs** are medications and other substances that change the way the body or brain functions. According to these definitions, all medications are drugs. Not all drugs, however, are medications. This is because there are two categories of drugs— legal drugs and illegal drugs (**Figure 10.1**).

Legal drugs are medications that can treat health conditions to improve a person's health and enhance wellness. You will be learning about legal drugs in this lesson. *Illegal drugs* are substances that are against the law to use because they can be harmful to a person's health. In the next lesson, you will learn about the types and effects of illegal drugs.

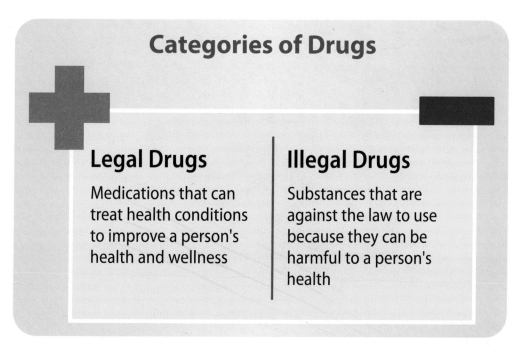

Categories of Drugs

Legal Drugs
Medications that can treat health conditions to improve a person's health and wellness

Illegal Drugs
Substances that are against the law to use because they can be harmful to a person's health

Figure 10.1
All medications are drugs, but certain drugs (such as illegal drugs) are not considered medications.

Types of Medications

There are two different types of medications people take to improve their health. These types include over-the-counter medications and prescription medications. Both types come in many different forms. For example, medications may come in liquid, pill, tablet, and capsule forms that you swallow. Creams, gels, and ointments are *topical* forms of medicine that work best if placed directly on an affected area, such as a rash on your feet. An *injection*, or shot, is yet another way to take medication. When you get an injection, a special needle is used to insert liquid medicine into your body. **Figure 10.2** shows the different forms of medications.

In addition to the many different forms of medications available, medicines also come in different doses and dosages. A *dose* refers to the amount of a medicine you take at one time. *Dosage* describes the number of times, or how often, you take the medicine.

Over-the-Counter Medications

Over-the-counter (OTC) medications are medicines people can purchase without a doctor's written order or prescription to treat the symptoms of many minor health conditions. Your parents may keep certain OTC medications in the house in case someone gets sick. These medications can treat headaches, fevers, and the common cold.

The most commonly used OTC medications are pain relievers, such as aspirin, acetaminophen, and ibuprofen. Other OTC medications include fever reducers, cold medicines, cough medicines, and certain allergy medications.

Figure 10.2
The form of medication a person needs depends on the type of condition being treated. *If you have a rash on your arm, what form of medication often works best to treat this condition?*

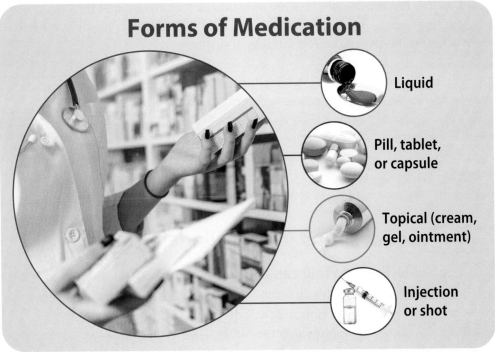

Forms of Medication

- Liquid
- Pill, tablet, or capsule
- Topical (cream, gel, ointment)
- Injection or shot

Left: Aleksandar Karanov/Shutterstock.com; Top to bottom: Africa Studio/Shutterstock.com; Triff/Shutterstock.com; Enriscapes/Shutterstock.com; studiovin/Shutterstock.com

Prescription Medications

Prescription medications are medicines that people can only purchase with a prescription from a doctor. Once a person has a prescription, he or she can take it to a pharmacy to get the medication. A *pharmacy* is a store that sells both over-the-counter and prescription medications. If a person needs more of the prescription medication, he or she must get approval for a refill from the doctor.

There are different types of prescription medications. Each different type has a different function. **Figure 10.3** shows different types of prescription medications and the functions of each.

Health Risks of Taking Medications

Taking over-the-counter and prescription medications can be beneficial to your health. Using these medications, however, can also carry some risks. These include side effects, drug interactions, and allergic reactions.

Types and Functions of Prescription Medications

Types	Functions
Antibiotics	Kill or slow the growth of bacteria
Anesthetics	Eliminate or reduce pain
Vaccinations	Work with the body's natural immune system to reduce the risk of developing an infection or disease
Opioids	Reduce pain, often after surgery
Depressants (also called *sedatives* or *tranquilizers*)	Reduce anxiety and help people relax, stay calm, and sleep
Stimulants (available both with a prescription and over-the-counter)	Increase energy, alertness, and attention

Figure 10.3 The types of medications listed in the table above can only be purchased by having a written prescription from a doctor. *What is the name of a store that sells both OTC and prescription medications?*

Side Effects

All medications, even OTC medications, can cause side effects. A **side effect** is a typically unpleasant and unwanted symptom that occurs from taking a medication. Side effects can be minor or severe. For example, minor side effects may include drowsiness, headache, nausea, or dry mouth. Side effects that are more serious include stomach bleeding, ulcers, suicidal thoughts, or abnormal heart rhythms. Some side effects may even cause permanent damage or death. Side effects are more likely to occur in certain situations, including when you do the following:

- start taking a new medication
- stop taking a medication that you have been taking for a while
- increase or decrease the amount of a medication you are taking

Before taking any new medication, always read the label on the medication bottle, which includes information about possible side effects. Knowing the side effects ahead of time allows you to better understand them if they occur. If you do not understand the possible side effects of a medication, ask your doctor or pharmacist to explain them to you.

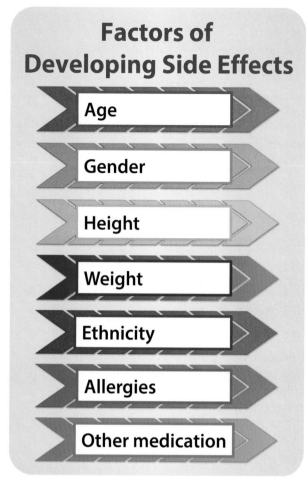

Factors of Developing Side Effects

- Age
- Gender
- Height
- Weight
- Ethnicity
- Allergies
- Other medication

Figure 10.4 Several factors can affect whether a person may be more likely than another to experience side effects from certain medications. *If you do experience side effects, what actions can your doctor recommend to reduce or eliminate the side effects?*

Several factors affect whether you will have side effects from a medication (**Figure 10.4**). You may not experience any side effects, however. If side effects do occur, ask your doctor if there is a way to reduce or eliminate them. Your doctor may suggest switching to a different medication or changing the dose or dosage of the medication you are taking.

Drug Interactions

Some medications cause health risks by interacting with other drugs, dietary supplements, foods, or drinks. These health risks can be minor. For example, you may need to take a medicine with food. If you take the medicine without eating anything, you may get an upset stomach. Other health risks from drug interactions are serious and can be life threatening.

Many medication labels include warnings to avoid mixing alcohol with medicines. This is because using alcohol while taking medication can make the medicine less effective. Mixing alcohol with medicines can also cause side effects, some of which can be very serious.

When your doctor prescribes a new medication, tell him or her about the medications you are already taking. This will help your doctor give you information on possible drug interactions. You can also learn about potential interactions by reading the label on the medication bottle or by asking the pharmacist (**Figure 10.5**).

Allergic Reactions

If a person is *allergic* to a substance, he or she has unpleasant, sometimes life-threatening symptoms related to the substance. When you think about allergies, you probably think about dust or pollen in the air, or food allergies such as a peanut or gluten allergy.

Figure 10.5 Over-the-counter medication labels will list any potential drug interactions. Read the label carefully before taking any medicines.

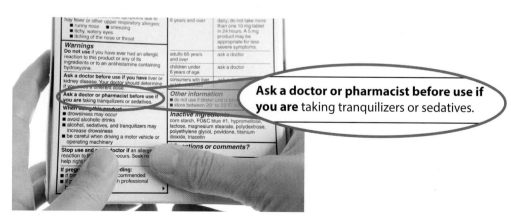

iStock.com/JulNichols

Some people are allergic to certain medicines. This means that a person has an allergic reaction after taking a medicine. In some cases, reactions can be minor, such as vomiting, nausea, or a rash. In other cases, reactions can be serious and even life threatening. For example, a person might experience swelling of the tongue or difficulty breathing.

People may not know they are allergic to a medication until they take it and have a reaction. If you have an allergic reaction after taking a medication, tell your parents immediately. Some reactions may require emergency medical care. Once you know you are allergic to a medicine, always be sure to tell the doctors and other healthcare professionals you see about this allergy.

Strategies for Using Medications Safely

Carefully reading and following prescription and over-the-counter usage instructions can help people make sure they are taking medications safely. The instructions should be on the medication label, box, or container. **Figure 10.6** shows the usage instructions on a prescription medication label and an over-the-counter label. Always make sure you understand the usage instructions before taking any medication. If you have any questions about a medicine, consult your doctor or pharmacist.

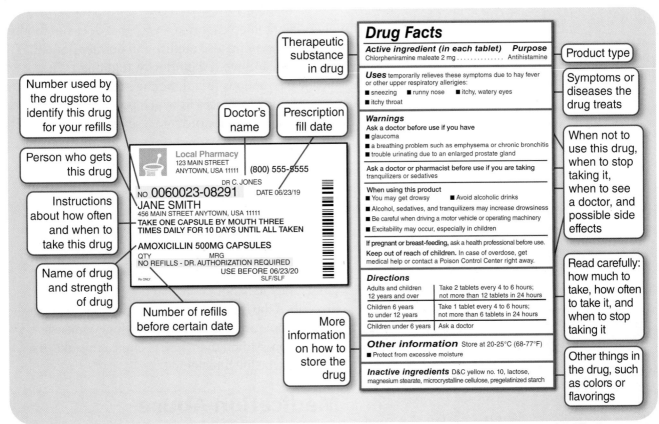

Courtesy of the US Department of Health and Human Services

Figure 10.6 Both prescription and OTC labels provide instructions about when to use the drug, when not to use the drug, when to stop taking it, and possible side effects. *Who should you consult if you have any questions about a medicine?*

Other strategies for using medications safely include the following:

- Follow the directions for taking a medication exactly as written. Pay attention to any warnings printed on the label.
- Use OTC medications that have only the ingredients needed to treat the condition or symptoms.
- Check the expiration date. Just as food items can go bad, medications can go bad. Expired medications will be less effective.
- Store medications carefully in a dry, cool area on high shelves or in locked cabinets where children cannot reach them.
- Do not give OTC medications intended for adults to infants or children (**Figure 10.7**).
- Never use a medication prescribed for someone else or let someone else use a medication prescribed for you. Prescriptions are given specifically for one person, based on that person's symptoms, age, weight, and height, and cannot be used safely by anyone else.
- See a healthcare professional if a health problem does not go away after using OTC medication.
- Never take more than the recommended dosage of a medication. Doing so can lead to accidental **overdose**, or taking too much of a medication. An overdose can pose dangerous risks to your health and may even lead to death.

Medication Misuse

Medication misuse involves taking medication in a way that does not follow the medication's instructions. People may misuse medication unintentionally because they forgot or did not understand what their doctor told them. They might misunderstand the label or instructions for taking the medication.

Medication misuse may also include instances in which people stop taking a medication before they should. Perhaps a doctor ordered a seven-day supply of medication, but the person feels better in five days and stops taking the medicine. Even though the person feels better, the person should take the medicine for all seven days. Taking someone else's prescription medicine and offering someone your prescription medicine are other forms of medication misuse.

Medication misuse is typically the result of honest mistakes. People who misuse medications often misunderstand instructions or forget to check them. They may not know that only the person prescribed the medication should take that medicine. These people are not necessarily trying to misuse medication. Although misuse is often a mistake, the results can be life threatening.

Medication Abuse

Medication abuse involves taking a drug in a way other than its intended use. Unlike medication misuse, which is often unintentional, medication abuse is *intentional*, meaning that people do it

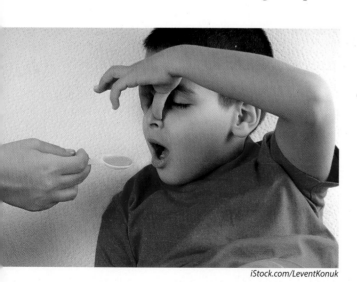

iStock.com/LeventKonuk

Figure 10.7
There are OTC medications specifically intended for children's use.

on purpose. The most commonly abused prescription medications are opioids, depressants, and stimulants (**Figure 10.8**). Medication abuse is a growing problem among young people that can result in many negative long-term health effects.

Young people may abuse prescription and OTC drugs to achieve effects similar to those experienced with many illegal drugs. They may also abuse these drugs to lose weight, fit in with their peers, or even study more effectively. Some young people will share a prescription drug with their friends just for fun. Taking someone else's prescription, however, is actually against the law. Medicines are only safe when taken for their intended purpose, in the recommended amounts, and by the person who has a prescription.

Medication abuse can negatively affect a person's physical, mental, social, and emotional health. A person who abuses medications may also experience problems at home, at school, at work, or with family and friends. Later in this chapter, you will learn more about the consequences of drug abuse.

Health Effects of Prescription Medications

Drug	Health Effects
Opioids (codeine, hydrocodone, morphine, oxycodone)	Dizziness, nausea, vomiting, lack of coordination, low blood pressure, confusion, sweaty and clammy skin, coma, death (especially when combined with alcohol or depressants)
Depressants (antianxiety medications, sleep medications)	Slowed and slurred speech, poor concentration, lack of coordination, confusion, lowered inhibition, depression, chronic fatigue, difficulty sleeping, coma, death (often by overdose)
Stimulants (ADHD medication, energy pills, weight-loss supplements)	Increased blood pressure and heart rate, low-quality sleep, decreased appetite (which could lead to malnutrition), increased body temperature, depression, feelings of hostility, paranoia, irregular heartbeat, heart attack, stroke

Figure 10.8 Abusing prescription medications has a number of negative consequences for a young person's health, including a high rate of dependence and addiction.

Lesson 10.1 Review

1. _____ are drugs and medicines used to treat symptoms of an illness or to cure, manage, or prevent a disease.
2. What is a store that sells both over-the-counter and prescription medications?
3. **True or false.** People who take the same medication experience the same side effects.
4. List three strategies for using medications safely.
5. **Critical thinking.** List three examples of ways a person can misuse medication. Explain whether each example is on purpose, on accident, or both.

Hands-On Activity

Create a list of risky behaviors related to medication use and misuse. Write each risky behavior on a sticky note, and arrange the notes in order from *least* risky to *most* risky. On each note, justify your ranking. With a partner, compare answers and discuss why you ranked the risky behaviors in a particular order. Based on collaboration with your partner, change your ranking order if needed and add to your list of reasons. Lastly, choose one of the behaviors and create an illustrated digital poster to raise awareness of the negative long-term effects of this behavior.

Illegal Drugs

Key Terms 📱

illegal drugs substances that are against the law to use because they can be harmful to a person's health

marijuana drug made up of dried parts of the cannabis plant

cocaine drug that usually comes in the form of white powder made from the leaves of the coca plant

methamphetamine stimulant that speeds up brain functions

hallucinogens drugs that alter the way people view, think, and feel about things, causing hallucinations

heroin drug similar to painkillers that has dangerous side effects and is very addictive

club drugs several different types of drugs that young people may abuse at parties, bars, and concerts

inhalants chemicals that people breathe in to experience some type of high

drug abuse continued use of a drug despite negative or harmful outcomes

drug addiction complete dependence on a drug

Learning Outcomes

After studying this lesson, you will be able to

- **give examples** of common types of illegal drugs.
- **describe** the short- and long-term health effects of illegal drugs.
- **explain** why some young people use drugs.
- **describe** the physical, mental, emotional, and social consequences of drug abuse and addiction.
- **recognize** the signs of drug abuse and drug addiction.

Graphic Organizer 📱

Negative Effects of Drugs

As you read this lesson, use a table like the one shown below to list the types of illegal drugs and include a list of negative side effects. Highlight the negative effects the illegal drugs have in common. An example is provided for you.

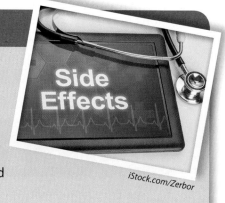

iStock.com/Zerbor

Drug Name	Negative Effects
Inhalants	Slurred speech, memory problems, lack of coordination, muscle spasms and tremors, dizziness, hallucination

In the previous lesson, you learned that *medications* are substances used to treat symptoms of an illness or to cure, manage, or prevent a disease. In this lesson, you will be learning about drugs that are not medications. They are *illegal drugs*.

Jamal, from the first lesson, does not mess around with illegal drugs. He is even generally pretty careful with the prescription medications he uses. His cousin became addicted to cocaine when he was younger, and Jamal remembers the way the drug took over his cousin's life. She sold all of her things to make money to buy more drugs, and she stopped going to school or hanging out with her friends. Eventually, she got arrested. Jamal never wanted that for himself, so he promised that he would never take illegal drugs.

Types of Illegal Drugs

Illegal drugs are substances that are against the law to use because they can be harmful to a person's health. People often use illegal drugs to experience a *high*, which is an elevated mood or rush of positive emotions. In contrast, some drugs make people feel relaxed. Most drugs, however, can be very dangerous. In this section, you will learn about some common types of illegal drugs and the harmful effects they can have on all aspects of a person's health.

Marijuana

According to the National Institute on Drug Abuse, marijuana is the most commonly used illegal drug in the United States. **Marijuana** is a drug made up of dried parts of the cannabis plant (**Figure 10.9**). People who use marijuana usually smoke it as a cigarette (a joint) or in a pipe. Others may mix marijuana into food or brew it as a tea. Slang terms for marijuana include *weed*, *pot*, *Mary Jane*, and *grass*.

The active ingredient in marijuana is a mind-altering chemical called *THC*. Upon entering the bloodstream, THC travels to the brain and other organs. THC affects the parts of the brain that control pleasure, memory, thinking, concentration, sensory and time perception, and movement.

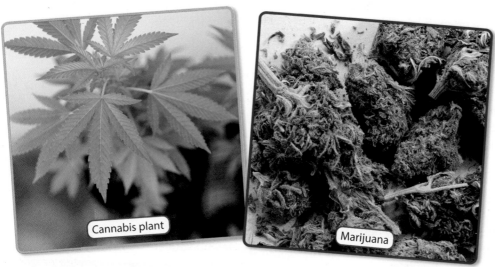

Figure 10.9
Parts of the cannabis plant are dried to create the drug marijuana. *What is the name of the mind-altering chemical that is the active ingredient in marijuana?*

Cannabis plant

Marijuana

Cannabis plant: iStock.com/MStudioImages; Marijuana: Courtesy of the Department of Justice, Drug Enforcement Administration

Marijuana can be manufactured to have up to four times the concentration of THC. This is called *marijuana concentrate*, or *THC extraction*. Slang terms for marijuana concentrate include *wax*, *honey oil*, and *dabs*. Marijuana concentrate is similar in appearance to honey or butter, and is usually smoked.

Negative Health Effects

People who use marijuana experience many negative health effects. They have overall poorer physical, mental, social, and emotional health. They also experience more problems at school, home, or work. Marijuana use has a wide range of short-term negative health effects, which may include the following:

- difficulty thinking and problem solving
- problems with memory and learning
- anxiety and panic attacks
- loss of coordination
- delayed reactions to situations

CASE STUDY

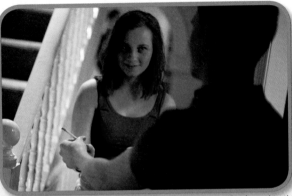

iStock.com/sturti

Raquel's Risky Behavior

Raquel did not think it was that big of a deal—just a couple hits of marijuana. She felt so free. All her thoughts and worries disappeared. She laughed with her friends that day, but mostly just chilled. When Raquel returned home, her parents were still yelling at each other, and her responsibilities as a big sister felt overwhelming.

Days passed and Raquel remembered craving the feeling of getting high. Tension continued to escalate in her family, and her grades were dropping. She promised herself that she would never smoke again. Raquel's cousin used to make straight A's in high school and had such a promising future until he started smoking marijuana all of the time. Raquel was not sure why he smoked so much considering he did not have any of the problems as she did. Raquel thought to herself, "I have real problems, and it feels like no one sees me or hears my voice."

Raquel resisted for weeks, and then gave in and smoked with a group of friends—once again, feeling free and happy. She smoked about once a week during the school year. Her home life never got better, and her grades continued to decline throughout the school year.

Finally, school was out for the summer. Raquel's parents allowed her to attend a graduation party

with a small group of friends. While at the party, one of Raquel's friends pulled out a handful of pills and offered them to the group. None of the girls seemed interested. Neither was Raquel—although she was a little curious. Her friend said it was Xanax and that the pill would make her feel relaxed. Raquel had promised herself that she would never move onto another drug.

Thinking Critically

1. How is drug use molding Raquel's future?

2. If you were Raquel's friend, what advice would you give her to cope with her stressful family life? List at least four healthy strategies that Raquel could use to relieve stress and anger.

3. Do you think Raquel will take the Xanax? Why or why not? Defend your answer.

4. Predict whether you think that knowing the consequences will help Raquel to stop using drugs. Defend your answer.

The effects of marijuana on learning and memory can last for days or weeks after the immediate effects of the drug wear off. This is because the chemical THC remains in the body for days or weeks after using marijuana. Due to the high concentration of THC in marijuana concentrate, the negative health effects can be more intense.

Marijuana use can also lead to long-term negative health effects. People who use marijuana show a substantial increase in heart rate, which can cause heart problems. Because people tend to smoke marijuana, they can develop the same respiratory problems that affect tobacco smokers. Minor respiratory problems include daily cough, more frequent chest illnesses, and an increased risk of lung infection.

Legalization of Marijuana

Until recently, marijuana was illegal to sell, buy, and use across the United States. Today, a number of states and the District of Columbia allow adults with a doctor's prescription to legally buy and use marijuana in that state for medical purposes only. Marijuana can ease the symptoms of various medical conditions, including seizures, muscle spasms, and the nausea caused by chemotherapy treatments for cancer.

In 2014, Colorado voted to allow people older than 21 years of age to buy a limited amount of marijuana for recreational or nonmedical use. During the 2016 election, California, Nevada, Maine, and Massachusetts also legalized recreational marijuana use and sale. People who purchase marijuana legally in these states cannot take the marijuana into a state where it is illegal. If they do, they are breaking the law.

Although some states have legalized marijuana, many other states, along with the federal government, still classify marijuana as an illegal drug. This is because the use of marijuana, even for medical purposes, can still pose health risks. Therefore, there is much debate on both federal and state levels of government about legalization of marijuana. Research about medical uses for marijuana is ongoing.

Cocaine

Cocaine is a white powder that comes from the leaves of the coca plant (**Figure 10.10**). People who use cocaine do so by inhaling the substance through the nose. Others may dissolve the cocaine in water and inject it into a vein. Some people may process this illegal drug into a solid form, known as *crack cocaine*, which they smoke in a pipe. Slang terms for cocaine include *blow, coke, crack, candy, rock,* and *snow.*

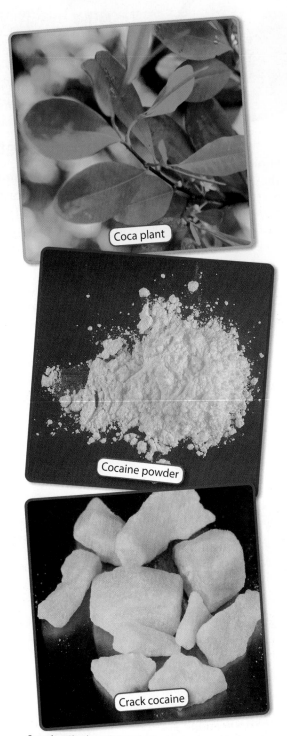

Coca plant

Cocaine powder

Crack cocaine

Coca plant: iStock.com/mtcurado; Cocaine powder and crack cocaine: Courtesy of the Department of Justice, Drug Enforcement Administration

Figure 10.10 The leaves of the coca plant are manufactured into a white powder, called *cocaine,* or into a solid form, which is known as *crack cocaine.*

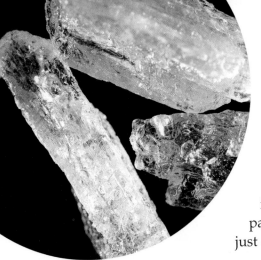

Courtesy of the Department of Justice, Drug Enforcement Administration

Figure 10.11
The clear crystal chunks of crystal meth is a form of methamphetamine that is very powerful and addictive.

Cocaine causes a fast, intense high. The high wears off quickly, however, and the user feels nervous and depressed. Cocaine is addictive because its high does not last very long. A person is likely to use cocaine more than once to achieve that intense high again. The more a person uses cocaine, the more dangerous it becomes.

Cocaine can have both short- and long-term negative effects on the body. These side effects include high body temperature, increased heart rate, high blood pressure, headaches, abdominal pain and nausea, paranoia, and loss of sense of smell. Using cocaine just one time can lead to sudden death due to a heart attack or stroke.

Methamphetamine

Methamphetamine is a manmade stimulant that speeds up brain function. *Crystal meth* is a form of methamphetamine that people create and use to get high (**Figure 10.11**). This drug consists of clear crystal chunks. Crystal meth is usually smoked, but people may also inhale it through the nose, inject it into a vein, or swallow it. Slang terms for this drug include *meth, ice, crank, crystal,* and *speed*.

Crystal meth is a very powerful and extremely addictive illegal drug. People who use this drug quickly become physically and psychologically addicted to its use. This means their bodies and minds crave the drug.

People who use crystal meth feel energized. They are often able to engage in continuous activity without stopping for sleep. Users also experience irregular heartbeats, sweating, blurred vision, and dizziness. Crystal meth has many short- and long-term negative health effects, which are similar to those of cocaine. These include violent and unpredictable behavior, mood swings, problems with memory, and paranoia. Users sometimes develop a condition known as "meth mouth," which consists of broken or rotten teeth (**Figure 10.12**). Using too much crystal meth at one time can result in brain damage, coma, stroke, and death.

Hallucinogens

Hallucinogens are drugs that alter the way people view, think, and feel about situations, thereby causing hallucinations. *Hallucinations* are things that seem real, such as a sound, image, or smell, but do not really exist. The most common hallucinogen is *LSD*, which is a colorless, odorless substance that is often soaked into pieces of paper. People lick or swallow this paper to take the drug. People may also swallow hallucinogens as pills or tablets.

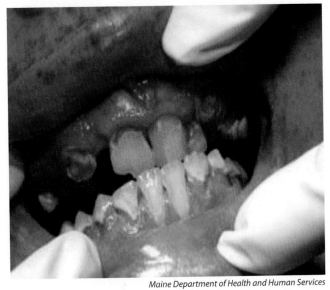

Maine Department of Health and Human Services

Figure 10.12 One of the more visible side effects of abusing crystal meth is damaged, blackened teeth. **What is the nickname for this condition?**

People who use hallucinogens experience negative short-term health effects. These include trouble sleeping, panic, increased blood pressure and breathing rate, and paranoia. Long-term negative health effects include memory loss, difficulties with speech and thinking, and seizures. People may also experience *flashbacks*, or recurring thoughts of certain effects of these drugs. Flashbacks can happen suddenly, without warning, within a few days, or more than a year after using the drugs. In some cases, even a single use of a hallucinogen can lead to death.

Opiods (Heroin)

The drug known as **heroin** is made from morphine, a substance that comes from the opium poppy plant found in Asia, Mexico, and South America (**Figure 10.13**). Pure heroin is a white powder, but other forms of the drug are dark brown or black. People usually inject, snort, or smoke heroin. Slang terms for heroin include *smack*, *horse*, and *junk*. A *speedball* is the term used when people mix heroin with crack cocaine.

Morphine is also an opioid prescription pain medication. The effects of morphine are similar to the effects of heroin. People who abuse prescription medications that contain morphine may be more likely to try heroin. In fact, the National Institute on Drug Abuse reports that nearly 80 percent of Americans using heroin abused prescription opioids before trying heroin.

Once a user takes heroin, the drug rapidly enters the brain and changes back into morphine. Users feel a sudden, intense "high" that quickly wears off. Many negative short-term health effects soon follow the high. These include dry mouth, flushed skin, problems thinking, and semiconsciousness. Heroin is highly addictive and people experience constant cravings for the drug, making it difficult to stop using heroin.

People who become addicted and try to stop using heroin experience severe withdrawal symptoms. These symptoms can begin within a few hours after taking the drug. Symptoms may include vomiting, cold flashes, uncontrollable leg movements, muscle aches, sleep problems, and severe cravings for the drug.

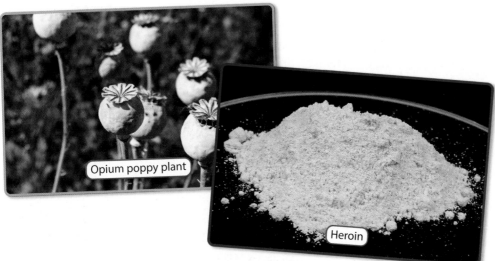

Opium poppy plant

Heroin

Figure 10.13
The legal drug morphine and the illegal drug heroin can both be made from the opium poppy plant. *What percentage of heroin users abused prescription opioids like morphine before trying heroin?*

Opium poppy plant: DNetromphotos/Shutterstock.com; Heroin: Courtesy of the Department of Justice, Drug Enforcement Administration

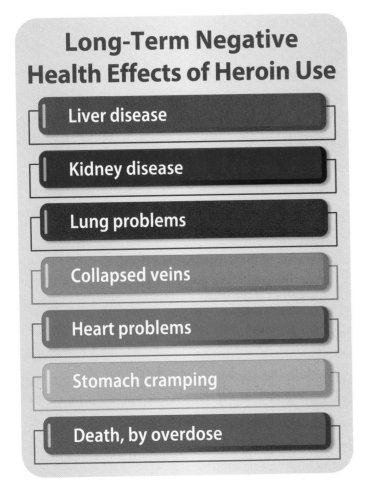

Long-Term Negative Health Effects of Heroin Use

- Liver disease
- Kidney disease
- Lung problems
- Collapsed veins
- Heart problems
- Stomach cramping
- Death, by overdose

Figure 10.14 Heroin use can cause negative health effects in many parts of the body, including the heart, lungs, kidneys, and stomach.

Many long-term negative health effects occur from using heroin (**Figure 10.14**). Death can occur, even after one use, if a person takes too much heroin. This is because the heroin causes a person's breathing to slow or stop. The lack of oxygen to the brain can cause a coma, permanent brain damage, or death.

Heroin purchased on the street is often mixed with other chemicals that can cause negative health effects, which include permanent damage to the brain, lungs, liver, and kidneys. Users who inject heroin and share needles with others have an increased risk of contracting HIV and hepatitis C.

Club Drugs

The term **club drugs** refers to several different types of drugs young people may abuse at parties, bars, and concerts. These drugs include Rohypnol® (*roofies*), GHB (gamma hydroxybutyrate), and MDMA (*ecstasy*, or *Molly*). Club drugs often come in capsule, tablet, liquid, or powder form. Some types may also be ground and inhaled or injected into the body.

Club drugs often have no smell or taste. Sometimes, people have used these drugs to slip them into someone else's food or drink without the person knowing. This can lead to highly dangerous situations. For example, these drugs are known as *date rape drugs* because criminals sometimes use them to commit sexual assaults. Club drugs have many short- and long-term health effects (**Figure 10.15**).

Figure 10.15 Some criminals use club drugs to help them commit sexual assaults. *What is another name for club drugs when this type of dangerous situation occurs?*

Effects of Club Drugs	
Rohypnol	Rohypnol makes people unable to move or respond to events that are happening. After the drug wears off hours later, the person cannot remember what happened. Short-term health effects include headaches, nausea, dizziness, and confusion. Long-term effects may include breathing problems and depression. Rohypnol is addictive.
GHB	GHB is a drug that slows the processes in the brain. It causes an intense high and hallucinations. Short-term health effects include dizziness, nausea, and vomiting. The drug may cause unconsciousness. Using GHB can result in death.
MDMA	MDMA is a manmade chemical that is the main ingredient in ecstasy. MDMA increases activity of chemicals in the brain that increase heart rate and blood pressure and affect a person's mood, sleep, and other functions. Short-term side effects include muscle tension, nausea, dizziness, and high body temperature. MDMA can be addictive and may lead to permanent brain damage, organ failure, or death.

Anabolic Steroids

Anabolic steroids are artificial hormones, meaning they were created in a lab. Some steroids imitate *testosterone* (the male sex hormone), which helps build muscle in the body.

Doctors may prescribe steroids to treat hormonal issues or muscle disorders. These are legal uses of steroids. Some people, however, use anabolic steroids illegally to gain strength and increase muscle size. Common ways to take anabolic steroids include swallowing, injecting, or applying them as a gel, cream, or patch. Steroid use can be addictive.

Common short-term effects of using steroids include extreme irritability and mood swings that could lead to violence, delusions, and impaired judgment. Long-term effects of anabolic steroid abuse may lead to liver damage, stroke, heart attack, and kidney problems or failure. Some other effects of steroid use are specific to gender, which include the following:

- Men experience shrinking of the testicles, baldness, development of breasts, and increased risk of prostate cancer.
- Women experience growth of facial hair, baldness, changes in or disruption of the menstrual cycle, and a deepened voice.

Inhalants

Inhalants are chemicals that people breathe in to experience some type of high. Common inhalants are often substances found in the home (**Figure 10.16**). These substances are inhaled into the nose or mouth in several ways. Chemical fumes may be sniffed or snorted from a container, which is called *huffing*. Chemicals can also be sprayed directly into the nose or mouth. Slang terms for inhalants include *whippets, poppers*, and *snappers*.

Inhalants cause a high that lasts just a few minutes, so people tend to use them more than once to maintain the feeling. Inhaling chemicals can decrease the body's supply of oxygen. This damages the body's cells, especially brain cells. Other side effects of using inhalants include slurred speech, memory problems, lack of coordination, muscle spasms and tremors, dizziness, and hallucinations.

Inhalant use can also cause serious, permanent side effects. These include hearing loss and damage to the brain, central nervous system, liver, and kidneys. Using inhalants—even once—can cause death due to heart failure or suffocation.

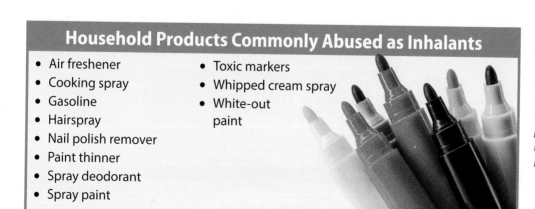

Household Products Commonly Abused as Inhalants

- Air freshener
- Cooking spray
- Gasoline
- Hairspray
- Nail polish remover
- Paint thinner
- Spray deodorant
- Spray paint
- Toxic markers
- Whipped cream spray
- White-out paint

Lunatictm/Shutterstock.com

Figure 10.16 Products commonly found in households can be very dangerous when used for purposes other than their intended uses. *Why do people abuse common household products as inhalants?*

Why Do Some Young People Use Illegal Drugs?

Choosing to live a drug-free lifestyle can be challenging for young people, especially when their environment exposes them to drugs and the pressures of trying them (**Figure 10.17**). For example, if a young person's family member, friend, or role model uses drugs, he or she may copy that behavior.

Often, young people have an incorrect picture of how drugs will make them feel or affect their lives. For example, young people may believe that drugs will help them think more clearly, become popular, and be better artists or athletes.

During the adolescent years, peers have a strong influence on a young person's drug use. Young people may feel pressured to try drugs if they attend parties where drugs are present. They may not want to feel left out, or they may think they will enjoy the party more if they try drugs. Young people whose friends use drugs are more likely to use drugs.

Young people may also believe that drugs can help them feel better. For example, young people who have mental health problems, such as depression or anxiety, may use drugs to cope with their symptoms (**Figure 10.18**). The only way to successfully treat their conditions, however, is to seek professional help.

In Lesson 10.3, you will learn strategies you can use to refuse drugs. It is important to remember that trying a drug just one time can cause serious health problems. That single use can also lead to long-term drug abuse and addiction.

Figure 10.17
The people and communities in a young person's life have the biggest influence on whether or not he or she decides to try drugs.

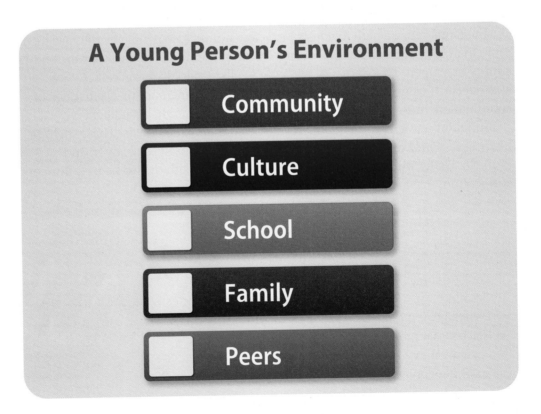

A Young Person's Environment

- Community
- Culture
- School
- Family
- Peers

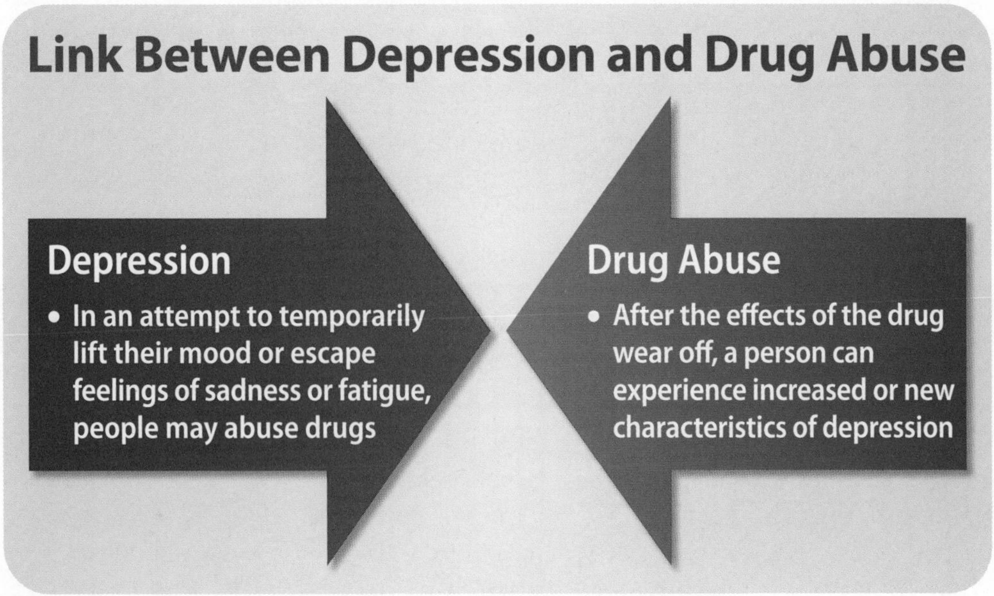

Link Between Depression and Drug Abuse

Depression
- In an attempt to temporarily lift their mood or escape feelings of sadness or fatigue, people may abuse drugs

Drug Abuse
- After the effects of the drug wear off, a person can experience increased or new characteristics of depression

Figure 10.18
People who are depressed may use drugs to treat their mental health condition, but drugs can increase feelings of despair, exhaustion, and sadness. *What is the only way to successfully treat a mental health condition?*

Drug Abuse

Drug abuse is the continued use of an illegal drug despite negative or harmful outcomes. Some outcomes of drug abuse affect a person's health. The types of health outcomes a person faces will depend on which drug a person takes. Certain health outcomes affect everyone who abuses drugs, regardless of the specific drug. These outcomes include the following:

- Because drug use *impairs*, or weakens, the ability to think clearly and carefully, people under the influence of drugs are more likely to engage in risky, unsafe behaviors. These behaviors can result in injury and other negative outcomes.
- People who use a needle to inject drugs have an increased risk of contracting serious diseases, such as HIV or hepatitis C.
- Drugs change brain functions and can impair a person's ability to drive safely. If a person tries to drive while under the influence of a drug, he or she is likely to have an accident. This can result in injury to or death of oneself and others.
- An overdose may result from taking too much of a drug at one time, causing life-threatening health risks. A person who overdoses on a drug may do so on purpose or by accident.

In addition to these negative health outcomes, people who abuse drugs experience other problems. These include the following:

- legal problems, such as a criminal record
- academic problems, such as being suspended or expelled from school
- work problems, such as a habit of taking time off, failing drug tests, and getting fired
- financial problems
- social problems, such as losing friends

The Consequences of Drug Use

GAME OVER

YOUR SCORE: 0

— GAME RECAP —

LEGAL PROBLEMS
- A criminal record
- Possible jail time

ACADEMIC PROBLEMS
- Suspension
- Expulsion
- Inability to focus
- Slacking on homework

SOCIAL PROBLEMS
- Losing friends
- Isolation
- Estrangement from family

WORK PROBLEMS
- Bad habits such as taking time off
- Failing drug tests
- Termination

Start Over

Drug Addiction

Drug addiction is a complete dependence on a drug. If a person is addicted to a drug, he or she has a physical and psychological need for the drug. This means that the person's mind and body both crave the drug. **Figure 10.19** shows characteristics of drug addiction.

No one who starts using drugs plans to become addicted to them. Unfortunately, many people who use drugs become addicted and spend years trying to break their habit. As you learned in earlier chapters, addiction to tobacco and alcohol follow certain stages—experimentation, regular use, tolerance, and dependence. Drug addiction also follows these stages.

Young people may think it is harmless to experiment with drugs, but this is very untrue. Experimentation can lead to regular use, which often results in developing a tolerance for a drug. After people develop a tolerance to a drug, they often become dependent on a drug. This means they are physically and psychologically addicted to the drug.

Drug addiction is a disease. Just as other diseases require treatment, overcoming drug addiction often requires professional help. People with a drug addiction cannot just fix themselves. They need the help of family, friends, and professionals to end their dependence on drugs and return to their normal lives.

Characteristics of Drug Addiction

- Using the drug to feel "normal" or function "normally"
- Having intense cravings for the drug
- Spending excessive amounts of money on the drug
- Failing to fulfill responsibilities at school or in the family
- Withdrawing from social activities
- Experiencing withdrawal symptoms when trying to stop using the drug

Figure 10.19 Characteristics of drug addiction include using the drug to function "normally," such as someone who takes caffeine pills to stay up late studying.

Lesson 10.2 Review

1. _____ is a drug that comes from the cannabis plant, and the drug _____ comes from the coca plant.
2. Which type of drug involves experiencing sounds, images, or smells that do not really exist?
3. Nearly 80 percent of Americans using _____ abused prescription opioids first.
4. **True or false.** The health outcomes a person will face due to drug abuse are the same for all drugs.
5. **Critical thinking.** Name three types of illegal drugs and explain the negative short- and long-term health effects associated with each.

Hands-On Activity

The decision to use drugs can cost you more than you know—so much more than just money. In small groups, choose one of the illegal drugs described in Lesson 10.2. Research how this drug can negatively affect social, mental and emotional, and physical health, along with the monetary costs of the drug or addiction over time and the legal consequences. Use presentation software to create your group's report. Include pictures that support your findings, and be sure to credit the sources. Present your report to the class.

Preventing and Treating Drug Abuse and Addiction

Key Terms ☞

public service announcement (PSA) message that is shown in the media to support public health

AWARxE Prescription Drug Safety Program organization that spreads awareness of the growing prescription drug abuse problem

relapse occurrence when a person takes a drug again after deciding to stop

rehabilitation program treatment for drug addiction that may involve detoxification, medications, or time spent in a rehabilitation facility

residential treatment program plan for helping people get through the early stages of breaking an addiction in an inpatient environment with lots of support and few distractions

outpatient treatment program provides drug education or counseling without requiring a hospital stay

skills-training program plan that teaches people skills for dealing with peer pressure and for handling stressful life events without relying on drugs

sober living communities alcohol- and drug-free living environments that reduce some of the temptation and pressure people may feel to use alcohol and drugs

Learning Outcomes

After studying this lesson, you will be able to

- **explain** strategies for preventing drug abuse and addiction.
- **demonstrate** refusal skills to resist peer pressure to use drugs.
- **describe** several treatment methods for drug abuse and addiction.
- **explain** how you can help someone who is addicted to drugs.

Graphic Organizer ☞

Prevent Drug Addiction

This lesson is about preventing drug abuse and addictions. After reading this lesson, write two summary statements for each of the headings found in the graphic below. Team up with a partner and discuss each other's lists.

illustratorkris/Shutterstock.com

Preventing Drug Abuse and Addiction
- •
- •

Strategies for Refusing Drugs
- •
- •

Treating Drug Abuse and Addiction
- •
- •

Helping Someone Who Is Addicted to Drugs
- •
- •

n the previous lessons, you learned about the negative health effects associated with medication abuse and illegal drug use. Despite the negative effects, people continue to abuse drugs. Because medications are also drugs, the use of the terms *drug abuse* and *drug addiction* in this lesson will include medications and drugs.

The best way to avoid drug abuse and addiction is never to abuse medications or try illegal drugs, like Jamal from the previous lessons. Strategies exist to prevent drug abuse and refuse drugs. In this lesson, you will learn about those prevention strategies. Despite the peer pressure, Jamal is always open and honest with his friends about not wanting to do illegal drugs. Because they are his friends, they respect Jamal's choices and do not bully him.

In this lesson, you will learn how people like Jamal's cousin can get help to treat a drug addiction. When her family found out about her drug addiction, they looked into rehabilitation programs for her. You will also learn how you can help and support someone who is trying to stop using or abusing drugs. Jamal and his family only want to show his cousin that they want what is best for her and to support her in her recovery.

Preventing Drug Abuse and Addiction

Drug addiction is a preventable disease. People who never try drugs cannot abuse them and become addicted to them. It is especially important to prevent young people from using drugs. Drug use changes brain function, and a young person's brain is still developing (**Figure 10.20**). Preventing early drug use can help prevent serious health consequences. Unfortunately, many young people do not understand how quickly drug abuse can lead to addiction. Educating young people about the hazards of drug use can help prevent drug abuse and addiction.

Schools play a role in preventing drug abuse and addiction. Many schools have established substance-abuse prevention programs to help educate students about the dangers of using tobacco, alcohol, and drugs. Studies show that drug use is lower among students who participate in school-based substance-abuse prevention programs. These programs explain the short- and long-term effects of drug use. In addition, school policies and regulations exist to eliminate drug use on school property.

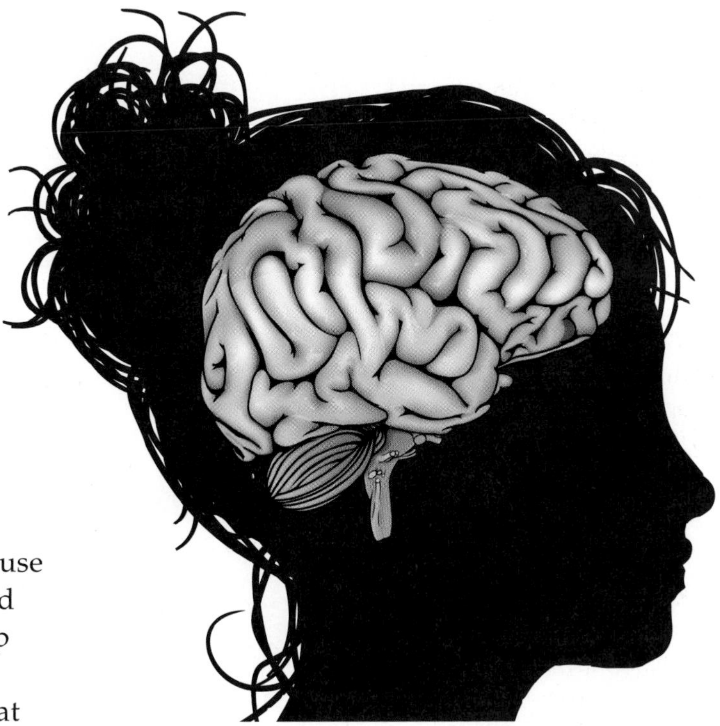

Christos Georghiou/Shutterstock.com

Figure 10.20 Since the part of the brain that regulates emotions and impulses does not stop developing until about age 25, young people are more likely to engage in dangerous, risky behaviors such as doing drugs.

Certain government groups and programs exist to increase public awareness of drug abuse and addiction. For example, the CDC and the National Institute on Drug Abuse (NIDA) create public service announcements (PSAs) for TV, radio, and the Internet. A **public service announcement (PSA)** is a media message to support public health. You may have seen some PSA videos on TV, in movie previews, or on the Internet.

The **AWARxE Prescription Drug Safety Program** spreads awareness of the growing problem of prescription drug abuse. The program teaches people valuable skills, such as how to use and store medications safely, and how to dispose of medications safely (**Figure 10.21**). If followed, the tips in this program can help keep prescription drugs away from young people.

Figure 10.21
In addition to the AWARxE program, many community resources help prevent medication misuse by collecting and safely disposing of unused or expired medications.

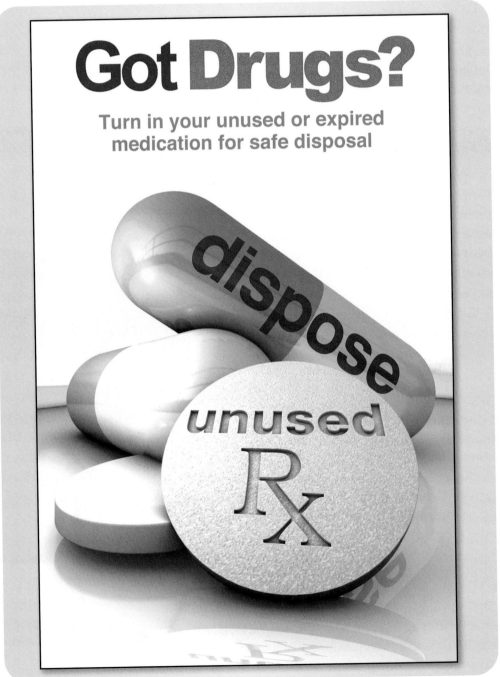

Courtesy of the Department of Justice, Drug Enforcement Administration

Drug Facts

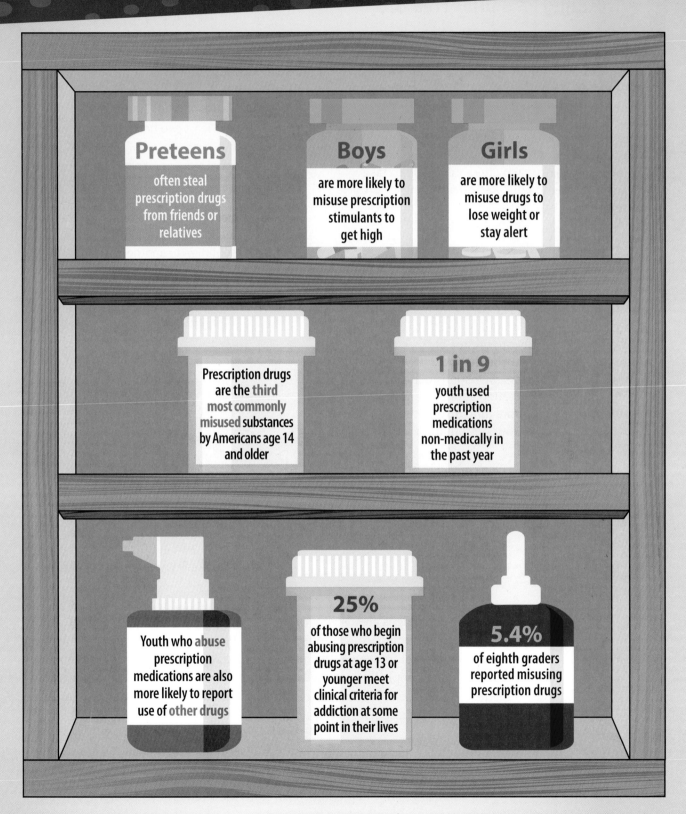

Preteens often steal prescription drugs from friends or relatives

Boys are more likely to misuse prescription stimulants to get high

Girls are more likely to misuse drugs to lose weight or stay alert

Prescription drugs are the **third most commonly misused** substances by Americans age 14 and older

1 in 9 youth used prescription medications non-medically in the past year

Youth who **abuse** prescription medications are also more likely to report use of **other drugs**

25% of those who begin abusing prescription drugs at age 13 or younger meet clinical criteria for addiction at some point in their lives

5.4% of eighth graders reported misusing prescription drugs

Bottles top, bottom: Krylovochka/Shutterstock.com; Bottles middle, bottom middle: Neonic Flower/Shutterstock.com

Advocating for a Drug-Free Life

Students often receive their drug education from teachers and parents. Your ability to advocate for the benefits of a drug-free life can positively influence your peers and others. In fact, your peers may be more likely to listen to you than to some adults. The power of positive peer pressure and peer education can make such a difference in the decision making of young people. This activity requires you to take a leadership role to educate and advocate for drug-free youth.

Educating Your Peers

Be an advocate for a healthy drug-free life by creating a drug-awareness presentation to educate your peers about the negative consequences of using drugs. To create your presentation, divide into groups of three and choose a drug that will be the focus of your group presentation. Then, assign responsibilities to each group member for creating your presentation. Refer back to the chapter and do additional research as needed. Your presentation should do the following:

- identify the drug name and at least two slang names for it
- use appropriate, educational images throughout the presentation (and properly cite sources)

- explain two or more harmful short-term and two or more harmful long-term effects of the drug
- identify two or more convincing ways to refuse a drug
- express at least three ways to get "high on life" without the use of drugs
- summarize at least two benefits of remaining drug-free
- share personal reasons for choosing to be drug-free

After your group finishes creating the presentation, practice and then present it to the class. With teacher and administration approval, deliver your presentation to another classroom of peers, too.

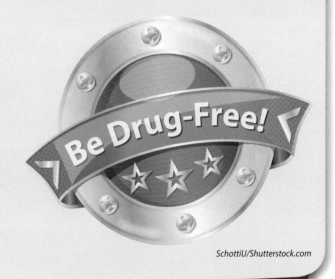

SchottiU/Shutterstock.com

Media campaigns are also important for preventing drug abuse and addiction. The "Above the Influence" campaign seeks to help young people stand up to peer pressure and other influences that may lead them to use drugs. This campaign reaches young people through TV commercials, Internet advertising, and social media. "Above the Influence" encourages young people to stay true to themselves and stand up to those who may want them to try drugs.

Strategies for Refusing Drugs

As you learned in Chapter 8, refusal skills are strategies you can use to stand up to pressures and influences that want you to engage in unhealthy behaviors.

Knowing how to respond and what to say if someone offers you drugs can help you avoid them. For example, one good strategy for refusing drugs is to be direct and say in a firm, but polite way, "No thanks, I don't use drugs." Another strategy is to provide an excuse, such as "I don't want to try drugs because my parents will kill me if I do."

If you continue to feel pressure to use drugs, you might ask the person pressuring you why it is so important to him or her that you use drugs. Remember that real friends respect each other's choices. Let the person know that you need him or her to respect your decision not to try drugs. If the person refuses to accept this, you may need to stop spending time with that person.

You may feel pressured to use drugs because it seems like everyone is doing it, but this is not true. Many young people have never tried drugs and have committed to living a drug-free lifestyle (**Figure 10.22**). A good rule is to make friends with people who share your values. You may want to make new friends by getting involved in activities that promote health and wellness.

Treating Drug Abuse and Addiction

There are two types of treatment for drug addiction—medicinal and behavioral. These types are often both used to treat a patient. *Medicinal treatment* may include medications that help lessen withdrawal symptoms a person experiences as he or she stops using a drug. *Behavioral treatment* focuses on teaching people how to live without drugs. This includes how to handle cravings, how to avoid situations that might trigger the desire for a drug, and how to prevent or handle relapses.

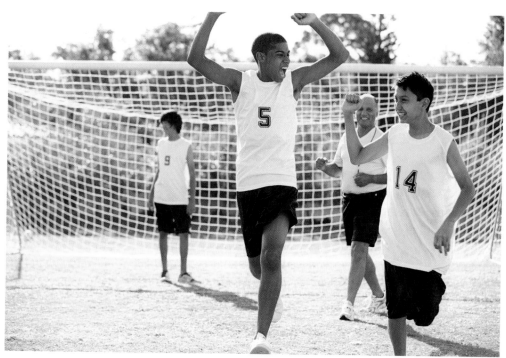

Figure 10.22
Doing drugs can impact your ability to do well in school, in sports, and in other areas of your life. *What is a good way to make friends with people who share your values about health?*

Monkey Business Images/Shutterstock.com

A **relapse** occurs when a person takes a drug again after deciding to stop. A person's drug addiction can be very strong, so a relapse may occur. It is important for the person to have a good support system, as well as professional help, if a relapse occurs.

A **rehabilitation program** can help treat drug abuse and addiction (Figure 10.23). This may involve detoxification, medications to lessen the impact of withdrawal symptoms, or time spent at a rehabilitation facility. Even after breaking the addiction to drugs, many people struggle with managing their addiction throughout their lives. The following programs are available to help treat drug abuse and addiction:

- **Residential treatment programs.** The goal of a **residential treatment program** is to help people get through the early stages of breaking an addiction in an inpatient environment with lots of support and few distractions. The term *inpatient* means that a person stays at a healthcare or rehabilitation facility while receiving treatment. These programs often begin with a process called *detoxification*, which clears all drugs from a person's body. Medications may be needed to help lessen the withdrawal symptoms that occur. These programs may last for weeks or for months.

- **Outpatient treatment programs.** An **outpatient treatment program** may provide drug education or counseling without requiring a hospital stay. Some programs may provide services similar to those offered in residential treatment programs.

- **Skills-training programs.** These programs help people recognize and avoid situations that lead them to use drugs. A **skills-training program** teaches people skills for dealing with peer pressure and for handling stressful life events without relying on drugs.

Figure 10.23
Each type of rehabilitation program has a slightly different approach to helping a person overcome his or her drug abuse and addiction. *What term describes when a person takes a drug again after deciding to stop?*

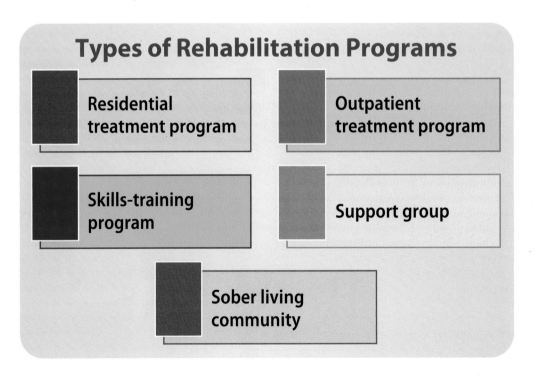

Types of Rehabilitation Programs

Residential treatment program

Outpatient treatment program

Skills-training program

Support group

Sober living community

- **Support groups.** People who are trying to overcome a drug addiction can come together and discuss the challenges they face (**Figure 10.24**). Sharing struggles with people who understand can help those trying to break a drug addiction. Narcotics Anonymous is an example of a support group for drug abuse.
- **Sober living communities. Sober living communities** are alcohol- and drug-free living environments. These environments reduce some of the temptation and pressure to use alcohol and drugs that people may feel. These communities also provide social support for remaining drug free.

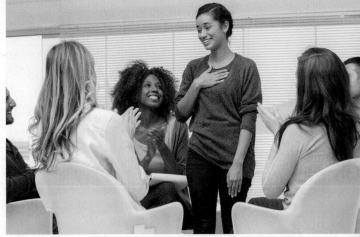

wavebreakmedia/Shutterstock.com

Figure 10.24 Sometimes, people come together in a group to overcome a challenge together, sharing advice and emotional support. ***What is an example of a drug abuse support group?***

The Substance Abuse and Mental Health Services Administration (SAMHSA) provides a locator tool people can use to find treatment options. It may also be helpful to talk to a trusted adult, such as a parent, doctor, school counselor, or school nurse.

Helping Someone Who Is Addicted to Drugs

Drug addiction is a serious and sometimes scary situation. If you want to help someone you know who is addicted to drugs, you should first get support for yourself. Talk to a parent, doctor, school counselor, or school nurse. These trusted adults can often provide advice and guidance for helping someone who is addicted to drugs.

How do you know if someone is abusing drugs or addicted to drugs? Possible warning signs that someone may be using drugs are shown in **Figure 10.25**.

If you know that your friend is addicted to drugs, express your concern for his or her health. People with an addiction can often feel alone and isolated. Tell your friend that you care about him or her, and that you will be available to help.

Warning Signs That Someone May Be Using Drugs
- Loss of interest in school
- Change in mood or personality
- Trouble concentrating in class
- Change in sleeping habits
- Change in eating habits
- Hanging out with a new group of friends who use drugs
- Stealing money or selling belongings to get money for drugs

Figure 10.25 Being alert to the warning signs of potential drug abuse and addiction can increase the chances that you can help a friend or loved one get the help he or she needs.

Knowing that you care and are concerned can help the person understand the seriousness of the problem. Offer to help the person find someone to talk to about the addiction. A person must want to break his or her addiction. You may need to wait for your friend to admit he or she has a problem.

Once a friend has decided to stop using drugs, you can support him or her in various ways. You can offer to go with your friend to a meeting with a counselor. Offer your friend encouragement and praise for staying drug-free. Your friend may want to avoid parties where drugs are present. To support your friend, you can avoid those parties and spend time with him or her. In addition, you may want to attend a support group for relatives and friends of someone with a drug addiction. This can help you get the support you need.

If you notice your friend starting to relapse and use drugs again, talk to a trusted adult. This does not mean you are a tattletale or a snitch. Instead, this means you are concerned about your friend and want him or her to get help.

Lesson 10.3 Review

1. Why are young people more vulnerable to changed brain function due to drug use?

2. **True or false.** Most young people have tried or would like to try drugs.

3. When a person takes a drug again after deciding to stop, it is called a(n) _____.

4. Which type of rehabilitation program helps people recognize and avoid situations that lead them to use drugs?

5. **Critical thinking.** What can you do to help someone who is addicted to drugs? Explain actions you can take before the person gets help, once the person decides to get help, and if you notice a relapse.

Hands-On Activity

Standing up to peer pressure can be very difficult; practicing what you will say in difficult situations can help. Imagine that you are at a party and someone is pressuring you to take a drug. You are immediately uncomfortable and want to say *no*. With a partner, practice your refusal responses to the following pressure lines using the skills you have learned:

Take the pill. My mom takes them for her back pain and she is fine.	Everybody smokes. One hit of marijuana is not a big deal.	If you want to hang out with us, you have to smoke this.	Pop this Molly and you will feel so good.

Once you and your partner are confident with your responses, choose one or two to role-play for the class. What suggestions does the class have for making your refusals stronger?

Summary

Lesson 10.1 Medications

- *Medications* are drugs and medicines used to treat symptoms of an illness or to cure, manage, or prevent a disease. *Drugs* are medications and other substances that change the way the body or brain functions. Medications can be prescription medication or over-the-counter (OTC) medication.
- Medications can cause side effects. Some medications can also cause health risks by interacting with other drugs, dietary supplements, foods, or drinks. Some people are allergic to certain medications.
- Carefully reading and following usage instructions can ensure that people are taking medications correctly. *Medication misuse* involves taking medication in a way that does not follow the instructions, which can be on accident. *Medication abuse* is purposely taking a drug in a way other than its intended use.

Lesson 10.2 Illegal Drugs

- *Illegal drugs* are against the law to use because they can be harmful to a person's health. Illegal drugs include: marijuana, cocaine, methamphetamine, hallucinogens, heroin, club drugs, anabolic steroids, and inhalants.
- Although illegal drugs cause serious and life-threatening risks, some young people still choose to use them. Young people can be influenced by their community, culture, school, family, friends, peers, and the media. Role models young people look up to can also influence their attitudes about drug use.
- *Drug abuse* is the continued use of an illegal drug despite negative or harmful outcomes, which can affect a person's physical health as well as cause legal, academic, work, financial, and social problems.
- Complete dependence on a drug is *drug addiction*. Experimentation can quickly lead to an addiction. Withdrawal from a drug may be so severe that a person gives up on quitting.

Lesson 10.3 Preventing and Treating Drug Abuse and Addiction

- School and government programs increase awareness of health effects of drug use, drug abuse, and addiction. PSA videos help teach young people to stand up to peer pressure.
- Refuse drugs by saying "no" in a direct and firm, but polite, way. Real friends will respect your choices and will not pressure you to do something you do not want to do.
- Medicinal treatment uses medications to lessen withdrawal symptoms. Behavioral treatment teaches people how to live without drugs. Most treatments use both methods.
- Types of rehabilitation programs include residential treatment programs, outpatient treatment programs, skills-training programs, support groups, and sober living communities.
- If you know a person who is addicted to drugs, express your concern and offer to find help. Wait for your friend to admit he or she has a problem. Support your friend through treatment. If you notice a relapse, talk to a trusted adult.

Check Your Knowledge ⇗

Record your answers to each of the following questions on a separate sheet of paper.

1. **True or false.** All drugs are medications, but *not* all medications are drugs.
2. Which type of medications can be purchased without a doctor's written order?
3. An unpleasant, sometimes life-threatening symptom related to a substance in a medicine is called a(n) _____ reaction.
4. What is the term for unintentionally taking a medication or drug in a way that does *not* follow the proper instructions?
5. Which of the following is a potential health effect of marijuana use?
   A. Improved memory.
   B. Anxiety and panic attacks.
   C. Improved coordination.
   D. Clear problem solving.
6. What is involved in the condition "meth mouth" from the use of crystal meth?
7. **True or false.** All use of anabolic steroids is illegal.
8. A person who has a physical and physiological need for a drug has a(n) _____ _____.
9. What is the name for a media message that supports public health, such as an anti-drug commercial?
10. What are the two types of treatment for drug addiction?
11. **True or false.** In a residential treatment program, a person will stay at a healthcare or rehabilitation facility while receiving treatment.
12. Which of the following is a sign of drug abuse and addiction?
    A. Regular sleeping habits.
    B. Changing eating habits.
    C. Interest in school.
    D. Steady personality.

Use Your Vocabulary ⇗

AWARxE Prescription Drug Safety Program	legal drugs	prescription medications
club drugs	marijuana	public service announcement (PSA)
cocaine	medication abuse	rehabilitation program
drug abuse	medication misuse	relapse
drug addiction	medications	residential treatment program
drugs	methamphetamine	side effect
hallucinogens	outpatient treatment program	skills-training program
heroin	overdose	sober living communities
illegal drugs	over-the-counter (OTC) medications	
inhalants		

13. Classify each of the terms above into the categories *drug use* and *drug abuse and addiction*. Pair up with a classmate and compare how you classified the terms.
14. Choose one of the terms on the list above. Then, use the Internet to locate photos that visually show the meaning of the term you chose. Share the photo and meaning of the term in class. Ask for clarification if necessary.

Think Critically

15. **Identify.** Marijuana and over-the-counter and prescription drugs are widely abused drugs among teens. Identify reasons the use of these drugs are so popular.

16. **Draw conclusions.** What are reasons some teens choose to abstain from drug use while others choose to use drugs?

17. **Analyze.** What do you think causes some people to get addicted to drugs while others use, but are able to quit?

18. **Make inferences.** Since drug use is illegal, should schools allow random drug testing among students with legal consequences for positive results? Defend your answer.

DEVELOP Your Skills

19. **Decision-making skills.** Imagine it is Friday night, and you are home with your family watching a movie. Several of your friends are at a party, and one of your friends posts a picture on Instagram with the following caption:

    "Come over! No adults are here, just us and these really cute boys. Everyone brought pills and alcohol. I even took a Xanax and drank a little."

    You are immediately concerned about her safety. What should you do? Write a paragraph describing how you would respond to this situation.

20. **Communication skills.** Imagine that you attend a "punch-bowl party" where kids are taking pills from a large bowl and ingesting them. The pills are multicolored without any identifying marks. You have no idea what kind of pills are in the bowl. Your best friend tells you that she is going to close her eyes, select two, and swallow them. How would you respond to convince her not to do it? Write your response in essay form. Then, share and discuss your responses with the rest of the class.

21. **Advocacy, access information, and technology skills.** In groups of three, review Lesson 10.3 and do additional research on ways to help a friend who is using or addicted to drugs. Then, create a public-service announcement (PSA). Use school-approved video creation software to create a video highlighting at least six ways to help and be a supportive friend. In addition, include information on local resources available in your community, and add pictures or video footage that support the content in your video PSA. Share your video in class or post it to the class website for peer and teacher review.

22. **Technology skills.** Some people have to take medicine weekly, daily, or even several times throughout the day. Research what kind of apps are available for people who take medicine. Choose one and create a presentation about your app highlighting three appealing features and two benefits to using the app. Present it to the class.

Protecting Your Physical Health and Safety

Warm-Up Activity

Reducing Risks

As you grow up, you will become more and more responsible for managing your health, safety, and environment. Part of managing these factors is identifying and reducing *risks*, or potential threats. For example, during the winter season, your classmates may catch the flu. When you hang out with friends at the mall, a stranger may make you uncomfortable. You may cough when there is smog in the air. In all of these situations, you can take certain actions to reduce your risks.

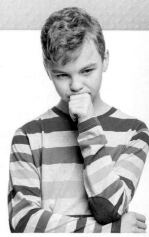

VaLiza/Shutterstock.com

The pictures below illustrate situations that have different risks. Look at these pictures and work with a partner to list actions you could take to reduce the risks present. Write these actions on a separate piece of paper. After reading this unit, revisit your list and add or change actions based on what you learned.

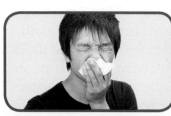
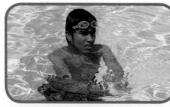
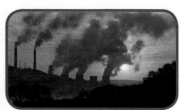
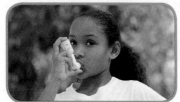
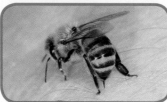
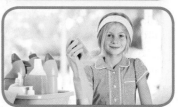

Left to right: leungchopan/Shutterstock.com; juan carlos tinjaca/Shutterstock.com; Tatiana Grozetskaya/Shutterstock.com; sirtravelalot/Shutterstock.com; Mirko Graul/Shutterstock.com; Africa Studios/Shutterstock.com

Chapter 11

Understanding and Preventing Diseases

Essential Question

What causes communicable and noncommunicable diseases, and how can you prevent them?

Video ↗

Access the Chapter 11 video to start thinking about chapter topics.

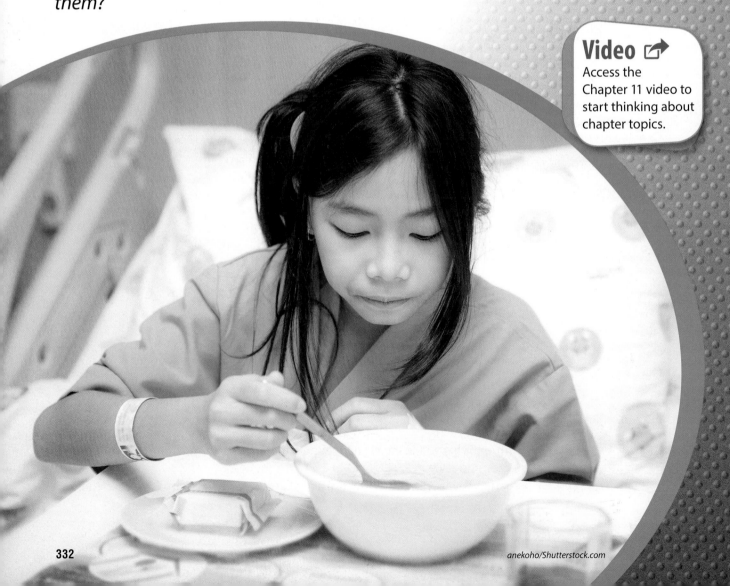

anekoho/Shutterstock.com

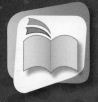

Reading Activity

Skim through this chapter and list all of the headings you see. Then, compose a "topic sentence" for each heading. After you read this chapter, write a new topic sentence for each section, outlining the main points you learned.

How Healthy Are You?

In this chapter, you will be learning about diseases and how to prevent them. Before you begin reading, take the following quiz to assess your current disease prevention habits.

Healthy Choices	Yes	No
Do you regularly wash your hands with soap and water?		
Do you practice respiratory etiquette, including covering your mouth and nose with a tissue or your sleeve when coughing or sneezing?		
Do you store the appropriate foods in the refrigerator or freezer to slow or stop the growth of microorganisms?		
Do you make sure that any meat you eat has been cooked thoroughly?		
Do you wash fruits and vegetables before eating, peeling, or cutting open?		
Do you receive the recommended vaccines, including an annual flu vaccine?		
Do you eat a healthy diet, engage in regular physical activity, and avoid tobacco and alcohol to prevent heart disease?		
Do you know the preventable risk factors for different types of common cancers?		
Do you get regular screenings and physical examinations to increase the possibility of treating diseases in their early stages?		
Are you aware that abstinence is the only 100 percent effective method for preventing STIs?		
Do you know of community resources that are available for the treatment of STIs?		
Are you aware of the hazards associated with unsterilized needles?		

Count your "Yes" and "No" responses. The more "Yes" responses you have, the more healthy disease prevention habits you exhibit. Now, take a closer look at the questions with which you responded "No." How can you make these healthy habits part of your daily life? Think about how implementing these ideas can help improve your physical health and wellness.

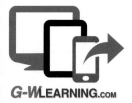

While studying this chapter, look for the activity icon to

- **practice** key terms with e-flash cards and matching activities.
- **reinforce** what you learn by completing graphic organizers, self-assessment quizzes, and review questions.
- **expand** knowledge with interactive activities and activities that extend learning.

communicable disease
condition someone can develop after coming into contact with humans, animals, or plants infected with the disease; also called *infectious disease*

pathogens microorganisms that cause communicable diseases

method of transmission
way a disease gets from one organism to another; may be direct or indirect

influenza viral infection of the respiratory system; also known as *the flu*

mononucleosis common viral infection that spreads through kissing or by sharing certain objects; also known as *mono* and *the kissing disease*

tonsillitis bacterial or viral infection that affects the tonsils

conjunctivitis viral or bacterial infection that causes inflammation of part of the eye; also known as *pinkeye*

antibiotics substances that target and kill pathogenic bacteria

Learning Outcomes

After studying this lesson, you will be able to

- **understand** the nature of communicable diseases.
- **explain** the types of pathogens that can make you sick.
- **describe** the different methods of disease transmission.
- **understand** common communicable diseases.
- **describe** treatment methods for communicable diseases.

Graphic Organizer 👉

Understanding Communicable Diseases

Create a graphic organizer like the one below to increase your knowledge and awareness about pathogens that cause communicable diseases. As you read this lesson, list three key points about each type of pathogen identified in the organizer. Then, list a disease that each may cause.

Africa Studio/Shutterstock.com

Bacteria
1.
2.
3.

Viruses
1.
2.
3.

Fungi
1.
2.
3.

Protozoa
1.
2.
3.

The term *communicable* means "able to be transmitted." If a disease is *communicable*, that means it can be transmitted to you. In other words, a **communicable disease** (also called an *infectious disease*) is a condition you can develop after coming into contact with humans, animals, or plants infected with the disease.

Twelve-year-old Dakota knows that communicable diseases like the flu are different from diseases, such as heart disease, that he might inherit from his parents or grandparents. A communicable disease is one that he can "catch." When his friend Tavon came to school with the flu last month, for example, Dakota ended up sick, too. Dakota cannot, however, catch heart disease.

In this lesson, you will learn about the causes of communicable diseases. You will also learn about common communicable diseases that you may encounter in your life. Finally, you will learn possible treatment methods for communicable diseases.

Understanding Communicable Disease

Common living things that you can see are called *organisms*. You, your teacher, your dog, and the trees outside are all examples of organisms. Many living things, however, are too small to see with the naked eye. These *microorganisms* are so small that you cannot even see them without the use of a microscope. Certain microorganisms, known as **pathogens**, can cause communicable diseases (**Figure 11.1**). The term *pathogen* is a more scientific way of describing *germs*.

Pathogens are everywhere. They are so small, however, that you cannot see them. Pathogens are only visible with a microscope, which magnifies them, or creates a bigger image of them. While most people are unfamiliar with pathogens, these microscopic organisms influence human lives in many ways. Pathogens include bacteria, viruses, fungi, and protozoa.

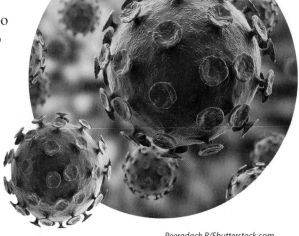

Peeradach R/Shutterstock.com

Figure 11.1
Pathogens, pictured here, are disease-causing microorganisms. Specific pathogens cause different communicable diseases. *Can you see microorganisms with the naked eye? Why or why not?*

Bacteria

Bacteria are single-celled organisms that live in almost every place where life can thrive. Bacteria even live inside the human body. In fact, so many bacteria live in the body that, of the several trillions of cells that make up your body, 90 percent are bacterial cells.

You may find it scary that bacteria are nearly everywhere. The good news is that most bacteria are helpful. For example, the bacteria found in your body help the digestive system function efficiently. These bacteria also prevent harmful bacteria from thriving in your body. The bad news is that certain varieties of bacteria can cause different kinds of illnesses. Some of these illnesses may be minor while others can be quite serious and even deadly.

One type of bacteria that can cause disease is E. coli. *E. coli* bacteria typically live in healthy people's and animals' intestines. There are different varieties of E. coli bacteria, however. Some varieties are harmless while others can cause food poisoning.

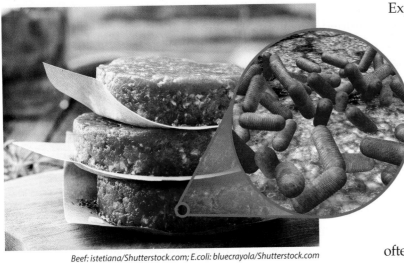

Beef: istetiana/Shutterstock.com; E.coli: bluecrayola/Shutterstock.com

Figure 11.2 Undercooked ground beef can contain *E. coli*. If consumed, E. coli can cause food poisoning.

Exposure to harmful E. coli bacteria can occur from eating contaminated food, such as undercooked ground beef, or drinking contaminated water (**Figure 11.2**). If you get sick from food poisoning, you may develop symptoms such as diarrhea, nausea, fever, and vomiting.

Another common type of bacteria, *S. aureus*, is present in about 30 percent of people's nasal passages. The bacteria S. aureus often does not cause any harm. It can, however, spread to others through contact with contaminated hands. Sometimes, S. aureus causes *staph infections* (skin and soft tissue infections).

Anyone can get a staph infection, especially if you have a cut or scratch. People with chronic diseases and weakened immune systems are at greater risk of developing a more serious staph infection.

Viruses

Viruses are very different from bacteria or cells in your body. Viruses are much smaller than bacteria, and they are completely incapable of doing anything cells can do on their own. Viruses depend entirely on other cells for reproduction and growth. In fact, every virus must live inside a cell and use that cell's resources and energy to grow and reproduce.

Viruses must be inside another living organism to thrive. Though viruses can stay on surfaces for a short time, they will die quickly if they do not find an organism in which to live. Once inside the body, a virus invades a person's cells and multiplies quickly. The result of a virus multiplying is an illness (**Figure 11.3**).

Fungi

Fungi (singular—*fungus*) are multi-celled, plant-like microorganisms that thrive in damp, warm places. These microorganisms are much more complex than bacteria and viruses. Examples of fungi include mushrooms, molds, and yeast. A fungus cannot produce its own food, so it receives nourishment from plants, foods, and animals.

Figure 11.3 Some common viral illnesses are influenza, the common cold, measles, chicken pox, West Nile virus, and mumps.

Common Illnesses Caused by Viruses

Influenza (the flu)	Common cold	Measles	Chicken pox	West Nile virus	Mumps

Like bacteria, few fungi cause disease, and many are beneficial. For example, the mold known as *Penicillium notatum* makes the life-saving drug penicillin, an antibiotic that controls bacterial infections. Other fungi, however, damage crops and stored foods. A few fungi cause disease in humans. Ringworm, athlete's foot, and jock itch are common fungal infections. People with weakened immune systems may be more likely to contract a fungal infection.

Protozoa

Protozoa are single-celled organisms that live nearly everywhere, and only a few cause diseases. Many kinds of protozoa form the basis of food chains, providing nutrients for other organisms. Certain protozoa, however, cause some of the world's most feared diseases. These include *malaria*, a dangerous flu-like illness, and *dysentery*, a severe intestinal infection. Protozoa thrive in moist environments, and typically spread through contaminated water.

Common Communicable Diseases

For a disease to be *communicable*, it must be able to transmit from one source to another. Pathogens causing communicable diseases may travel by various methods of transmission (**Figure 11.4**). A **method of transmission** is simply the way a disease gets from one organism to another. Methods of transmission are either direct or indirect, depending on how the transmission occurs.

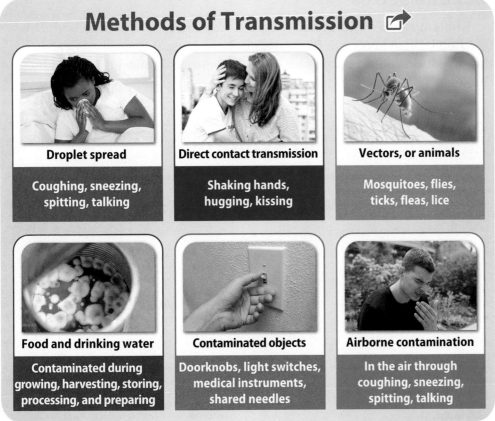

Methods of Transmission

Droplet spread
Coughing, sneezing, spitting, talking

Direct contact transmission
Shaking hands, hugging, kissing

Vectors, or animals
Mosquitoes, flies, ticks, fleas, lice

Food and drinking water
Contaminated during growing, harvesting, storing, processing, and preparing

Contaminated objects
Doorknobs, light switches, medical instruments, shared needles

Airborne contamination
In the air through coughing, sneezing, spitting, talking

Figure 11.4
Communicable diseases are spread among people, animals, and objects. Different diseases spread through different methods of transmission. For example, the common cold is transmitted through droplet spread and direct contact. West Nile virus is usually transmitted through mosquitoes acting as vectors. *Which method of transmission involves medical instruments and shared needles?*

Left to right: Andrey_Popov/Shutterstock.com; Olesya Kuznetsova/Shutterstock.com; frank60/Shutterstock.com; Jana Behr/Shutterstock.com; Alexey Rotanov/Shutterstock.com; Michael Moloney/Shutterstock.com

Direct transmission is the movement of a pathogen from an infected person to a susceptible person. A person is *susceptible* to a disease if he or she is likely to be easily affected or harmed by it. If a person has a weak immune system, he or she may be more susceptible to a disease than someone with a healthy immune system. *Indirect transmission* is the movement of a pathogen to a susceptible person through a source that acts only as a disease carrier. In this case, the carrier is simply moving a pathogen from one source to another.

There are many examples of communicable diseases, and most are not serious or life threatening. You will likely encounter one or more communicable diseases during your life. Some common communicable diseases include influenza, mononucleosis, tonsillitis, and conjunctivitis. Sexually transmitted infections (STIs) are also communicable diseases. (You will learn about STIs in Lesson 11.2.)

Influenza

Influenza, also known as *the flu*, is a viral infection of the respiratory system. This means the virus infects the nose and lungs, but it also causes symptoms throughout the body. The flu moves from person to person through droplet spread, and sometimes through contact with an object touched by an infected person. **Figure 11.5** shows common flu symptoms. The best treatment for the flu is to get lots of rest and drink plenty of liquids.

Mononucleosis

Mononucleosis, also called *mono*, is a very common viral infection. This infection is often known as *the kissing disease* because it typically spreads through direct contact such as kissing. Mononucleosis may also spread by sharing objects such as cups, toothbrushes, and lip gloss.

Figure 11.5
Common symptoms of the flu are headache, fever, stuffy nose, sore throat, muscle aches, and dry cough. *How does the flu move from person to person?*

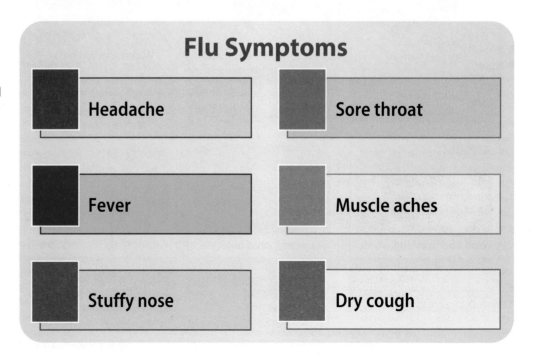

Flu Symptoms

Headache

Sore throat

Fever

Muscle aches

Stuffy nose

Dry cough

Symptoms of mononucleosis include fatigue, fever, sore throat, loss of appetite, and sore muscles. Some people experience mild symptoms. Others experience no symptoms at all. A person experiencing any combination of these symptoms should see a healthcare provider for diagnosis and treatment.

Tonsillitis

A virus or bacterium may cause **tonsillitis**, which is an infection that affects the tonsils (**Figure 11.6**). The tonsils usually protect the body from infection. Sometimes, however, the tonsils become infected.

Symptoms of tonsillitis include sore throat, fever, painful swallowing, and vocal changes. If you think you have tonsillitis, you should contact a doctor. Often, the best treatment for tonsillitis is getting lots of rest and drinking plenty of fluids.

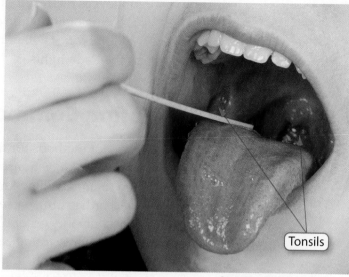

BravissimoS/Shutterstock.com

Figure 11.6 Tonsillitis is an infection of the tonsils, which are located at the back of the throat. When the tonsils are infected, they become *inflamed*, or swell and turn red.

Conjunctivitis

Conjunctivitis, also known as *pinkeye*, is a viral or bacterial infection that causes inflammation of the conjunctiva in the eye. The *conjunctiva* is the tissue that covers the eye and inner surface of the eyelid. Inflammation of the conjunctiva results in itchiness and a red or pink appearance, which gives this condition its name (**Figure 11.7**). Pinkeye may also cause swelling of the affected eye and *discharge*, or liquid that leaks from the eye.

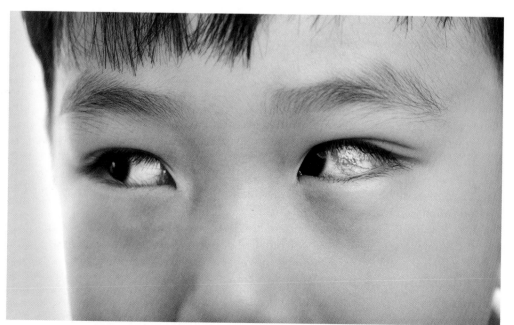

Figure 11.7 Itchiness and red or pink eyes are symptoms of pinkeye. *What does the conjunctiva cover?*

kdshutterman/Shutterstock.com

If pinkeye is the result of a bacterial infection, treatment typically involves the application of antibiotic drops to the affected eye. If the infection is viral, however, antibiotics will not work. A viral infection will run its course and go away as the body fights it.

Treating Communicable Diseases

Treatment methods for infections vary depending on the type of infection. To treat bacterial infections, many doctors prescribe antibiotics such as penicillin or amoxicillin. **Antibiotics** are substances that target and kill *pathogenic*, or harmful, bacteria.

While antibiotics generally work well to treat bacterial infections, they do not work against viruses, fungi, and protozoa. Medications cannot treat a virus, but some medications can help treat the symptoms of a viral infection, such as a fever and body aches. The best treatment methods for viral infections include rest, good nutrition, and fluids to strengthen the body so it can fight the virus.

To treat fungal infections, doctors often prescribe antifungal ointments or creams that are applied directly to the infected area. Doctors may also prescribe medications to treat infections caused by protozoa. These medications are determined on a case-by-case basis, depending on the type of illness, the person's symptoms, and his or her overall health.

Lesson 11.1 Review

1. What is a pathogen?
2. **True or false.** Bacteria are multi-celled, plant-like microorganisms that thrive in damp, warm environments.
3. List two methods of disease transmission.
4. List four communicable diseases.
5. **Critical thinking.** What are antibiotics? For what communicable diseases are antibiotics most effective?

Hands-On Activity

Put a small amount of hand lotion on your hands. Before spreading it into your hands, dump a small amount of single-colored glitter on the lotion. Now, rub the lotion into your hands as usual. Your classmates should do the same, but with a different color glitter. Go on with your class period as usual (passing out papers, sharing writing utensils, working together, etc.). Try not to pay any attention to the glitter on your hands.

At the end of class, take notice of how many different colored glitters are on your belongings and your person. How does this relate to the spreading of communicable diseases? What is the most important health behavior an individual should participate in to lessen the spread of communicable diseases?

Sexually Transmitted Infections (STIs)

Learning Outcomes

After studying this lesson, you will be able to

- **understand** how people contract sexually transmitted infections (STIs).
- **describe** the most commonly reported STIs.
- **identify** potential STI resources.
- **explain** treatment methods for STIs.

Graphic Organizer

STI Cause and Effect

As you read this lesson, use a graphic organizer like the one below to take notes about the most common STIs. Identify whether the cause of the STI is a bacteria, virus, or protozoa. Then, identify the effects and possible treatments for each STI. An example is provided for you.

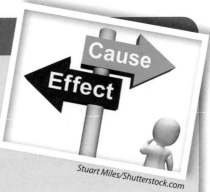

Stuart Miles/Shutterstock.com

STI	Cause	Health Effects	Treatment
Chlamydia	Bacteria	Silent disease with few or no symptoms; progresses quietly to severe bacterial infection; can cause infertility	Antibiotics prescribed by doctor

Key Terms

sexually transmitted infections (STIs) communicable diseases spread from one person to another during sexual activity

chlamydia bacterial infection known as a "silent" disease because it has few or no symptoms

gonorrhea bacterial infection that primarily affects the genitals, rectum, and throat

syphilis bacterial infection divided into stages that causes extremely serious health problems and disability

trichomoniasis curable infection caused by protozoa that is more common among young women than men

genital herpes viral infection that results in sores on the genitals

human papillomavirus (HPV) most commonly contracted STI that causes genital infections and sometimes cancer

abstinence commitment to refrain from sexual activity; only method that is 100 percent effective in preventing STIs

latex condom device that provides a barrier to microorganisms that cause STIs

ommunicable diseases spread from one person to another during sexual activity are **sexually transmitted infections (STIs)**. When discussing STIs in his health class, Dakota from the previous lesson asked the question, "Am I at risk of contracting an STI?" The answer for him is *no* because Dakota does not engage in sexual activity. The answer would be *yes*, however, for a young person who is sexually active.

In this lesson, you will learn how people contract STIs. You will also learn about the most common STIs (**Figure 11.8**). Treatments for these conditions will be discussed as well.

How People Contract STIs

Just as with other communicable diseases, bacteria, viruses, and protozoa cause STIs. These microorganisms live in and on the surfaces of the reproductive organs. Depending on the type of STI, these microorganisms may also reside in the mouth, rectum, blood, and other bodily fluids of an infected person.

Engaging in sexual activity one time with just one infected sexual partner is all it takes to contract an STI. People with more sexual partners have greater chances of getting an STI. Although it is possible for a person with certain *oral* (appearing on the mouth) STIs to transmit the infection by kissing, other STIs are not transmitted this way. Casual contact with an infected person, such as using the same toilet seat, does not transmit STIs.

Common STIs

As you learned in Figure 11.8, the most commonly reported STIs include chlamydia, gonorrhea, syphilis, trichomoniasis, genital herpes, and human papillomavirus. As you read the following sections, you will learn about the signs, symptoms, and treatments for each of these STIs. You will learn about HIV/AIDS in the next lesson.

Chlamydia

Chlamydia, a common STI caused by bacteria, is a "silent" disease because it has few or no symptoms (**Figure 11.9**). If symptoms do occur, they are often mild, such as nausea or a burning sensation during urination.

Figure 11.8
The most commonly reported STIs are chlamydia, gonorrhea, syphilis, trichomoniasis, genital herpes, and human papillomavirus (HPV). Of these, the most common is HPV.

Most commonly reported STIs

- Chlamydia
- Gonorrhea
- Syphilis
- Trichomoniasis
- Genital herpes
- Human papillomavirus

Figure 11.9
A staggering one million cases of chlamydia go undiagnosed each year. This is partly because chlamydia can be a "silent" disease that has no symptoms.

This lack of symptoms is dangerous because chlamydia poses a serious threat to the reproductive health of women. The "silent" nature of the disease allows it to quietly progress to a severe bacterial infection of the female reproductive organs. This condition, called *pelvic inflammatory disease (PID)*, can cause *infertility*, or the inability to have children. Chlamydia can be treated and cured with prescription antibiotics.

Gonorrhea

Gonorrhea is a bacterial infection that primarily affects the genitals, rectum, and throat. According to the CDC, gonorrhea is a very common STI, especially among people between 15 and 24 years of age. Like chlamydia, gonorrhea causes few or no symptoms in many people. Symptoms, however, do develop in some cases of gonorrhea (**Figure 11.10**). Doctors often prescribe two kinds of antibiotics to treat gonorrhea.

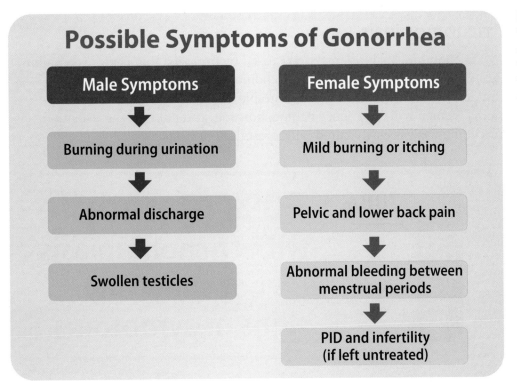

Possible Symptoms of Gonorrhea

Male Symptoms	Female Symptoms
Burning during urination	Mild burning or itching
Abnormal discharge	Pelvic and lower back pain
Swollen testicles	Abnormal bleeding between menstrual periods
	PID and infertility (if left untreated)

Figure 11.10
While most cases of gonorrhea present few or no symptoms, the symptoms that do develop vary between males and females.

Syphilis

Syphilis is a bacterial infection that causes extremely serious health problems and disability. This STI progresses through several stages, which include the following:

- **Primary syphilis stage.** During this first stage, sores develop at the site of the infection. Direct contact with a syphilis sore during sexual activity is what causes the spread of syphilis. The sores are not painful, do not itch, and heal after a few weeks.
- **Secondary syphilis stage.** The secondary stage of syphilis develops days, weeks, or even months after the primary stage. In the secondary stage, a red or copper-color rash appears, mainly on the palms of the hands and soles of the feet, but sometimes elsewhere. The rash heals, but the person remains infected and enters the next syphilis stage (**Figure 11.11**).
- **Latent syphilis stage.** During the latent syphilis stage, a person is still infected, but there are no signs or symptoms of the disease.
- **Late-stage syphilis.** In this final stage of syphilis, an internal infection that does not include obvious external signs is present. It is characterized by damage to the brain in the form of *dementia* (deteriorating mental function), paralysis, and fatal damage to the heart, liver, and blood vessels.

Syphilis is most treatable during the early stages. Antibiotics can most effectively cure syphilis in its primary and secondary stages. Even if late-stage syphilis is cured, the organ damage remains permanent.

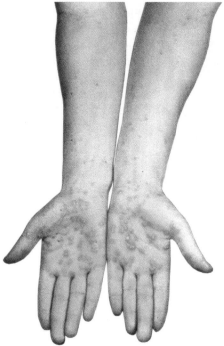

Courtesy of the Centers for Disease Control and Prevention

Figure 11.11 The secondary stage of syphilis includes a red or copper-color rash. This rash will go away on its own, but that does not rid a person of the syphilis infection. *During the secondary stage of syphilis, where does the rash typically develop?*

Trichomoniasis

Trichomoniasis is an infection caused by protozoa that is more common among young women than men. Trichomoniasis often has no symptoms, and it is considered to be the most curable common STI (**Figure 11.12**). Some women will experience itching, burning, and pain during urination. Trichomoniasis is easily cured with prescription drugs.

Figure 11.12 When an STI shows no symptoms, infection can go undiagnosed and untreated. This means that people are more likely to infect their sexual partners.

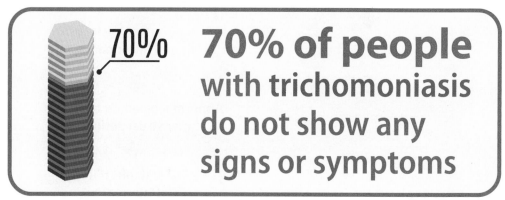

70%

70% of people with trichomoniasis do not show any signs or symptoms

bbgreg/Shutterstock.com

Because men often have no symptoms, their infection may go undiagnosed and untreated, making it easy to reinfect their partners. Therefore, both partners must be treated to control reinfection.

Genital Herpes

Two kinds of herpes simplex virus (HSV) cause infections: *HSV type 1* and *HSV type 2* (**Figure 11.13**). **Genital herpes** is very common in the United States among men and women between 14 and 49 years of age.

A person infected with genital herpes usually has mild or no symptoms. Blisters arise at the site of infection, burst, and heal after a few weeks. Typically, these blisters return, but in a milder form, sometimes with swollen lymph nodes and fever. This recurrence of genital herpes is called an *outbreak*. No cure exists for herpes, but medication can control the frequency and severity of outbreaks.

Herpes Simplex Viruses That Cause Genital Herpes

HSV-1
- Cold sores on mouth and lips and genital infections
- Transmitted by kissing or through sexual activity

HSV-2
- Genital infections only
- Transmitted only through sexual contact

Figure 11.13 The two kinds of herpes simplex virus (HSV) are caused by different types of direct contact and cause different infections. *Which type of HSV causes genital infections only?*

Human Papillomavirus

A **human papillomavirus (HPV)** infection is the most commonly contracted STI. HPV is a virus that infects cells in skin and membranes, causing them to grow abnormally. At least 40 kinds of HPV can cause genital infections. Some types can cause cancer.

Almost all sexually active people carry HPV at one time or another. Luckily, most HPV infections do not cause health problems because the body fights and eliminates the viruses. Some types of HPV, however, cause genital warts, and other types can cause cervical cancer (**Figure 11.14**).

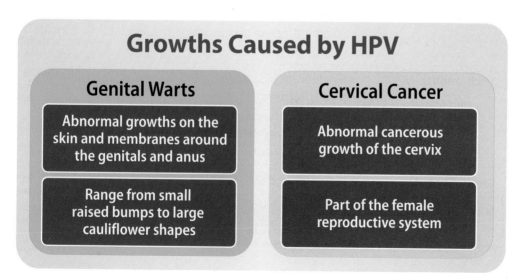

Growths Caused by HPV

Genital Warts
- Abnormal growths on the skin and membranes around the genitals and anus
- Range from small raised bumps to large cauliflower shapes

Cervical Cancer
- Abnormal cancerous growth of the cervix
- Part of the female reproductive system

Figure 11.14
The body easily fights and eliminates most types of HPV. Some types of HPV, however, can cause genital warts or cervical cancer.

If a person develops visible genital warts from an HPV infection, the doctor may prescribe skin treatments, prescription medication, or surgical removal. Treatments for cancer caused by HPV vary depending on the severity and location of the cancer.

A vaccine exists to reduce the risk for HPV infection. The vaccine is recommended for girls and boys from 11 to 12 years of age. The vaccine is given in three shots over a six-month period of time. If people do not get all of the vaccine at this age, they can still receive the vaccination between 13 and 26 years of age.

Preventing STIs

STIs have many unpleasant symptoms (**Figure 11.15**). Although treatments exist for these conditions, it is easier to prevent STIs than it is to treat them. Two of the most effective methods for preventing STIs include abstinence and the use of latex condoms.

Figure 11.15
While it is possible that an STI will not show any noticeable symptoms, most STIs show some symptoms. *Which STI is characterized by hair and weight loss in later stages?*

Sexually Transmitted Infections	
Name	**Symptoms**
Chlamydia	• Vaginal or penile discharge, painful urination, fever • If left untreated, may damage reproductive organs and cause sterility
Gonorrhea	• Vaginal or penile discharge, painful or frequent urination, fever, abdominal pain • If left untreated, may damage reproductive organs and cause sterility
Pelvic inflammatory disease (PID)	• Discharge, abdominal pain, fever, painful urination • If left untreated, may cause sterility
Syphilis	• Early stage: small, painless sore on affected area • Later stages: body rash, fever, hair and weight loss, headache, sore muscles • If left untreated, may cause permanent internal damage and death
Trichomoniasis	• For men: itching and burning in the urethra, discharge from the penis • For women: yellow-green vaginal discharge with a foul odor, burning, itching, and pain during urination and sexual intercourse
Genital herpes	• Sores around the affected area with pain and itching
HPV	• Warts on genitals, painful urination • Cervical and other types of cancer

Practicing Abstinence

Because people contract STIs through sexual activity, the most effective way to prevent STIs is to practice abstinence. Sexual **abstinence** is the commitment to refrain from sexual activity. Abstinence is the only 100 percent effective method for preventing STIs. If a person does not engage in sexual activity, he or she will not contract an STI.

There are certain obstacles, such as peer pressure, that may prevent people from practicing abstinence. Friends or partners may try to persuade a person to engage in sexual activity. The use of alcohol and drugs can also be a barrier that prevents people from practicing abstinence. Alcohol and drugs impair judgment and lower *inhibition* (feelings of restraint), so their use is an important factor in early and unwanted sexual activity. By avoiding risky situations that may include drugs and alcohol, a person can make responsible decisions involving his or her choice to maintain abstinence.

Committing to abstinence may require a person to use refusal skills. As you learned in Chapter 8, refusal skills can help someone stand up to peer pressure. Planning and even practicing refusal skills for refusing sex, drugs, and alcohol can help people become familiar with words and actions they can use if risky situations occur (**Figure 11.16**).

Planning and Practicing Refusal Skills

Practice

- Before you are presented with a risky situation, consider the words you might use.
- What if you are invited to an unsupervised party where alcohol or drugs may be present?
- What if your boyfriend or girlfriend is pressuring you to have sex?

Refuse

- Verbally refuse the risky behavior. Be assertive and honest. Keep your response short, clear, and simple.
- If verbally refusing is not enough, walk away from the situation.

Seek Advice

- Remember that you do not need to face this stress alone.
- Find guidance for handling specific situations from a parent, teacher, counselor, or other trusted adult.

Figure 11.16
You can decrease your chances of being pressured or convinced to participate in risky behaviors by preparing your refusal skills in advance.

Using Latex Condoms

Although abstinence is the only method that is 100 percent effective for preventing STIs, a correctly used latex condom can also reduce the chances of contracting STIs. A **latex condom** is a device that provides a barrier to microorganisms that cause STIs. Condoms made of other materials are not effective prevention methods.

To be effective, a latex condom must be applied correctly, must fit well, must be used for each sex act from beginning to end, and must be removed correctly. A condom can be used only once, and a new one must be used each time a person has sex. Any condom that has expired, has holes or tears, or has dried out must be thrown away because it will not work. In fact, a person should only use condoms he or she has recently purchased or has received from a reliable source, such as a clinic nurse. Condoms may become damaged if stored in places that become very cold or hot, such as in a car, or where they could be crushed, such as in a wallet.

Treatment of STIs

Many STIs are easily treated, especially in their early stages. For example, bacterial STIs are treatable, even curable, with antibiotics prescribed by a doctor. Being cured, however, does not mean that people cannot contract those STIs again. Even after receiving treatment, exposure to an STI will result in another infection.

Viral infections cannot be treated with antibiotics, but they can be controlled with a number of antiviral medications. Viral infections are not curable, however. Antiviral medications simply control the virus, sometimes greatly reducing the severity and frequency of symptoms. **Figure 11.17** shows treatments of STIs.

STI Resources

If a person suspects he or she might have an STI, community resources are available to help. Doctors can provide tests to determine whether the person has an STI, and treatment if necessary. Public health departments often provide diagnosis, treatment, and prevention programs. Private and nonprofit organizations may also offer assistance. Some schools may even provide sexual health and wellness programs.

Those who need additional emotional support may find counseling services and support groups in their communities. People may also find support through their friends and family. People can learn more about resources available to them by searching the Internet or by asking a doctor or nurse. Getting help when necessary is a good way to promote overall health and well-being.

Treatment for STIs

Chlamydia	Prescribed antibiotics
Gonorrhea	Prescribed antibiotics
PID	Prescribed antibiotics; in severe cases, surgery
Syphilis	Prescribed antibiotics or penicillin injection
Trichomoniasis	Prescription antibiotics
Genital herpes	No cure, but prescribed medication can control breakouts and symptoms
HPV	No cure, but prescribed medication can ease symptoms

Figure 11.17
While bacterial infections are treatable and usually curable with antibiotics, viral infections such as genital herpes and HPV cannot be cured. Treatment options for viral infections include easing symptoms and controlling breakouts.

Lesson 11.2 Review

1. _____ are communicable diseases spread from one person to another during sexual activity.
2. **True or false.** Gonorrhea is the bacterial infection that can cause pelvic inflammatory disease (PID) and lead to infertility.
3. What causes the spread of syphilis?
4. Name two ways to help prevent STIs.
5. **Critical thinking.** Are all STIs curable? Explain your response.

Hands-On Activity

Interview an important, trusted adult in your life about his or her knowledge of sexually transmitted infections. Be sure to prepare quality, in-depth questions in advance. Compare his or her answers to the information provided in the text. Did your trusted adult provide accurate information? Would you consider this person a good resource for sexual health information? How did you feel talking with this person about STIs? Why did you feel that way? What other questions do you have now about STIs?

HIV/AIDS

Key Terms

human immunodeficiency virus (HIV) virus that infects and kills cells, weakening the body's immune system; leads to AIDS

acquired immunodeficiency syndrome (AIDS) often fatal disease in which the body cannot fight infections and diseases

HIV-positive status determined by a laboratory test that indicates the presence of HIV antibodies in a person's blood

opportunistic infections conditions that occur when pathogens take advantage of a weakened body; the cause of death in HIV/AIDS cases

long-term non-progressors HIV-positive people whose infection progresses to AIDS slowly

anti-retroviral therapy (ART) treatment for HIV/AIDS in which a cocktail of three drugs is given to interfere with HIV reproduction

Learning Outcomes

After studying this lesson, you will be able to

- **distinguish** between HIV and AIDS.
- **understand** the transmission of HIV.
- **describe** the signs and symptoms of HIV/AIDS.
- **explain** testing procedures for diagnosing HIV/AIDS.
- **identify** treatment methods for HIV/AIDS.

Graphic Organizer

KWL Chart: Learning About HIV/AIDS

Create a chart like the one shown below. Before you read the lesson, outline what you know and what you want to know about understanding HIV/AIDS. After reading the lesson, outline what you have learned. An example is provided for you.

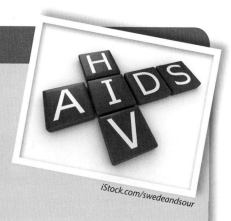

iStock.com/swedeandsour

K **What I Know**	**W** **What I Want to Know**	**L** **What I Have Learned**
HIV infects and kills cells, weakening the body's immune system	Does everyone infected with HIV develop AIDS?	AIDS is a condition in which the body cannot fight infections/disease; can develop later after HIV onset

n Lesson 11.2, Dakota learned about common sexually transmitted infections. Many of those STIs can pose serious health risks if left untreated. Another STI that can have serious health consequences is HIV/AIDS.

HIV/AIDS continues to be the leading infectious cause of death worldwide, killing about two million people each year. It affects men, women, and children of all ages and races and people of all countries. Learning this, Dakota became interested in putting together a school advocacy program that would help inform his classmates and peers about the transmission, health effects, prevention, and treatment of HIV/AIDS.

In this lesson, you will learn about HIV/AIDS. Like Dakota, you will also learn about the transmission of, signs and symptoms of, testing for, and prevention and treatment of HIV/AIDS.

Understanding HIV and AIDS

To understand HIV and AIDS, you must first know what each term means (**Figure 11.18**). **Human immunodeficiency virus (HIV)** infects and kills cells, weakening the body's immune system. At a certain point, the HIV infection completely wears down the immune system. This leads to **acquired immunodeficiency syndrome (AIDS)**, an often fatal disease in which the body cannot fight infections and diseases.

AIDS can develop later, perhaps many years after the onset of the HIV infection. In other words, *HIV* refers to the virus and *AIDS* refers to the disease. Therefore, people transmit HIV, not AIDS. The title of this lesson uses the term *HIV/AIDS* to recognize the relationship between HIV and AIDS.

A person is **HIV-positive** if a laboratory test detects the presence of HIV *antibodies* in the person's blood. *Antibodies* are proteins the body's immune system produces to detect and destroy certain harmful substances, such as HIV. If HIV antibodies are in a person's blood, the person's blood must contain HIV. Being HIV-positive means that a person is infected with HIV, but it does not necessarily mean that a person has AIDS.

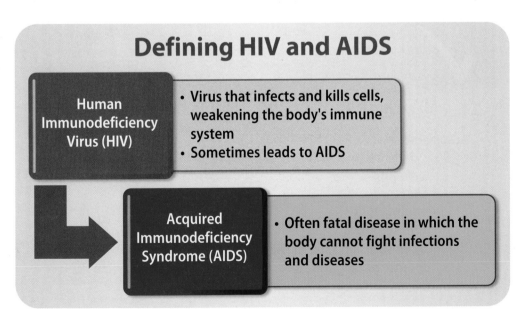

Defining HIV and AIDS

| Human Immunodeficiency Virus (HIV) | • Virus that infects and kills cells, weakening the body's immune system
• Sometimes leads to AIDS |

| Acquired Immunodeficiency Syndrome (AIDS) | • Often fatal disease in which the body cannot fight infections and diseases |

Figure 11.18
HIV is a virus that infects cells and weakens the body's immune system. Sometimes, perhaps many years after the onset of HIV, the body develops AIDS, in which the body cannot fight infections and diseases. *Can HIV be cured with antibiotics? Why or why not?*

HIV Transmission

There are certain ways HIV can and cannot be transmitted (**Figure 11.19**). HIV is found in bodily fluids, including blood, semen, vaginal fluids, and breast milk. HIV is not found in tears, saliva, or sweat. HIV can be transmitted through sexual intercourse. Babies born to HIV-positive mothers can become infected, and mothers can transmit the virus in their breast milk. The virus can also be transmitted through contaminated needles used for drugs, tattoos, or body piercings. At one time, HIV was often transmitted in *blood transfusions*, or procedures in which people receive donated blood. In the United States, however, the blood supply is now screened for HIV, so transfusions are usually very safe.

HIV is *not* transmitted by mosquitoes or by kissing, spitting, shaking hands, sharing food, or using the same toilet seat. Healthy, intact skin provides an effective barrier to HIV infection. HIV transmission is possible through open sores on skin, in the mouth, or on genitals.

Certain factors increase the risk for HIV transmission. People who abuse injected drugs are more likely to share hypodermic needles, increasing their risk of exposure to HIV-positive blood. Having other STIs also increases the risk for developing HIV. Sores and inflammation associated with other STIs damage the intact skin that protects against HIV infection. This means a person with STIs is more at risk for HIV infection.

Signs and Symptoms of HIV/AIDS

Following HIV infection, the infected person may develop minor symptoms that are not recognized. In some people, these symptoms do not occur for months. Early symptoms resemble a flu-like illness with fatigue and swollen, painful lymph nodes. HIV infection may not develop into AIDS for two years or more.

Figure 11.19
HIV can be transmitted in certain bodily fluids such as blood and semen, but not through other fluids such as saliva or sweat.

HIV Transmission

HIV can be found in
- blood (including needles for drugs, tattoos, or piercings)
- semen
- vaginal fluids
- breast milk
- open sores on skin, in the mouth, or on genitals

HIV is *not* found in
- tears
- saliva (kissing, spitting, sharing food)
- sweat
- mosquitoes
- healthy, intact skin (for shaking hands, using the same toilet seat, etc.)

AIDS develops when the immune system becomes disabled. This decline in immunity can be measured with blood tests that show a greatly reduced number of important immune system cells called *T-helper cells* or *CD4 cells*. HIV specifically destroys these immune system cells (**Figure 11.20**).

When the virus sufficiently disables the immune system, unusual or normally harmless pathogens continuously assault the body, causing **opportunistic infections**. These infections occur when pathogens take advantage of a weakened body. Opportunistic infections are the cause of death in HIV/AIDS cases. The presence of opportunistic infections is a sign of HIV/AIDS.

One opportunistic infection, caused by a fungus called *Pneumocystis*, is a form of pneumonia that healthy immune systems easily beat. A yeast infection of the mouth, called *thrush*, also takes advantage of the weakened immune system. *Tuberculosis*, a bacterial lung infection, is often associated with AIDS. In addition to these infections, people with AIDS may develop a blood vessel tumor called *Kaposi's sarcoma*. Other signs and symptoms of AIDS include severe weight loss, diarrhea, fever and chills, and nausea.

According to medical research, HIV/AIDS develops differently and at different rates for all affected people. In some people, HIV infection quickly leads to AIDS, while others do not progress to AIDS for decades (**Figure 11.21**). HIV-positive people whose infection progresses to AIDS slowly are **long-term non-progressors**. Medical researchers may study long-term non-progressors to help explain how the body successfully fights HIV.

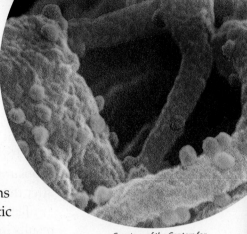

Courtesy of the Centers for Disease Control and Prevention

Figure 11.20
HIV (shown here in green) weakens the body's immune system by infecting and killing cells (shown in red). *Which immune system cells are destroyed by HIV?*

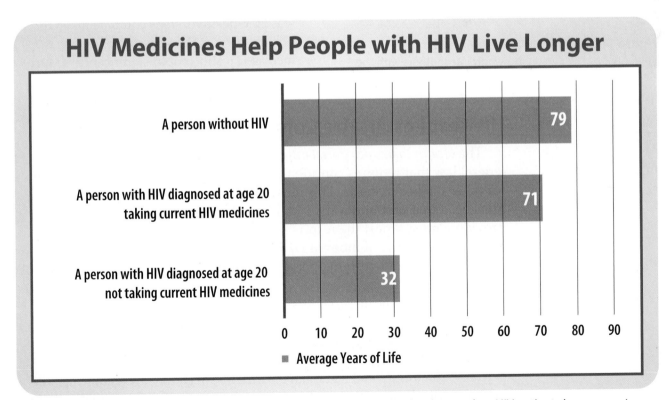

Figure 11.21 People with HIV who take proper medications are able to live longer than HIV patients in years past.

Testing for HIV/AIDS

HIV/AIDS testing is critical for personal and community health. The HIV test examines a blood sample for the presence of HIV antibodies. Recall that the presence of HIV antibodies means the presence of HIV. A person may not develop HIV antibodies until weeks or months after exposure to HIV. Therefore, if a person gets a negative blood test, and he or she suspects exposure to HIV within the past three months, HIV testing should be repeated after three more months have passed.

Test results are available in a few days, or the rapid version of the test gives results in 20 minutes. Though tests are typically performed in doctors' offices and hospital labs, they may be done in other locations as well. HIV test sites can be found by searching the Internet or by contacting the Centers for Disease Control and Prevention (CDC).

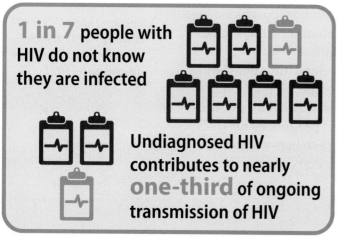

Telman Bagirov/Shutterstock.com

Figure 11.22 Sexually active people who have undiagnosed HIV can unknowingly infect others with the virus.

A home version of the HIV test is available without a prescription at drugstores. The test is inexpensive, fast, painless, and private. If the home test indicates HIV infection, the person should see a doctor for a test to confirm the results.

HIV testing is the key to controlling HIV/AIDS transmission within society. Sexually active people should be tested every year and every time they switch sexual partners. Sadly, some people with HIV do not know they are infected (**Figure 11.22**). If each affected individual knew he or she was HIV-positive, steps could be taken to prevent further transmission of the virus. Increased testing could significantly reduce HIV transmission.

HIV Test Results Are Confidential and Private

The *Health Insurance Portability and Accountability Act (HIPAA)* is a federal law that requires confidentiality for HIV test results, just as it does for other medical records. This means the results of a person's HIV test must be kept secret under the law. If an HIV test is positive, healthcare providers must report the results to the state. This is because the states track and study the number of HIV cases. The results, however, are reported with no identifying personal information to protect the identity of the individual.

Although healthcare providers and states must keep HIV test results private, HIV-positive individuals are encouraged to share their results with certain people. HIV/AIDS is easily transmitted between sexual partners, so HIV-positive individuals should share their test results to protect their partners. Some cities and states have partner-notification laws requiring HIV-positive individuals or their doctors to notify sexual partners or needle-sharing partners (**Figure 11.23**).

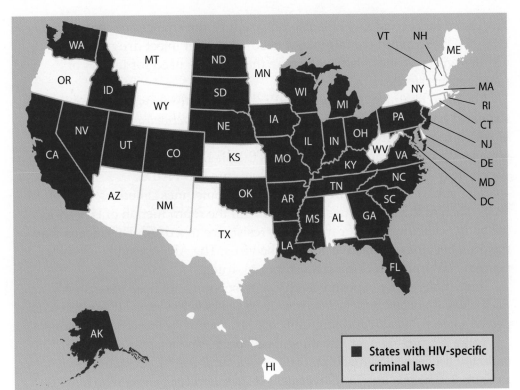

Figure 11.23 Many states throughout the United States have passed laws requiring HIV-positive individuals to disclose information about their disease to sexual partners.

Legend: States with HIV-specific criminal laws

Paul Stringer/Shutterstock.com

Protecting HIV-Positive Individuals from Discrimination

HIV-positive individuals often face discrimination in society and in their workplaces. *Discrimination* is the unfair treatment of a certain group of people. Some employers might refuse to hire HIV-positive people, worrying that they will take many sick days. Others might make assumptions about an HIV-positive person's lifestyle and disapprove of his or her situation. This can also lead to discrimination. The federal government seeks to prevent this type of discrimination.

Two important laws protect the rights of HIV-positive people. The *Americans with Disabilities Act (ADA) of 1990* and the *Rehabilitation Act of 1973* prohibit discrimination against people with HIV/AIDS. This means that people with HIV/AIDS cannot be denied jobs, benefits, education, services, or other rights because of their HIV/AIDS status. These laws also protect the families of people living with HIV/AIDS.

Preventing and Treating HIV/AIDS

People contract HIV/AIDS through sexual activity or through the use of contaminated needles. The same methods used to prevent other STIs also help prevent HIV/AIDs. This means that abstinence is the only method that is 100 percent effective in preventing HIV/AIDS (**Figure 11.24**).

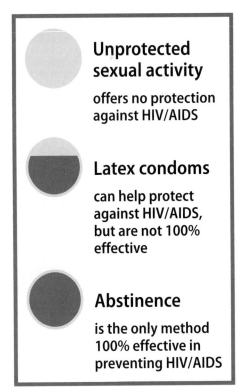

Unprotected sexual activity

offers no protection against HIV/AIDS

Latex condoms

can help protect against HIV/AIDS, but are not 100% effective

Abstinence

is the only method 100% effective in preventing HIV/AIDS

Figure 11.24 There are many methods to prevent STIs, but abstinence is the only method that is 100 percent effective.

The use of latex condoms will also help reduce the chances of contracting HIV/AIDS. To avoid contaminated needles, do not inject drugs or share needles with anyone. Also, make sure that needles used for tattoos or piercings are sterile.

The main treatment method for HIV/AIDS is **anti-retroviral therapy (ART)**, so named because HIV is a type of virus known as a *retrovirus*. The specific aim of ART is to reduce the number of viruses in the body so the immune system remains strong. ART also greatly reduces the likelihood of HIV transmission. It should be noted, however, that ART *does not* cure HIV/AIDS.

ART consists of a mixture of three drugs, sometimes called a *cocktail of drugs*. Each of the three drugs interferes with the reproduction of HIV inside the body. Sometimes, HIV can develop resistance to a drug. This means that the drug becomes ineffective against the virus. The ART cocktail is designed to prevent HIV from developing resistance to drugs.

Immediately after exposure to HIV, a person may not need to begin ART. Each case differs and depends on how long a person has been HIV-positive. The person's general health and immunity are also factors in prescribing treatment.

There is a pre-exposure treatment, called *pre-exposure prophylaxis (PrEP)*, that may prevent HIV infection. PrEP uses a similar ART cocktail known as *Truvada*. The pre-exposure treatment is intended for people who have a high risk of HIV infection. This might include HIV/AIDS researchers who study the virus in a laboratory or doctors and nurses who work closely with HIV-positive patients.

Lesson 11.3 Review

1. **True or false.** The presence of HIV antibodies in the blood indicates a person is HIV-positive.

2. Each of the following is a bodily fluid source of HIV *except* _____.
   A. blood
   B. semen
   C. saliva
   D. breast milk

3. List two types of opportunistic infections.

4. What type of test indicates a person is HIV-positive?

5. **Critical thinking.** What is discrimination? What laws protect the rights of HIV-positive people against discrimination in the workplace?

Hands-On Activity

Create a Venn diagram. Label one of the circles "People living *with* HIV/AIDS" and the other "People living *without* HIV/AIDS." Complete the Venn diagram. List examples of everyday activities that these groups of people can and cannot do. The center, where the circles overlap, indicates what activities both groups of people can or cannot do. When complete, review your information. Draw conclusions about what people living with HIV/AIDS can and cannot do. What do your conclusions show about misconceptions people may have about those who are living with HIV/AIDS?

Noncommunicable Diseases

Learning Outcomes

After studying this lesson, you will be able to

- **understand** terms associated with noncommunicable diseases.
- **explain** the risk factors for noncommunicable diseases.
- **identify** five common noncommunicable diseases that are important health concerns in the United States.
- **describe** risks that noncommunicable diseases pose to your health.

Graphic Organizer

Risk Factors for Noncommunicable Diseases

Create a graphic organizer like the one below to take notes as you read this lesson. In the large circle on the left, write "Noncommunicable Diseases." In the circles on the right, list the types of noncommunicable diseases you learn about in this lesson. In the space around each circle, list two risk factors (lifestyle, heredity, or environment) that can increase the likelihood for developing that disease.

klenger/Shutterstock.com

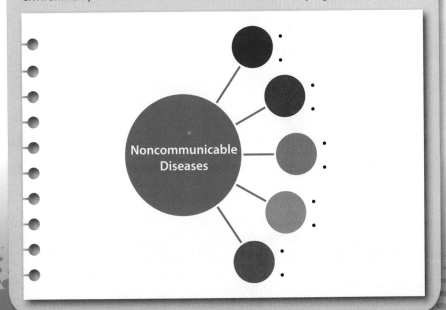

Noncommunicable Diseases

Key Terms

noncommunicable diseases medical conditions that cannot be spread through person-to-person contact, but develop as a result of heredity, environment, and lifestyle factors; also known as *noninfectious diseases*

heart attack medical emergency in which flow of blood to the heart is restricted, causing the heart to beat irregularly and inefficiently

stroke medical emergency in which blood flow to part of the brain is interrupted, injuring or killing brain cells

cancer complex disease that typically involves an uncontrolled growth of abnormal cells

tumor mass of abnormal cells

diabetes mellitus disease resulting from the body's inability to regulate glucose; commonly known as *diabetes*

arthritis condition that results in inflammation of the joints, causing pain and stiffness

autoimmune disease condition that causes the body's immune system to attack and damage the joints

What Is a Noncommunicable Disease?

Communicable disease
- Infectious disease
- A disease that can be spread

Noncommunicable disease
- Noninfectious disease
- A disease that cannot be spread

Figure 11.25 Noncommunicable diseases are different from communicable diseases in that they are not caused by pathogens and cannot be spread among people, objects, and animals.

Recall in the first lesson of this chapter, Dakota and Tavon both developed cases of the flu, which is a communicable disease that people can "catch." In this lesson, you will learn how people develop noncommunicable diseases. *Noncommunicable diseases* are diseases that cannot be transmitted (**Figure 11.25**). Tavon, for example, has asthma, which is not something that Dakota can catch from him.

In developed countries such as the United States, more people die from noncommunicable diseases than from communicable diseases. If these diseases are not transmitted, how do they develop? Understanding noncommunicable diseases is important to reducing the number of deaths they cause.

Understanding Noncommunicable Disease

Noncommunicable diseases, also called *noninfectious diseases*, cannot be spread through person-to-person contact. Instead, a person may inherit the possibility of developing a noncommunicable disease. A person's environment and lifestyle choices may also contribute to its development. **Figure 11.26** shows common noncommunicable diseases.

Many noncommunicable diseases are *chronic* illnesses. This means they are long-term diseases that may not heal for years. In fact, they might even cause permanent disability or health complications.

Figure 11.26 Common noncommunicable diseases include heart disease, stroke, cancer, high blood pressure, lung diseases, and arthritis. *Can noncommunicable diseases spread between people? Why or why not?*

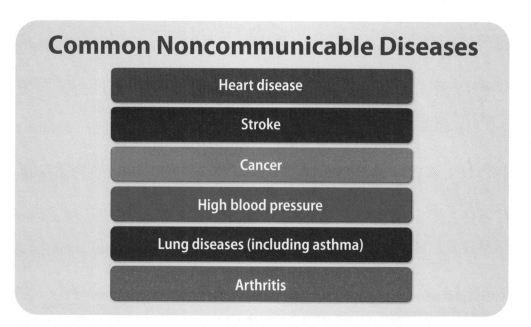

Common Noncommunicable Diseases

- Heart disease
- Stroke
- Cancer
- High blood pressure
- Lung diseases (including asthma)
- Arthritis

When evaluating a patient with a noncommunicable disease, doctors may give a prognosis. A *prognosis* is a prediction (educated guess) of how likely a person is to recover from the disease. A prognosis means something is likely to happen, but it is not a sure guarantee that it will. Prognosis includes the chances for full recovery, disability, or death. Diseases that will end in death are *terminal*.

Sometimes, a disease enters *remission*, which is a time without signs and symptoms associated with that disease. Remission may last for weeks, years, or an indefinite period. The term *relapse* refers to the recurrence of a disease, in which signs and symptoms return after a period of remission (**Figure 11.27**). Certain cancers can return after remission in an even more severe way than before. A *complication* is a new problem or second disease that arises in a person already suffering from one disease. For example, a serious complication of diabetes is loss of eyesight.

Risk Factors for Noncommunicable Diseases

Noncommunicable diseases develop as a result of heredity, environmental, and lifestyle factors. *Heredity* is the passing of characteristics or diseases from one generation to the next. Heredity and family history are important factors in a person's risk of developing noncommunicable diseases. For example, the risk for heart disease and cancer are often passed from one generation to another. If a person has parents or grandparents who develop these diseases, he or she may have a greater risk of developing them as well. Family history of a disease is not, however, a guarantee that someone will develop that disease.

Environment can play a role in the development of some noncommunicable diseases. Living in a major city with high pollution can increase your risk of developing chronic lung diseases. Exposure to secondhand smoke may also increase your risk of developing breathing problems.

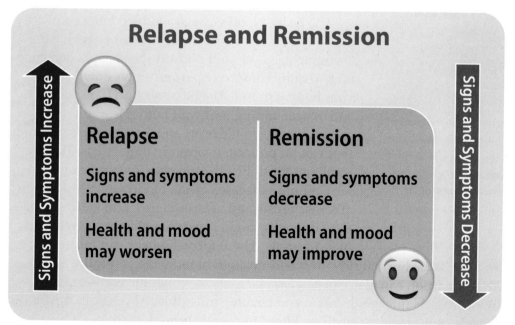

Relapse and Remission

Signs and Symptoms Increase

Relapse

Signs and symptoms increase

Health and mood may worsen

Remission

Signs and symptoms decrease

Health and mood may improve

Signs and Symptoms Decrease

Figure 11.27
Some noncommunicable diseases have symptoms that come and go. Symptoms subside during remission and return during relapse. *Does relapse occur before or after remission?*

ober-art/Shutterstock.com

Risk Factors for Noncommunicable Diseases

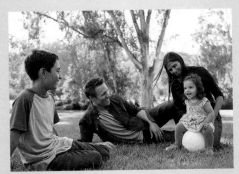

Heredity

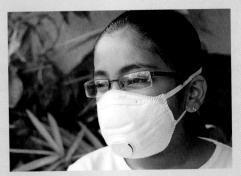

Environment

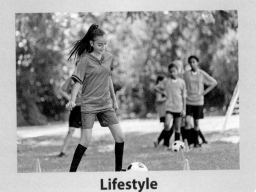

Lifestyle

Top to bottom: Monkey Business Images/Shutterstock.com; iStock.com/VikramRaghuvanshi; iStock.com/Steve Debenport

Figure 11.28 Heredity, environment, and lifestyle choices all contribute to a person's likelihood of having a noncommunicable disease. *Is diet a hereditary, environmental, or lifestyle-related risk factor?*

A person's lifestyle choices and behaviors can increase his or her risk of developing a noncommunicable disease. For example, behaviors such as using tobacco, being physically inactive, and eating an unhealthy diet can lead to breathing problems, heart disease, and cancer.

In most cases, a combination of lifestyle factors, environment, and heredity determine a person's overall risk for developing certain types of noncommunicable diseases (**Figure 11.28**). As a result, you can often reduce your risk of developing these diseases. Although family history is an important risk factor, behavior and environment also contribute to a person's risk. Changing your lifestyle and behaviors can potentially reduce your risk of developing certain noncommunicable diseases.

Common Noncommunicable Diseases

Heart disease, cancer, chronic lung disease, diabetes, and arthritis are important health concerns in many countries, including the United States. In the following sections, you will learn about the risks these diseases pose to your health. Gaining knowledge about these diseases can help you make lifestyle choices that promote optimal health both now and in the future.

Heart Disease

The heart, blood vessels, and blood make up the body's *circulatory system*. The heart adapts to the changing needs of your body. It speeds up when your body requires more oxygen and slows down when your body is at rest. The blood vessels transport blood and oxygen throughout your body. Heart disease causes damage to the heart and blood vessels, meaning they cannot perform their normal functions. This can result in serious health outcomes, including death.

Common diseases of the blood vessels include atherosclerosis and arteriosclerosis. In *atherosclerosis*, fatty deposits called *plaque* develop in the walls of blood vessels. These fatty deposits can build up and block the normal flow of blood through blood vessels (**Figure 11.29**). This condition can also cause *arteriosclerosis*, in which the walls of the blood vessels thicken, harden, and become inflexible. As a result, the blood vessels cannot stretch to allow blood to pump through them.

Atherosclerosis ↗

Normal artery

Atherosclerosis increasing

— Plaque increasing

Plaque buildup narrows the artery

Atherosclerosis

Atherosclerosis with blood clot

Artery blocked, heart attack occurs

© Body Scientific International

Figure 11.29
Atherosclerosis refers to the narrowing of blood vessels. Plaque builds up in the walls of blood vessels, restricting blood flow. Complete blockage of blood flow in coronary arteries (blood vessels that deliver blood to the heart) can lead to a heart attack.

Atherosclerosis and arteriosclerosis can result from tobacco use, physical inactivity, and an unhealthy diet. The nicotine in tobacco can change the blood vessels, making them more likely to develop fatty deposits. Physical inactivity and an unhealthy diet can lead to obesity, which contributes to heart disease in various ways.

The blockage of important blood vessels can stop the flow of blood to the heart. When blood flow to the heart stops, and the heart cannot get enough oxygen, a **heart attack** occurs. During a heart attack, the heart beats irregularly and inefficiently, and pain arises partly because the heart is not receiving enough oxygen. A heart attack is a medical emergency and immediate help can save lives.

A blockage of blood vessels can also cause a **stroke**. During a stroke, blood flow to a part of the brain is interrupted, injuring or killing brain cells (**Figure 11.30**). A stroke can result in paralysis, inability to speak, and mental disability. Lifestyle choices that contribute to atherosclerosis increase a person's risk of experiencing a stroke.

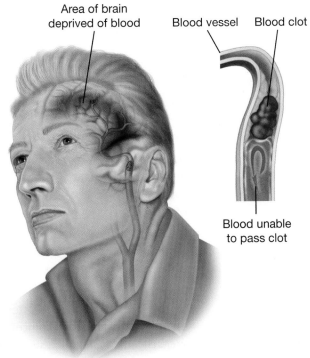

Area of brain deprived of blood

Blood vessel

Blood clot

Blood unable to pass clot

Figure 11.30
Complete blockage of a blood vessel in the brain can deprive part of the brain of blood and oxygen. Without oxygen, cells in the brain die or are injured. This event is called a *stroke.*

© Body Scientific International

There are several treatment options for heart disease. One option is surgery to insert a *stent,* a small tube made of a fine mesh that pushes aside fatty deposits. Doctors may also prescribe blood-thinning medications to increase blood flow.

Cancer

Cancer is a complex disease, with different forms of the disease having different characteristics. All forms of cancer involve an uncontrolled growth of abnormal cells. Healthy cells control their growth, dividing only when needed. Cancerous cells divide rapidly and produce abnormal cells that do not function like normal cells. Scientists call a mass of abnormal cells a **tumor.**

CASE STUDY

Sawyer Copes with Cancer

Sawyer is a middle school student who loves school. Her teachers often describe her as someone who "loves learning and works hard to achieve her goals." Sawyer always tries to answer questions in class, even when she is not sure of an answer. If she answers incorrectly, Sawyer does not get upset, but considers it a learning opportunity.

Sawyer also gets along well with her classmates. She is kind to others and always willing to help when needed, but is not bossy, mean, or snobby. Her classmates think she is friendly and enjoy working with her.

Although she is not perfect, Sawyer is aware of good health behaviors and she tries to take care of herself. She eats healthy foods, gets enough sleep, does not let stress overwhelm her, and gets some sort of physical activity every day. When she is sick, she stays home to recover and keeps her germs to herself.

It came as a shock to everyone when Sawyer was out of school for an extended length of time. People were starting to spread rumors about her being kicked out, about her moving, or about her being very sick. Unfortunately, the last rumor was true. Sawyer was diagnosed with cancer. Not a cancer that had anything to do with choices she or her family made; just a cancer that happens. Fortunately, Sawyer's cancer was detected early. She has been receiving treatments in a nearby city that

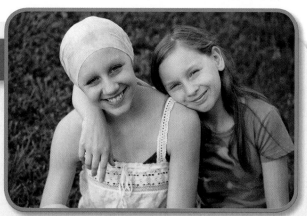

iStock.com/jessicaphoto

make her feel terrible, but she remains optimistic about her future. Despite her illness, and the fact that she does not feel great, Sawyer wants to come back to school, and she does.

Thinking Critically

1. What should Sawyer do to ensure her mental, physical, and social health throughout her illness and treatment?

2. How should Sawyer's classmates and friends treat Sawyer? What questions could they ask Sawyer to help them better understand the situation?

3. If you were Sawyer, what would you do? How much information about your illness would you want your classmates to know?

4. Why do you think remaining optimistic and hopeful are important characteristics during treatments for noncommunicable diseases such as cancer?

Tumors fall into two categories—malignant and benign. *Malignant* tumors are cancerous, while *benign* tumors are not.

There are more than 100 forms of cancer, but certain forms are more common than others. Cancers of the skin, lung, breast, and colon are some of the most common types of cancer (**Figure 11.31**). Together, these four types of cancer make up most of the reported cases in the United States.

As with other noncommunicable diseases, heredity, environment, and lifestyle are all risk factors that can increase a person's chances of developing cancer. For example, some people inherit the risk of developing cancer from their parents and grandparents. Environmental exposure to carcinogens, such as those found in tobacco smoke, may also increase your risk of developing cancer. Physical inactivity can lead to obesity, which can cause certain types of cancer. Making healthy lifestyle choices and forming healthy habits now can reduce your risk of developing cancer later in life.

Common Types of Cancer

Skin Cancer
- Caused by UV radiation, which comes from sunlight and tanning beds
- Melanoma is a very serious type that spreads from skin cells to other cells in the body if it is not caught early
- Can monitor changes in the skin with the ABCDE method (assymetry, border, color, diameter, evolution)

Lung Cancer
- Leading cause of cancer death in the United States
- Main cause is tobacco smoke
- Symptoms include a cough that gets worse with time, chest pain, difficulty breathing, coughing blood, fatigue, and weight loss

Breast Cancer
- Group of diseases that affect breast tissue
- More common in women
- Risk for developing breast cancer increases with age
- Signs and symptoms include a lump in the breast or armpit, thickening or swelling of breast tissue, and irritation or pain in breast tissue or nipple

Colon Cancer
- Second leading cause of cancer death in both men and women
- Polyps (abnormal growths) develop in the colon or rectum and can become cancerous
- Sometimes, no symptoms may be present

Figure 11.31
Skin cancer, lung cancer, breast cancer, and colon cancer are very common in the United States. Each type has unique causes, signs, symptoms, and treatment. *Which type of cancer is the leading cause of cancer death in the United States?*

Early detection of cancer allows for early treatment and better chances for recovery and survival. There are common signs and symptoms of cancer, which are summarized by the acronym *C.A.U.T.I.O.N.* (**Figure 11.32**).

People who have cancer often see a doctor who specializes in cancer care, called an oncologist, for treatment. Cancer treatment may include three specific methods, which include the following:

- **Surgery.** Doctors remove the cancerous tissue from a person's body.
- **Radiation therapy.** Machines deliver powerful X-rays to the part of the person's body affected by cancer. The goal is to shrink cancerous tissues or eliminate them completely. Side effects include fatigue, nausea, and vomiting.
- **Chemotherapy.** Medicines are delivered to patients through an IV, by mouth, or by injection to kill cancer cells. Side effects include weight loss, hair loss, nausea, and loss of appetite.

A combination of treatments is often more effective than any one treatment. For example, chemotherapy and radiotherapy both shrink the amount of cancerous tissue in a person's body. Surgery is more likely to be effective if the cancer is confined to a small area. Therefore, a patient may receive chemotherapy or radiotherapy before surgery, to make the surgery simpler.

Figure 11.32
The C.A.U.T.I.O.N. system is used to detect changes in the body that may signal cancer.

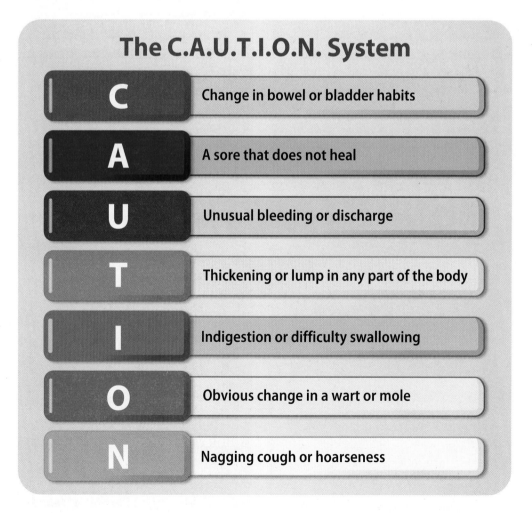

The C.A.U.T.I.O.N. System

C Change in bowel or bladder habits

A A sore that does not heal

U Unusual bleeding or discharge

T Thickening or lump in any part of the body

I Indigestion or difficulty swallowing

O Obvious change in a wart or mole

N Nagging cough or hoarseness

Chronic Respiratory Diseases

The *respiratory system* includes the nose, throat, voice box, windpipe, and lungs. Chronic respiratory diseases cause damage to these structures, meaning that they no longer work properly. Although respiratory diseases can damage all structures of the respiratory system, not just the lungs, they are often called *chronic lung diseases* for short. Examples of chronic lung diseases include chronic obstructive pulmonary disease (COPD) and respiratory allergies.

Chronic Obstructive Pulmonary Disease (COPD)

Chronic obstructive pulmonary disease (COPD) is a group of lung diseases that limit the amount of air that can flow through the lungs. These diseases include emphysema, chronic bronchitis, and asthma. (To review information on emphysema and chronic bronchitis, see Chapter 8.) *Asthma* is a chronic disease in which a person's airways constrict and fill with mucus, making it difficult to breathe (**Figure 11.33**). Membranes in the airways also swell, blocking airflow even more and trapping stale air in the lungs. This triggers the wheezing that often occurs in asthma. Asthma cannot be cured, but medications can reduce the amount and severity of attacks.

People with COPD often experience common symptoms. These symptoms include breathlessness, as well as a cough that lasts a long time and produces a lot of mucus. Causes of COPD include tobacco use, air pollution, and exposure to dusts or chemicals in the workplace. Goals of COPD treatment include managing the condition and its symptoms, as well as preventing the condition from getting worse.

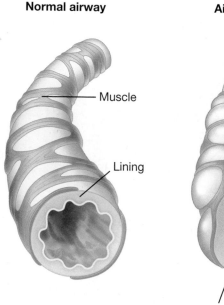
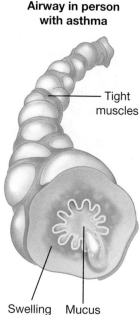

Normal airway

Muscle

Lining

Airway in person with asthma

Tight muscles

Swelling   Mucus

© *Body Scientific International*

Figure 11.33
In asthma, a person's airways swell and become clogged with mucus. The buildup of mucus makes breathing difficult. *Is asthma a long-term or short-term disease?*

Respiratory Allergies

Respiratory allergies are those that specifically affect a person's ability to breathe. The main example of a respiratory allergy is *allergic rhinitis*, commonly known as *hay fever*. Hay fever occurs when someone breathes in a substance that he or she is allergic to, known as an *allergen*. This causes inflammation and swelling inside the nose. Indoor and outdoor allergens can cause hay fever (**Figure 11.34**). Hay fever usually goes away on its own, but it can cause irritating symptoms that may require medication.

Diabetes

Diabetes mellitus, commonly referred to as *diabetes*, is a disease that results from the body's inability to regulate glucose. *Glucose* is a sugar found in foods that the body converts into energy. In someone who does not have diabetes, glucose enters the bloodstream through food. The pancreas, an organ that helps with digestion, creates a hormone called *insulin* that transports glucose to the body's cells. Diabetes disrupts this process.

There are two types of diabetes—type 1 diabetes mellitus (often called *juvenile diabetes*) and type 2 diabetes mellitus. Each type disrupts the body's use of glucose in a different way. Both types result in high blood sugar, which can lead to other health problems. Some potential long-term health problems of diabetes may include heart disease, nerve damage, vision damage, hearing impairment, foot damage, and kidney damage.

Figure 11.34
Three common causes of hay fever are tree, grass, and weed pollen; animal dander; and dust. *What is an allergen?*

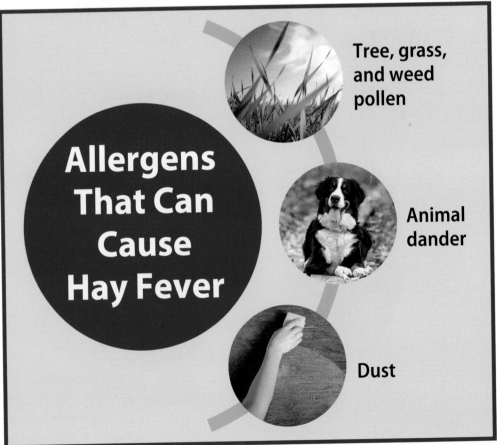

Top to bottom: tomertu/Shutterstock.com; DragoNika/Shutterstock.com; Photographee.eu/Shutterstock.com

Diabetes by the Numbers

Type 2 Diabetes

is the most common type of diabetes, and often does not have any symptoms

Diabetes is the

7th leading cause of death

in the United States

85% of people with type 2 diabetes are overweight or obese

About **1/3** of all people with diabetes do not know that they have the disease

An estimated **30 million Americans** have diabetes

Map: chrupka/Shutterstock.com; Girl: Visual Generations/Shutterstock.com; Speech bubble: Vector.design/Shutterstock.com; Scale: VAZZEN/Shutterstock.com; Tombstone: jabkitticha/Shutterstock.com; Diabetes test: HelgaMariah/Shutterstock.com

Type 1 Diabetes Mellitus

In *type 1 diabetes mellitus*, the pancreas cannot produce insulin. This is a result of the immune system attacking the pancreas and destroying cells that make insulin. This means there is no insulin to transport glucose to the body cells. Instead, glucose stays in the blood, resulting in a high blood sugar level. Type 1 diabetes usually first appears between 10 and 14 years of age.

The main risk factor for type 1 diabetes is family history of the condition. The most common symptoms of type 1 diabetes include excessive urination, thirst, hunger, and weight loss (**Figure 11.35**).

People with type 1 diabetes treat the condition by regularly checking their blood sugar level and giving themselves injections of insulin. Diabetics must also control the amount of sugar in their blood by controlling the amount of food and the sugars they eat. Moderate physical activity also helps regulate blood sugar.

Type 2 Diabetes Mellitus

Type 2 diabetes mellitus develops later in life and is associated with obesity. In this condition, the pancreas creates insulin, but the body does not respond to it normally. Although insulin is present, it does not transport glucose to the body's cells. The pancreas continues to create insulin, however, because it detects the high blood sugar level in the body. This can wear out the pancreas, resulting in an inability to produce enough insulin to meet the body's needs..

Symptoms of type 2 diabetes include excessive urination, thirst, and fatigue. Risk factors for type 2 diabetes include a family history of diabetes, advanced age, obesity, and a physically inactive lifestyle.

Treatment for type 2 diabetes includes eating a balanced diet, managing weight, and taking medications to assist cells with insulin usage. Some people also need insulin if they cannot control their diabetes with diet and weight loss.

Figure 11.35
Diabetes causes symptoms in multiple systems of the body, including the central nervous system, respiratory system, digestive system, and urinary system. It also causes changes in the eyes and breath. Across all systems, it causes weight loss.

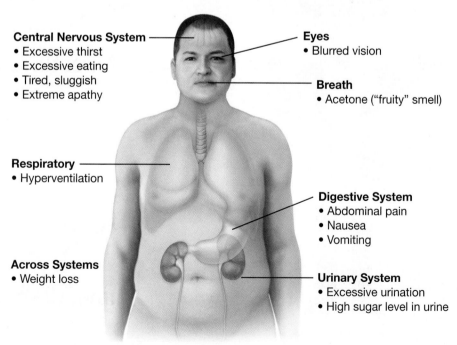

Central Nervous System
• Excessive thirst
• Excessive eating
• Tired, sluggish
• Extreme apathy

Eyes
• Blurred vision

Breath
• Acetone ("fruity" smell)

Respiratory
• Hyperventilation

Digestive System
• Abdominal pain
• Nausea
• Vomiting

Across Systems
• Weight loss

Urinary System
• Excessive urination
• High sugar level in urine

© *Body Scientific International*

Arthritis

Arthritis means inflammation of the joints. People with arthritis move slowly and stiffly because of the inflammation of their joints. Multiple joints within the body can be affected by arthritis (**Figure 11.36**). Two common types of arthritis include osteoarthritis and rheumatoid arthritis. Each type of arthritis has different causes, treatments, and outcomes.

Osteoarthritis is the most common form of arthritis among older adults. It is caused by the wearing down of cartilage that normally pads the surfaces of bones that meet at the joints. The bones then come into contact with each other, triggering pain, swelling, and stiffness. Osteoarthritis can be treated with anti-inflammatory medicine, pain relievers, and mild exercises. Severely damaged joints may require surgery or replacement with an artificial joint.

Rheumatoid arthritis occurs in adults of all ages and affects many joints, the eyes, and the heart. Rheumatoid arthritis is an **autoimmune disease**—a condition that causes the body's immune system to attack and damage the joints. The same joints often swell painfully on opposite sides of the body. The pain and swelling often come and go, repeatedly becoming worse, then improving. Over time, the damage from this disease causes crippling deformities in the joints.

Treatment for rheumatoid arthritis includes anti-inflammatory medication, pain relievers, and mild exercises. Certain medications target the immune system and block its attack on the joint tissues.

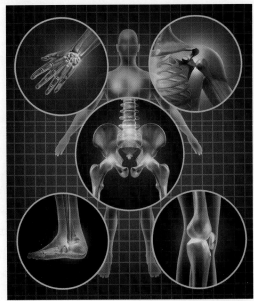

Lightspring/Shutterstock.com

Figure 11.36 Arthritis can cause inflammation in many different joints and often affects joints in the hands, shoulders, back, hips, knees, and feet. *How does arthritis affect the movement of joints?*

Lesson 11.4 Review

1. List three factors that contribute to the development of a noncommunicable disease.
2. The heart, blood vessels, and blood make up the body's _____ system.
   - **A.** respiratory
   - **B.** circulatory
   - **C.** reproductive
   - **D.** lymphatic
3. A mass of abnormal cells is called a(n) _____.
4. What is arthritis?
5. **Critical thinking.** Contrast the risk factors for type 1 diabetes and type 2 diabetes.

Hands-On Activity

With a partner, choose one noncommunicable disease discussed in this chapter. Review information about the disease's causes, signs and symptoms, and treatments. Then, create a flowchart that illustrates this information. Your flowchart should start with the causes of the disease and end with treatment options. For each step in the flowchart, include a related image. Share your completed flowchart with the class.

11.5

Preventing Diseases

Key Terms 🔗

respiratory etiquette
practice of covering your mouth and nose with a tissue while coughing or sneezing, or sneezing into your sleeve

food sanitation food safety practices that maintain the safety of food you handle and eat; includes refrigerating and freezing certain foods, cooking meat thoroughly, and washing vegetables and fruits

vaccine substance that contains a dead or nontoxic part of a pathogen that is injected into a person to train his or her immune system to eliminate the live pathogen

Learning Outcomes

After studying this lesson, you will be able to

- **demonstrate** proper hand washing to prevent communicable diseases.
- **describe** respiratory etiquette practices to prevent communicable diseases.
- **give examples** of food sanitation practices that maintain the safety of food you handle and eat.
- **explain** the purpose of vaccines in disease prevention.
- **summarize** how to reduce your risk of noncommunicable diseases.

Graphic Organizer 🔗

Focus on Disease Prevention

Create a table like the one shown below. Include as many rows as you need. As you read this lesson, list the ways to prevent or reduce the risk of communicable and noncommunicable diseases. Identify as many details as you need for each prevention method. (An example is provided for you.) When you finish reading the lesson, team up with a classmate to discuss each other's lists. What items do you need to add?

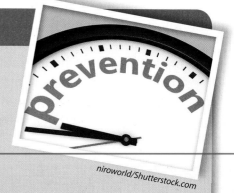

niroworld/Shutterstock.com

Preventing Communicable Diseases	Preventing Noncommunicable Diseases
Cover your mouth and nose with a tissue while coughing or sneezing.	Eat a healthy diet to reduce the risk of heart disease, cancer, and diabetes.

n the previous lessons, you learned how diseases develop. Some diseases develop after contact with pathogens, like the flu that Dakota and Tavon had. Others, such as Tavon's asthma, develop due to family history, behavior, and environment. No matter what the cause, prevention methods exist for all types of disease. In this lesson, you will learn steps you can take to prevent communicable diseases. You will also learn about lifestyle changes that can help prevent and manage noncommunicable diseases.

Preventing Communicable Diseases

As you learned, microorganisms called *pathogens* cause communicable diseases. Bacteria, viruses, and other pathogens can travel from person to person, animal to person, or object to person (**Figure 11.37**). How can you protect yourself from something you cannot even see? The task may seem impossible, but you can use a few simple actions to ensure microorganisms do not make you sick. You can prevent communicable diseases by washing your hands frequently, using respiratory etiquette, practicing food sanitation, and getting regular vaccines.

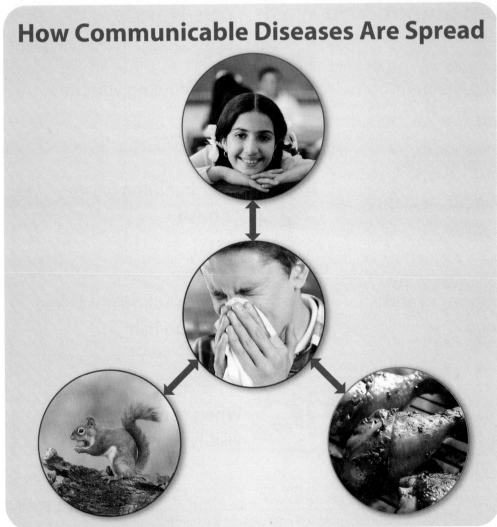

How Communicable Diseases Are Spread

Figure 11.37
Communicable diseases can be transmitted among people, objects, and animals. *What are disease-causing microorganisms called?*

Top to bottom: Zurijeta/Shutterstock.com; Billion Photos/Shutterstock.com; Mircea Costina/Shutterstock.com; amenic181/Shutterstock.com

Hand Washing

What have you touched today? Nearly everything you touch, from doorknobs to your dog, contains pathogens that transfer to your hands. Now think about everything you do with your hands. When you eat with dirty hands, pathogens you pick up from other objects enter your body with the food. Washing your hands on a regular basis, and in certain situations, can eliminate pathogens and prevent communicable diseases. **Figure 11.38** lists occasions to wash your hands.

Hand washing is the most important method of preventing many communicable diseases. Washing your hands is a simple action you can take to prevent germs on your hands from making you sick. Always use running water and soap to wash your hands. Rub your hands together, scrubbing every surface, for 20 seconds. To make sure you are washing your hands for at least 20 seconds, hum or sing the "Happy Birthday" song twice. After 20 seconds of scrubbing, rinse your hands under warm running water. Then air-dry your hands or pat them dry with a clean towel.

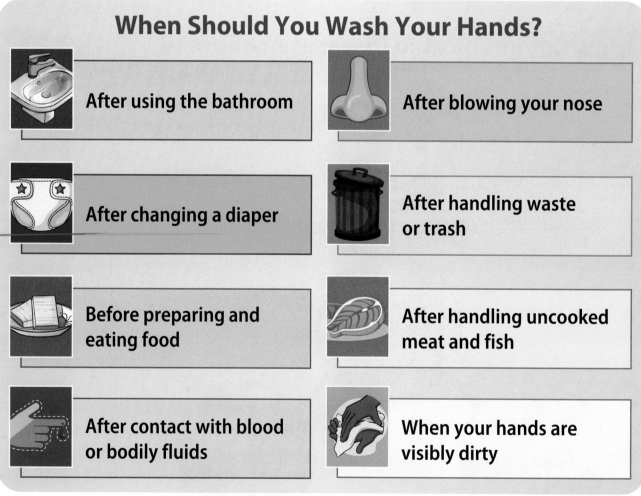

When Should You Wash Your Hands?

After using the bathroom

After blowing your nose

After changing a diaper

After handling waste or trash

Before preparing and eating food

After handling uncooked meat and fish

After contact with blood or bodily fluids

When your hands are visibly dirty

Left, top to bottom: Codrut Crososchi/Shutterstock.com; Panda Vector/Shutterstock.com; ogieurvil/Shutterstock.com; Jemastock/Shutterstock.com; Right, top to bottom: Top Vector Studio/Shutterstock.com; Anahit/Shutterstock.com; SofiaV/Shutterstock.com; Luciano Cosmo/Shutterstock.com

Figure 11.38 Washing your hands on all of these occasions will help prevent the transmission of communicable diseases.

How to Wash Your Hands

1. Wet hands

2. Use soap

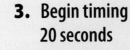

3. Begin timing 20 seconds

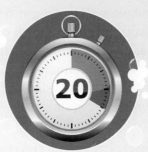

4. Or you could hum "Happy Birthday" twice

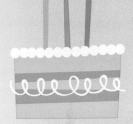

5. Rub palm to palm

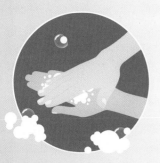

6. Back of hands

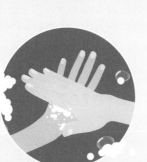

7. Rub fingernails

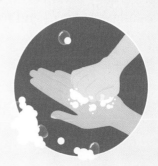

8. Fingers interlaced

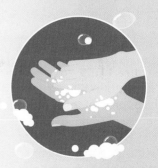

9. Base of thumbs

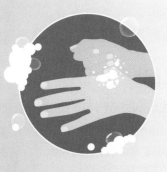

10. Rub wrists

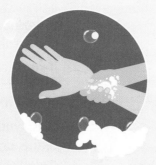

11. Rinse hands

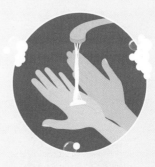

12. Dry hands

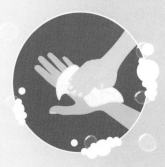

Washing hands: Pro_Vector/Shutterstock.com; Birthday cake: vannilasky/Shutterstock.com; Timer: Aleksandr Bryliaev/Shutterstock.com

Alcohol-based hand rubs, or hand sanitizers, are very effective when soap and water are unavailable. Visibly dirty hands, however, need to be washed first for the alcohol rubs to work. Alcohol-based sanitizer dispensers are often located in stores and other public places. Although use of hand sanitizers is convenient, prolonged use can dry out a person's skin.

Respiratory Etiquette

In Lesson 11.1, you learned that communicable diseases, such as the common cold and flu, can infect people through droplet spread. Droplet spread occurs when pathogens travel in droplets of fluid created by coughing, sneezing, and talking. Doctors recommend that people practice respiratory etiquette to prevent spreading diseases through droplet spread. **Respiratory etiquette** is the practice of covering your mouth and nose with a tissue while coughing or sneezing, or sneezing into your sleeve (**Figure 11.39**). Use respiratory etiquette when you are sick to help the people around you avoid getting sick.

Food Sanitation

The indirect transmission of pathogens through contaminated food, water, and surfaces can cause some dangerous communicable diseases. You can adopt certain food safety practices, known as **food sanitation**, to maintain the safety of the food you handle and eat. Food sanitation practices include refrigerating and freezing certain foods, cooking meat thoroughly, and washing vegetables and fruits (**Figure 11.40**).

Figure 11.39
Respiratory etiquette helps prevent the spread of communicable diseases through droplets in the air. *What are some examples of diseases that can infect people through droplet spread?*

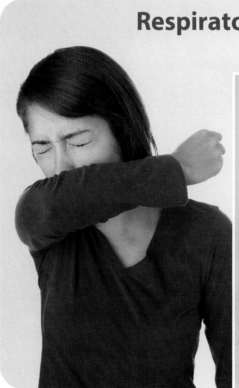

Respiratory Etiquette

- **Cover your mouth and nose when you sneeze or cough. This prevents droplets from spreading.**
- **Cover your nose and mouth with a tissue when coughing or sneezing. Do not reuse or store the tissue.**
- **If you have no tissues, cough or sneeze into your upper arm, sleeve, or elbow, not your hands.**
- **Wash your hands after using a tissue, or after sneezing and coughing into your hands.**

iStock.com/sebarnes

Food Sanitation Practices

Figure 11.40
Practicing good food sanitation includes refrigerating and freezing perishables, cooking meat thoroughly, and washing vegetables and fruits.

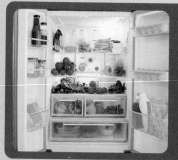

Refrigerate and Freeze Perishables

Refrigeration and freezing slow or stop the growth of pathogens. Food that can spoil should be kept cold or frozen. Remember, however, that refrigerating and freezing foods does not kill pathogens.

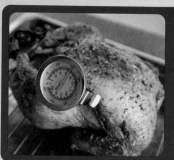

Cook Meat Thoroughly

Cooking meat thoroughly will kill pathogens. Instant meat thermometers have a scale noting safe temperatures for various types of meat. Always use a meat thermometer or cook meat until its juices no longer run pink.

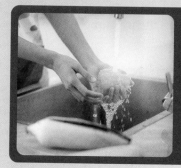

Wash Vegetables and Fruits

The outer coverings of fruits and vegetables often contain pathogens. Therefore, it is important to wash vegetables and fruits under running water before eating. Fruits you peel or cut open should be washed before cutting.

Top to bottom: Andrey_Popov/Shutterstock.com; Africa Studio/Shutterstock.com; Pumz/Shutterstock.com

Vaccines

Vaccination is the only proven method of successfully getting rid of an infectious disease. For example, the highly contagious, deadly viral infection *smallpox* was eliminated by vaccination. In the next few years, vaccines will probably conquer *polio*, which has caused paralysis in many people throughout history.

A **vaccine** is a substance that contains a dead or nontoxic part of a pathogen that is injected into a person to train his or her immune system to eliminate the live pathogen. A doctor or another healthcare worker will administer a vaccine through an injection. When injected into a person, the vaccine causes an immune response in the body. This means the injected person's body produces white blood cells, proteins, and chemicals that fight infections. The vaccine is the body's first encounter with the pathogen. The body's immune response to the vaccine is like a rehearsal for when the body encounters the real pathogen.

Common Vaccines for Adolescents

Vaccine	Effect
Human papillomavirus (HPV) vaccine	The HPV vaccine helps prevent cancers caused by HPV, the most common STI. It is recommended for boys and girls around age 11 or 12.
Influenza (flu) vaccine	The flu vaccine (commonly called the *flu shot*) is given yearly and protects against infection with the flu. If a vaccinated person does get the flu, his or her symptoms are milder.
Meningococcal vaccine	Meningococcal vaccines protect against diseases caused by the *Neisseria meningitidis* bacteria. These bacteria can cause severe infections around the brain and spinal cord. The vaccine is recommended at age 11 or 12 and again at age 16.
Tdap vaccine	The Tdap vaccine protects against three diseases: tetanus, diphtheria, and pertussis (also called *whooping cough*). The vaccine is recommended around age 11 or 12.

Figure 11.41 Most vaccines are given during childhood. The vaccines in this table are recommended for adolescents. *Which vaccine is given yearly?*

The dead pathogen or part of a pathogen in the vaccine cannot cause an illness, but it makes the person's body familiar with the illness. After getting a vaccine, a person's body will recognize the pathogen included in the vaccine. If a person encounters the real, disease-causing pathogen, his or her immune system will respond strongly and quickly. When exposed to a pathogen after vaccination, the body knows how to react to the pathogen.

Because vaccination activates the immune system, it is also called *immunization*. Vaccines are safe and effective, and they prevent many types of communicable diseases (**Figure 11.41**). Some vaccines are effective for nearly a lifetime, others for many years. Some vaccines require follow-up injections, called *boosters*, to restimulate the immune system.

Preventing Noncommunicable Diseases

Pathogens do not cause noncommunicable diseases. Instead, family history and lifestyle choices contribute to the development of noncommunicable diseases. People cannot avoid conditions such as heart disease, cancer, chronic respiratory disease, and diabetes through hand washing or food sanitation. Making healthy lifestyle choices early in life can help you prevent noncommunicable diseases (**Figure 11.42**).

Figure 11.42
Your health now impacts your health in the future.

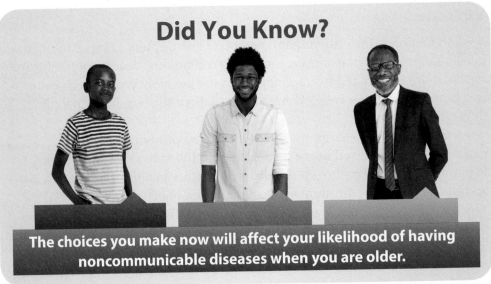

Did You Know?

The choices you make now will affect your likelihood of having noncommunicable diseases when you are older.

Left to right: iStock.com/Yuri_Arcurs; Rawpixel.com/Shutterstock.com; Rawpixel.com/Shutterstock.com

Love Your Heart

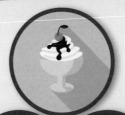

EAT LESS SUGARY AND SALTY FOODS

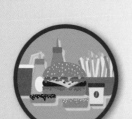

LIMIT INTAKE OF FATTY FOODS

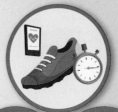

ENGAGE IN CARDIO EXERCISE FOR AT LEAST 30 MINUTES FIVE DAYS PER WEEK

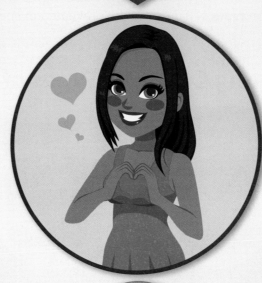

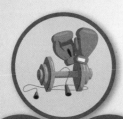

FOCUS ON MUSCLE STRENGTHENING EXCERCISES TWO DAYS PER WEEK

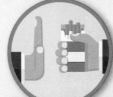

AVOID SMOKING AND OTHER USES OF TOBACCO

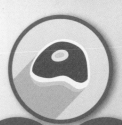

TRY EATING SOME MEALS WITHOUT MEAT

Girl: Kakigori Studio/Shutterstock.com; Icons, clockwise from top: PureSolution/Shutterstock.com; Elegant Solution/Shutterstock.com; Macrovector/Shutterstock.com; hvostik/Shutterstock.com; Elegant Solution/Shutterstock.com; Vadim Ermak/Shutterstock.com

Heart Disease

Heart disease occurs as a result of damage to structures such as the blood vessels. The best method of prevention is making lifestyle choices that protect your blood vessels and heart. One important lifestyle choice is eating a healthy diet. Including more fruits and vegetables and fewer processed foods in your diet can improve heart health. Engaging in regular physical activity can also help you avoid heart disease. Getting regular exercise will keep your heart in shape and working properly.

Maintaining a healthy weight also reduces the risk of heart disease. Eating a healthy diet and being physically active can help you manage your weight. In addition, avoiding tobacco and alcohol increases heart health. Making these healthy lifestyle choices can reduce your risk of developing heart disease.

Cancer

Maintaining a healthy lifestyle is also important for preventing cancer. To reduce your risk for cancer, be sure to maintain a healthy weight and eat a healthy diet. Physical activity is also important. In addition, each of the common types of cancer can be prevented in specific ways (**Figure 11.43**).

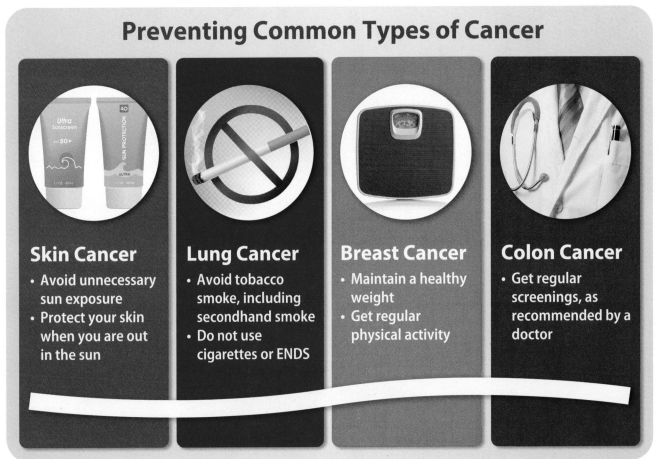

Preventing Common Types of Cancer

Skin Cancer
- Avoid unnecessary sun exposure
- Protect your skin when you are out in the sun

Lung Cancer
- Avoid tobacco smoke, including secondhand smoke
- Do not use cigarettes or ENDS

Breast Cancer
- Maintain a healthy weight
- Get regular physical activity

Colon Cancer
- Get regular screenings, as recommended by a doctor

Figure 11.43 Though heredity and environment still play a role, lifestyle choices can help prevent common types of cancer.

Family History

Noncommunicable diseases are caused by lifestyle choices, your environment, and the genes passed down to you by your biological parents. Your genes determine many of your traits, including your eye color, hair color, and likelihood of having certain noncommunicable diseases. Because of this, some noncommunicable diseases run in families. For example, if your grandfather had heart disease, you may be at an increased risk for having heart disease when you are older.

To see what noncommunicable diseases run in a family, doctors often ask questions about *family history*, which is a biological family's history of disease. A family history typically includes information about your biological parents, siblings, and extended family, and should list diseases such as heart disease, cancer, diabetes, and asthma.

Charting Your Family's History of Disease

Knowing your family's history of noncommunicable diseases can help you take action to prevent diseases in your future. For example, if your family has a history of type 2 diabetes, you can reduce your risk factors for that disease. To chart your family history, begin by meeting with your parents or guardian. Draw a family tree like the one below and fill in the names of your biological parents, siblings, and grandparents. If you do not have access to this information, talk with your teacher. For each person on your family tree, write down any noncommunicable diseases the person has or had. Talk with your parents about the noncommunicable diseases that run in your family and make a list of five actions you could take to reduce your risk of these diseases in the future.

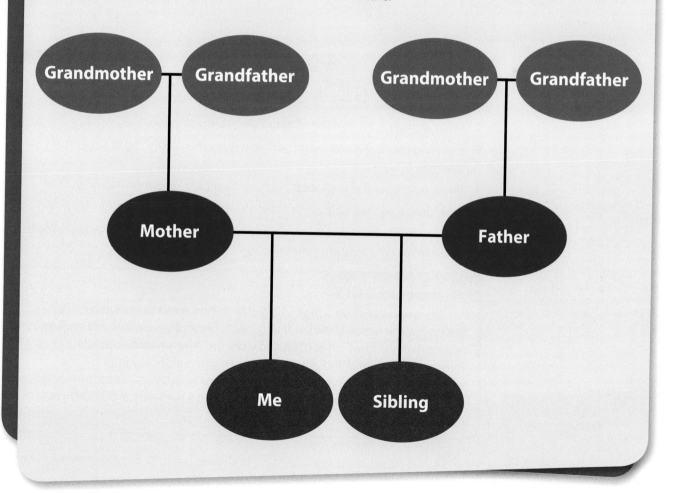

Chronic Respiratory Diseases

Chronic respiratory diseases include bronchitis, emphysema, and asthma. The main causes of bronchitis and emphysema include tobacco smoke and pollutants in the home or workplace. You can reduce your risk of developing bronchitis or emphysema by avoiding these substances. In addition, early detection of bronchitis and emphysema can prevent these diseases from getting worse and leading to COPD. Once a respiratory disease is detected, a person who smokes should stop smoking immediately and reduce exposure to substances that cause COPD.

Most doctors and scientists do not know the cause of asthma, so people cannot prevent development of the disease. People can manage the symptoms of asthma, however. For example, people can manage asthma by avoiding substances or situations that trigger asthma attacks. In addition, medicine can reduce asthma attacks and improve a person's breathing.

Diabetes

Risk factors for type 2 diabetes include having a physically inactive lifestyle and being overweight or obese. The best way to prevent diabetes is to avoid these risk factors. Maintaining a healthy weight can help reduce your risk of developing diabetes. Eating a healthy diet and getting regular physical activity can help you manage your weight.

Lesson 11.5 Review

1. What are four ways to prevent communicable diseases?
2. Covering your nose and mouth with a tissue when coughing or sneezing is an example of _____ _____.
3. What are three food sanitation practices that help keep food safe to eat?
4. How does a vaccine help prevent illness?
5. **Critical thinking.** Name three ways to help prevent noncommunicable diseases and explain why they are helpful.

Hands-On Activity

Disease prevention is highly linked to the choices a person makes. Review the lesson and make a list identifying which prevention choices you engage in appropriately and which you need to work on. Why are some behaviors easy for you to do while others are not? How can you realistically improve your disease prevention behaviors? What support or help do you need from others to do this? Who can provide that support? Write a summary explaining your answers.

Summary

Lesson 11.1 Communicable Diseases

- Pathogens are microorganisms that cause communicable diseases. They are only visible with a microscope. Bacteria, viruses, fungi, and protozoa are pathogens that cause communicable diseases.
- Pathogens that cause communicable diseases travel by various methods of transmission from one organism to another. Methods of transmission may be direct or indirect.
- Communicable diseases include influenza, mononucleosis, tonsillitis, and conjunctivitis.
- Treatment with antibiotics is effective against most pathogenic bacteria, but is not effective against viruses, fungi, and protozoa.

Lesson 11.2 Sexually Transmitted Infections (STIs)

- Sexually transmitted infections are communicable diseases that spread from one person to another during sexual activity. Common STIs include chlamydia, gonorrhea, syphilis, trichomoniasis, genital herpes, and human papillomavirus (HPV).
- Abstinence is the only 100 percent effective method for preventing STIs.
- Many STIs are easily treated and curable, but people can contract STIs again.

Lesson 11.3 HIV/AIDS

- Understanding the relationship between HIV and AIDS is important. Infection with HIV does not necessarily mean that a person has AIDS.
- HIV is found in bodily fluids such as blood, semen, vaginal fluids, and breast milk, but not in tears, saliva, or sweat. Early HIV symptoms are similar to flu-like illness.
- Testing for the presence of HIV antibodies involves examining a sample of blood.
- Anti-retroviral therapy (ART) is the main treatment for HIV/AIDS, but is not a cure.

Lesson 11.4 Noncommunicable Diseases

- Noncommunicable diseases, or noninfectious diseases, do not spread from person to person. They are often the result of heredity, environment, and lifestyle choices.
- Noncommunicable diseases include heart disease, cancer, chronic respiratory diseases, diabetes, and arthritis.
- Understanding the risks of noncommunicable diseases helps you make lifestyle choices to promote optimal health.

Lesson 11.5 Preventing Diseases

- Preventing communicable diseases involves taking actions to ensure microorganisms do not make people sick. Prevention methods include hand washing, respiratory etiquette, and food sanitation.
- Vaccines prevent communicable diseases by stimulating the immune response. The immune response is like a rehearsal for an encounter with the real pathogen.
- Lifestyle choices such as a healthy diet and regular physical activity help prevent noncommunicable diseases.

Check Your Knowledge ↗

Record your answers to each of the following questions on a separate sheet of paper.

1. Describe the difference between communicable and noncommunicable diseases.
2. What communicable disease is also known as *pinkeye*?
3. What does *method of transmission* mean?
4. What is the most commonly contracted STI?
5. What is the most effective way to prevent STIs?
   A. Latex condom.
   B. Respiratory etiquette.
   C. Sexual abstinence.
   D. Hand washing.
6. **True or false.** AIDS is the virus that causes the disease HIV.
7. What is the main treatment method for HIV/AIDS?
8. List three actions you can take to help prevent heart disease.
9. Which noncommunicable disease is characterized by the uncontrolled growth of abnormal cells?
10. **True or false.** Improper hand washing and heredity are risk factors for noncommunicable diseases.
11. **True or false.** Refrigerating and freezing certain foods is an example of a food sanitation practice.
12. What is respiratory etiquette?

Use Your Vocabulary ↗

abstinence	food sanitation	mononucleosis
acquired immunodeficiency syndrome (AIDS)	genital herpes	noncommunicable diseases
	gonorrhea	
antibiotics	heart attack	opportunistic infections
anti-retroviral therapy (ART)	HIV-positive	pathogens
	human immunodeficiency virus (HIV)	respiratory etiquette
arthritis		sexually transmitted infections (STIs)
autoimmune disease	human papillomavirus (HPV)	
cancer		stroke
chlamydia	influenza	syphilis
communicable disease	latex condom	tonsillitis
conjunctivitis	long-term non-progressors	trichomoniasis
diabetes mellitus		tumor
	method of transmission	vaccine

13. On a separate sheet of paper, list words that relate to each of the terms above. Then, work with a partner to explain how these words are related.
14. Read the text passages that contain each of the terms above. Then, write the definitions of each term in your own words. Double-check your definitions by re-reading the text and using the text glossary.

Think Critically

15. **Cause and effect.** What dangers, to self and others, does a person create by coming to school sick with a communicable disease?

16. **Identify.** What agencies and resources are available in your community for accessing sexual healthcare services (such as STI testing)? Identify at least two.

17. **Analyze.** Why is HIV/AIDS testing critical for personal and community health?

18. **Draw conclusions.** What prevention behaviors can help prevent more than one noncommunicable disease? Which behaviors do you believe are the most important for maintaining health? Why?

DEVELOP Your Skills

19. **Teamwork and advocacy skills.** Practicing health-enhancing behaviors and avoiding health risks are important to everyone, especially for preventing STIs and HIV/AIDS. In small groups, review the information on practicing abstinence. Then, as a group, write a script for a role-play scenario in which a person makes responsible decisions to maintain abstinence. Include refusal skills and other healthy behaviors in your role-play. After reviewing your role-play with your teacher, present it to the class to advocate for abstinence.

20. **Communication and advocacy skills.** Illustrate how to use healthy behaviors to prevent or reduce the risk of one noncommunicable disease discussed in the chapter. Use a school-approved software application to create a digital poster *or* digital public service announcement to get the word out to those you know.

21. **Literacy and accessing information skills.** Read a story (such as a novel, short story, or children's book) about a middle-school student facing one of the diseases discussed in the chapter. Complete a book report that assesses the accuracy of the information about the disease. Also, include the take-home message, theme, or moral of the story, and a recommendation for reading. Share your report with a classmate.

22. **Goal-setting skills.** To improve your personal hand-washing behavior, set a SMART goal for yourself. Create a plan of small steps to achieve this goal. Implement your plan and keep track of your progress in a journal. Write a reflection on the process after achieving your goal. How realistic was your goal? What strategies helped you?

23. **Communication and accessing information skills.** Imagine you are a writer for a middle-school newspaper or website. Write an editorial targeted at middle-school students. Choose a topic based on what you have read in the chapter. Be sure the information is relevant and interesting to your audience. Likewise, be sure that the information you provide is accurate. Use other valid and reliable sources to help formulate your writing. Be sure to cite your sources.

Preventing and Responding to Accidents and Injuries

Essential Question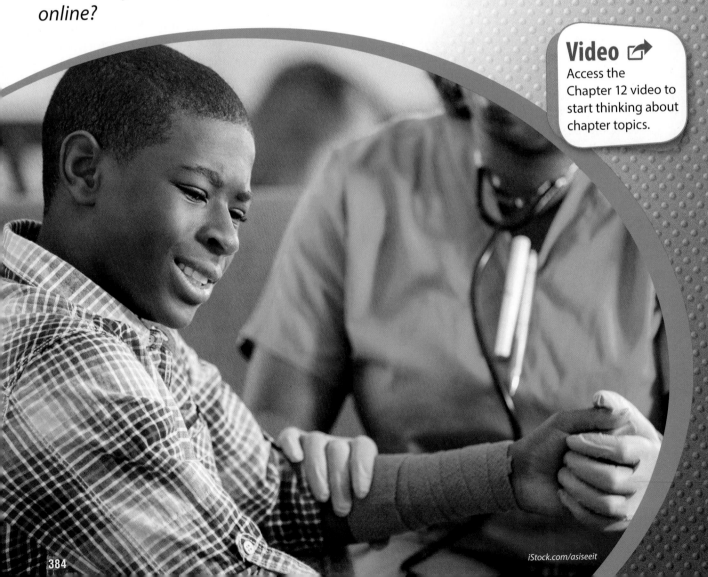

How can you protect yourself at home, in the community, and online?

Lesson 12.1 Staying Safe in the Home

Lesson 12.2 Staying Safe in the Community and Online

Lesson 12.3 Knowing Basic First Aid

Video ↗

Access the Chapter 12 video to start thinking about chapter topics.

iStock.com/asiseeit

How Healthy Are You?

In this chapter, you will be learning about preventing and responding to accidents and injuries. Before you begin reading, take the following quiz to assess your current accident and injury prevention habits.

Healthy Choices	Yes	No
Do you know the phone number for the Poison Control Center?		
Do you and your family have an established emergency evacuation plan in case of a fire?		
Do you and your family have a first-aid kit and other emergency supplies stored in your home and in any vehicles?		
Do you practice caution with strangers and get away from any stranger who makes you uncomfortable?		
Do you use the Privacy settings on any social media accounts you have to protect your personal information?		
Do you take precautions as a pedestrian to make yourself visible and safe from getting hit by a car?		
Do you always wear a helmet when riding a bike and follow all traffic rules?		
Do you know what to do in the case of cuts, scrapes, severe bleeding, bites, stings, electrical shocks, and burns?		
Would you immediately call 911 if someone stopped breathing (including choking) or their heart stopped?		

Count your "Yes" and "No" responses. The more "Yes" responses you have, the more healthy accident and injury prevention and response habits you exhibit. Now, take a closer look at the questions with which you responded "No." How can you make these habits part of your daily life? Think about how implementing these ideas can help improve your overall health.

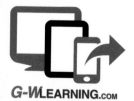

G-WLEARNING.com

While studying this chapter, look for the activity icon ➦ to

- **practice** key terms with e-flash cards and matching activities.
- **reinforce** what you learn by completing graphic organizers, self-assessment quizzes, and review questions.
- **expand** knowledge with interactive activities and activities that extend learning.

Staying Safe in the Home

Key Terms 📲

precautions actions you take to prevent something bad from happening

poisonous able to cause illness or death upon entering the body

fire triangle model to help you remember the elements that are needed for a fire to occur; elements include fuel, heat, and oxygen

flammable easily set on fire

extinguish put out

escape plan strategy that outlines safe routes and procedures for leaving the house in the event a fire occurs

emergency preparedness knowing how to respond to a specific type of emergency

natural disasters events or forces of nature that usually cause great damage

Learning Outcomes

After studying this lesson, you will be able to

- **give examples** of ways to prevent falls in the home.
- **explain** how to prevent illness or injury from potentially hazardous products in the home.
- **describe** how the presence of weapons in the home increases the risk of serious injuries.
- **create** an escape plan for leaving your home in case of a fire.
- **develop** an emergency preparedness plan for your family.
- **identify** ways to remain safe when staying home alone.

Graphic Organizer 📲

Black Jack/Shutterstock.com

Safety at Home

Before reading this lesson, draw or create a floor plan of the place you live. An example floor plan is shown below. Label each room and leave enough space to take notes. As you read this lesson, list potential safety hazards you observe in each room. Then, identify safety precautions you can take to avoid these hazards.

Dining room

Kitchen

Fire hazard
* Conduct inspection
* Practice escape plan

Bathroom

Foyer

Parents' bedroom

My bedroom

Dr Project/Shutterstock.com

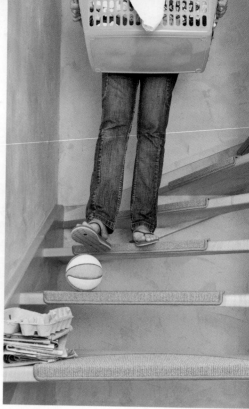

Throughout her day, 13-year-old Jada may encounter unsafe situations. It is important for Jada to understand these potential situations and learn practices she can use to ensure her personal safety. For example, Jada and her family are very careful to avoid overloading electrical outlets. They regularly check smoke detectors and fire extinguishers to make sure they are working properly. They even have an escape plan in the event a fire occurs. Jada's family also stores various supplies such as flashlights and a first-aid kit in case of emergencies.

The safety practices Jada and her family take to prevent something bad from happening are known as **precautions**. Jada and her family take precautions to remain safe in their home. In this lesson, you will learn about simple safety precautions you and your family can take to protect yourselves from unsafe situations in the home.

iStock.com/Wicki58

Figure 12.1 Activities and situations you encounter every day can cause falls. *What fall hazards are present in this photo?*

Fall Prevention

Most falls people experience are likely to happen at home while doing regular daily activities (**Figure 12.1**). Some falls may be a result of hazards in the environment. Other falls may occur because of a person's physical or medical condition. A simple fall can result in a broken bone, a head injury, or another medical condition.

The following steps can help reduce the risk of falls in your home:

- Clear the floors and stairs of clutter.
- Keep electrical cords and telephone lines away from walkways.
- Cover slippery floors with nonslip rugs.
- Install handrails for stairs, in bathtubs, and near toilets for older adults.
- Use stepstools or ladders to reach high cabinets or shelves.
- Ensure good lighting by replacing burned lightbulbs and using night-lights.
- Repair or replace worn carpet edges and seams.

Poisoning Prevention

Many chemicals in household products are poisonous and can be hazardous if used incorrectly. A **poisonous** substance can cause illness or death upon entering the body. Poisonous substances around the home may include cleaning products, garden and yard products, automotive chemicals, gasoline, and carbon monoxide. *Carbon monoxide* is a toxic, odorless, invisible gas produced during the burning of gasoline, natural gas, oil, kerosene, charcoal, and other fuels. Understanding which products are potentially hazardous can help prevent poisonings in the home (**Figure 12.2** on the next page).

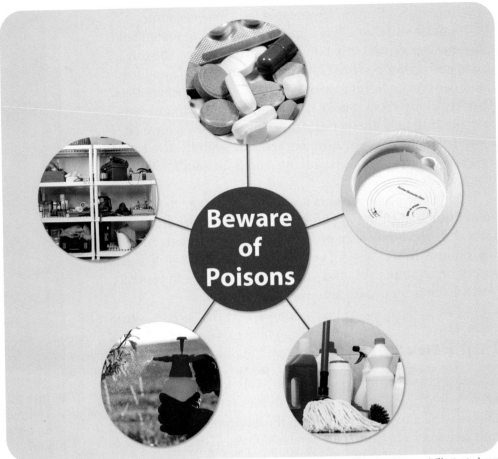

Clockwise, starting at top: Nataliya Turpitko/Shutterstock.com; Leena Robinson/Shutterstock.com; goir/Shutterstock.com; encierro/Shutterstock.com; Africa Studio/Shutterstock.com

To prevent illness or injury from potentially hazardous products, read and follow label directions for safe use. Store all chemicals in original containers in a locked area that children and pets cannot access. When using a chemical, wear protective equipment required by the label directions. This equipment might include goggles, gloves, or a mask. Dispose of chemicals as described on the label. If poisoning does occur, call the Poison Control Center (800-222-1222) immediately.

Weapons Safety

Your parent or guardian may keep a gun or other weapon in the home for hunting or personal safety. Weapons, however, can pose serious dangers to children who find them. Accidents involving weapons can seriously injure or kill someone.

To help prevent accidents in homes that contain weapons, adults should keep guns and other weapons locked in a safe place that is out of reach of children. When storing a gun, adults should remove the ammunition (bullets) and keep it in another locked place away from the gun.

If you happen to see a gun, leave the area without touching the gun. Find a trusted adult to tell right away. It is very important to report any weapon you find, as well as any person who was using or playing with the weapon. These safety rules apply whether you are inside your own home, in a friend's home, or at school (**Figure 12.3**).

What Should You Do If You See a Gun?

Leave the area without touching the gun ▶ **Tell** a trusted adult about the gun ▶ **Report** anyone who was using or playing with the gun

Fire Prevention and Safety

A fire in the home is a dangerous emergency that can be deadly. Fortunately, there are steps you can take to help prevent a fire. If a fire does break out, you and your family need to know how to exit the home safely. The following steps can help you prevent fires and remain safe if one does occur:

- **Step 1.** Know how a fire starts by understanding the fire triangle.
- **Step 2.** Conduct a fire safety inspection within the home and address any concerns.
- **Step 3.** Have an escape plan in place and practice it so everyone knows what to do.

Understand the Fire Triangle

Before you can learn how to prevent a fire, you must know how a fire starts. There are three elements needed to start a fire. These elements include fuel, heat, and oxygen. The **fire triangle**, also known as the *combustion triangle*, is a model that can help you remember these elements (**Figure 12.4**). When fuel, heat, and oxygen are present in the right amounts, a chemical reaction occurs that can start a fire.

The fuel in the fire triangle refers to the material that is burning. Materials that are easily set on fire are **flammable**. Examples of flammable materials include wood, oils, paper, fabrics, and some liquids. When a heat source, such as a match, comes in contact with flammable materials, a fire starts. To stay burning, the fire needs oxygen.

To **extinguish** (put out) the fire, you need to remove one of the elements in the fire triangle. For example, putting a fire blanket over the flames will remove the oxygen from the fire and cause the fire to stop burning. When firefighters use water to put out the fire, they are removing the heat, which cools down the fire and extinguishes it.

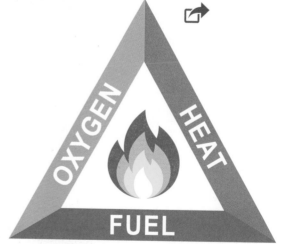

BALRedaan/Shutterstock.com

Figure 12.4 The fire triangle consists of the three elements needed to start a fire: fuel, heat, and oxygen. Knowing how to use a fire extinguisher can help you put out a fire.

Conduct a Fire Safety Inspection

Now that you understand how fires start, you can inspect your home to make sure the environment is safe and no fire hazards are present (**Figure 12.5**). Properly installed smoke detectors on every level of the home, including the attic and basement, can reduce your risk of injury and death from fire. Smoke detectors should be installed outside all sleeping areas, in the kitchen, and near the furnace. Test smoke detectors monthly and replace the batteries at least yearly to make sure they are working properly.

Everyone in the family who is old enough should know the location of fire extinguishers in the home and learn how to use them. Fire extinguishers can control small fires and prevent them from causing damage or injury. A fire extinguisher should be available near the furnace, in the garage, and in the kitchen for grease and cooking fires. There are different types of fire extinguishers, so be sure to check fire extinguisher labels carefully. Fire departments often provide training on how to properly use fire extinguishers.

Have an Escape Plan

A fire may break out in your home despite your best prevention efforts. This is why families should have an escape plan in place. An **escape plan** outlines safe routes and procedures for leaving the house in the event a fire occurs.

Because you never know where the fire may start, an escape plan should show two ways to exit each room of the home. If one exit becomes blocked or is too dangerous to pass through, you still have another way out.

Figure 12.5
Use this checklist to check for potential fire hazards in your home. Then, work with your parents or guardian to address any areas of concern that you note during your inspection.

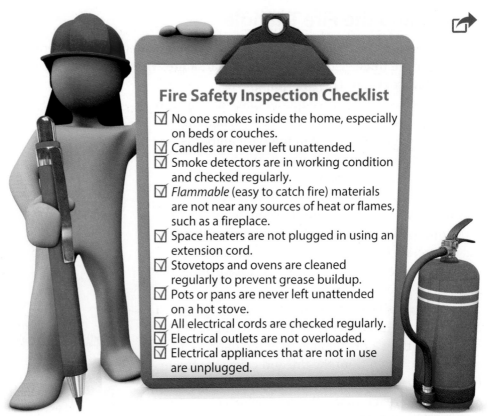

Fire Safety Inspection Checklist

☑ No one smokes inside the home, especially on beds or couches.
☑ Candles are never left unattended.
☑ Smoke detectors are in working condition and checked regularly.
☑ *Flammable* (easy to catch fire) materials are not near any sources of heat or flames, such as a fireplace.
☑ Space heaters are not plugged in using an extension cord.
☑ Stovetops and ovens are cleaned regularly to prevent grease buildup.
☑ Pots or pans are never left unattended on a hot stove.
☑ All electrical cords are checked regularly.
☑ Electrical outlets are not overloaded.
☑ Electrical appliances that are not in use are unplugged.

style-photography/Shutterstock.com

Part of the plan should identify who will assist babies and young children so everyone gets out safely. The plan should also include a place outside for all family members to meet once they are safely out of the home (**Figure 12.6**).

Once your family has an escape plan, arrange to practice the plan before a fire occurs. This way all family members can learn the plan without the stress of an actual emergency. The more you and your family practice, the more you increase your chances of everyone getting out of the home safely.

As your family practices the escape plan, make sure everyone knows how to respond to the sound of the smoke alarm. You may want to have a family member time how long it takes everyone to exit the home. As you leave the home, there are certain procedures you should follow to stay safe. These emergency evacuation procedures include the following:

- During a fire, feel doors with the back of your hand to determine if they are hot before opening them. If the door is hot, escape through a window.
- Check that all bedrooms in your home have a window that opens. Windows should be easy to unlock and open quickly.
- If you can, alert people in your home about the fire. Get out of the building and call 911 from a neighbor's home or a cell phone.
- Crawl near the floor to escape dangerous smoke, toxic fumes, and heat, which will rise toward the ceiling.
- If your clothing catches fire, stop, drop, and roll to put out the flames (**Figure 12.7**).
- Once outside, never reenter a burning building.

What Is in an Escape Plan?

EXIT

What are two ways to exit each room?

Who will assist babies and young children?

Where will we meet outside?

Figure 12.6 An escape plan should answer the three questions shown here. *Why is it important to identify two ways to exit each room?*

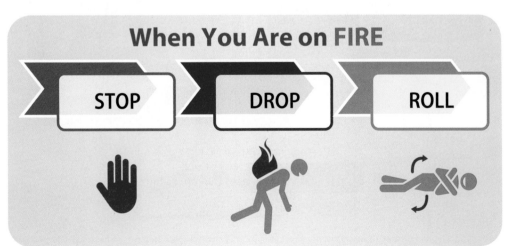

When You Are on FIRE

STOP → DROP → ROLL

Figure 12.7 Stop, drop, and roll if your clothing catches fire. Rolling will help smother the flames.

Emergency Preparedness

In addition to a house fire, families should prepare for other types of disasters. **Emergency preparedness** involves knowing how to respond to a specific type of emergency.

Depending on where you live, you may experience one or more types of natural disasters. **Natural disasters** are events or forces of nature that usually cause great damage. Examples of natural disasters may include tornadoes, floods, hurricanes, earthquakes, and winter storms (**Figure 12.8**). Other emergencies may include power failure, landslide, wildfire, and terrorism. With some simple preparation and the appropriate supplies, you and your family can be ready to deal with natural disasters and other emergencies.

Most emergencies you might experience include similar problems, such as exposure to the elements, loss of power, lack of sanitation, and lack of access to food or water. Planning for these problems is part of *emergency preparation*. In emergencies, people also need to communicate and receive emergency information. Doing so improves your chances of staying safe during a disaster.

Figure 12.8
Natural disasters can cause emergency situations and result in injuries, loss of power, exposure to the weather, and lack of food or water. *What natural disasters pose a risk to your community?*

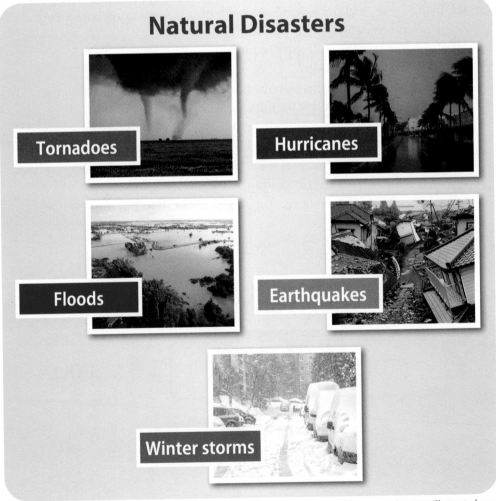

Natural Disasters

Tornadoes

Hurricanes

Floods

Earthquakes

Winter storms

Top row: Eugene R Thieszen/Shutterstock.com, Miami2you/Shutterstock.com; Middle row: wachira tasee/Shutterstock.com; austinding/Shutterstock.com; Bottom: Tainar/Shutterstock.com

Are You Prepared?

Tornadoes
- Take shelter in a safe, interior room with no windows on the lowest level of your home or below ground.
- Do not open windows.
- If outdoors, take cover in a vehicle or seek shelter in the nearest building.
- Do not hide under a bridge or overpass. You are safer in a low, flat area.

Hurricanes
- Build and store an emergency kit that can sustain you and your family for 3-5 days.
- Have an emergency plan in the case of evacuations.
- As a storm approaches, promptly follow instructions from public safety officials.

Winter Storms
- Stock up on food and water before the storm begins.
- Make sure you have a fully stocked first-aid kit.
- Stay indoors.

Earthquakes
- Practice "Drop, Cover, and Hold On."
- Stay indoors until the shaking stops.
- Cover your head.
- If outdoors, stay away from buildings, tall trees, and power lines.
- Move around as little as possible. Most earthquake injuries are from people moving around or falling.

Floods
- Move immediately to or stay on higher ground.
- Evacuate if directed.
- Avoid walking or driving through flood waters.

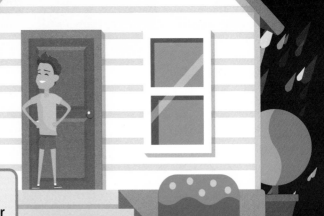

Keeping emergency supplies on hand can help you stay safe during many kinds of emergencies (**Figure 12.9**). Store emergency supplies in an easily accessible area of your home or car, and make sure everyone in your family knows where to find them.

After assembling emergency supplies, write an emergency plan. Different emergencies require different actions. Regardless of the type of emergency, an emergency plan should answer the following questions:

- Where will you take shelter during this emergency? For example, plan to go to a basement or a sturdy inner room, such as a bathroom, during a tornado. If you live in an area affected by hurricanes, know evacuation routes and shelters.
- How will you communicate with your family? Do you know how to reach a parent or guardian at work? Can you designate a contact person who lives outside of the area to relay information to all family members? How and where will you meet if family members are separated?
- Whom will you contact for emergency assistance, and how will you contact them? For example, know how to contact the police, fire department, and paramedics in an emergency.
- What supplies and equipment will you need to get through the emergency? Where will the supplies be located? What do you need to do to make sure these supplies are available?
- How will you learn when the danger has passed?

Figure 12.9
Emergency supplies may include a multi-tool or pocketknife, flashlights, masks, lanterns, matches, a first-aid kit, candles, nonperishable food, bottled water, a battery-powered radio, batteries, and blankets. *What other supplies could be helpful in an emergency?*

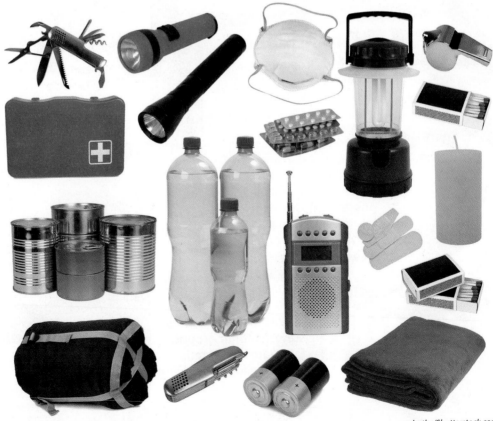

photka/Shutterstock.com

Safety When Home Alone

A major milestone occurs in a child's life when his or her parents or guardian decides that the child is responsible enough to stay home alone for a short period of time. Some cities and states have laws indicating that children cannot be legally left home alone until they are at least 11 years old. Laws vary from state to state, however, and some responsible children may be able to stay home alone for short periods at an earlier age.

BUILDING Your Skills

Planning for an Emergency

Dangerous weather or a house fire can cause an emergency quickly and unexpectedly. Having an emergency plan can help minimize the chaos and panic that accompany emergency situations and increase the chance of survival. An effective emergency plan should do the following:

- Identify a dangerous situation.
- List the needed emergency supplies and where they are located.
- Provide a detailed plan for responding to the emergency. The plan should answer questions such as the following: Where will you take shelter? With whom will you communicate (for example, family, friends, and emergency services)? How will you communicate? How will you know when the emergency has ended?

Write Your Family's Emergency Plan

Complete the first few steps of this activity with members of your family. After creating an emergency plan, share it with a partner, give feedback, and present it to the class. To create a family emergency plan, use the following steps:

1. With your family, consider the likelihood of the following dangerous situations: floods, tornadoes, hurricanes, winter storms, power failures, landslides, house fires, wildfires, earthquakes, and terrorist attacks. Choose two situations.

2. Refer to the information in this lesson and work with your family to create emergency plans for the two situations. Illustrate the emergency plans with pictures of emergency supplies and plan details.

3. Bring your emergency plan to class and share it with a partner. Your partner should also share his or her emergency plan. Exchange feedback and make changes or additions to your plans as needed.

4. Present your plans to the class.

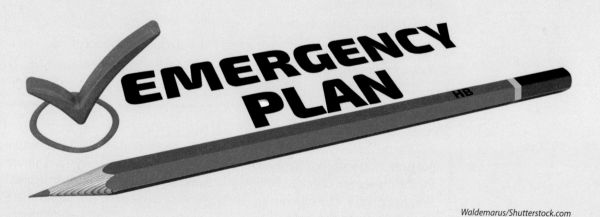

Waldemarus/Shutterstock.com

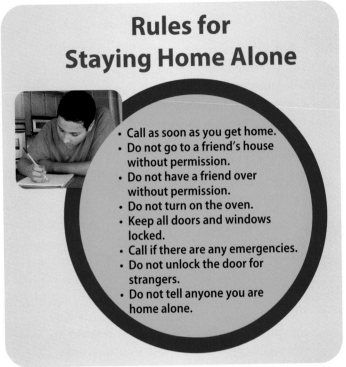

Rules for Staying Home Alone

- Call as soon as you get home.
- Do not go to a friend's house without permission.
- Do not have a friend over without permission.
- Do not turn on the oven.
- Keep all doors and windows locked.
- Call if there are any emergencies.
- Do not unlock the door for strangers.
- Do not tell anyone you are home alone.

Rob Marmion/Shutterstock.com

Figure 12.10 Some examples of rules for staying home alone are shown here. Marco's parents set these rules to keep Marco safe.

Your parents or guardian will probably set rules for you to follow when staying home alone (**Figure 12.10**). It is important that you follow these rules. The rules your parents or guardian set are meant to keep you safe and to prevent accidents from occurring. If you are staying home alone after school, your parent or guardian may expect you to call and check in as soon as you safely arrive home. Other rules may involve whether you can leave to go to a friend's house or whether you can have friends come over to visit. There may also be rules about whether you can do any cooking.

When you stay home alone, you need to know about fire safety, emergency preparedness, and first aid. You also need to know whom you can call if you need help. Other precautions you can take when staying home alone include making sure that all doors and windows are locked. Never unlock the door for strangers, including delivery people. Do not tell anyone on the phone or on public websites (including social media), that you are home alone. Instead, say that your parent or guardian is home, but is busy. You will learn about other safety precautions in the next lesson.

Lesson 12.1 Review

1. Safety practices that you use to prevent something bad from happening are called _____.
2. Which of the following is a fall risk?
   - **A.** Good lighting.
   - **B.** Electrical cords.
   - **C.** Handrails.
   - **D.** Dry floor.
3. What should you do if a poisoning occurs?
4. **True or false.** When you are home alone, you should unlock the door for delivery people.
5. **Critical thinking.** Name one natural disaster that is a hazard in your area of the country and then identify two emergency supplies you should have to respond to this disaster.

Hands-On Activity

For this activity, sit down with your family and discuss the fire-prevention measures you and your family members already take. As a family, read aloud the fire inspection checklist in Figure 12.5 and review the family escape plan. Take five photos illustrating your family's fire-prevention measures and share your photos with the class.

Staying Safe in the Community and Online

Learning Outcomes

After studying this lesson, you will be able to

- **describe** safety precautions you can take to stay safe at school.
- **give examples** of ways you can stay safe in public places.
- **demonstrate** how to protect your privacy and safety online.
- **explain** precautions you can take to stay safe on the road.
- **identify** ways to stay safe while participating in outdoor activities.

Key Terms ☛

strangers people whom you do not know

identity theft stealing and using someone's personal identifying information, often for financial gain

hackers people who illegally access data in your computer

pedestrians people walking, running, or bicycling along a road

Graphic Organizer ☛

A Safe Day

In a table like the one below, list your activities for each day. Include activities like going to school, spending time on social media, and swimming. As you read this lesson, identify the risks associated with your daily activities. List precautions pertaining to each activity.

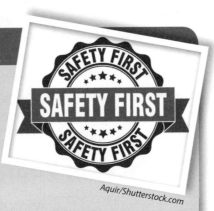

Aquir/Shutterstock.com

Day	Activities	Precautions
Monday	School Video-call with Beverley	Follow P.E. rules Ask permission to share our photo online
Tuesday		
Wednesday		
Thursday		
Friday		
Saturday		
Sunday		

Although your community is likely a safe place, it may also contain potential dangers. You may face hazards in familiar places, such as your school, or in unfamiliar public places. When doing outdoor activities, you need to know how to keep yourself safe. Being part of an online community also has risks you need to be aware of so you can protect yourself (**Figure 12.11**).

Remember in the first lesson how Jada's family takes precautions against emergencies. Jada extends these precautions into her community as well. She always wears her helmet when riding her bike and she watches for vehicles when crossing any street. Jada also spends a lot of time online. She uses the security and privacy settings on all of her profiles and she does not talk online to people she does not know.

When you encounter hazards within your community, you need to know how to respond. Luckily, in this lesson you will learn about certain precautions you can take to stay safe.

Staying Safe at School

Your school may feel like a very safe place, and it probably is safe most of the time. There are times, however, when you might encounter hazards, or dangers, at your school. Someone may try to start a fight with you. Another student may bring a weapon into the school. You may experience an injury during sports practice or physical education (P.E.) class.

Figure 12.11
It is important to get out of the house and engage in your community at school, in public, outdoors, and online. Keep in mind, however, that all of these settings have certain dangers. To keep yourself safe, you should know about these dangers and act safely.

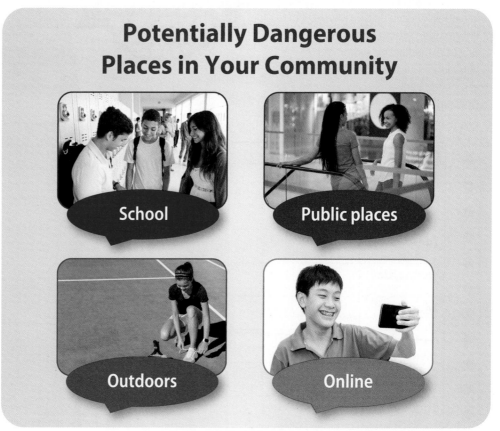

Potentially Dangerous Places in Your Community

School

Public places

Outdoors

Online

Top left to right: Monkey Business Images/Shutterstock.com; Mangostar/Shutterstock.com;
Bottom left to right: Maridav/Shutterstock.com; Studio concept/Shutterstock.com

Schools have safety rules and procedures in place to protect you from school-related hazards. You have a responsibility to follow these safety rules and procedures whenever you are on school property. You also have a responsibility to alert school staff to unsafe conditions and emergencies that may exist, such as the presence of weapons. If you are uncomfortable about anything you see at school or during extracurricular activities, tell a teacher, counselor, dean, or school security officer (**Figure 12.12**). By alerting the appropriate staff to potential risks, you may be able to reduce the risk of an accident or injury occurring.

During sporting events and P.E. classes, follow rules to help protect your safety and the safety of other students. To reduce the risk of sports-related injuries, use safety equipment, such as helmets and kneepads, whenever necessary. Always be respectful of your fellow students and use gym equipment appropriately.

School personnel and parents can also play a role in keeping schools safe. Principals and school administrators set the rules you should follow at school. Teachers and parents can reinforce these rules. Ultimately, however, you are responsible for keeping yourself and others safe at school.

Staying Safe in Public Places

As you get older, you may enjoy spending time with your friends in public places rather than staying at home. Your parents may drop you off at the mall or the park to hang out with your friends. These are examples of public places, which include anywhere that is not your home or a friend's home. Spending time outside and in public places like the mall can be fun, but dangers also exist.

When you are in public places, you are often around people you do not know. These people are **strangers**. Someone who is a stranger could be a danger to you. The rules in **Figure 12.13** can help you stay safe in public places.

iStock.com/asiseeit

Figure 12.12
If you encounter a dangerous or uncomfortable situation at school, be sure to tell a trusted adult at the school. These adults have the responsibility to act on situations that put students at risk. *Should you tell trusted adults at school about unsafe situations during extracurricular activities? Why or why not?*

Staying Safe in Public Places
- Tell your parents or guardian where you are going, how you will get there, and when you will be home.
- Take identification and only enough money for your needs. Carry a charged cell phone to call for a ride or help if needed.
- Travel in well-lit areas and with other people whenever possible.
- If you do not know someone, do not go anywhere with the person or accept money or gifts from him or her.
- If a stranger makes you or your friends uncomfortable, get away from the person and go tell a trusted adult right away.
- If a thief confronts you and wants your purse or phone, hand the items over without fighting.

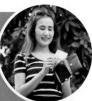
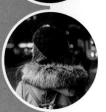
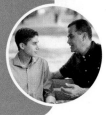

Figure 12.13
In public places, you will encounter many different types of people, including strangers who may be dangerous. It is important to take precautions to protect yourself before going out in public.

Top to bottom: iStock.com/Jillwt; iStock.com/finwal; iStock.com/Aldo Murillo

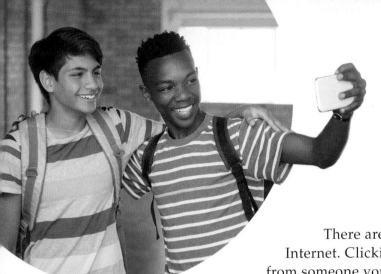

iStock.com/Wavebreakmedia

Figure 12.14 📤
Just because a friend takes a picture with you does not mean he or she wants that picture posted online. Be sure to ask friends before sharing their pictures. Also, keep in mind that pictures can help others identify your location. *Why should you be careful about sharing pictures that identify your location?*

Staying Safe on the Internet

Spending time on the Internet can be lots of fun. You can look up almost any information online. You can keep in touch with friends or talk to new people. You can play games, listen to music, or watch videos.

There are risks, however, to spending time on the Internet. Clicking on a certain website or opening an e-mail from someone you do not know can lead to getting a virus on your computer, smartphone, or tablet. Sharing your passwords or too much personal information can enable someone to commit identity theft. **Identity theft** is the stealing and using of someone's personal identifying information, often for financial gain. Identity theft happens when someone uses information about you without your permission. A person who gains access to personal information about you, such as your birthdate, address, or Social Security number, can open a credit card or buy a phone in your name. You could then be legally required to pay those bills.

To protect your privacy and safety online, use the following guidelines:

- Never give your personal information to anyone without getting your parents' or guardian's permission. If you want to give out another person's personal information, ask that person's permission first. Be aware that sharing photos and personal information, such as your name, home address, or school's name, can identify you and let others, including people you do not know, find you (**Figure 12.14**).

- If you would like to upload photos or videos of yourself or anyone else to social media, or share personal information like your name or birthday, make sure that your profiles are set to "Private" to ensure that only people you approve can see this content. Do not upload photos or videos of another person to social media without that person's permission.

- Do not share any inappropriate photos, messages, or videos online, even in what might seem like a private message. Photos or messages sent to one person are easily saved and shared with other people. Taking, sending, or forwarding inappropriate content can result in consequences at school, humiliation with peers, and even trouble with the law. If you receive an inappropriate message or if someone shares an inappropriate photo of you, tell a trusted adult.

- Do not get together in person with someone you met online without your parents' or guardian's permission. Even if you have permission, have your parent or guardian accompany you and meet your online friend in a brightly lit, public location.

- If someone says something or sends you a picture that makes you feel uncomfortable, threatened, or unsafe, leave the conversation and ask a trusted adult for help. Block this person from contacting you in the future. If you are being bullied online, you should also tell a trusted adult (**Figure 12.15**). (You will learn more about cyberbullying in Chapter 15.)

- Do not post anything online that you would not want everyone to see. Although it seems like you can keep certain photos or messages private, there is always the risk that someone will leak this information. Even if you delete the original post, the Internet will keep a copy of what you shared. If you want something kept private, do not post it online.

- Keep all of your passwords private. Do not share them even with friends. Do not open or click on links in suspicious e-mail or text messages. These may contain viruses that can harm your computer, smartphone, or tablet or allow hackers into your personal accounts. **Hackers** are people who illegally access data in your computer.

- Only download applications and software from reliable, credible websites. If you are unsure whether a website is credible, ask a trusted adult. Sometimes downloads can carry viruses that can infect your computer, smartphone, or tablet.

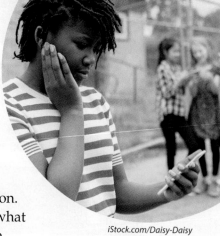

iStock.com/Daisy-Daisy

Figure 12.15
Being bullied online is just as serious as being bullied in person. Always tell a trusted adult if someone is bullying you or making you uncomfortable online.

CASE STUDY

Brianna's Online Relationship

Now that Brianna is 13 years old, her parents are giving her more and more freedom. This year, Brianna's parents let her begin using social media, and according to Brianna, life is *finally* getting interesting. Brianna likes to send her friends funny pictures and follow their lives.

Last week, Brianna met a boy named James on social media. James lives in her city and messages her throughout the day. Brianna likes James and feels like he really understands her. She has told her friends about James, but has not told them everything because James wants to keep their relationship private. Brianna wants to tell her parents, but they seem too busy.

Brianna decides that she will tell her parents after she meets James. After all, she may not like him when they meet. Brianna makes plans to meet James in her neighborhood park and tells her friend Addison about her plan. Addison tells Brianna that James sounds a bit weird, but Addison does not really know James. Brianna feels nervous just thinking about the day she and James will meet.

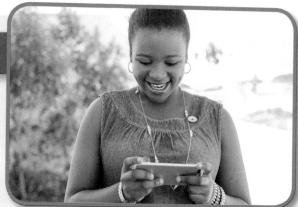

John Warner/Shutterstock.com

Thinking Critically

1. List the benefits and risks of Brianna meeting James in person.

2. If you were Addison, what advice would you give Brianna about talking with and meeting James? What should you do to help keep Brianna safe?

3. Are there any red flags that Brianna and James may not have a healthy relationship? If so, what are they?

4. If Brianna is going to meet James in person, how should she do so safely?

Staying Safe on Social Media

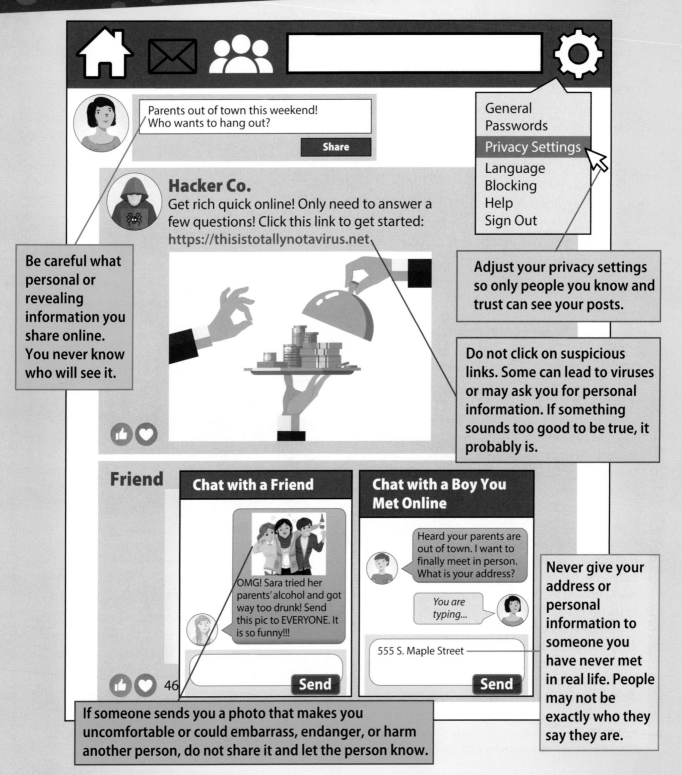

Be careful what personal or revealing information you share online. You never know who will see it.

Hacker Co.
Get rich quick online! Only need to answer a few questions! Click this link to get started: https://thisistotallynotavirus.net

General
Passwords
Privacy Settings
Language
Blocking
Help
Sign Out

Adjust your privacy settings so only people you know and trust can see your posts.

Do not click on suspicious links. Some can lead to viruses or may ask you for personal information. If something sounds too good to be true, it probably is.

Parents out of town this weekend! Who wants to hang out?
Share

Friend

Chat with a Friend

OMG! Sara tried her parents' alcohol and got way too drunk! Send this pic to EVERYONE. It is so funny!!!

Send

46

Chat with a Boy You Met Online

Heard your parents are out of town. I want to finally meet in person. What is your address?

You are typing...

555 S. Maple Street

Send

Never give your address or personal information to someone you have never met in real life. People may not be exactly who they say they are.

If someone sends you a photo that makes you uncomfortable or could embarrass, endanger, or harm another person, do not share it and let the person know.

Staying Safe on the Road

Did you know that motor vehicle crashes are the leading cause of death among young people? In fact, motor vehicle crashes account for about 70 percent of the deaths associated with unintentional injuries. Many of these deaths occur among pedestrians involved in the accidents. **Pedestrians** are people walking, running, or bicycling along a road (Figure 12.16). To protect yourself and remain safe, there are certain precautions you can take while walking, running, and riding your bike. You can also take precautions to stay safe while riding in a car or school bus.

Pedestrian Walking and Running Safety

Pedestrians have the "right of way" when walking or running along a road. This is the legal right of a pedestrian to move before a vehicle moves, in certain situations. For example, if a vehicle comes to a stop sign, and pedestrians are waiting at the corner, the pedestrians have the right of way to cross the street first. The driver must respect that right and allow the pedestrians to cross.

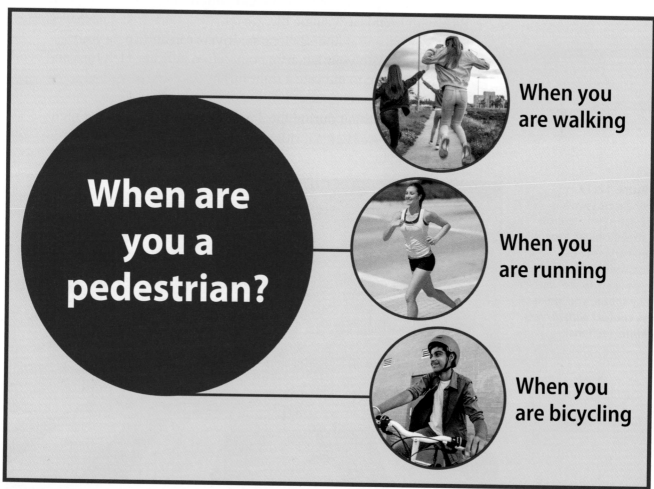

When are you a pedestrian?

When you are walking

When you are running

When you are bicycling

Top to bottom: iStock.com/golero; iStock.com/nycshooter; iStock.com/kate_sept200

Figure 12.16 Whenever you go for a walk or a bike ride in your community, you are a pedestrian.

As a pedestrian, however, you also have responsibilities. These include the following:

- Always assume that drivers cannot see you. Drivers should stop for pedestrians, but that does not mean they always do.
- Walk where drivers would expect you to walk, which is on sidewalks, if possible.
- If walking on the road, always walk facing traffic, not in the direction of traffic.
- Make eye contact with drivers at intersections to make sure they see you.
- Obey all traffic signals and use specific crosswalk areas at intersections, where it is safer for you to cross (**Figure 12.17**).
- If you must walk at night, wear bright clothing or carry a flashlight.

Pedestrian Bicycling Safety

Riding a bicycle is an inexpensive form of transportation and a fun way to get physical activity. Use the following guidelines to remain safe while riding a bicycle:

- Always wear a properly fitted helmet.
- Know and obey all traffic rules.
- Ride on the right side of the road and with traffic, never facing traffic.
- Ride with friends in a single file.
- Signal your turns at intersections so drivers can anticipate your movements. With your left arm, point left to indicate a left turn and bend your forearm up to indicate a right turn.
- Always stop at red lights.
- Wear bright clothing during the day and reflective clothing at night.
- Use front and rear lights if riding after dark.

Figure 12.17
Using a crosswalk is the safest way to cross a street. Drivers expect pedestrians to use crosswalks and are more likely to see you. *Why should you make eye contact with drivers at intersections?*

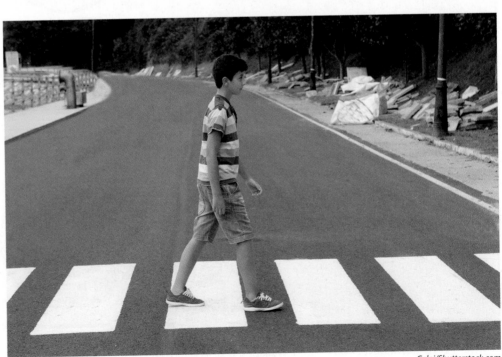

Gelpi/Shutterstock.com

Vehicle Safety

Although you cannot drive yet, you probably spend a lot of time as a passenger in a car. The most important safety precaution you can take in the car is to wear a seatbelt (**Figure 12.18**).

Another safety precaution you can take is to avoid distracting the driver. Any distractions in the car, such as noisy passengers, can make it difficult for the driver to concentrate. This increases the risk of an accident. Texting while driving is another distraction that can cause accidents. If you see the driver texting, ask him or her to stop and pay attention to the road to stay safe.

Perhaps you take the school bus each morning and afternoon. If so, there are specific precautions to take when riding the school bus. Only get on the bus once the bus has stopped and the driver says it is safe. Always listen to instructions from the bus driver. Wear your seatbelt if the bus has seatbelts, and avoid distracting the bus driver.

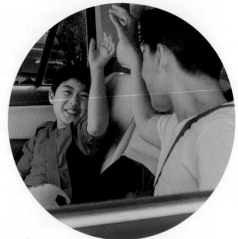

iStock.com/SolStock

Figure 12.18
When used properly, seatbelts can reduce crash-related injuries and deaths by half.

Staying Safe in the Water

In the summer when the weather is hot, people often like to engage in water-related activities such as swimming in the local public swimming pool. Sailing, water-skiing, and spending time at the beach are also fun water-related activities (**Figure 12.19**). This means that water-related accidents can occur.

Figure 12.19
Water-related activities are fun, but pose safety risks.

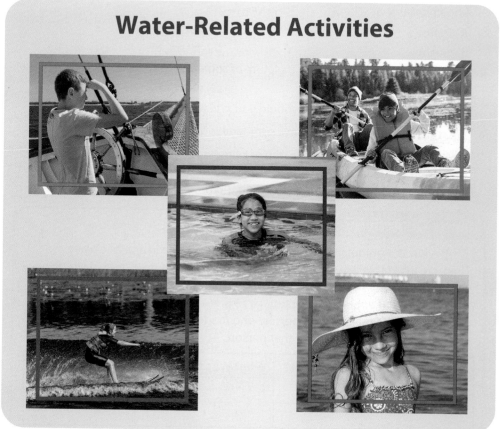

Water-Related Activities

Clockwise from top: iStock.com/arkanex; Monkey Business Images/Shutterstock.com; Katya Shut/Shutterstock.com; ChrisVanLennepPhoto/Shutterstock.com; photonewman/Shutterstock.com

You can prevent accidents by learning and practicing the following water-safety tips:

- Never leave children alone in or near water of any kind—including ponds, lakes, swimming pools, and beaches—even when lifeguards are on duty. This also means never leaving children alone in bathtubs. A drowning can occur in minutes when someone stops paying attention or turns away.
- Teach children how to swim.
- Wear a life jacket when swimming.
- Never swim alone or in unsupervised areas.
- Do not dive in shallow water.
- Check the weather and avoid getting in the water if a storm is coming.
- Do not swim in a river after a storm because currents may be stronger.
- Check the water temperature and avoid swimming in really cold water.
- If you believe someone is drowning, call 911 or tell someone to call right away. The American Red Cross recommends that untrained rescuers avoid entering the water. Drowning people panic and will push you down. They can even drown you. Instead, rescuers should reach for the drowning person or throw him or her a flotation device, life jacket, rope, or any object that will float.

Lesson 12.2 Review

1. You should tell your _____ if you see something that is unsafe or that makes you uncomfortable at school.

   A. friend
   B. sibling
   C. teacher
   D. classmates

2. **True or false.** It is okay to post a picture of someone to social media without that person's permission.

3. When you are riding a bicycle, should you ride with traffic or facing traffic?

4. What should you do if you believe someone is drowning?

5. **Critical thinking.** Give some examples of messages, photos, or videos that would be inappropriate to share online. Explain why these examples are inappropriate and discuss the consequences of sharing them.

Hands-On Activity

Review the guidelines in this lesson for staying safe in a public place. Then, create a table like the one shown below. Over the next three days, pay attention to safety mistakes you and others make in public. Identify at least five safety mistakes and list precautions to prevent them. Share your findings with the class. If you know the person who made the mistake, share the recommended precaution with that person.

Safety Mistake	Who Did It?	What Was the Risk?	Precautions

Knowing Basic First Aid

Learning Outcomes

After studying this lesson, you will be able to

- **identify** items needed in a first-aid kit.
- **describe** the three steps you should take after determining that you can help someone in need of first aid.
- **summarize** ways to provide treatment for various common injuries.
- **explain** what a medical emergency is and how you should respond to one.

Key Terms ☞

first aid treatment given in the first moments of an accident or injury—usually before medical professionals arrive on the scene

first-aid kit container that includes the supplies needed to treat most types of minor injuries

bystander someone who is at an event or incident, but is not directly involved

standard precautions infection control practices that apply when giving first aid to any person under any circumstances

anaphylaxis allergic response in which fluid fills the lungs and air passages narrow, restricting breathing

medical emergency urgent, life-threatening situation

cardiopulmonary resuscitation (CPR) emergency procedure that uses chest compressions to restore heartbeat; may also involve mouth-to-mouth breathing

automated external defibrillator (AED) rescue device that delivers a controlled, precise shock to the heart

Graphic Organizer ☞

First-Aid Guidelines

Skim this lesson and find pictures or illustrations online of the injuries and emergencies described. Arrange the images like in the example below. As you read this lesson, take notes underneath each image.

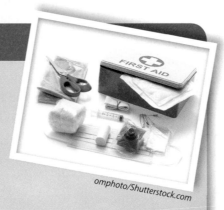

omphoto/Shutterstock.com

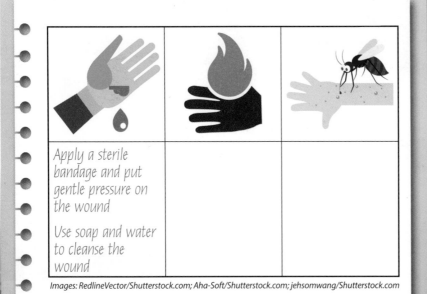

Apply a sterile bandage and put gentle pressure on the wound		
Use soap and water to cleanse the wound		

Images: RedlineVector/Shutterstock.com; Aha-Soft/Shutterstock.com; jehsomwang/Shutterstock.com

Despite your best efforts to stay safe, accidents and injuries can still occur. When an accident or injury does happen, a person with first-aid skills can help the injured person. **First aid** is treatment given in the first moments of an accident or injury—usually before medical professionals arrive on the scene. First-aid skills allow you to provide treatment for a person while you are waiting for emergency medical professionals to arrive. The first aid given right after an injury occurs could actually help save a life.

Jada from the previous lessons takes first aid very seriously. She knows that professional organizations such as the American Red Cross and the American Heart Association offer basic first-aid certification classes. She takes these classes to learn how to administer first aid properly (**Figure 12.20**). Even before she took one of these classes, there were basic first-aid skills she had learned. This lesson will discuss some of those basic first-aid skills.

Keep a First-Aid Kit on Hand

To administer first aid, you need to have certain supplies on hand. A **first-aid kit** contains the supplies needed to treat many types of minor injuries. You can put together your own kit or purchase a ready-made kit at most drugstores or from the American Red Cross. The American Red Cross suggests keeping a first-aid kit in the home and in vehicles. When spending time doing outdoor activities, such as hiking or camping, it is a good idea to carry a first-aid kit with you. Keep the first-aid kit out of reach and out of sight of small children, and away from family pets. **Figure 12.21** shows supplies often included in a first-aid kit.

Figure 12.20
First-aid classes teach students the basics of delivering first aid. These basics usually include wound care, the five-and-five method for choking, and cardiopulmonary resuscitation (CPR).

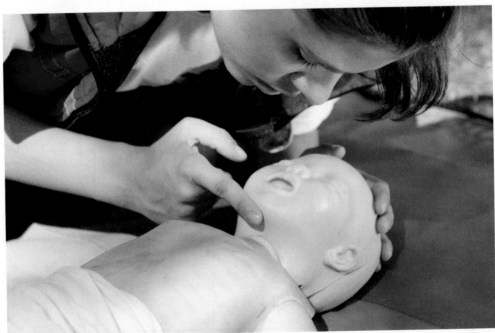

First-Aid Kit Essentials

Figure 12.21
A first-aid kit should include the essentials shown here and any additional supplies you need for yourself or your family. *Where in your home should you keep a first-aid kit?*

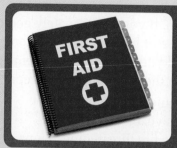

Resources

- First-aid manual
- Phone numbers for the Poison Control Center, family doctor, police department, and fire department

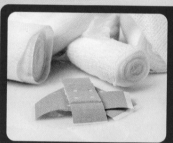

Supplies for Treating Wounds

- Gauze pads and assorted bandages
- Medical tape
- Cotton balls and cotton swabs
- Scissors

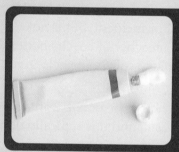

Supplies for Preventing Infections

- Antibiotic ointment (cream)
- Antiseptic wipes
- Hand sanitizer
- Disposable latex or synthetic gloves

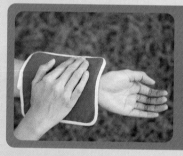

Supplies for Treating Various Injuries

- Elastic wrap
- Instant cold packs
- Tweezers
- Sterile eyedrops or eyewash solution
- Oral thermometer (nonmercury/nonglass)

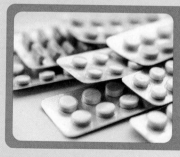

Over-the-Counter Medications

- Pain relievers such as ibuprofen or acetaminophen
- Hydrocortisone cream
- Antihistamine medications

Top to bottom: Mega Pixel/Shutterstock.com; Henrik Dolle/Shutterstock.com; nokwalai/Shutterstock.com; Chutima Chaochaiya/Shutterstock.com; DedMityay/Shutterstock.com

Determine If You Can Help

Before administering any first aid, you need to check the scene to determine if you can safely help the injured person. If you cannot safely get to the person because of his or her location, or because of hazardous conditions, call 911 immediately. Do not risk becoming injured yourself. If you can remain safe and provide help, then stay calm and perform the following three steps:

1. **Check the victim's condition.** Do a very quick assessment of the situation. Is the person awake and responsive, or is the person unresponsive? Does the injury appear to be life threatening? Signs of a life-threatening injury may include the following:

   - severe bleeding
   - labored or no breathing
   - *shock*—a life-threatening condition in which the vital organs do not receive enough blood and oxygen
   - unconsciousness—the person passes out and cannot be awakened

   Do not move the person unless you must leave a dangerous situation.

2. **Call 911.** As soon as you can, call 911 or your local emergency services, or tell a bystander to call while you perform first aid (**Figure 12.22**). A **bystander** is someone who is at an event or incident, but is not directly involved. If you are at school, tell a teacher or coach about the emergency. These trusted adults may be able to call 911 or help give first aid while you call 911.

3. **Give first aid.** If possible, ask the victim whether he or she wants to receive first aid. This is called *obtaining consent*, and it is typically done for legal reasons. Under the law, you may perform first aid without consent if the victim is unconscious or if the victim is a child.

Figure 12.22 Communicating appropriately with 911 dispatchers can help them understand the situation better and get aid to you faster. *What should you tell a 911 dispatcher about the victim?*

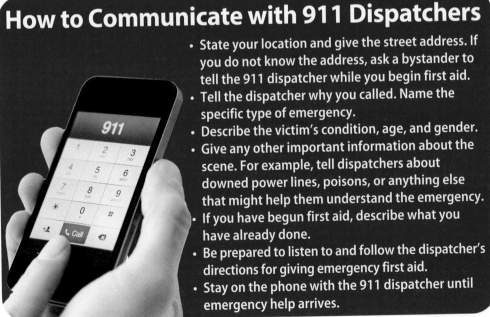

How to Communicate with 911 Dispatchers

- State your location and give the street address. If you do not know the address, ask a bystander to tell the 911 dispatcher while you begin first aid.
- Tell the dispatcher why you called. Name the specific type of emergency.
- Describe the victim's condition, age, and gender.
- Give any other important information about the scene. For example, tell dispatchers about downed power lines, poisons, or anything else that might help them understand the emergency.
- If you have begun first aid, describe what you have already done.
- Be prepared to listen to and follow the dispatcher's directions for giving emergency first aid.
- Stay on the phone with the 911 dispatcher until emergency help arrives.

iStock.com/TommL

Provide Treatment for Common Injuries

By learning and practicing first-aid skills, you will be able to remain calm, think clearly, and act rationally during the stress of helping an injured person. By studying Chapter 7, you have already learned how to treat sprains and know what to do if a bone becomes fractured or dislocated. In the following sections, you will learn about standard precautions and basic first-aid treatments for some other common injuries.

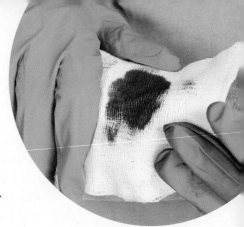

Joe Belanger/Shutterstock.com

Figure 12.23
Bodily fluids such as blood can contain pathogens, which are microorganisms that cause disease.

Standard Precautions

A person giving first aid is often at risk for infection. This is because first-aid procedures often bring a person in contact with bodily fluids (**Figure 12.23**). People who perform first aid should follow standard precautions to protect themselves from infection.

Standard precautions are infection control practices based on universal precautions. Standard precautions were developed by the Centers for Disease Control and Prevention (CDC). Like universal precautions, standard precautions protect from bloodborne infections, such as HIV. Standard precautions, however, also protect from infections transmitted by respiratory droplets.

Standard precautions apply when giving first aid to any person under any circumstances. An example of a standard precaution is to wear protective gloves when there is a risk of contact with blood or bodily fluids that may contain blood. Washing hands with soap and water after giving first aid is another example of a standard precaution.

Cuts, Scrapes, and Puncture Wounds

A person who gets a minor cut or scrape often does not need to receive professional medical treatment. Some bleeding may occur, but the bleeding will often stop on its own. If the bleeding does not stop, follow the steps in **Figure 12.24**.

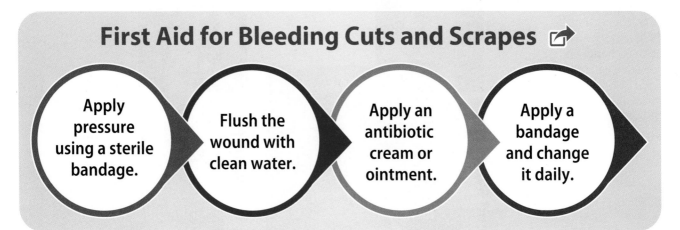

First Aid for Bleeding Cuts and Scrapes ↗

Apply pressure using a sterile bandage. → Flush the wound with clean water. → Apply an antibiotic cream or ointment. → Apply a bandage and change it daily.

Figure 12.24   These steps can help you care for a cut or scrape that does not stop bleeding. If the cut is deep enough that it does not easily press together, however, you should seek medical attention. You should also seek medical attention if the bleeding does not stop after these steps. ***Should you apply antibiotic ointment before or after flushing the wound?***

Deep cuts usually require stitches provided by a medical professional. A cut is considered deep if the edges of the cut do not easily press together by applying gentle pressure. Some cuts are so deep that they expose the dermis or fatty tissue. People with deep cuts, scrapes, and puncture wounds may also need a vaccine to prevent *tetanus*, a serious bacterial infection associated with these types of wounds.

Puncture wounds—such as penetrating wounds from nails, thorns, or other sharp objects—usually bleed a small amount and appear to close up right away. The object that caused the puncture, however, can introduce bacteria deep into the tissues where it can become trapped and cause infections.

Severe Bleeding

The most important part of first aid for severe bleeding is the application of pressure to the wound. Other steps slow blood loss by careful positioning of the body. Following are steps to take when providing first aid to someone experiencing severe bleeding:

1. Apply pressure to wound or squeeze arterial pressure points.
2. Position the wound higher than the heart.
3. Dress the wound.
4. Keep the victim calm.
5. Treat the victim for shock (**Figure 12.25**).

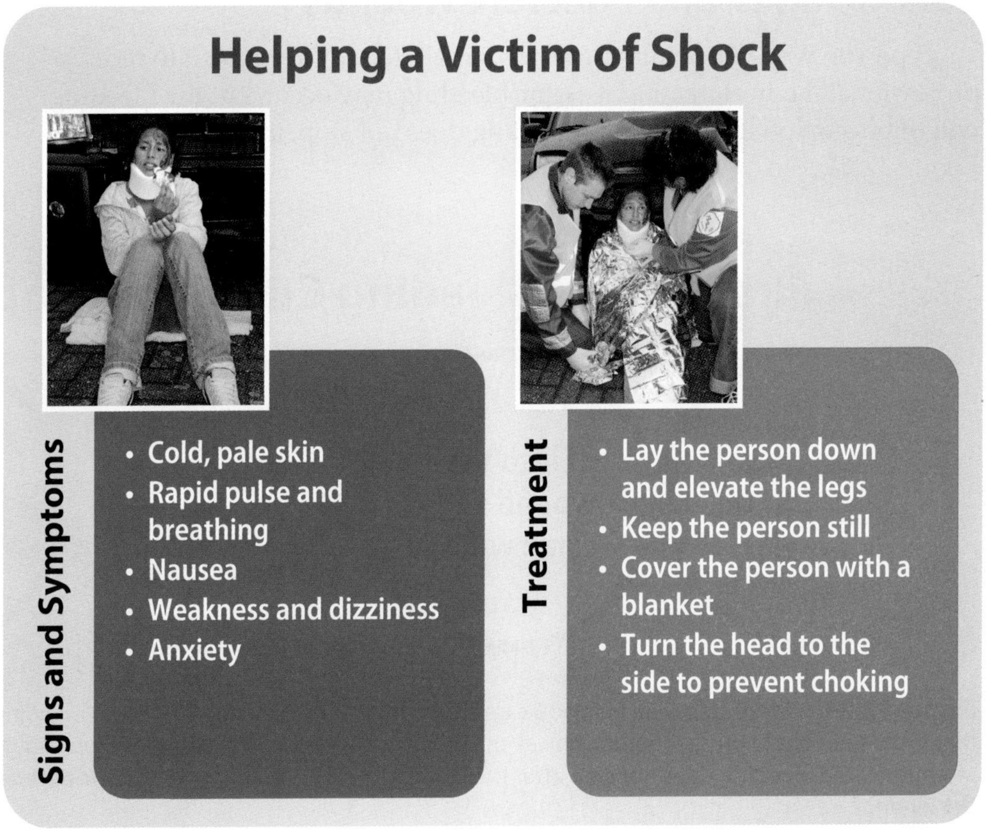

Figure 12.25
Shock is a life-threatening condition that can result from severe bleeding or trauma. Treating a victim for shock can help the victim stay calm and warm.

Helping a Victim of Shock

Signs and Symptoms
- Cold, pale skin
- Rapid pulse and breathing
- Nausea
- Weakness and dizziness
- Anxiety

Treatment
- Lay the person down and elevate the legs
- Keep the person still
- Cover the person with a blanket
- Turn the head to the side to prevent choking

Anneka/Shutterstock.com

Bites and Stings

People may experience bites from domestic animals, such as dogs or cats. Wild animals, such as raccoons, may also bite people. Common biting and stinging insects include bees, wasps, mosquitoes, and some types of ants.

All animal bites require a doctor's attention. Bite wounds that break or puncture the skin carry the risk of infection. The most dangerous of these infections is the *rabies virus*, which infects the nerves, brain, and spinal cord. The disease is fatal if not treated immediately, before the virus reaches the brain and symptoms begin. Until you see the doctor, you can wash the bite wound with soap and water, cover it with a clean bandage, and elevate the affected area.

Mild reactions to insect bites are common, and often include swelling or itching at the site of the bite. Treat these reactions with cool cloths, calamine lotion, or over-the-counter hydrocortisone cream if the itching is severe.

More severe reactions are typically associated with stings from bees, wasps, yellow jackets, and fire ants. The venom of these insects triggers pain, swelling, and redness. Some people develop *hives*—a swollen, fluid-filled skin rash (**Figure 12.26**). Treat these stings with cold compresses or ice, pain reliever, elevation of the stung area, and rest. Use tweezers to remove any stingers stuck in the skin, wash the area, and apply hydrocortisone cream to relieve swelling and itching.

A few people experience an extremely severe, life-threatening allergic reaction to insect stings, called *anaphylaxis*. **Anaphylaxis** is an allergic response in which fluid fills the lungs and air passages narrow, restricting breathing. This type of reaction requires immediate emergency care or the person could die. People who have such severe allergic reactions often have medication such as the EpiPen® (**Figure 12.27**).

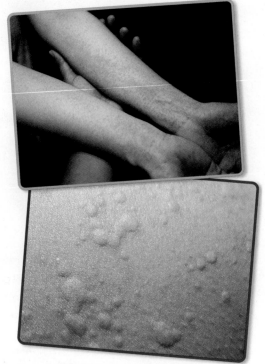

Chatchai.wa/Shutterstock.com; lpen/Shutterstock.com

Figure 12.26 Hives can break out in response to venom or as an allergic reaction.

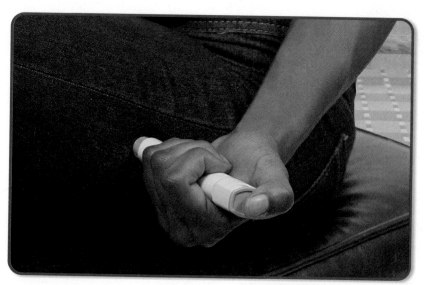

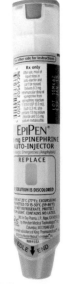

Figure 12.27 EpiPens® help treat allergic reactions and are important in emergency situations. *Why is anaphylaxis an emergency situation?*

EpiPen® in use: Bob Byron/Shutterstock.com; Goodheart-Willcox Publisher

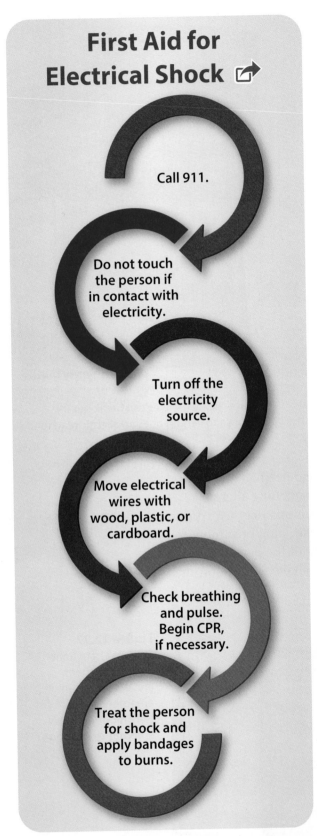

First Aid for Electrical Shock

Call 911.

Do not touch the person if in contact with electricity.

Turn off the electricity source.

Move electrical wires with wood, plastic, or cardboard.

Check breathing and pulse. Begin CPR, if necessary.

Treat the person for shock and apply bandages to burns.

Figure 12.28 These steps can help you care for someone after electrical shock. *When should you call 911 if someone experiences electrical shock?*

Electrical Shock

Electrical shock occurs when the body is in contact with an electrical current. The shock could come from fallen power lines, which is a hazard that accompanies severe weather. People also get shocked when standing in flooded streets or basements. In these situations, the water conducts electricity to the body from electrical wires, outlets, or downed power lines.

An electrical shock may cause burns, internal injuries, cardiac arrest, or even death. Use the first-aid steps in **Figure 12.28** to treat electrical shock while waiting for emergency medical help to arrive.

Burns

Burns are common injuries that range from mild to life threatening. Causes of a burn can include exposure to any source of heat and energy such as fire, burning or smoldering materials, steam, hot surfaces, or extremely hot gases and liquids. Chemicals, electric current, and the sun are also possible causes of burns.

All types of burns can seriously damage skin. Dangerous complications from burns include infection, shock, dehydration, pain, and immobility of the affected body part. First aid is essential for all burns. To give appropriate first aid, you need to identify whether the burn is a first-, second-, or third-degree burn (**Figure 12.29**).

Respond to Medical Emergencies

A **medical emergency** is an urgent, life-threatening situation. Examples of medical emergencies may include a person choking or requiring cardiopulmonary resuscitation (CPR). When medical emergencies such as these arise, call 911 right away. Then, follow emergency first-aid treatment. These medical emergencies require an immediate first-aid response. Otherwise, the victim could die.

Types of Burns

First-Degree Burns 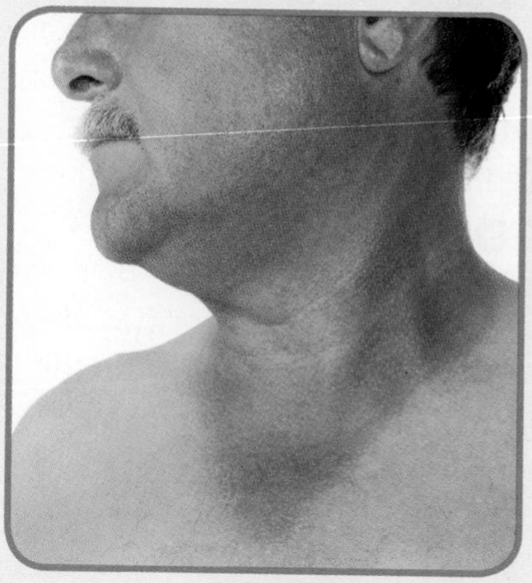	Second-Degree Burns 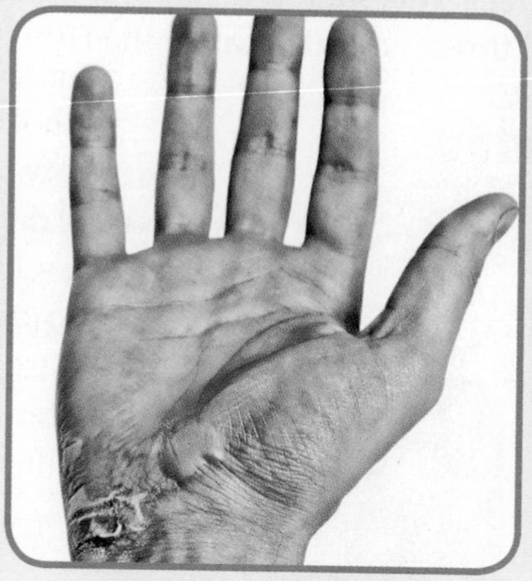	Third-Degree Burns 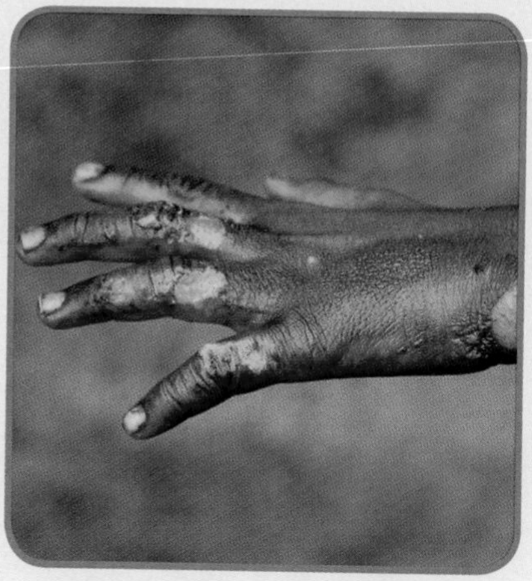

Suzanne Tucker/Shutterstock.com

nikkytok/Shutterstock.com

Naiyyer/Shutterstock.com

First-Degree Burns
- Damage only the outer layer of skin
- Cause redness, swelling, and pain
- Treatment includes holding the burned skin under cool water, covering the burn, and taking pain reliever

Second-Degree Burns
- Affect the second layer of skin
- Cause blisters, redness, and swelling
- Burns affecting less than 3 inches can be treated like first-degree burns
- Burns affecting more than 3 inches are medical emergencies and should be treated like third-degree burns

Third-Degree Burns
- Affect all layers of skin and underlying tissue
- Are medical emergencies
- To respond, call 911 immediately and check the person's breathing and pulse, elevate the burned body part, cover the burn, and treat for shock until help arrives
- Do not remove burned clothing or immerse burns in cool water

Figure 12.29 First-, second-, and third-degree burns require different care.

Choking

Choking is a medical emergency in which an object, such as a piece of food, blocks the airway. This means that a choking person cannot breathe. Choking may occur when people chew their food too quickly or when young children put objects in their mouths.

Many people instinctively grab their throats with both hands when they are choking, but there are other signs as well. If you know these signs, you can quickly recognize when someone is choking and provide help. The following are signs of choking:

- inability to breathe normally
- inability to talk or make noise
- inability to cough or expel air forcefully
- blue skin, lips, and nails

The American Red Cross recommends the *five-and-five method* for helping a person who is choking (**Figure 12.30**). This method involves a series of back blows alternating with abdominal thrusts, which force air out of the choking person's lungs. This should help push the stuck object out of the airway. Abdominal thrusts are also called the *Heimlich maneuver*.

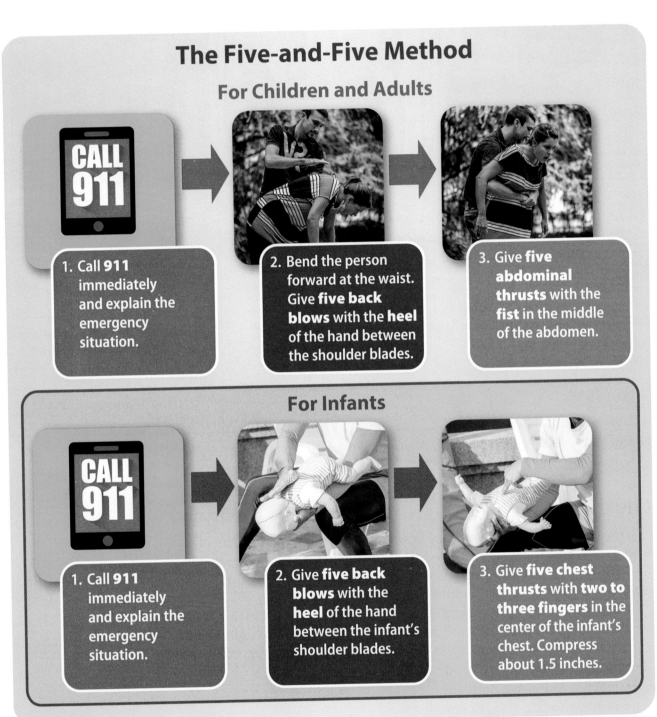

The Five-and-Five Method

For Children and Adults

CALL 911

1. Call **911** immediately and explain the emergency situation.

2. Bend the person forward at the waist. Give **five back blows** with the **heel** of the hand between the shoulder blades.

3. Give **five abdominal thrusts** with the **fist** in the middle of the abdomen.

For Infants

CALL 911

1. Call **911** immediately and explain the emergency situation.

2. Give **five back blows** with the **heel** of the hand between the infant's shoulder blades.

3. Give **five chest thrusts** with **two to three fingers** in the center of the infant's chest. Compress about 1.5 inches.

Top left to right: gst/Shutterstock.com; pixelaway/Shutterstock.com; Bottom: narin phapnam/Shutterstock.com

Figure 12.30 If a person is choking, use the five-and-five method to give aid. After you call 911, perform steps 2 and 3 and continue them, if necessary, until help arrives. *Which part of your hand should you use to give back blows?*

Cardiopulmonary Resuscitation (CPR)

Your heart beats and your lungs breathe in air to keep you alive. Medical emergencies in which a person's heart stops beating or the victim stops breathing are life threatening. In these situations, first aid and medical care must begin as soon as possible to restore breathing and heartbeat. The main technique used to restore breathing and heartbeat is cardiopulmonary resuscitation, or *CPR*.

Cardiopulmonary resuscitation (CPR) is an emergency procedure that uses chest compressions to restore heartbeat. Full CPR involves mouth-to-mouth breathing, or *rescue breaths*. *Hands-Only*™ *CPR* only involves chest compressions. The American Heart Association (AHA) and the American Red Cross recommend that rescuers use Hands-Only™ CPR for adults in most cases. This is because rescue breaths require training, and almost anyone can perform chest compressions without training. Hands-Only™ CPR delivers blood circulation to victims who suffer cardiac arrest. Cardiac arrest describes a condition in which the heart stops beating. **Figure 12.31** describes how to perform Hands-Only™ CPR for adults.

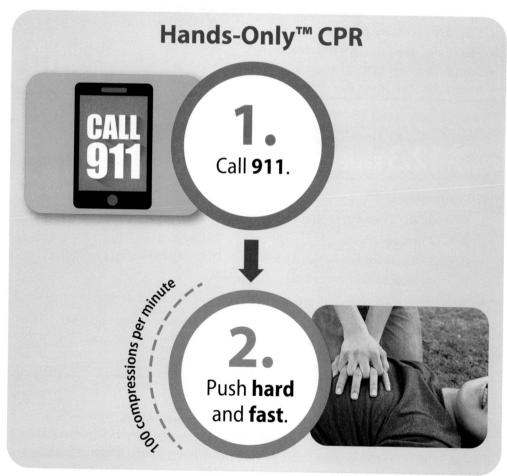

Hands-Only™ CPR

CALL 911

1.
Call **911**.

100 compressions per minute

2.
Push **hard** and **fast**.

Figure 12.31
Hands-Only™ CPR is used to help adults who are not breathing and whose hearts are not beating. To deliver 100 compressions per minute, you can push to the song "Stayin' Alive" by the Bee Gees.

Top to bottom: gst/Shutterstock.com; Sajee Rod/Shutterstock.com

Do not slow down or stop performing CPR until emergency services arrive, or an **automated external defibrillator (AED)** is available and ready for use. This rescue device delivers a controlled, precise shock to the heart and gives automated instructions (**Figure 12.32**). An AED can restore a person's heartbeat after cardiac arrest. Hands-Only™ CPR and AEDs can be used even by people with little or no training.

Figure 12.32
An AED can be found in most public places. AEDs usually give automated instructions for their use. The steps for using an AED are listed here.

Using an Automated External Defibrillator (AED)

After calling 911, adults trained in using an AED can use the following steps if an infant, child, or adult is unconscious and not breathing. If the person is an infant or child, obtain parental consent, if possible.

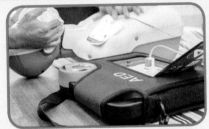
narin phapnam/Shutterstock.com

- **Step 1.** Turn on AED.
- **Step 2.** Wipe bare chest dry.
- **Step 3.** Attach pads.
  For infants and children younger than eight years of age: Use *pediatric pads* if possible. Place one pad on the upper-right side of the chest and the other pad on the left side of the chest. If the pads touch (because the infant or child is too small), place one pad in the middle of the chest and one pad in the middle of the back.
  For children older than eight years of age and adults: Place one pad on the upper-right side of the chest and the other pad on the left side of the chest.
- **Step 4.** If necessary, plug in connector.
- **Step 5.** Tell everyone to stand clear.
- **Step 6.** Deliver shock.
- **Step 7.** Perform about five cycles of CPR.

Lesson 12.3 Review

1. Where should a first-aid kit be kept?
2. Which of the following should you do first when you see that someone is injured?
   - **A.** Give first aid.
   - **B.** Check the scene to make sure it is safe.
   - **C.** Call 911.
   - **D.** Check the victim's condition.
3. Which type of burn affects all layers of the skin?
4. **True or false.** The five-and-five method is used to help people who are choking.
5. **Critical thinking.** Give one example of a time you were injured and received first aid. How does the first aid you received compare to the first-aid guidelines in this chapter?

Hands-On Activity

In groups of three, choose one of the injuries or emergencies discussed in this lesson and create a real-life scenario involving it to role-play. One group member should be the victim, and the other two group members should respond correctly to the situation. Use items and materials in the classroom as first-aid equipment and write scripts for each group member. Perform the role-play for the class.

Summary

Lesson 12.1 Staying Safe in the Home

- Falls are dangerous accidents. You can help prevent them by reducing fall risks in the environment.
- Poisonous substances include chemicals found outside and in the home, gasoline, and carbon monoxide. If a poisoning occurs, you should call the Poison Control Center (800-222-1222) immediately.
- All weapons should be kept in a locked safe place away from children. Ammunition should be stored separate from a gun.
- Knowing how fires start and being aware of fire hazards can help prevent fires. Your family should establish an escape plan in case a fire does occur.
- Emergency preparedness involves knowing how to respond to an emergency. You can prepare by gathering emergency supplies and making an emergency plan.
- Always follow your parents' or guardian's rules when home alone and do not open the door for strangers.

Lesson 12.2 Staying Safe in the Community and Online

- Always follow safety rules at school. If you encounter unsafe or uncomfortable situations at school, you should tell a teacher, counselor, dean, or school security officer.
- In public places, pay attention to your surroundings and never go with or accept gifts from strangers.
- To remain safe online, never share your personal information or inappropriate content. Ask a person's permission before sharing a photo or video of him or her. If you receive a message or photo online that makes you uncomfortable, tell a trusted adult.
- When walking on the road, walk facing traffic. When riding a bike on the road, ride with traffic. When in a vehicle, never distract the driver.
- To be safe in the water, swim only in supervised areas and do not dive in shallow water. If you see someone drowning, call 911 immediately.

Lesson 12.3 Knowing Basic First Aid

- A first-aid kit contains supplies for treating minor injuries and should be kept in the home and in vehicles.
- Before giving first aid, always check the scene and check the victim's condition. If the injury is life threatening, call 911. Follow standard precautions to prevent infection.
- Cuts, scrapes, and puncture wounds need to be cleaned and bandaged. If wounds are deep, they may require professional treatment or a vaccine. If wounds bleed severely, applying pressure and dressing the wound can help. All animal bites and some insect bites and stings require a doctor's attention. Electrical shock is always an emergency, as are third-degree burns. First- and second-degree burns that are minor can be treated with cool water, bandages, and pain reliever.
- You can use the five-and-five method when a person is choking. If a person's heart and breathing stop, performing Hands-Only™ CPR can save the person's life.

Check Your Knowledge ⤴

Record your answers to each of the following questions on a separate sheet of paper.

1. If you find a gun in an unsecured area, what should you do?
2. **True or false.** During a fire, you should crawl on the floor to escape dangerous smoke.
3. What is emergency preparedness?
4. **True or false.** If a thief demands your phone, you should refuse to hand it over.
5. **True or false.** Deleting a photo online completely removes it from the Internet.
6. How should you signal that you are turning left when riding a bike?
   A. Bending your forearm.
   B. Pointing left.
   C. Waving your left arm.
   D. Veering left.
7. Which of the following is a good water-safety practice?
   A. Diving in shallow water.
   B. Wearing a life jacket.
   C. Swimming in an unsupervised area.
   D. Swimming in cold water.
8. Which of the following is a sign of a life-threatening injury?
   A. Shock.
   B. Minor bleeding.
   C. Swelling.
   D. Bruising.
9. How should you provide first aid to someone experiencing severe bleeding?
10. What happens during anaphylaxis?
11. When should you call 911 if you find someone who is *not* breathing and whose heart is *not* beating?
    A. After giving five abdominal thrusts.
    B. Immediately.
    C. After giving one cycle of CPR.
    D. After finding an AED.
12. What is Hands-Only™ CPR?

Use Your Vocabulary ⤴

anaphylaxis	escape plan	medical emergency
automated external defibrillator (AED)	extinguish	natural disasters
	fire triangle	pedestrians
bystander	first aid	poisonous
cardiopulmonary resuscitation (CPR)	first-aid kit	precautions
	flammable	standard precautions
emergency preparedness	hackers	strangers
	identity theft	

13. Draw a cartoon for one of the terms above. Use the cartoon to express the meaning of the term. Share your cartoon with the class. Explain how the cartoon shows the meaning of the term.
14. Working in pairs, locate a small image online that visually describes or explains each of the terms above. Create flash cards by writing each term on a note card. Then, paste the image that describes or explains the term on the opposite side. Pair up with another team and review each other's flash cards.

Think Critically

15. **Cause and effect.** What are the consequences of being unprepared for an emergency? Give examples of consequences for at least three emergency situations.

16. **Draw conclusions.** In a small group, discuss whether a middle school student is old enough and responsible enough to stay home alone.

17. **Compare and contrast.** Compare and contrast a safe and unsafe school environment. Give examples of how the school environment can positively or negatively impact a middle-school student's physical and emotional health.

18. **Identify.** What are some ways that middle school students can have fun on social media without putting their personal safety at risk?

DEVELOP Your Skills

19. **Access information and communication skills.** Talk with your parents or guardian about expectations and rules for staying home alone. Create a *Guide to Staying Home Alone* that lists at least five safety rules for staying home alone. Use pictures to illustrate each rule and display your guide in a visible place in your home.

20. **Refusal and communication skills.** Imagine that you are flirting with someone you met on social media. You have been talking with this person for three weeks and enjoy your online relationship. One day, this person sends the following message to you. How would you respond to protect your personal safety?

> You are amazing. Tell me more about yourself. I want to know everything about you.

21. **Decision-making skills.** Imagine that you are seeing a movie with two friends. The movie is not very good, so you and your friends decide to walk to the mall 10 blocks away. To save time, your friends plan to walk behind buildings and on side streets. When you reach the lobby of the theater, however, you notice how dark it is outside. List the pros and cons of each decision you could make and write a summary describing the pros and cons, safety risks and precautions, and what you would do.

22. **Advocacy.** Think about the personal safety threats that endanger students in your school and create a personal safety flyer highlighting one safety threat. Include at least five safety tips related to the threat and at least two pictures to support your content. If you have permission, hang your flyer on a wall in your school.

23. **Teamwork and technology skills.** As a class, divide into three groups and assign each group one lesson in this chapter. In your group, review your assigned lesson and outline the most important ideas and safety practices. Ask your teacher if you are not sure which ideas and safety practices are most important. Create a multimedia presentation that uses text, photos and illustrations, and music to summarize the main points in the lesson. Present your interactive summary to the class and answer any questions your classmates have.

Chapter 13

Protecting Environmental Health

Lesson 13.1 Common Hazards in the Environment

Lesson 13.2 Pollution Prevention and Greener Living

Essential Question

How is your health influenced by the environment in which you live?

Video ↗

Access the Chapter 13 video to start thinking about chapter topics.

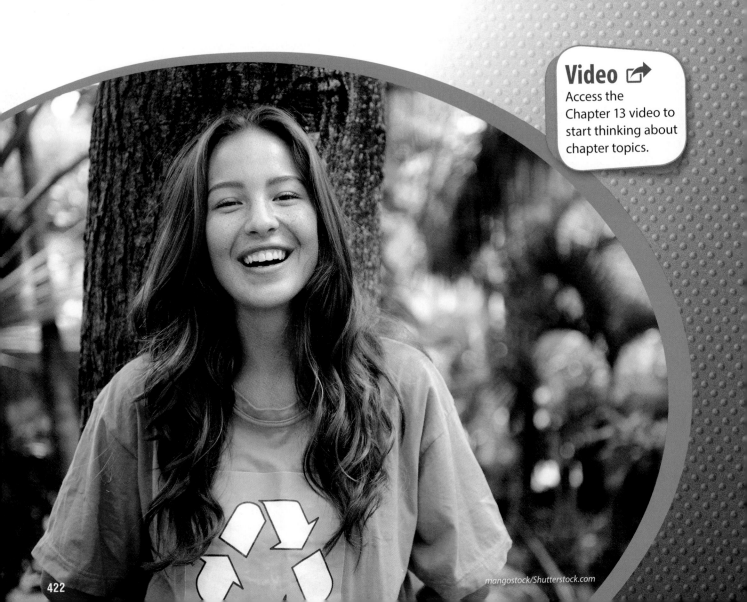

mangostock/Shutterstock.com

Reading Activity

Write the Learning Outcomes for this chapter on a piece of paper and then, beneath each outcome, rewrite it as a question. While reading the chapter, take notes about information relating to these outcomes. After reading, refer to your notes and write two or three sentences answering each outcome's question.

How Healthy Are You?

In this chapter, you will be learning about environmental health. Before you begin reading, take the following quiz to assess your current environmental health habits.

Healthy Choices	Yes	No
Do you know how to properly dispose of products that contain chemicals and pollutants?		
Do you know what to do if you or someone you know has been in contact with a harmful substance?		
Do you know what the symbols on packages of chemicals mean? Do you make sure to read these labels carefully before using or storing chemicals?		
Do you limit your exposure to high levels of noise, such as through headphones?		
Do you use a reusable bottle instead of disposable plastic bottles?		
Do you reduce the amount of energy you use by turning off the lights when you leave a room or by turning off the water while you brush your teeth?		
Do you recycle items made from paper, aluminum, glass, or plastic?		
Do you safely dispose of hazardous materials such as aerosol cans, batteries, or medical waste?		
Do you use energy-efficient, green, and biodegradable products as much as possible?		
Do you do your best to reuse materials or make green choices away from home and on the road, as well as in your home?		

Count your "Yes" and "No" responses. The more "Yes" responses you have, the more healthy environmental habits you exhibit. Now, take a closer look at the questions with which you responded "No." How can you make these healthy habits part of your daily life? Think about how implementing these ideas can help improve your overall health.

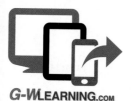

While studying this chapter, look for the activity icon to

- **practice** key terms with e-flash cards and matching activities.
- **reinforce** what you learn by completing graphic organizers, self-assessment quizzes, and review questions.
- **expand** knowledge with interactive activities and activities that extend learning.

www.g-wlearning.com/health/

Common Hazards in the Environment

Learning Outcomes

After studying this lesson, you will be able to

- **describe** different types of air pollution and their effects.
- **assess** causes of water pollution and ways to keep water safe.
- **identify** types of chemicals that are harmful to the environment.
- **explain** how to handle chemicals safely.
- **recognize** the health dangers of noise pollution and how to avoid them.

Graphic Organizer 👉

Pollution Basics

Find or take photos that illustrate the following types of pollution: air pollution, water pollution, chemicals, and noise pollution. Under each photo, draw two circles labeled *Sources* and *Effects*. An example is shown below. As you read this lesson, identify the sources and effects of the different types of pollution. Write them next to the appropriate circles.

Bankolo5/Shutterstock.com

Left to right, top to bottom: cubicidea/Shutterstock.com; Mjosedesign/Shutterstock.com; Makc/Shutterstock.com; grmarc/Shutterstock.com

Ten-year-old Diego lives in a city with his family, and he has experienced more than a few hazards in his home environment. He can visibly see and smell the smog from cars. Even indoors, Diego experiences tobacco smoke and dust in many different locations. Diego has asthma and has had a hard time breathing lately, even when he is not having an asthma attack. To improve Diego's health and wellness, Diego's parents have started to discuss moving to an area with cleaner air and less pollution. Air pollution is one of a few hazards in your environment that will be covered in this lesson.

The Environment

When you think about health, you probably think about the actions you take to stay healthy. How and when you exercise, the food you eat, and how much sleep you get all have important effects on your health. Your health is also influenced by the environment in which you live, however.

Humans all live on planet Earth, and depend on the planet's resources to survive (Figure 13.1). You may not even think about what Earth provides, including the food you eat, the water you drink, and the air you breathe.

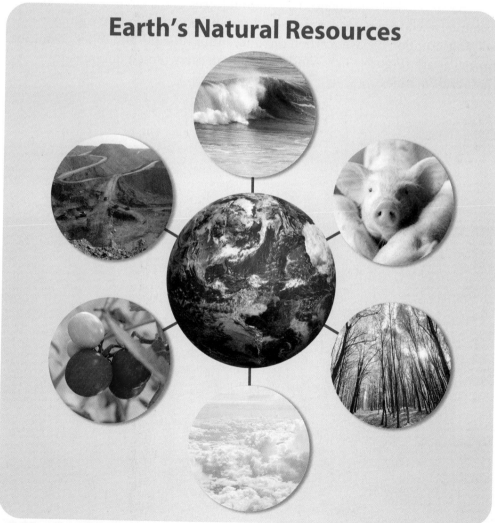

Earth's Natural Resources

Figure 13.1
Water, animals, trees, air, other plants, and fossil fuels are some examples of Earth's natural resources.

Unfortunately, people do not always treat their environment with the care it deserves. Human activities can harm the environment and affect people's health. This harm can lead to hazards like air pollution, water pollution, and chemicals.

The field of *environmental health* examines how factors in the natural environment, such as air, water, and soil, impact your health. Environmental factors also include spaces made by people, such as homes, apartments, schools, and offices.

Air Pollution

Humans survive by breathing in air. Air contains oxygen, which people need to survive. Air also contains other gases, including nitrogen, argon, and carbon dioxide. Sometimes, air contains other substances, known as **pollutants**, which contaminate the environment and can harm people.

Outdoor Air Pollution

The air outside is influenced by natural forces in the environment. For example, a wildfire releases smoke and carbon monoxide into the air. A volcanic eruption releases carbon dioxide, sulfur dioxide, and other chemicals, as well as ash (**Figure 13.2**). Wind currents can carry these pollutants for thousands of miles.

Figure 13.2
A volcanic eruption is one example of a natural cause of air pollution. When a volcano erupts, it releases pollutants into the air, and wind can carry these pollutants miles from the eruption. *What pollutants does a volcanic eruption release?*

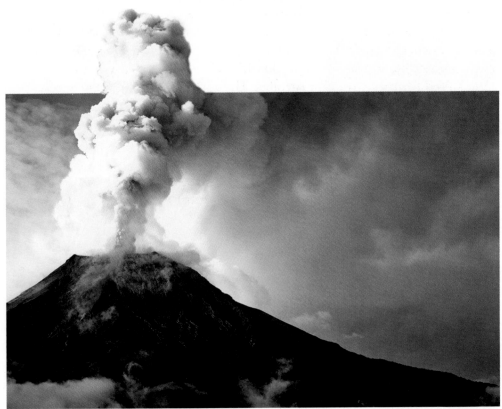

Kali Guerra/Shutterstock.com

The air outside is also affected by human activity. You might have seen pictures of smog hanging over a big city. **Smog** is a fog that has mixed with smoke and chemical fumes (**Figure 13.3**). Car exhaust is a major cause of smog in cities. The burning of coal, oil, and gas to power cars and produce electricity also pollutes the air. Even tractors on farms create dust clouds when plowing the fields.

When polluting gases are released into the air, they mix with water, oxygen, and other chemicals to form acids. These acids then fall to the ground, as rain, snow, hail, fog, or even dust. Any form of precipitation that includes particles containing acid is known as **acid rain**.

Another source of air pollution is *particulate matter*, which is made up of tiny particles and drops of liquid. These tiny particles and liquids that float in the air can include chemicals, metals, and dust. Some particulate matter is natural. One example is pollen from flowers and trees carried on the wind. Particulate matter can also be created by human actions, such as cooking on a grill or burning fuel in a power plant.

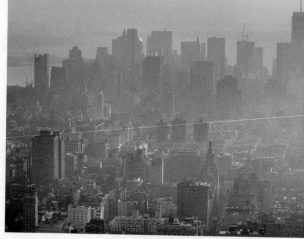

Venturelli Luca/Shutterstock.com

Figure 13.3 Smog sometimes hangs over densely populated areas such as cities. *What are the components of smog?*

Indoor Air Pollution

Indoor air can also contain pollutants. Indoor pollution can be caused by many different factors, including sources such as paint, tobacco smoke, cleaning products, pet dander, and dust (**Figure 13.4**).

Some of these pollutants can be seen or smelled. For example, you can see smoke from cigarettes and smell some cleaning products. Other types of pollutants, however, are so small and have no odor that you cannot see or smell them. For example, very tiny bugs, called *dust mites*, are one of the most common causes of indoor air pollution. Dust mites live in mattresses, upholstered furniture, rugs, or curtains. They survive by eating the tiny pieces of dead skin you flake off. These bugs are found in about 80 percent of the homes in the United States. Dust mites are not dangerous, but their bodies and waste matter can trigger allergic reactions and asthma in humans.

Sources of Indoor Air Pollution

Figure 13.4 Tobacco smoke, pet dander, and dust are three substances that can pollute the air indoors.

Left to right: Greentellect Studio/Shutterstock.com; bstecko/Shutterstock.com; narin phapnam/Shutterstock.com; February_Love/Shutterstock.com; Evg Zhul/Shutterstock.com; struvictory/Shutterstock.com

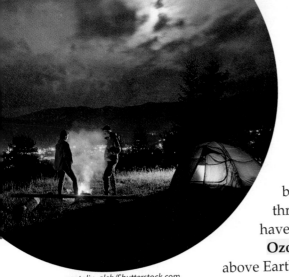

anatoliy_gleb/Shutterstock.com

Figure 13.5
Particulate matter, such as the particles found in smoke, can irritate the eyes, nose, and throat.

Effects of Air Pollution

Breathing in pollutants can create health problems. In some cases, it can cause very serious problems, such as cancer and heart disease. Air pollution can also make current health problems worse. For example, smog can make it very difficult for people with respiratory disease to breathe.

Particulate matter can get into people's lungs and bloodstream. Larger particles can irritate the eyes, nose, and throat. You have probably experienced this type of irritation if you have sat close to a charcoal grill or beside a campfire (**Figure 13.5**).

Ozone is a gas made up of oxygen that naturally exists high above Earth's atmosphere. It helps protect people from the damaging ultraviolet (UV) rays produced by the sun. Some kinds of air pollution caused by humans can damage this ozone layer, which increases the amount of UV rays reaching Earth. UV rays can cause skin cancer. Too much UV radiation may also damage plants, including crops grown for food. Ozone poses other dangers, too. Ozone close to the ground can cause respiratory problems and environmental harm. Ground-level ozone is usually caused by chemical reactions between different pollutants in the air.

Air pollution also has an effect on Earth's climate. Earth's atmosphere is made up of different gases, including nitrogen, oxygen, and carbon dioxide. These gases trap the energy produced by the sun, which warms Earth. As a result, Earth maintains a balanced and stable temperature over time.

When these gases build up in the atmosphere, however, they trap more heat near the surface of Earth. The effects of this buildup can change climates around the world. Many scientists have concluded that the buildup of gases released by burning fuels to produce energy has resulted in climate change. Climate change can lead to shifts in weather patterns. These changes can lead to more major disasters, such as hurricanes, heat waves, droughts, and flooding. Scientists also warn that rising temperatures will melt ice on Earth's surface. This melting ice can raise sea levels and threaten flooding in coastal areas (**Figure 13.6**).

Figure 13.6
The buildup of gases in Earth's atmosphere may lead to rising temperatures, which could melt ice on the planet's surface. *What are two potential consequences of ice on Earth's surface melting?*

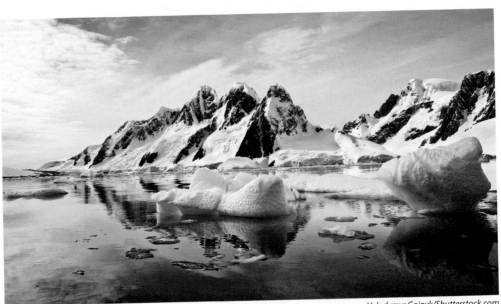

Volodymyr Goinyk/Shutterstock.com

Water Pollution

Humans need water to drink in order to survive. More than two-thirds of Earth's surface is covered by water, but most of this water is in the ocean. People cannot use salty ocean water for drinking. They need freshwater for drinking.

Only about three percent of the water on Earth is freshwater. Most of this freshwater is frozen in the polar ice caps and glaciers. This leaves only about one percent of the water on Earth available to use as drinking water. Usable sources of freshwater are found in lakes, rivers, and reservoirs. There is also freshwater inside Earth. These combined sources provide the freshwater needed for farms, homes, businesses, factories, and communities. Unfortunately, if this water becomes polluted, it is no longer safe for humans to drink.

A number of factors can pollute the water. Water can be polluted by human-made products, such as chemicals and pollutants, but also by natural disasters.

Human Causes of Water Pollution

The products that people use in their daily lives can end up in the water supply. When rain or melted snow is not absorbed on Earth's surface, it becomes runoff, travels over the ground, and picks up loose soil and pollutants (**Figure 13.7**). These pollutants can include the following:

- pesticides and fertilizers from lawns and fields
- oil, grease, and chemicals from cars, trucks, and other vehicles
- metals and chemicals from factories and construction sites

Runoff travels to bodies of water, such as ponds, lakes, streams, and rivers. People can then wash their food in, bathe in, or drink the water. Exposure to chemicals and pollutants through these activities can make people sick.

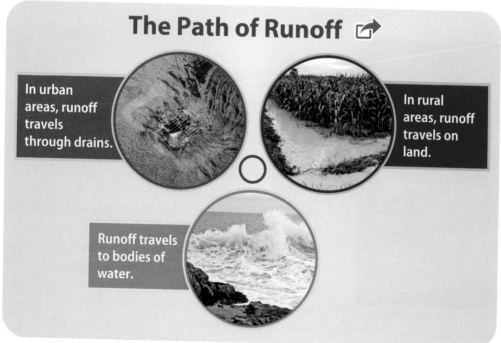

The Path of Runoff

In urban areas, runoff travels through drains.

In rural areas, runoff travels on land.

Runoff travels to bodies of water.

Figure 13.7
Rain or melted snow that is not absorbed on Earth's surface becomes runoff. In urban areas, runoff travels through drains. In rural areas, runoff travels on land. In both situations, runoff can pick up pollutants before reaching bodies of water.

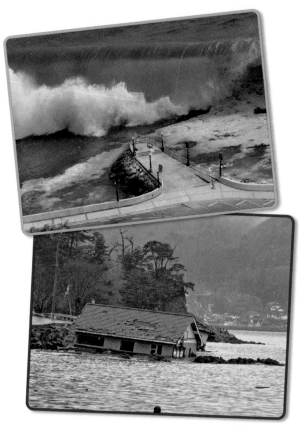

Christian Vinces/Shutterstock.com; mTaira/Shutterstock.com

Figure 13.8 Natural disasters can cause tsunamis, which may damage surrounding land and crops as well as people's property and homes.

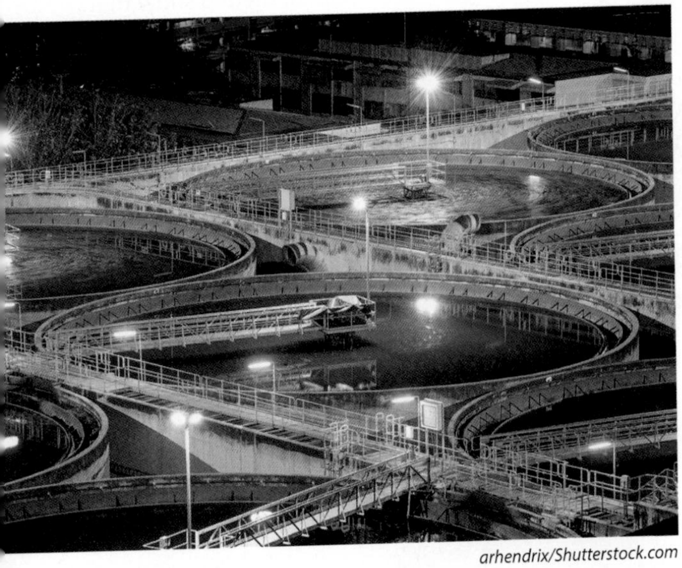

arhendrix/Shutterstock.com

Figure 13.9 A water treatment plant removes pollutants from water and cleans it before people drink it.

Water pollution can also occur when people do not properly dispose of products containing chemicals and pollutants. These products include paint cans, batteries, and medicines. There are special rules for disposing of these products to help prevent water pollution. Sometimes, however, people do not know these rules or do not follow them.

Natural Causes of Water Pollution

Major natural disasters, such as hurricanes, typhoons, and earthquakes, can cause water pollution. During hurricanes and floods, pollutants that are usually stored in landfills or other disposal areas are swept into waterways. Examples are raw sewage, fertilizers, chemicals, and oil. Earthquakes can trigger tsunamis, or tidal waves, which flood an area with salt water (**Figure 13.8**). This water can destroy farmland and crops.

Tiny organisms, such as bacteria, viruses, and parasites, can live in the water supply. Even though you cannot see these organisms, drinking water that contains them can make people sick. In the case of a disaster, the water supply of a whole town or area can be dirtied. In some cases, people can even die from drinking this water.

Water Treatment

People use water every day—to drink, to take a shower, and to wash clothes and dishes. This water comes from natural bodies of water, such as streams, ponds, and rivers.

Drinking water in the United States is treated in a water treatment plant. This process takes between 8 and 16 hours. The process involves removing pollutants from the water and cleaning the water before people use it and before it returns to the environment. All water people use goes through a treatment plant before it is used in homes, farms, or industries (**Figure 13.9**). This water is also tested to make sure it is safe to use. This process is designed to protect people from drinking polluted water that can cause diseases and other health problems.

Chemicals

Chemicals are substances that have specific properties or characteristics. Some chemicals are found in nature. For example, vitamin C (ascorbic acid) is a chemical naturally found in some fruits. Other chemicals are made by people. For example, aspirin (acetylsalicylic acid) is a chemical made by people from substances found in tree bark. People use chemicals every day, in many different ways. You are exposed to chemicals through items you eat and drink, but also through the air you breathe and even through the objects you touch.

Types of Chemicals

Many chemicals are safe for people to use, at least in reasonable amounts. Minerals, such as iron, are naturally occurring chemicals that your body needs to stay healthy. Some kinds of chemicals, however, are *toxic*, meaning they can have harmful effects (**Figure 13.10**). People can get sick from coming into contact with these chemicals by touching them, eating or drinking something that contains them, or inhaling them. It is important to know what these chemicals are and where they are found so you can be safe. These chemicals include the following:

- **Mercury.** Mercury is found in fish and household products such as batteries, paint, glass thermometers, and compact fluorescent light bulbs. Eating fish with high levels of mercury and disposing of mercury-containing products inappropriately can have harmful effects. Natural events, such as forest fires, and the burning of fossil fuels can also release mercury into the air.
- **Lead.** Lead was used in household products such as paint, gasoline, and pesticides before 1978. It was used in water pipes before 1986. Exposure to lead-based products and water containing lead can harm people's health. Trained people can test homes for lead and recommend steps to take to remove it.

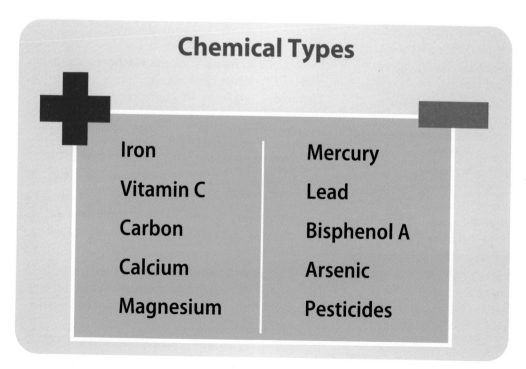

Chemical Types

Iron	Mercury
Vitamin C	Lead
Carbon	Bisphenol A
Calcium	Arsenic
Magnesium	Pesticides

Figure 13.10
Chemicals are in everything, and not all chemicals are bad for health. In fact, the chemicals in the left column of this chart are essential to health. *What does it mean for a chemical to be toxic?*

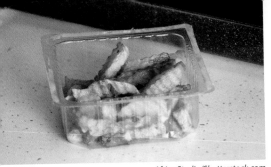
Africa Studio/Shutterstock.com

Figure 13.11 Plastic containers release chemicals into whatever substance they are holding, including food and drinks. Therefore, when people eat or drink items from a plastic container, they ingest the chemicals found in this plastic. Thus, toxic chemicals in plastics can cause great harm. *What is the name of the chemical found in many plastics?*

- **Bisphenol A (BPA).** BPA is a chemical found in many plastics. Scientific research shows that BPA may pose health risks (**Figure 13.11**). Many plastic products, such as water bottles and food containers, are now labeled *BPA-free* to show that this chemical is not used in this product.

- **Arsenic.** Arsenic naturally occurs in rocks, soil, water, and air. It can lead to water pollution when rain or melted snow runs over the ground. Arsenic can also be released from mining and is used in some products that protect wood against termites. Exposure to arsenic can cause serious health conditions.

- **Pesticides.** Pesticides are chemicals that control, or kill, weeds, bugs, and rodents. Pesticides can cause harm if they are ingested with food. Water can also carry pesticides from lawns, gardens, and farms into nearby bodies of water.

Whether a chemical is harmful to your health depends on a number of factors. These factors include how you are exposed to the chemical, how long you are exposed to it, and the amount of the chemical to which you are exposed.

CASE STUDY

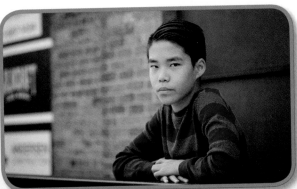
Torgado/Shutterstock.com

Seiji's Paint Job

For months, Seiji has been telling his parents he wants to paint his bathroom. Seiji's bathroom has the same light-blue wallpaper it had when he and his parents moved into the old apartment. Seiji liked the wallpaper when he was younger, but now he wants the bathroom to be darker. Last week, Seiji's parents finally agreed to let him remove the wallpaper and paint the bathroom.

Seiji and his father work together to remove the wallpaper from Seiji's bathroom, and Seiji enjoys working with his father. The wallpaper-removal process produces a lot of dust, and underneath the wallpaper, Seiji and his father discover peeling, yellow paint. Seiji and his father do not feel well that evening, but they decide to wait until the morning to see if they feel better.

The next morning, both Seiji and his father have headaches and feel tired. Seiji's father says they should not continue working on the bathroom until professionals come to test the bathroom for lead paint. Seiji is glad his father cares about his health, but is disappointed he and his father will not finish painting over the weekend. When Seiji tells his

teacher about the paint job, his teacher tells him that lead exposure can have very harmful effects. That makes Seiji feel a little better about the delay.

Thinking Critically

1. Why do you think Seiji's father suspected that the peeling paint underneath the bathroom's wallpaper might contain lead?

2. Should Seiji go into his bathroom before the professionals come to test the paint? Why or why not?

3. If Seiji told you he was disappointed his father delayed their painting project, what would you say to him? How would you explain to Seiji that his father is looking out for his safety?

Certain groups of people have an increased risk of harm due to chemical exposure (**Figure 13.12**). Exposure to toxic chemicals can lead to nausea and vomiting, skin or eye problems, and cancer. Exposure to some chemicals, such as pesticides (which are poisons), can cause death.

If you are worried that you have been exposed to a dangerous chemical, talk with your doctor, school nurse, or another trusted adult. You can also call the Poison Control Center at (800) 222-1222. This resource is very helpful if you think you or someone you know has been in contact with a harmful substance.

Safe Chemical Use

To prevent harm from toxic chemicals, use household chemicals, such as paint and cleaning supplies, properly. Make sure to read warning labels carefully before using any kind of chemical. Other strategies for protecting yourself—and the environment— from chemicals include the following:

- Start by learning the symbols placed on the packages of chemicals (**Figure 13.13**). These symbols explain how the chemicals may impact a person's health and whether they can hurt the environment.

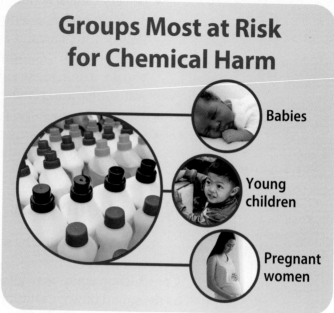

Groups Most at Risk for Chemical Harm

Babies

Young children

Pregnant women

Chemicals: Sfocato/Shutterstock.com; Top to bottom: Tatiana Katsai/Shutterstock.com; Titikul_B/Shutterstock.com; Africa Studio/Shutterstock.com

Figure 13.12 Exposure to chemicals is particularly dangerous for babies and young children. This is because babies' and young children's bodies are still growing. Women who are pregnant need to avoid exposure to chemicals, which can cause health problems for the fetus.

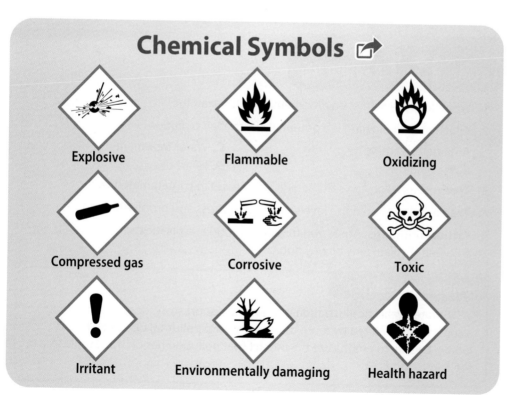

Chemical Symbols

Explosive

Flammable

Oxidizing

Compressed gas

Corrosive

Toxic

Irritant

Environmentally damaging

Health hazard

Figure 13.13 By recognizing the chemical symbols on packaging, you can understand the warnings about health risks associated with chemicals in different products. *Look at the packaging of a cleaning product you use regularly. What chemical symbols are on the packaging?*

Rainer Lesniewski/Shutterstock.com

- Be very careful about mixing different chemicals together. For example, mixing bleach and ammonia produces a highly toxic gas.
- Protect your skin and eyes from chemical exposure. Wear gloves and other protective equipment, depending on the type of chemical product you are using. Make sure to wash your hands carefully with soap and water after using chemical products.
- When using chemical products, work outside or leave windows open.
- Store and dispose of chemical products properly. Keep them away from items used in cooking and eating. Do not move chemicals into new containers.

Noise Pollution

You are surrounded by sounds. People listen to music, television shows, and radio broadcasts. Cars, trucks, trains, and planes make sounds. Construction equipment generates sound, too. Some sounds are natural, such as the sound of waves hitting the shore or birds calling to one another.

When do these sounds become a problem? When do sounds become noise? *Noise* is sound that a person does not want to hear or is bothered by. Noise can be more than simply bothersome. It can affect a person's health.

High levels of noise over a period of time can lead to a loss of hearing. That is one reason that doctors warn about high volume levels when listening to music over earphones. Some studies have found that one in five teens suffers from some hearing loss. Other health effects of noise include stress, high blood pressure, problems sleeping, and lower productivity at work.

Experts recommend that the volume be set at no more than about 60 percent of full volume when listening to a device through earphones. Wearing earplugs when operating loud equipment like power mowers also helps.

Lesson 13.1 Review

1. What does the field of environmental health examine?
2. Which of the following is a potential effect of air pollution?
   A. Easier breathing.
   B. Hearing loss.
   C. Water treatment.
   D. Heart disease.
3. **True or false.** You can see bacteria and viruses in contaminated water.
4. **True or false.** High noise levels can lead to stress and problems sleeping.
5. **Critical thinking.** Should you microwave food in a plastic container that is *not* BPA-free? Explain why or why not.

Hands-On Activity

Create a realistic illustration, shadow box, short story, or song describing a community affected by more than one type of pollution discussed in this lesson. Be sure to emphasize the impact that pollution has on the people in the community.

Pollution Prevention and Greener Living

Learning Outcomes

After studying this lesson, you will be able to

- **give examples** of federal and state laws that protect the environment.
- **describe** what the environmental protection hierarchy is and how to use it.
- **determine** strategies you can use to reduce energy consumption and conserve natural resources at home.
- **identify** ways to be green at school.
- **explain** green choices people can make when traveling.

Graphic Organizer

Living Greener Every Day

Think about the places you visit every day—for example, your school, your home, or the park. List these places on a piece of paper, as shown below. As you read this lesson, take notes about environmental laws that affect each location and about strategies you can use to preserve the environment in each place you visit. An example is provided for you.

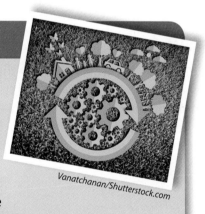

Vanatchanan/Shutterstock.com

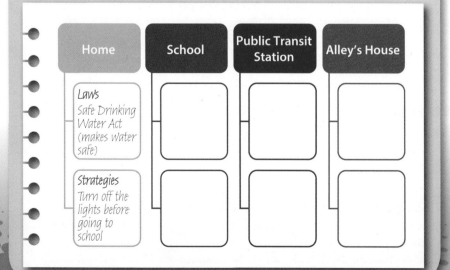

Home	School	Public Transit Station	Alley's House
Laws Safe Drinking Water Act (makes water safe)			
Strategies Turn off the lights before going to school			

Remember Diego from the first lesson. Because of the direct impact pollution has had on his life, Diego wants to live as green as he can. Diego carries a reusable water bottle instead of disposable cans or bottles, turns off any lights he is not using, and reuses items whenever possible. To avoid wasted food, Diego is careful at restaurants to order only the amount of food he can eat and to take home any leftovers to eat later. He also set up a carpool with a few of his friends at school to help minimize car exhaust pollution. You will learn about these and more ways to prevent pollution and live greener in this lesson.

Society's Actions to Protect the Environment

Federal and state governments have passed laws to promote a safe environment. The *Environmental Protection Agency (EPA)* is the federal government agency that sets rules and regulations to protect people's health and the environment in the United States (**Figure 13.14**). These rules put into practice laws passed by Congress. They are based on scientific research.

States have their own laws aimed at protecting the environment. Each state has departments with power to enforce those laws.

Clean Air Act

The *Clean Air Act* is a federal law that regulates air pollution levels to protect people's health. This law sets specific limits on the amounts and types of pollution that power plants can release into the air. It also regulates the amounts and types of pollution produced by motor vehicles. This law has had a major impact on reducing air pollution.

Figure 13.14
When federal and state governments pass environmental safety laws, the EPA regulates and enforces these laws.

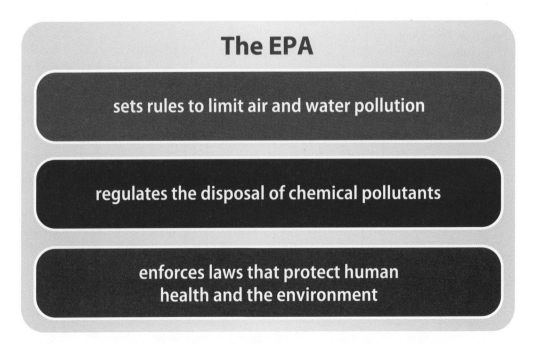

The EPA

sets rules to limit air and water pollution

regulates the disposal of chemical pollutants

enforces laws that protect human health and the environment

The EPA works with state and local agencies to create a measure of air pollution. This measure is called the **Air Quality Index (AQI)**. The AQI tells you about five major air pollutants (**Figure 13.15**). Large cities are required to report the AQI every day. Many smaller communities do as well. This index is available on the Internet or through a free e-mail or app.

People can use the AQI to protect themselves. If air pollution is high in an area one day, people can spend more time inside. This is especially important for people with allergies or asthma. If air pollution levels are high, stay indoors during the afternoon, when ozone levels are typically the highest.

Safe Drinking Water Act

The *Safe Drinking Water Act* requires that drinking water is tested for over 90 different pollutants. This testing includes metals, such as lead. It also includes pollutants that could spread diseases, such as *E. coli* and salmonella. Water systems are continually tested to make sure they meet safe standards.

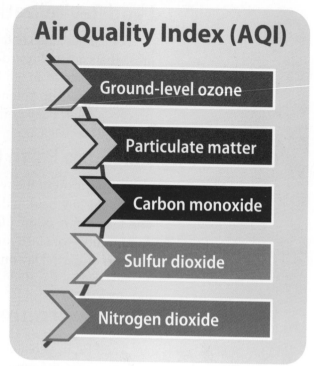

Air Quality Index (AQI)

Ground-level ozone

Particulate matter

Carbon monoxide

Sulfur dioxide

Nitrogen dioxide

Figure 13.15 The five major air pollutants identified in the AQI are ground-level ozone, particulate matter, carbon monoxide, sulfur dioxide, and nitrogen dioxide. *Which law has had a major impact in reducing air pollution?*

Resource Conservation and Recovery Act

The *Resource Conservation and Recovery Act* provides rules and regulations about managing hazardous waste. For example, some chemicals can cause harm if they are simply dumped in the trash. Some trash contains dangerous chemicals. If those chemicals are not in a special container, they can leak into the ground or water (**Figure 13.16**). There are now specific rules about disposing of such waste.

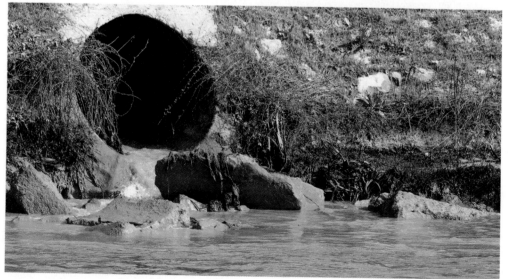

Figure 13.16 Hazardous waste in people's garbage can contaminate the water people use for cleaning, cooking, and drinking. *Which law provides rules and regulations about managing hazardous waste?*

Sinisha Karich/Shutterstock.com

Land Revitalization Program

Sometimes land contains hazardous waste that can hurt people's health. These areas that contain hazardous waste are called *brownfield sites*. A **brownfield site** may be the site of an old factory or gas station. The EPA's Land Revitalization Program cleans up potentially contaminated land so that it is safe to use. This process removes any polluting substances and creates more usable land.

Celebrate Earth Day

People around the world celebrate Earth Day on April 22 each year. Earth Day events are held to demonstrate support for protecting the environment and taking care of the planet. Join an Earth Day celebration in your school or community—or start your own. You can find lots of ideas for activities to do in support of Earth Day online.

The Environmental Protection Hierarchy

The EPA has created a graphic called the *environmental protection hierarchy*. It shows four different ways of protecting the environment. The higher up in the hierarchy, the better the approach (**Figure 13.17**).

Reduction

The best strategy for protecting the environment is to *reduce* trash and pollution. This eliminates the source, or cause, of pollution. For example, many people buy bottled water and then throw out the plastic container.

Figure 13.17
Ways to protect the environment include a reduction of trash and pollution, recycling and reusing items and materials, treatment of waste to make it less dangerous, and disposal of hazardous materials. *What is the most preferred way to protect the environment?*

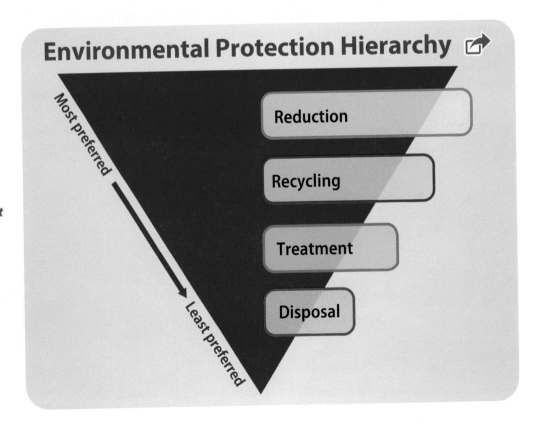

Environmental Protection Hierarchy

Most preferred

Least preferred

Reduction

Recycling

Treatment

Disposal

Instead, they could buy a reusable bottle and refill it. This approach would reduce the amount of plastic thrown away. Very simple strategies, such as turning off the lights when leaving a room and turning off the water when brushing teeth, reduce the amount of energy used.

Reducing the use of fossil fuels like oil, gas, and coal is another way to help the environment. These energy sources are called **fossil fuels** and were formed a very long time ago, when dinosaurs lived on Earth. Burning these fuels releases gases and particulate matter into the air. Many scientists also believe that they contribute to climate change. Driving electric or hybrid cars can reduce the amount of exhaust from fossil fuels.

Alternative sources of electric energy like solar power, wind power, and water power help as well. These sources of energy come from Earth's natural resources, such as wind, water, and sunlight. These types of energy are called **renewable energy** because they cannot be used up (**Figure 13.18**). People can use as much energy as possible from these sources, and never run out. Another advantage about this type of energy is that it does not cause pollution. That is why this type of energy is sometimes called *clean energy*. The more people can use renewable energy sources, the more they protect the environment.

Another way of reducing waste is to take care of your belongings, such as clothes and electronics, so they last longer. Buy used clothes or books instead of new ones. Shop at thrift stores, garage sales, and flea markets to save money and protect the environment at the same time. All of these strategies reduce the need to manufacture new products, which takes energy.

Recycling

The next best approach to reducing pollution is to *recycle* items you use, instead of just throwing them away. **Recycling** is a process in which used materials are turned into new products. This reduces the amount of trash sent to landfills.

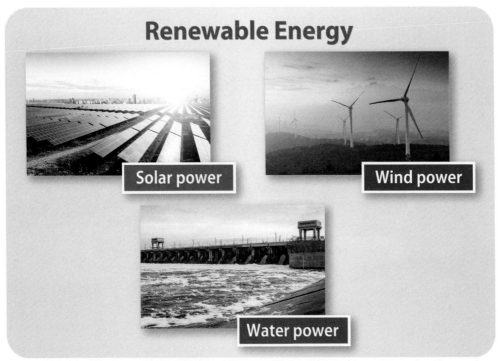

Figure 13.18
Earth's natural resources, such as sunlight, wind, and water, are sources of energy that cannot run out. They also do not cause pollution.

Left to right, top to bottom: Wang An Qi/Shutterstock.com; zhangyang13576997233/Shutterstock.com; Getmaneclnna/Shutterstock.com

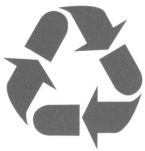

Figure 13.19
The symbol shown here can help you identify recycling receptacles when you are disposing of paper, plastic, glass, and aluminum items. *What happens in the process of recycling?*

Recycling conserves natural resources and saves energy. Recycling also helps limit the burning of fossil fuels, which contributes to climate change. Many items people use every day are recyclable, including newspapers and magazines, aluminum cans, glass bottles, and plastic containers (**Figure 13.19**).

Try to reuse products when you can. Instead of asking for a new plastic or paper bag every time you go shopping, carry a reusable bag. Buy rechargeable batteries, which you can reuse. When you are done using something, try to donate it so someone else can use it, too. For example, when you outgrow clothes, you could give them to a local homeless shelter or charitable organization.

Certain types of products need to be recycled in particular ways to protect the environment. These include electronic products, such as televisions and computers, and appliances, such as microwaves and refrigerators. These products can contain dangerous substances. It is important to recycle these products so that these substances do not pollute landfills. Many towns have special days in which these products can be dropped off for recycling. Some stores also collect these products for recycling.

Treatment

The third step in the hierarchy is *treating* substances that may be dangerous. This approach uses processes that make the substance less dangerous. For example, sewage is treated in water treatment plants to avoid the harmful effects of human waste entering the environment.

Disposal

Some products contain hazardous materials, and therefore are not able to be treated or recycled. These products need to be disposed of very carefully to avoid harming the environment. They cannot simply be placed in a trash can and then dumped in a landfill (**Figure 13.20**). Most communities provide specific instructions on how to carefully dispose of these products.

Figure 13.20
Products such as batteries, tires, aerosol cans, household chemicals, and medical waste require special disposal because they can harm the environment if dumped in a landfill.

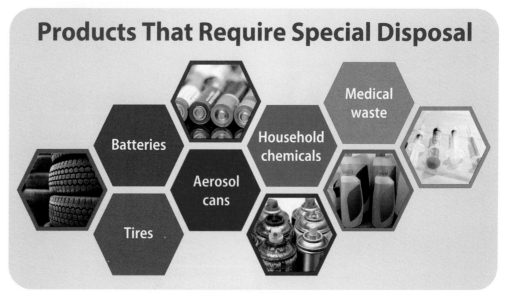

Products That Require Special Disposal

Batteries

Tires

Aerosol cans

Household chemicals

Medical waste

Greener Living

"Green" living means living in a way that protects the environment. It involves limiting or preventing actions that pollute and conserving resources. One goal of green living is to make choices that create **sustainability**, or actions that maintain the natural resources in the environment.

BUILDING Your Skills

Advocating for the Environment

One way to protect the environment is to advocate for it. An *advocate* is a person who stands up for what he or she believes is right. To be an advocate, a person must

- be passionate about a cause
- use his or her powers of persuasion to prove the importance of the cause
- inspire a behavior change among others

There are many ways to advocate for a cause, and one way is to create a campaign. You may have encountered campaigns before. For example, you have probably seen billboards, commercials, and T-shirts advertising a cause. You may have participated in awareness walks or worn a certain color ribbon for a meaningful day. All of these strategies aim to inspire awareness and action in certain people. You can create a campaign about a cause you care about, too.

Start a Campaign

The environment needs your help, so start a campaign to advocate for its health. First, form a small group to be your team. In your group, discuss environmental issues in your community (school, neighborhood, or town). Find an issue that you are all passionate about improving.

Once you have chosen an issue, research it. Become an expert on your chosen environmental topic. Remember that research should come from many sources, including books, online databases, and people. Research should also be reliable, so use trustworthy sources.

Next, create a campaign to promote your cause. Your campaign might be an event, a series of advertisements or messages, or a movement promoting change. Whatever the nature of your campaign, make sure your campaign is innovative, or new, and promotes your cause. While creating your campaign, keep in mind the multiple age levels in your community. Your campaign should appeal to all ages, from young children to older adults. Consider what each age group can do to help solve your issue and make sure each person knows what you are asking. Write down the details of your campaign and plan so you understand how to put the campaign into action. Then, with the help of your teacher, get your campaign out into the community.

As your campaign runs its course, be sure to "practice what you preach," or live out the cause you are promoting. After a while, observe the campaign's effect on your community and consider the following questions:

- What worked in your campaign? What did not work?
- Did people make changes in their behavior because of your campaign?
- Has the community environment improved because of your campaign? Is it too soon to tell? When will you know?
- What did you learn about yourself, about advocacy, and about your community during this campaign?

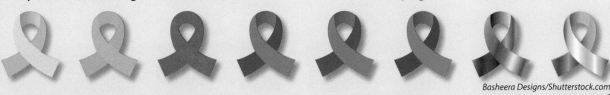

Basheera Designs/Shutterstock.com

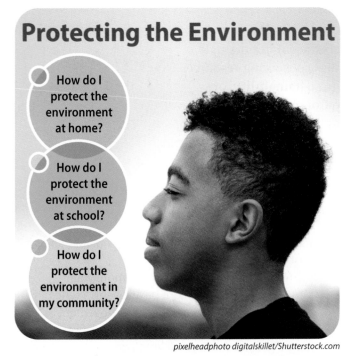

Protecting the Environment

- How do I protect the environment at home?
- How do I protect the environment at school?
- How do I protect the environment in my community?

pixelheadphoto digitalskillet/Shutterstock.com

Figure 13.21 Reflecting on actions you can take to protect your environment can help you make choices that will protect the planet for future generations. *What actions do you take to protect the environment at home, at school, and in your community?*

When people make responsible choices about using and consuming products, they help protect Earth so that these natural resources can last for many, many years. For example, sustainable gardening is a way of growing plants that reduces any negative impact on the environment. It includes such actions as avoiding the use of chemicals that can pollute the soil and capturing rain to water plants.

Making environmentally friendly choices helps to maintain the planet not just for the current generation, but also for future generations. People can take many different actions in their homes, schools, workplaces, and communities to help protect society and the environment (**Figure 13.21**).

Use Less Energy

Making small changes in your behavior can help reduce energy consumption and conserve natural resources. Following are some simple strategies for using fewer resources at home:

- Turn off lights when leaving a room.
- Use as little electricity as possible to heat and cool your home. Set the thermostat a bit higher in the summer and a bit lower in the winter to reduce the amount of energy used.
- Shut the refrigerator door as soon as you select what you need.
- Use light bulbs that run on less energy (**Figure 13.22**).

Figure 13.22 Energy-efficient light bulbs use less energy, which helps them last longer. By using less energy, these bulbs also produce less waste. *What is one way to tell if a product is energy efficient?*

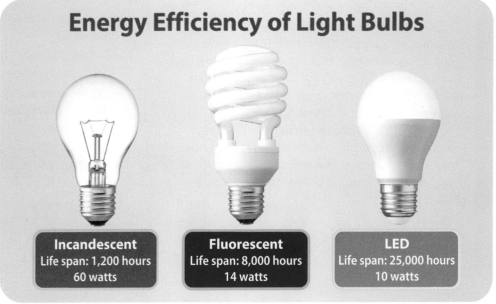

Energy Efficiency of Light Bulbs

Incandescent	Fluorescent	LED
Life span: 1,200 hours	Life span: 8,000 hours	Life span: 25,000 hours
60 watts	14 watts	10 watts

Somchai Som/Shutterstock.com

- Keep outside doors and windows shut when heating or cooling your home.
- Buy energy-efficient products. You can look for the *Energy Star symbol* to choose products that have energy efficiency. This symbol appears on products that use lower amounts of energy. These products save people money over time because they require less energy to run. They also reduce energy use, which saves energy and reduces pollution. The symbol is given to various products that use electricity, including computers and fans. It is also given to new buildings that meet standards for lower energy use.

Buy Green Products

Another approach to green living is to make wise purchases. **Green products** are goods that have a less harmful impact on the environment than traditional products. Green products could include any of the following features:

- made of recycled materials
- obtained from local stores or farms, meaning less energy was needed to transport them (**Figure 13.23**)
- made without harmful chemicals
- **biodegradable**, or able to break down without causing harm when thrown out

Reduce Food Waste

Another way to live greener is to reduce the amount of wasted food. Every year, Americans throw away more than 38 million tons of food. This includes food that has spoiled, but it also includes leftovers people just do not finish. Most of this food ends up in landfills. Being more mindful about your food choices can help reduce food waste and save money. You can reduce food waste in the following ways:

- Only buy as much food as you expect to eat.
- Store food carefully so that it stays fresh longer.
- Have a "leftovers night" each week.
- When eating out, take home food you do not finish to avoid it being thrown away.

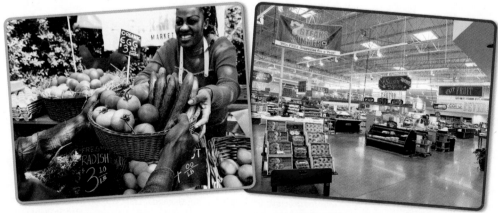

Figure 13.23
Locally grown food has had less exposure to potential contaminants in transport and is more likely to be fresh and full of nutrients than food shipped from far away.

Steps Toward a Greener Planet

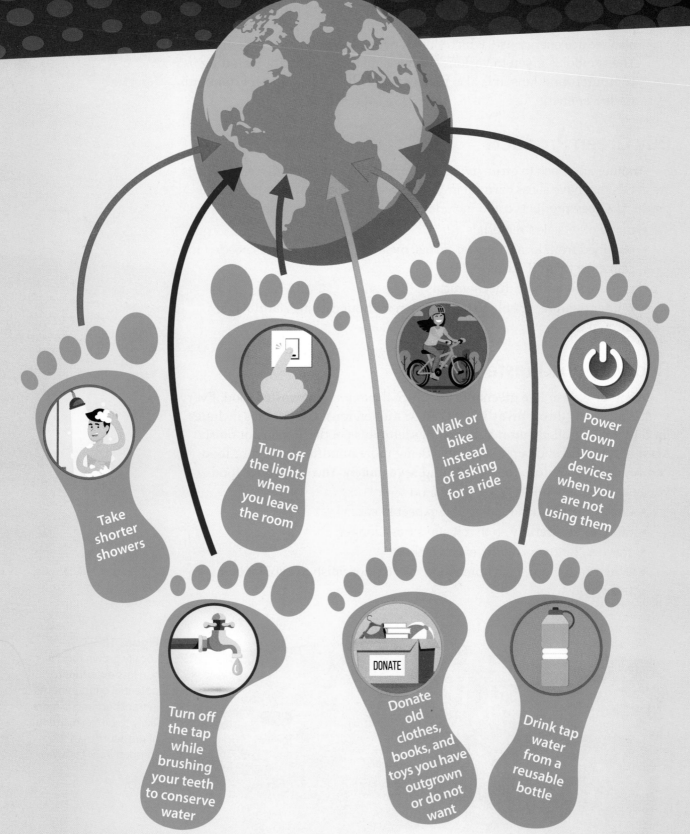

Earth: peiyang/Shutterstock.com; Footprints: Arcady/Shutterstock.com; Top to bottom, left to right: Boonyen/Shutterstock.com; Wor Sang Jun/Shutterstock.com;
bioraven/Shutterstock.com; Jane Kelly/Shutterstock.com; Marnikus/Shutterstock.com; Maike Hildebrandt/Shutterstock.com; Creative Stall/Shutterstock.com

Plant a Tree

Planting a tree is a pretty simple way to protect the environment (**Figure 13.24**). Trees beautify surroundings and provide shade. The shade trees provide can make a home cooler and reduce the demand for air-conditioning. Trees also absorb carbon dioxide and other gases (including carbon monoxide and sulfur dioxide) from the air, and release oxygen into the air. This helps air quality. Trees also help the environment by holding water in the soil, preventing it from running off.

Be Green Away from Home

There are many ways people can be green at school or work. Reusing materials is one approach. Instead of buying new notebooks, pens, and other supplies each new school year, reuse supplies from the previous year. If buying new items, look for those made from recycled products. Office workers can use paper that is no longer needed as note paper.

People can make green choices in the school or workplace cafeteria. Following are some easy ways to make environmentally friendly choices:

- If you bring lunch from home, use reusable containers instead of disposable ones.
- Bring drinks in a thermos or safe reusable water bottle.
- If you bring cans or bottles to school or work, recycle them.
- If you buy lunch, take only what you need. Extra napkins and ketchup packages simply add extra waste.

Some schools have a composting program to help reduce the amount of food waste. **Composting** involves gathering food scraps and yard waste into a bin and letting it decompose and then adding it to soil to help plants grow (**Figure 13.25**).

Benefits of Trees

Beautify surroundings
Provide shade
Absorb carbon dioxide
Release oxygen
Prevent runoff

John_T/Shutterstock.com

Figure 13.24 Planting trees is an easy, cheap activity that can have many benefits to the environment.

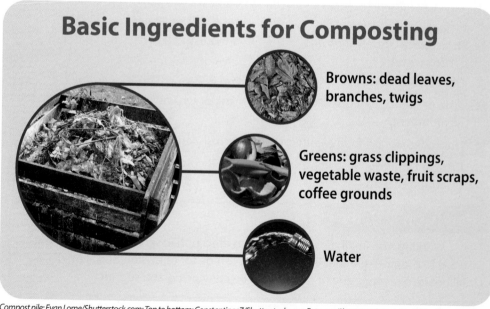

Basic Ingredients for Composting

Browns: dead leaves, branches, twigs

Greens: grass clippings, vegetable waste, fruit scraps, coffee grounds

Water

Figure 13.25
To create a compost pile, alternate layers of browns and greens in equal amounts. Add water to dry materials as they are placed in the bin to keep them moist. *What type of waste does composting help reduce?*

Compost pile: Evan Lorne/Shutterstock.com; Top to bottom: ConstantinosZ/Shutterstock.com; Fotocute/Shutterstock.com; Jim Barber/Shutterstock.com

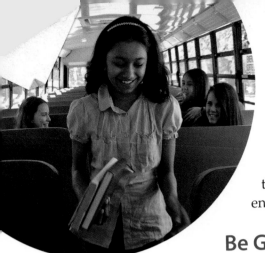

Figure 13.26
Taking the bus to school can help reduce energy consumed. The bus transports many people at once, which reduces the number of vehicles on the road.

If your school has this type of program, make sure to dispose of your food scraps properly so they are composted and not just thrown away. If your school does not have this type of program, maybe you could work with friends to start one.

Many people do not understand how their choices impact the environment, and how even small changes can help protect the planet. Educating people in your school or community about the benefits of reducing energy consumption can help protect the environment and improve overall health in your community.

Be Green on the Road

You can reduce energy consumed and pollution by making greener choices when you travel. For example, walking or biking to school is a greener choice than riding in a car (**Figure 13.26**). For longer distances, try to use public transportation, such as a subway, train, or bus. These forms of transportation take many people and use much less energy than if each person drove his or her own car.

Drivers can also make greener choices to help protect the environment. One way drivers can help the environment is to buy energy-efficient cars. Cars can differ a lot in how much gas they use. Cars with a high miles-per-gallon (MPG) use less gas than those with a low MPG. A high MPG car costs less to drive and reduces pollution. Although most cars run on gasoline, some newer cars use different forms of energy that are better for the environment. Electric cars do not use any gas and do not produce exhaust. Of course, they do use some energy—the electricity needed to recharge their batteries. Hybrid cars are powered with both gasoline and electricity. Driving these cars may save money because less money is spent buying gas.

Lesson 13.2 Review

1. Which Act requires large cities to report the AQI every day?
   - **A.** *Safe Drinking Water Act.*
   - **B.** *Resource Conservation and Recovery Act.*
   - **C.** *Clean Air Act.*
   - **D.** Land Revitalization Program.

2. List the four strategies of the environmental protection hierarchy.

3. **True or false.** Biodegradable products break down without causing harm to the environment.

4. How does storing food carefully to keep it fresh reduce waste?

5. **Critical thinking.** Research and describe your community's guidelines for disposing of batteries.

Hands-On Activity

Working in a small group, plan and create a public service announcement (PSA) to promote greener living. The PSA can be for television, social media, a billboard, or a magazine or newspaper. Be convincing and succinct.

Summary

Lesson 13.1 Common Hazards in the Environment

- The environment in which you live influences your health. The study of how factors in the natural environment impact your health is called *environmental health*. As a healthy environment can lead to better health, so can an unhealthy environment lead to poor health.

- Pollutants are substances that contaminate the environment and can harm people. Air pollution refers to the contamination of the air you breathe. Smog, acid rain, and particulate matter are examples of outdoor air pollution. Examples of indoor air pollution include tobacco smoke, paint, and dust. Air pollution can cause health problems in humans and is also believed to contribute to climate change.

- Polluted water poses major risks to human health. Sometimes, water pollution occurs because of human activity. For example, pesticides and chemicals that humans use can contaminate water. Water pollution can also be natural. Bacteria, viruses, and parasites can contaminate water and make people sick. To prevent water contamination, drinking water in the United States is treated according to a water treatment plan.

- Chemicals can also pollute the environment. Some chemicals are natural, while others are made by people. In large amounts, chemicals can harm health. For example, exposure to lead can have negative effects. Chemicals found in plastic can cause sickness. Identifying, storing, and disposing of chemicals safely can help prevent contamination.

- Noise pollution refers to noises you do not want to hear. High levels of noise can cause hearing loss and lead to stress. Listening to music at a moderate volume and wearing earplugs can help reduce noise pollution.

Lesson 13.2 Pollution Prevention and Greener Living

- The Environmental Protection Agency (EPA) sets regulations to help protect the environment. EPA initiatives include the *Clean Air Act, Safe Drinking Water Act, Resource Conservation and Recovery Act*, Land Revitalization Program, and Earth Day.

- The environmental protection hierarchy illustrates different ways of protecting the environment. The hierarchy's strategies are *reducing* trash and pollution, *recycling* items, *treating* dangerous substances, and *disposing* of hazardous materials carefully.

- Green living is living in a way that protects the environment. You can use many strategies to live more greenly. These include using less energy, buying green products, reducing food waste, and planting trees. You can make green choices away from home by reusing materials and educating others. You can make green choices on the road by using public transportation and energy-efficient cars.

Check Your Knowledge ⌕↱

Record your answers to each of the following questions on a separate sheet of paper.

1. **True or false.** Car exhaust is a major contributor to smog in cities.
2. How does runoff lead to the pollution of a water supply?
3. **True or false.** In the United States, drinking water travels from the water supply to your home without treatment.
4. Which of the following chemicals can be found in batteries, paint, and glass thermometers?
   - **A.** Mercury.
   - **B.** Arsenic.
   - **C.** Lead.
   - **D.** Aspirin.
5. Is it safe to move chemicals into different containers? Why or why not?
6. Which of the following is a health effect of noise pollution?
   - **A.** Low stress.
   - **B.** Deep sleeping.
   - **C.** High blood pressure.
   - **D.** High productivity at work.
7. Which EPA initiative cleans up brownfield sites so they are safe to use?
8. **True or false.** Burning fossil fuels releases gases and particulate matter into the air.
9. What is an example of a household product that requires special disposal?
10. **True or false.** Green products must be obtained from international sources.
11. How does planting a tree help the environment?
12. Which of the following is a good strategy for being green away from home?
    - **A.** Bring extra napkins for lunch.
    - **B.** Use disposable containers.
    - **C.** Drink out of plastic water bottles.
    - **D.** Recycle cans and bottles.
13. **True or false.** Using public transportation to get to school is a greener choice than riding in a car.

Use Your Vocabulary ⌕↱

acid rain	fossil fuels	renewable energy
air quality index (AQI)	green products	smog
biodegradable	ozone	sustainability
brownfield site	pollutants	
composting	recycling	

14. Write each of the terms above on a separate sheet of paper. For each term, quickly write a word you think relates to the term. In small groups, exchange papers. Have each person in the group explain a term on the list. Take turns until all terms have complete explanations.
15. With a partner, choose two of the terms above. Use the Internet to locate photos or graphics that show the meaning of these two terms. Print the photos or graphics and show them to the class. Explain how they show the meaning of the terms.

Think Critically

16. **Determine.** Describe how personal health and the health of a person's environment are connected.

17. **Cause and effect.** How have the use of technology and technological advances helped and harmed the environment?

18. **Make inferences.** Even though people are making changes to protect the environment, pollution still exists. As long as pollution is a problem, what behavior changes can you make to protect your personal health?

19. **Predict.** What effect could climate change have on human health?

20. **Identify.** Think about reasons that people do not make choices for greener living. List these reasons and share them with a partner. For each reason not to make greener choices, write a sentence in favor of making greener choices.

DEVELOP Your Skills

21. **Access information.** Working with a partner, research five local, state, national, and international agencies that promote environmental health and protection. Make a resource list that includes the name of each agency, the agency's mission or purpose, and the agency's contact information (for example, website address). Share your list with your classmates and create a class list to take home.

22. **Goal-setting skills.** Review this chapter's information about green living and brainstorm other ways middle school students can have a positive impact on the environment and human health. Identify one realistic action you can either add to or remove from your daily routine to improve environmental health. Write this action as a SMART goal and track your progress toward achieving it over one month. At the end of the month, review your actions, your feelings, and any impact on your environment.

23. **Leadership, decision-making, advocacy, and communication skills.** Identify one change you can make in your home or school that will promote environmental and human health. Will you need to purchase or subscribe to anything to make the change happen? What routines will need to change, and whom will they impact? Talk with your family or teacher about putting this change into action and then try it out.

24. **Literacy, communication, and technology skills.** Find and read a current news story about environmental health. Take notes as you read the news story and identify the most important ideas. Then, share the story with your classmates and use a meme, hashtag, or other online feature to highlight the most important ideas in the story.

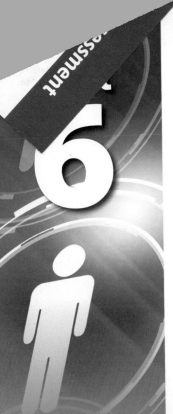

6

Social Health and Wellness

Chapter 14 Promoting Healthy Relationships

Chapter 15 Understanding Violent Behavior

Warm-Up Activity

Questions About Relationships

This unit will discuss what relationships are and what makes them healthy or unhealthy. Without talking with anyone else, answer the following questions on six separate sticky notes:

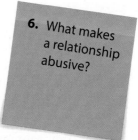

rui vale sousa/Shutterstock.com

1. What is a *relationship*?

2. What qualities are found in healthy relationships?

3. How can you strengthen a relationship?

4. How do you know when a relationship should end?

5. What makes a relationship unhealthy?

6. What makes a relationship abusive?

Squares: Brumarina/Shutterstock.com

When you are done answering these questions, post your answers on the wall. Everyone in the class should post their answers, and answers should be grouped by question. Walk around and read all of the answers to each question. For each question, write one statement summarizing the answers.

After reading the chapters in this unit, read these summary statements again and review how accurate they were. Enhance your statements to be more correct and complete.

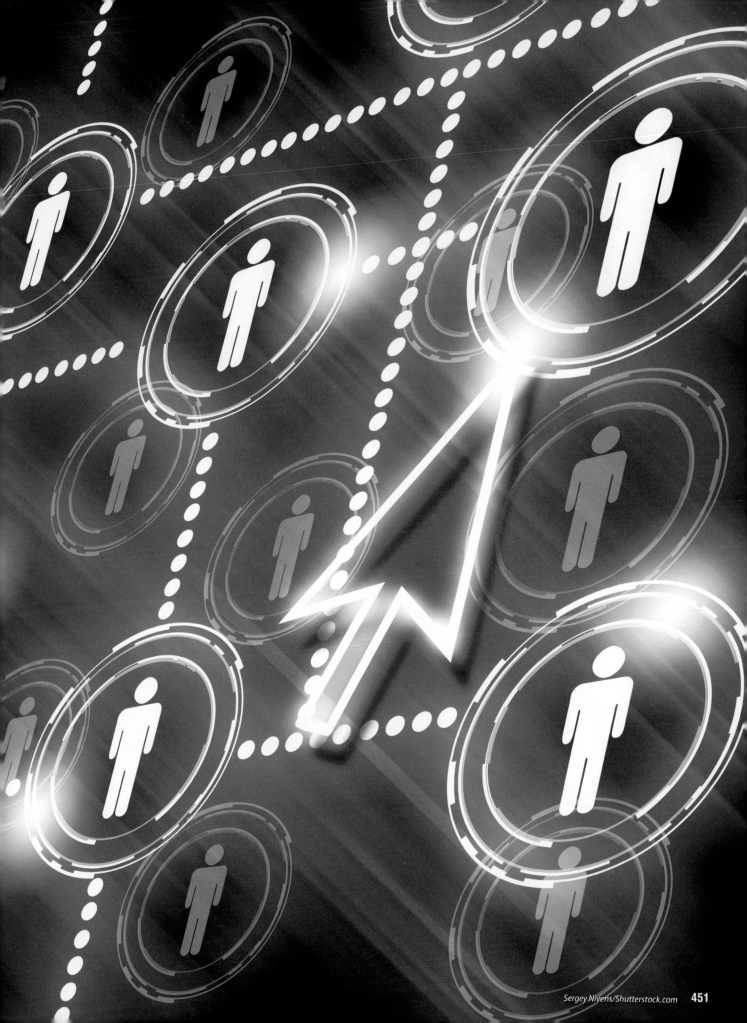

Chapter 14

Promoting Healthy Relationships

Essential Question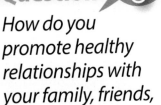

How do you promote healthy relationships with your family, friends, and dating partners?

Video ↗
Access the Chapter 14 video to start thinking about chapter topics.

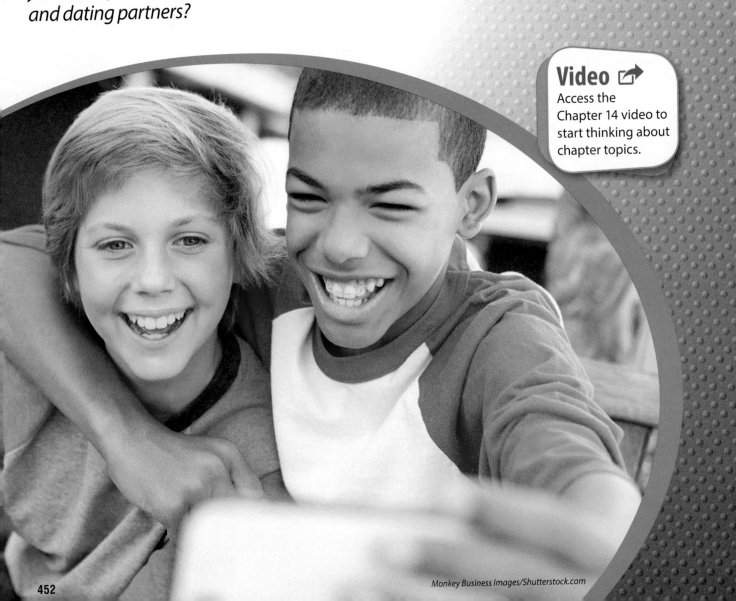

Monkey Business Images/Shutterstock.com

In groups of three, review healthy family relationships, friendships, and dating relationships. Assign each group member one of these types of relationships to review and summarize in two or three paragraphs. Then, discuss each summary with the group. After reading this chapter, draw connections between the types of relationships.

How Healthy Are You?

In this chapter, you will be learning about healthy relationships. Before you begin reading, take the following quiz to assess your current healthy relationship habits.

Healthy Choices	Yes	No
Do you have a social support system of people you can count on to help you in times of crises?		
Are you a patient and attentive listener?		
Can you clearly express to someone your wants, needs, opinions, and feelings?		
Are you able to prevent or resolve conflicts with parents and siblings?		
Do you and your friends avoid excluding other people from your group?		
Do you avoid interrupting, judging, or criticizing others when they are talking?		
Do you try not to rely too much on virtual interactions with your friends, choosing face-to-face interactions instead?		
Do you know the difference between casual dating and group dating?		
Are your relationships with others based on characteristics of honesty, trust, mutual respect, care, and commitment?		

Count your "Yes" and "No" responses. The more "Yes" responses you have, the more healthy relationship habits you exhibit. Now, take a closer look at the questions with which you responded "No." How can you make these healthy habits part of your daily life? Think about how implementing these ideas can help improve your relationships with others.

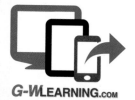

While studying this chapter, look for the activity icon to

- **practice** key terms with e-flash cards and matching activities.
- **reinforce** what you learn by completing graphic organizers, self-assessment quizzes, and review questions.
- **expand** knowledge with interactive activities and activities that extend learning.

www.g-wlearning.com/health/

What Is a Healthy Relationship?

Key Terms 📑

interpersonal skills abilities that help people communicate and relate in positive ways with others

communication process exchange of messages and responses between two or more people

feedback constructive response to a message to communicate that it was received and understood

verbal communication use of words to send a spoken or written message

nonverbal communication sending of messages through facial expressions, body language, gestures, tone and volume of voice, and other signals that do not involve the content of words

active listening way of paying attention to spoken messages with the goal of understanding the message and the speaker's feelings about it

peer mediation process in which specially trained students work with other students to resolve conflicts

Learning Outcomes

After studying this lesson, you will be able to

- **discuss** the importance of relationships for physical, emotional, and social health.
- **identify** the characteristics of a healthy relationship.
- **identify** signs of an unhealthy relationship.
- **explain** how to communicate effectively with others.
- **summarize** the process of negotiation to resolve conflicts.
- **describe** the purpose of peer mediation.

Graphic Organizer 📑

Visualizing Relationships

Before reading this lesson, skim the main headings and write each main heading in a different color on a separate piece of paper. As you read the lesson, take notes in the color you chose for each main heading, as shown below. After you finish taking notes for each section, draw a small illustration next to the section that will help you remember what you learned.

Alex Staroseltsev/Shutterstock.com

The Importance of Relationships	Communication Skills
Family relationships meet basic human needs	
Healthy Versus Unhealthy Relationships	**Conflict Resolution Skills**

Jemastock/Shutterstock.com

Relationships are an important part of every person's life, and as you grow up, you will form and maintain new types of relationships. For example, Kai is in eighth grade and is a very social person. For as long as he can remember, he has been close with his parents. He enjoys playing sports and video games with his younger brother. Since he started middle school, Kai has made many new friends. This year, he even likes a girl at school. Some of Kai's peers have stopped talking to their friends and lost friendships because of conflict. Kai does not want this to happen to him and his friends. Kai understands that his relationships are important to his health and well-being.

The Importance of Relationships

People live in social groups and have many relationships with other people. Most people live in families and have friends. Children and young people have relationships with other students, teachers, and adults. Adults have relationships with coworkers and members of groups to which they belong. All of these relationships help contribute to a person's health and well-being (**Figure 14.1**).

Some relationships meet basic human needs. Most of these relationships are in families, which are responsible for meeting the needs of members. Other relationships, however, also play a crucial role in your physical health.

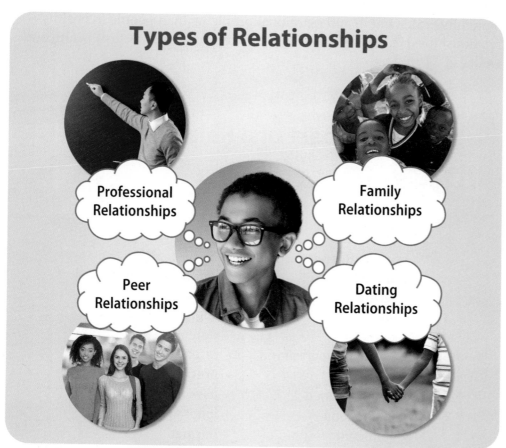

Types of Relationships

Professional Relationships

Family Relationships

Peer Relationships

Dating Relationships

Figure 14.1
All of your relationships impact your well-being. As you grow up, you will have more types of relationships and will get to know more diverse people. *Which type of relationship is responsible for meeting the needs of members?*

Center: LightField Studios/Shutterstock.com; Clockwise from top left: Africa Studio/Shutterstock.com; Monkey Business Images/Shutterstock.com; Diego Cervo/Shutterstock.com; Billion Photos/Shutterstock.com

Researchers have found that people with good social support are less likely to get sick than people who lack social support. People with good social support also tend to recover from illnesses faster and even live longer. Relationships filled with tension and conflict can have the opposite effects on health.

Relationships also meet the need to belong to a group and to feel connected with and loved by other people. Relationships impact you emotionally. A smile or a compliment from a friend or a classmate can lift your spirits. An argument with a sibling can make you feel angry or sad. Relationships allow you to learn more about yourself, receive and provide emotional support, and gain skills for communicating and resolving conflicts.

Different relationships satisfy different needs. When you were younger, most of your relationships were probably in your family. As you grow up, however, your social world is expanding to include other relationships, such as those with peers, teachers, and even dating partners.

Healthy Versus Unhealthy Relationships

The impact of relationships depends on how healthy the relationships are (**Figure 14.2**). For example, in healthy relationships, people receive support from family and friends when they go through times of crises. This support helps give people the strength they need to recover from the challenges they face. People in unhealthy relationships often do not receive the support they need. In turn, this can result in experiencing more physical, mental, and emotional problems than people in healthy relationships. Healthy relationships can improve all aspects of health and wellness.

Figure 14.2
A person with healthy relationships will experience more positive emotions and fewer negative emotions than a person with unhealthy relationships.

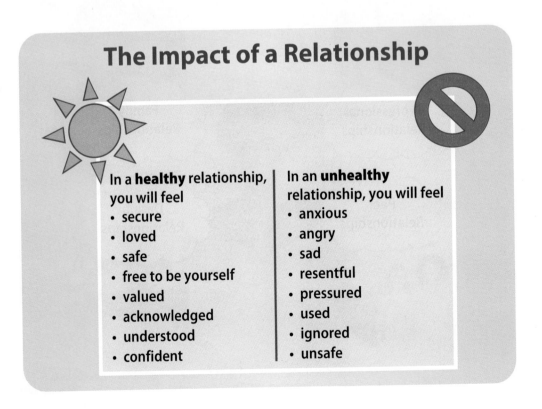

The Impact of a Relationship

In a **healthy** relationship, you will feel
- secure
- loved
- safe
- free to be yourself
- valued
- acknowledged
- understood
- confident

In an **unhealthy** relationship, you will feel
- anxious
- angry
- sad
- resentful
- pressured
- used
- ignored
- unsafe

As you form new relationships, you can ensure your own health by building *healthy relationships*. Healthy relationships have the following important characteristics:

- **Honesty.** Honesty means telling the truth about what you have done, what you want, and how you feel.
- **Trust.** Trust is believing that another person is not going to do or say something to hurt you.
- **Mutual respect.** Respect is knowing that each person has worth as a human being and has a right to have his or her feelings and desires recognized. Respect should be *mutual*, or go both ways.
- **Care and commitment.** You demonstrate care and commitment when you show concern for another person and work to make the relationship better.
- **Emotional control.** Controlling your emotions is an important part of building a healthy relationship. For example, controlling your anger can help you work through conflict in a positive way (**Figure 14.3**).
- **Understanding.** When you show understanding, you acknowledge and relate to the feelings and thoughts of another person.
- **Good interpersonal skills. Interpersonal skills** are abilities that help people communicate and resolve conflicts in positive ways. Healthy relationships are built using interpersonal skills.

Paying attention to these characteristics can help you build and maintain healthy relationships. If a relationship does not have these characteristics, it is unhealthy and needs to change (**Figure 14.4**).

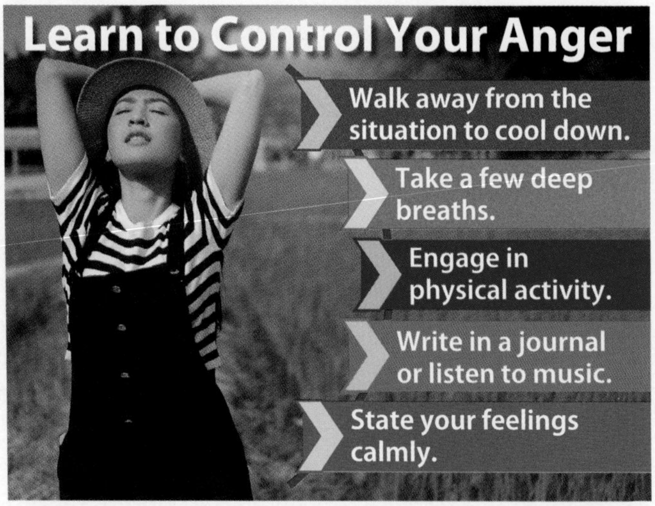

Learn to Control Your Anger

- Walk away from the situation to cool down.
- Take a few deep breaths.
- Engage in physical activity.
- Write in a journal or listen to music.
- State your feelings calmly.

eakkaluktemwanich/Shutterstock.com

Figure 14.3 Pausing and taking deep breaths can help you control anger in a relationship, which enables you to work through conflicts in a positive way. *Which skills help people communicate and resolve conflicts in positive ways?*

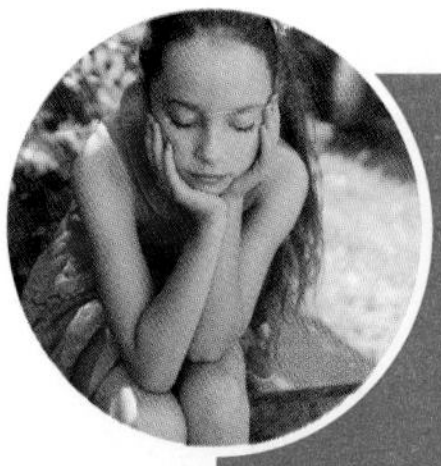

Signs of an Unhealthy Relationship

- You feel used, ignored, and unappreciated.
- One person is more interested in maintaining the relationship than the other person.
- You are subjected to angry outbursts.
- You feel you cannot say anything right.
- You and the other person are constantly fighting.
- You are made fun of or threatened.
- The other person is extremely jealous of you.
- The other person tells you to stay away from friends or family.
- The other person raises a hand as if to hit you.
- The other person has been violent toward you.
- You are being pressured to engage in activities that make you uncomfortable.

Figure 14.4 Some people may have trouble seeing the signs of an unhealthy relationship. This is especially true for people raised in environments without respect, kindness, or trust.

Katya Shut/Shutterstock.com

If a person in the relationship is not willing to invest in making the relationship better, the relationship may need to end. To build healthy relationships with others, you need to have good communication skills and conflict resolution skills.

Communication Skills

Effective communication is perhaps the most important part of a healthy relationship. The **communication process** involves the exchange of messages and responses between two or more people. Effective communication happens when the receiver understands the message and sends **feedback**—a constructive response—to communicate to the sender that the message was received and understood (**Figure 14.5**). The communication process continues with the further exchange of messages. Two types of communication are used to send messages: verbal and nonverbal communication.

Verbal Communication

Verbal communication involves the use of words to send a spoken or written message. You use verbal communication all the time—through everyday conversation, text messages, phone calls, e-mails, social media posts, letters, and notes. For example, telling a parent or guardian you will be home at a certain time is a form of verbal communication. Sending a text message to tell your parent or guardian when you do get home is another.

Figure 14.5
The communication process involves sending a message, such as a thought, idea, feeling, or information, to another person, called the *receiver*. *What is the term for a constructive response to a communicated message?*

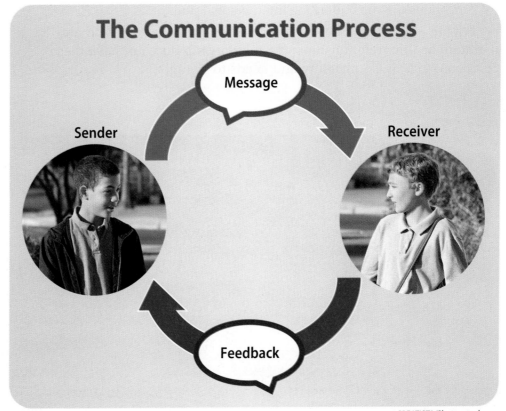

The Communication Process

Sender

Message

Receiver

Feedback

Nonverbal Communication

In many situations, communication involves more than just words. **Nonverbal communication** involves sending messages through facial expressions, body language, gestures, tone and volume of voice, and other signals that do not involve the content of words. Your nonverbal communication shows people whether you are paying attention and are interested in the conversation (**Figure 14.6**). These signals are an especially important part of showing respect for the person communicating with you.

Nonverbal communication includes the following:

- eye contact or lack of eye contact
- facial expressions, such as smiling, frowning, or eye rolling
- gestures, such as nodding, shaking the head, or moving the hands
- posture, such as leaning forward, facing away, or slumping in a chair
- tone of voice, such as encouragement, doubt, or sarcasm
- volume of voice, such as loudness showing anger or softness showing reluctance to speak
- pitch of voice, such as high-pitched excitement or low-pitched lack of interest

Ways to Communicate Effectively

In healthy relationships, people communicate their thoughts, values, and feelings. They know the other person in the relationship will listen to and support them. You can use the techniques in the next sections to communicate care, consideration, and respect for yourself and others. These techniques help ensure that people communicate clearly and effectively.

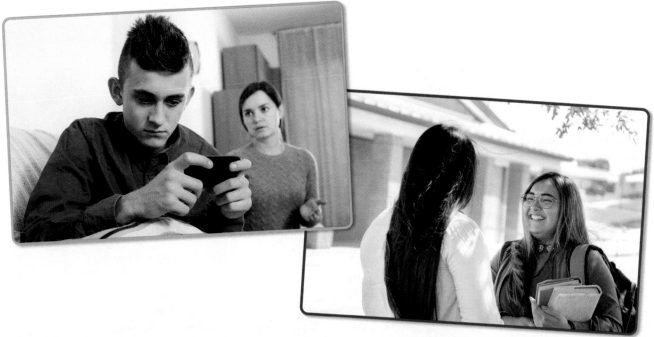

Left to right: Iakov Filimonov/Shutterstock.com; iStock.com/fstop123

Figure 14.6 In addition to the words you say, nonverbal cues can indicate either good communication or poor communication. *Which of the images shown here portrays good nonverbal communication?*

Use Active Listening

Good communication requires good listening skills. When you focus on what the other person is saying and listen, you work to understand his or her point of view and convey respect. **Active listening** is a way of paying attention to spoken messages with the goal of understanding the message and the speaker's feelings. Active listening involves the key steps shown in **Figure 14.7**.

Active listening is a great way to avoid misunderstandings. If you carefully listen to what others say, others will be more likely to do the same for you.

Clearly Express Your Needs and Preferences

To communicate effectively, people need to clearly, fully state their wants, needs, opinions, and feelings. Expecting the other person to be a mind reader is a sign of poor communication. Some people assume that others should be able to notice their subtle hints and know how they are feeling. This is a poor communication strategy. Instead, explain what you want the other person to understand.

Be Assertive

As you communicate with others, you may notice that people use different communication styles. There are three common communication styles, which include the following:

1. **Passive.** Passive communication does not clearly state needs, wants, and feelings. A passive communicator may seem to say "yes" to everything, speak very quietly, and let hurt feelings build up.

Figure 14.7
Giving the speaker your full attention and acknowledging his or her message with feedback are both important aspects to active listening. *What is a person attempting to understand with active listening?*

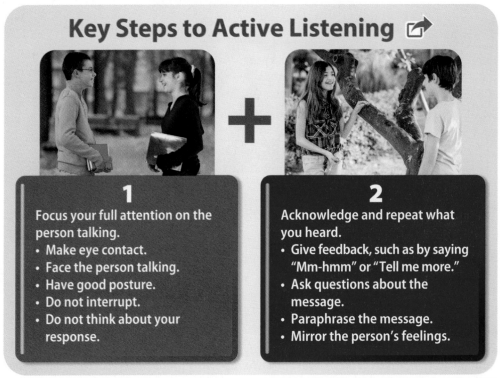

Key Steps to Active Listening

1
Focus your full attention on the person talking.
- Make eye contact.
- Face the person talking.
- Have good posture.
- Do not interrupt.
- Do not think about your response.

2
Acknowledge and repeat what you heard.
- Give feedback, such as by saying "Mm-hmm" or "Tell me more."
- Ask questions about the message.
- Paraphrase the message.
- Mirror the person's feelings.

Left to right: iStock.com/Vesnaandjic; iStock.com/Angelafoto

2. **Aggressive.** Aggressive communication makes demands of another person and insults others. A person with this communication style expresses needs and feelings in a way that disrespects others.

3. **Assertive.** Assertive communication clearly expresses feelings, needs, and goals in a way that shows respect to the other person.

BUILDING Your Skills

Be Assertive

You have probably encountered passive, aggressive, and assertive communication in your relationships and everyday life. For example, do you know people who say "yes" to activities they do not really want to do? Have you seen people get what they want by being mean and rude? Have you met some people who seem to get what they need without demanding it?

Not all of these styles are equally effective. Passive and aggressive communication can hurt your health and relationships. People with a passive style of communication often feel taken advantage of, and people with an aggressive style often have difficulty making lasting relationships. The assertive communication style is the healthiest for relationships.

Becoming more assertive can be challenging. Use the following tips to get started:

- Have good posture. Stand or sit up straight with your shoulders back and down.

- Make eye contact. Do not stare at the other person, but make sure you can tell what color his or her eyes are. Glance at the person's eyes periodically during the conversation.

- Use a strong, but not overly loud voice and say what you mean.

- Use I-statements instead of you-statements. For example, instead of saying, "You always steal my clothes," you could say, "I don't like it when you take my clothes without asking."

If being assertive does not come naturally to you, then just keep practicing. The more you use assertive communication, the more comfortable you will feel being assertive. As with most things in life, practice makes perfect.

Assert Yourself

You likely encounter plenty of opportunities to be assertive every day. For example, you can practice being assertive while talking to a teacher about a grade, disagreeing with a friend, or asking your parents or guardian for permission to go somewhere. The next time you encounter an opportunity to be assertive, practice your skills using the following steps:

1. Before starting the conversation, prepare yourself to act assertively. You could even write the word *assertive* on your hand as a reminder.

2. Remind yourself throughout the conversation to be assertive.

3. Once the conversation is over, think about how it went. Consider what you could do in the future to be even more assertive.

4. Repeat. The next time an opportunity presents itself, be assertive again.

thodonal88/Shutterstock.com

The best communication style for building healthy relationships is assertive communication. Assertive communication allows you to express how you feel and make yourself known. If you do not express your feelings and goals, you are not letting other people truly know you. Assertive communication also helps you express yourself respectfully, in a way that is understanding of others. Communicating in a way that disrespects others can hurt healthy relationships, but communicating assertively can help you build honest relationships based on trust and respect (Figure 14.8).

Use I-Statements

Effective communication uses I-statements to express feelings and desires. *I-statements* explain how the speaker feels without passing judgment on the receiver. An example of an I-statement is "I feel hurt when you ignore me in class."

Figure 14.8
The way you communicate with others—passive, aggressive, or assertive—can impact whether or not you form healthy relationships with them. *Which communication style shows respect to the other person while clearly stating feelings and needs?*

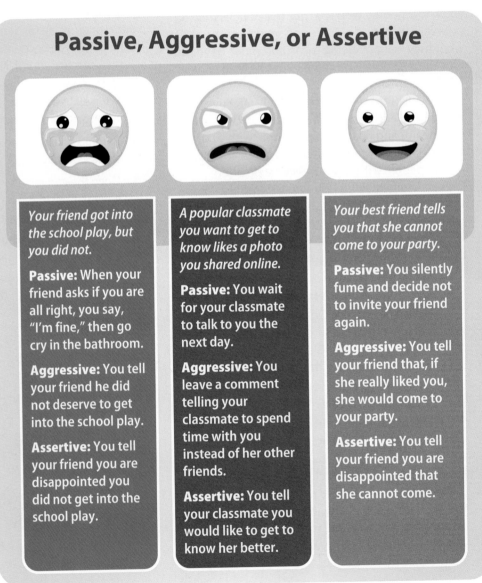

Passive, Aggressive, or Assertive

Your friend got into the school play, but you did not.

Passive: When your friend asks if you are all right, you say, "I'm fine," then go cry in the bathroom.

Aggressive: You tell your friend he did not deserve to get into the school play.

Assertive: You tell your friend you are disappointed you did not get into the school play.

A popular classmate you want to get to know likes a photo you shared online.

Passive: You wait for your classmate to talk to you the next day.

Aggressive: You leave a comment telling your classmate to spend time with you instead of her other friends.

Assertive: You tell your classmate you would like to get to know her better.

Your best friend tells you that she cannot come to your party.

Passive: You silently fume and decide not to invite your friend again.

Aggressive: You tell your friend that, if she really liked you, she would come to your party.

Assertive: You tell your friend you are disappointed that she cannot come.

Emojis: ChibVector/Shutterstock.com

This is more constructive than a you-statement, which makes assumptions about and blames the other person (for example, "You don't like me anymore"). Using I-statements to tell other people how you feel can help them understand your point of view without making them feel attacked (**Figure 14.9**).

Watch Your Nonverbal Communication

Be aware of the nonverbal messages you are sending. What messages do your facial expressions and body language communicate to others? For example, suppose you are having a conversation with your sister. As she speaks, you look down at your phone and periodically roll your eyes. These signals do not communicate active listening or respect for your sister. Making eye contact, nodding your head, and leaning forward would communicate that you value what she is saying.

Use Online Communication Wisely

Today, much communication happens online, through text messages, e-mails, or social media. You need to be careful when communicating through online messages. This type of communication lacks some of the nonverbal communication present in face-to-face contact. The shorter an online message is, the more incomplete it may be. When you use e-mails, text messages, or online posts, be sure that your message is clear and will not hurt another person. Remember that the other person is not receiving your body language or tone of voice.

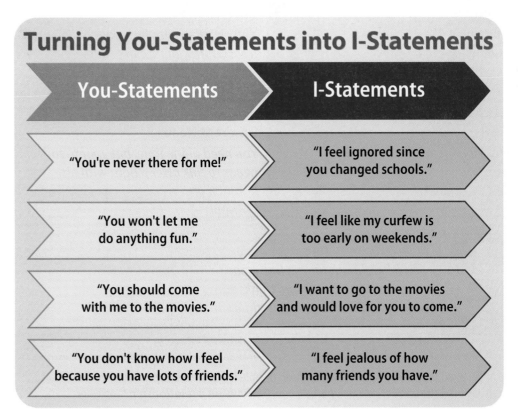

Turning You-Statements into I-Statements

You-Statements	I-Statements
"You're never there for me!"	"I feel ignored since you changed schools."
"You won't let me do anything fun."	"I feel like my curfew is too early on weekends."
"You should come with me to the movies."	"I want to go to the movies and would love for you to come."
"You don't know how I feel because you have lots of friends."	"I feel jealous of how many friends you have."

Figure 14.9
Using you-statements can make the other person feel blamed or judged, which can prevent positive communication. Instead, try to make I-statements.

Conflict Resolution Skills

Even with good communication, people can still have disagreements. These disagreements are called *conflicts* and are a normal part of life. Conflicts are present even in healthy relationships. **Figure 14.10** shows common sources of conflicts. What separates conflict in healthy relationships from conflict in unhealthy relationships is how conflict is resolved.

In disagreements of little importance, it may be best to simply accept differences between yourself and another person. There is no point arguing with a friend who does not like a food you enjoy eating, for example. Other conflicts, such as you and your friend disagreeing about which movie to see, are easy to settle with no hurt feelings. Many conflicts, however, are more complicated and are too serious to ignore.

Conflicts that are not resolved can be quite hurtful, can weaken feelings of trust, and can harm a person's mental and emotional well-being. Many people worry that addressing a conflict with another person can destroy a relationship or make conflict worse. In fact, working through a conflict can actually strengthen a relationship. The only way to settle a conflict is to address it. When people work together to resolve a conflict, they can end a hurtful situation and show their commitment to the relationship. When the conflict is settled, they can even feel closer to each other.

Common Sources of Conflict

Different Priorities
Your friend practices soccer instead of hanging out with you.

Different Values
You disagree with how your teacher treats a struggling classmate.

Different Goals
You want more independence, but your parents want to keep you safe.

Different Needs
You need alone time, but your friend needs to talk after a fight with his parents.

Misunderstandings
You tell a classmate you had a bad weekend, and your friend thinks you are complaining about your time with her.

Figure 14.10 Conflicts can arise, even in healthy relationships, when people have different priorities, values, goals, needs, or understandings of a situation. ***What effect can resolving a conflict have on a relationship?***

Negotiation

Settling a conflict requires negotiating skills. *Negotiating* is a process in which people work together (to think and talk) through a solution to a conflict. It involves preparing, keeping calm, stating your position, listening, compromising, and asking for help if needed (**Figure 14.11**).

Prepare

To prepare, agree with the other person on a time and place to discuss the situation. Meet when you both have enough time to focus on the issue. Choose a meeting place away from other people and distractions. Before the meeting, get yourself ready. Think about what you want, what reasons you have, and what the other person may want. Consider what you are willing to give up to satisfy the other person's goals.

Keep Calm

Intense feelings like frustration and anger can make a conflict worse. As a result, resolving conflict requires you to manage your emotions and share your feelings without letting them get out of control. If you feel anger building up, set that anger aside. Try taking several deep breaths or taking a break. Walk away and give yourself and the other person a chance to calm down.

State Your Position

When it is your turn to talk, state your position assertively. Speak honestly about your feelings, needs, and goals and do not behave passively or aggressively. Behaving passively can cause you to avoid the conflict and let it continue to build. Aggressive behavior can offend the other person and put him or her on the defensive. To state your position assertively, use I-statements instead of you-statements.

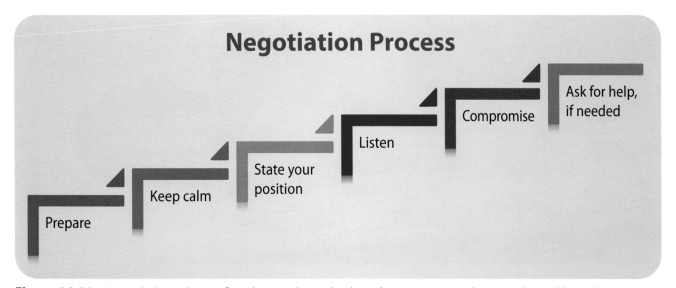

Figure 14.11 To work through a conflict, the people involved need to negotiate a solution to the problem. This involves time and effort.

Listen

Listen carefully to what the person is saying and try to understand his or her thoughts and feelings. Consider what good points the person is making and do not think about your response while the other person is talking (**Figure 14.12**). Also pay attention to the person's body language and tone of voice.

Compromise

In a *compromise*, each person gives up something he or she wants to reach a solution that is acceptable for everyone involved. For example, if you and your friends disagree about which movie to see, you could agree to see one movie this weekend and the other movie next weekend. Effective compromise is only possible if both sides are willing to be flexible.

Ask for Help

Sometimes a person is not ready to talk directly to the other person in a conflict. In that case, it might be best to talk to someone else first. Explaining the situation to an adult or another friend can help you work out how you feel and what you want. It can give you a new perspective on the problem and clarify what to do next.

Mediation

In some cases, a conflict is too serious or too difficult for the people directly involved to manage by themselves. In this situation, an outside individual can help the people or groups find a good solution.

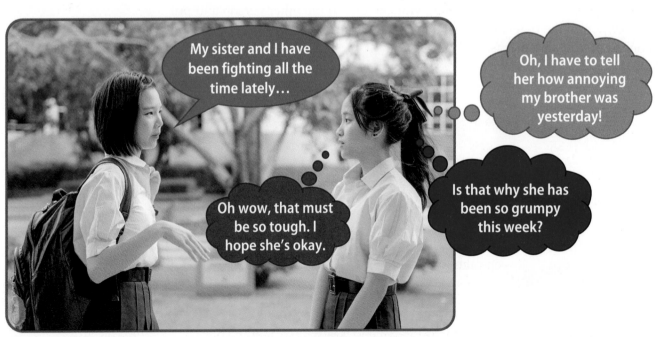

Crystal Home/Shutterstock.com

Figure 14.12 Thinking about what you want to say next and criticizing a person while he or she is speaking are examples of poor listening skills.

As you learned in Chapter 1, *mediation* is a strategy for resolving difficult conflicts by involving a neutral third party, or *mediator*. A neutral person is one who does not favor one side or another in a conflict.

Conflict resolution programs in many schools provide **peer mediation**, in which specially trained students work with other students to resolve conflicts (**Figure 14.13**). Peer mediators learn about conflicts and methods for resolving them. They work under the guidance of faculty advisors. When a conflict arises, the faculty member assigns a mediator to handle the situation. The mediator talks to the people involved in the conflict and sets up a meeting to work through a solution.

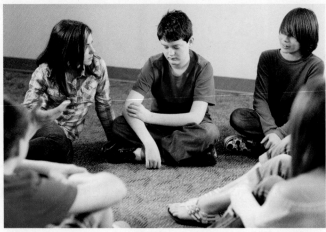

iStock.com/Alina555

Figure 14.13 In school peer mediation programs, students can help one another resolve conflicts in ways that maintain healthy relationships.

At the meeting, the mediator invites each person to state his or her view of the conflict. The mediator asks if those involved have thought of any possible solutions. If not, the mediator helps both people brainstorm possible solutions. The group discusses each alternative until both people agree on a solution.

Lesson **14.1** Review

1. What are three characteristics of a healthy relationship?
2. Which of the following is an example of nonverbal communication?

    A. E-mail. **C.** Text message.

    B. Posture. **D.** Phone call.

3. **True or false.** Active listening is thinking about your response while another person is talking.
4. What happens in a compromise?
5. **Critical thinking.** Explain why the assertive communication style is most effective for building healthy relationships.

Hands-On Activity

With a partner, review the information about I-statements in this lesson. Then, on a separate piece of paper, write five you-statements expressing negative emotions you have felt over the past year. Trade with your partner and rewrite your partner's you-statements into I-statements that would improve communication. Share the I-statements with your partner and discuss what each statement communicates.

Family Relationships

Key Terms

immediate family person's parents or guardians and siblings

socialize teaching children to behave in socially acceptable ways

traditions specific patterns of behavior passed down in a culture

rituals series of actions performed as part of a ceremony

sibling rivalry competition with a brother or sister

Learning Outcomes

After studying this lesson, you will be able to

- **analyze** the functions of the family.
- **explain** the role of community in supporting families.
- **identify** strategies to promote healthy relationships with parents or guardians and siblings.
- **describe** various changes that occur within families and ways to adjust to them.

Graphic Organizer

Healthy and Unhealthy Families

On a separate piece of paper, draw two pictures—one illustrating a healthy family and the other illustrating an unhealthy family— as in the example below. Then, as you read this lesson, organize your notes according to qualities that make families healthy and qualities that make families unhealthy. An example is provided for you.

Diversity Studio/Shutterstock.com

Healthy Family   **Unhealthy Family**

Provide for members' physical needs
Meet mental and emotional needs

Healthy and unhealthy families: Melinda Varga/Shutterstock.com

The very first relationships you had were probably with your family members. Most people spend lots of time with members of their **immediate family**, meaning their parents or guardians and siblings (**Figure 14.14**). Many people consider these family relationships to be among their closest.

For example, Kai's family has dinner together most nights, and Kai gets along well with his parents. Kai's little brother can get on his nerves, but Kai tries to walk away from the situation when he gets angry or upset. In this lesson, you will learn about different conflicts that can occur in family relationships and ways to prevent and resolve them.

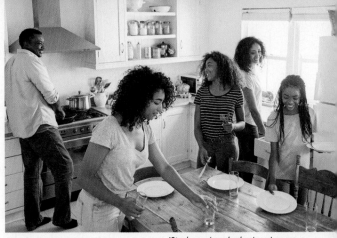

iStock.com/monkeybusinessimages

Figure 14.14 Most adolescents spend a lot of their time with immediate family, and have close relationships with their siblings and guardians.

Functions of Family Relationships

Family relationships have several unique functions that make them different from other relationships. Unlike other types of relationships, relationships in families have the responsibility of providing for members' physical needs, fulfilling members' mental and emotional needs, and educating and socializing children.

Provide for Physical Needs

Families typically provide for members' physical needs, including the needs for food, clothing, and a place to live. Families are also responsible for ensuring that members are healthy and safe (**Figure 14.15**).

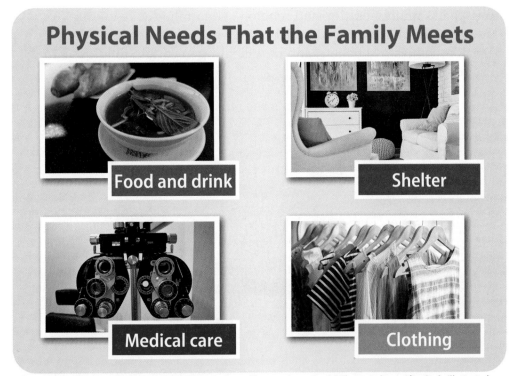

Physical Needs That the Family Meets

Food and drink

Shelter

Medical care

Clothing

Figure 14.15
It is the responsibility of your family to make sure that you have enough to eat and drink, clothes to wear, a safe place to live, and medical care.

Left to right: Dang Thach Hoang/Shutterstock.com; Photographee.eu/Shutterstock.com; Sarah P/Shutterstock.com; Africa Studio/Shutterstock.com

Your parents or guardians may take you to the doctor and dentist on a regular basis. They probably set rules—even rules you may not like—with the goal of keeping you safe and healthy.

As children grow older, they can take on tasks to help meet the family's physical needs. For example, doing some cleaning chores helps keep the home a healthy place to live. It also takes tasks away from parents or guardians who have to spend many hours a day working.

Meet Mental and Emotional Needs

Families also help meet members' mental and emotional needs, such as the needs for love, self-esteem, and emotional comfort. For example, your parents or guardians may attend your school performances and sporting events. They may celebrate your birthday and your achievements. The support and love you receive from your family members help you feel secure and good about yourself. Many people rely on their families for advice about how to solve problems or handle challenges.

Children can help meet the mental and emotional needs of adults in the family, too. When children show love for parents or guardians, those adults feel good. Children can provide words of support or encouragement when adults feel down.

Educate and Socialize Children

Families educate children by teaching them about the world and sending them to school. They also **socialize** children by teaching them to behave in socially acceptable ways (**Figure 14.16**). Children learn about culture, values, and **traditions** (specific patterns of behavior) through their families. They learn language from family members, as well as information about their families' culture and religion. All families have unique traditions, which may include celebrating special occasions, holding particular values and beliefs, and participating in certain religious **rituals**, or series of actions.

Figure 14.16
Families typically prepare their children for the outside world by teaching them lessons and sending them to school. *What are the specific patterns of behavior children learn through their families?*

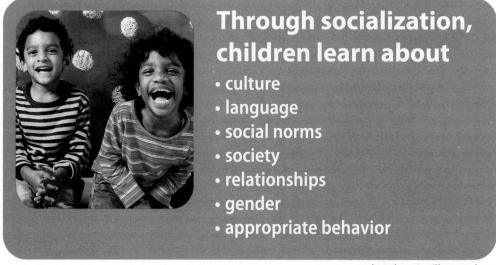

Through socialization, children learn about

- culture
- language
- social norms
- society
- relationships
- gender
- appropriate behavior

alexandre zveiger/Shutterstock.com

Families and the Community

Families live in larger social groups, or *communities*. Because of this, neighbors and even strangers can have an impact on family relationships. For example, they can give support to family members in times of trouble by providing meals when a parent is ill. Neighbors can be friends to family members and join with them in enjoyable social events.

A community is more than just a neighborhood, however. Families live in towns or cities, and these locations have institutions and services that can help families (**Figure 14.17**). State laws require that children receive certain vaccines to promote public health and prevent the spread of diseases. School officials take steps to remove students who threaten classmates, helping families meet the goal of keeping members safe.

It is important to have healthy relationships within your community. You can build healthy relationships in your community by treating other people with respect, being open and honest about what you think and feel, and being reliable and trustworthy.

Relationships with Parents or Guardians

Family relationships are some of the most important relationships you will have in your life. These relationships, however, can be difficult at times. For example, many children experience some conflict in their relationships with parents, guardians, or other caregivers. These conflicts can get worse as children grow older. Identifying common problems in these relationships and using certain strategies can help strengthen the relationship between caregivers and young people.

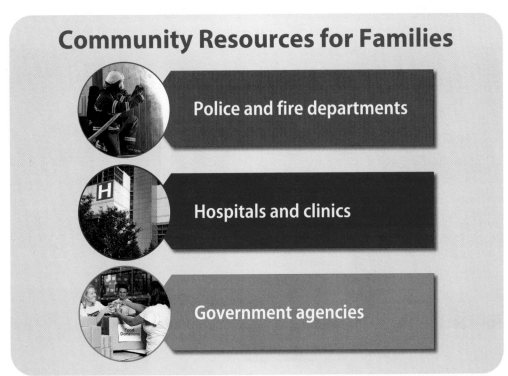

Community Resources for Families

Police and fire departments

Hospitals and clinics

Government agencies

Top to bottom: urbans/Shutterstock.com; Pete Spiro/Shutterstock.com; Monkey Business Images/Shutterstock.com

Figure 14.17
Police officers and firefighters protect people. Hospitals and clinics provide healthcare. Government agencies offer services to help families struggling economically.

Common Problems in Relationships with Parents or Guardians

Many problems between parents or guardians and young people result from conflicting goals. For example, one major goal young people have is to form a unique identity apart from family. Adolescence is a time of self-exploration. During this time, young people naturally push for more freedom, independence, and responsibility (**Figure 14.18**).

At the same time, parents' goals include keeping young people safe and healthy and teaching them how to function well in society. To do this, parents set rules that young people might find restrictive, or limiting. This is one reason why conflicts between parents and young people often escalate during adolescence.

Conflicts between parents and young people may also develop as a result of media influences like television and movies. Young people may see messages about living in families that conflict with the traditions or customs of their own families. These differences can be a source of conflict.

Maintaining Healthy Relationships with Parents or Guardians

Maintaining healthy relationships with parents or guardians takes effort. Fortunately, the following strategies for having healthy relationships and resolving conflicts with parents or guardians can help:

- Share your plans ahead of time. Make sure to get approval before you commit to do something with a friend. Answer any questions parents or guardians may have and revise the plan, if needed.
- Discuss family rules. If you disagree with a rule, calmly explain why you think the rule should change and give reasons for your suggested change (**Figure 14.19**). Your parents or guardian may agree to reconsider the rule.

Figure 14.18
During adolescence, young people want more independence, freedom, and responsibility, which can cause arguments with guardians or parents. *What type of identity do young people want to form during adolescence?*

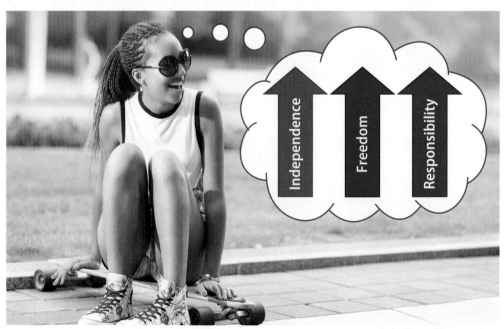

Dmitry Morgan/Shutterstock.com

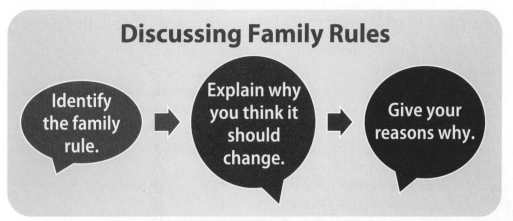

Discussing Family Rules

Identify the family rule. → **Explain why you think it should change.** → **Give your reasons why.**

Figure 14.19
If you think a family rule is unfair or unnecessary, the best response is to calmly discuss a possible change with your parent or guardian.

- Follow your family's rules, even if you disagree with them. Remember that parents and guardians may relax or lift these rules if you show responsible behavior and a willingness to obey limits. On the other hand, if you do not follow the rules, you may weaken your family's trust in you.
- Remain calm. When you have a disagreement, do not resort to yelling and do not walk away. Show your parents or guardians that you are capable of having a mature discussion and that you can be responsible.
- Spend time doing enjoyable activities with your family. You might suggest having a special family dinner one night a week or planning an outing. These types of activities can bring families together.

Relationships with Siblings

Sibling relationships are often the earliest friendships people have. Many siblings often fight and argue, however. Keeping these relationships healthy can lead to greater satisfaction as you grow older.

Common Problems in Sibling Relationships

Even siblings who are biologically related or who grow up in the same household may not share interests. Siblings may have different personalities, find different activities interesting, or have different ways of handling major life events (**Figure 14.20**). These differences can create conflict, especially when people spend a lot of time together.

Another source of problems among siblings is competition, which is called **sibling rivalry**. Examples of sibling rivalry include competing for a parent's attention or fighting over use of the television. When teasing is involved, feelings of competition may increase. Sibling rivalry may lead to negative feelings, such as resentment, anger, or jealousy.

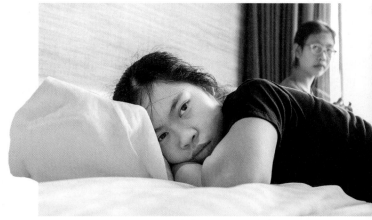

Chalermpon Poungpeth/Shutterstock.com

Figure 14.20 Siblings spend a lot of time together, which creates many opportunities for conflict since no two people are the same. *What is it called when siblings compete for material and nonmaterial items?*

Maintaining Healthy Relationships with Siblings

Effective strategies for keeping sibling relationships healthy include the following:

- Get away from tense situations and cool down. By taking a break from a heated situation, you will avoid making the argument worse.
- Express how you feel to your sibling. Communication is the first step in resolving conflict. Try to work with your sibling to find solutions to your disagreement, and show respect for your sibling's ideas.
- Talk to your parents or guardian about the conflict and see if they have advice for finding a good solution.
- Compromise when issues arise. Try to work out a solution that both you and your sibling think is fair (**Figure 14.21**). Together, you can develop specific rules for handling ongoing sources of conflict.
- Identify a personal space for each person. For example, if you share a bedroom with a sibling, talk to him or her about setting aside areas for each of you.
- Respect your sibling's space and privacy. Do not enter a sibling's room without knocking. If you share a room, respect your sibling's private space within that room.
- Find enjoyable ways of spending time with your sibling. This could include going for a bike ride or having a family game night.

Figure 14.21
When you disagree with a sibling, working out a solution that is fair to both parties can stop the disagreement before it causes a fight.

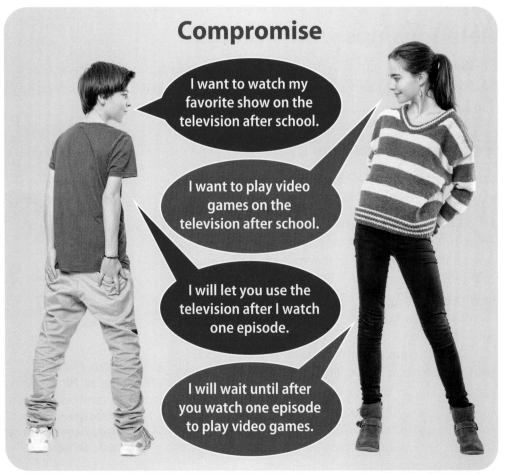

Armin Staudt/Shutterstock.com

Changes in Family Relationships

All families encounter changes over time. For example, a member may have a physical or mental illness, lose a job, or move to a new community. Change can create stress in a family and disrupt family relationships. These changes are a normal, although difficult, part of family life (**Figure 14.22**).

As you have read, even positive changes—such as a job promotion or starting middle school—can create stress. This is because new events lead to changes in how family members interact every day. For example, suppose a parent gets a big promotion at work. This may mean that the parent must work longer hours or travel more. Other family members may need to take on additional chores at home. Similarly, when a child starts attending middle school, family schedules may change to adjust to new school hours or travel times. Middle school students often have more homework than younger students. This can affect mental health and impact the whole family.

Some of the most challenging changes families experience are those that affect family structure—the addition or loss of a family member. These changes include the birth or adoption of a new family member, separation or divorce, remarriage, and the death of a family member. Although these events can be difficult, healthy families can work through them together. Sometimes, families even grow closer when dealing with changes such as these. Using good communication skills and effective strategies for maintaining family relationships will help members get through these challenging periods.

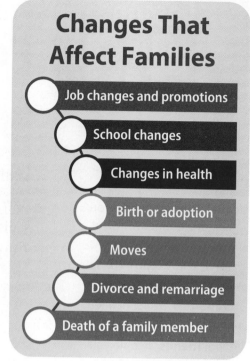

Changes That Affect Families

- Job changes and promotions
- School changes
- Changes in health
- Birth or adoption
- Moves
- Divorce and remarriage
- Death of a family member

Figure 14.22 Both positive and negative changes affect all families, and both can cause stress to the family members.

Lesson 14.2 Review 🔁

1. Name three unique functions that make family relationships different from other relationships.

2. **True or false.** Neighbors and strangers can influence family relationships.

3. If you disagree with a family rule, what should you do?

4. What is sibling rivalry?

5. **Critical thinking.** Why do even positive changes in families cause stress?

Hands-On Activity

Over several days, become an observer of your family's interactions. Pay attention to any signs of the conflicts discussed in this chapter and note how your family resolves these conflicts. Write a summary of your observations and then draw conclusions about your family's relationships. Identify healthy and unhealthy characteristics in your family's interactions. For each unhealthy characteristic, describe what you can do to make your family relationships healthier.

Peer Relationships

 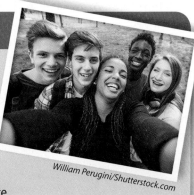
Learning Outcomes

After studying this lesson, you will be able to

- **distinguish between** different types of friendships.
- **explain** how to promote tolerance and celebrate diversity in relationships.
- **devise** a plan to use strategies for building and maintaining healthy friendships.
- **evaluate** common issues in friendships.
- **differentiate between** positive and negative types of peer pressure.

Graphic Organizer

Friendship Inventory

Take an inventory of your friendships by listing your closest peer relationships in the middle column of a table like the one shown below. As you read this lesson, identify each type of friendship and record the information after the person's name. In the left-hand column, write factors that could harm your friendships. In the right-hand column, write strategies for keeping your friendships healthy.

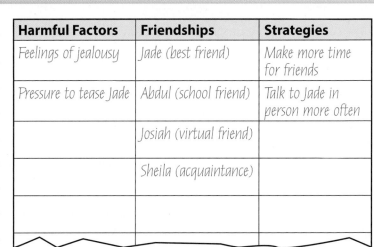

William Perugini/Shutterstock.com

Harmful Factors	Friendships	Strategies
Feelings of jealousy	Jade (best friend)	Make more time for friends
Pressure to tease Jade	Abdul (school friend)	Talk to Jade in person more often
	Josiah (virtual friend)	
	Sheila (acquaintance)	

Peer relationships are some of the most important relationships in your life. Close peer relationships, called *friendships*, develop because of mutual respect, care, trust, and affection. Friendships are especially important during adolescence, when relationships with peers can become the center of your world. As an example, consider Kai from the previous lessons. Kai loves talking with his friends. He spends a lot of time online joking with his classmates on social media. He has a best friend named Jacqueline, and they like to play soccer and video games. He avoids cliques because he would prefer to be friends and get along with everyone.

Types of Friendships

The most common type of peer relationship is friendship. The term *friendship* can include many different types of relationships (**Figure 14.23**). For example, you probably know the difference between your very closest friends and your more casual friends. Perhaps you have a single friend whom you consider your best friend. You may also have many **acquaintances**—people you know and interact with, but may not consider friends.

Living in a diverse culture, you are likely to meet people who see the world differently than you do. **Diversity** is present in a group of people with different backgrounds, including ages, genders, family traditions, ethnicities, and cultures.

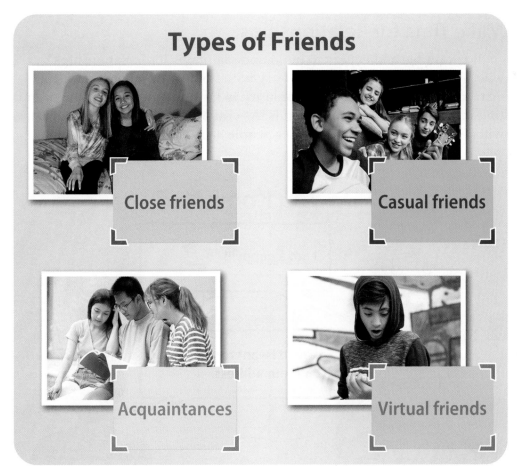

Types of Friends

Close friends

Casual friends

Acquaintances

Virtual friends

Figure 14.23
There are many different types of peer relationships that can all be considered friendships. *What is it called when you have a friendship with someone who has a different background than you?*

Left to right: May Hayward/Shutterstock.com; LightField Studios/Shutterstock.com; NiP photography/Shutterstock.com; HBRH/Shutterstock.com

Diverse groups include people with different gender identities and sexual orientations as well. In healthy relationships, people respect others for who they are. They celebrate differences and avoid making assumptions based on **stereotypes**, or oversimplified ideas about a group of people. Diversity in a culture can broaden people's knowledge. Ideally, people challenge and learn from others, while respecting others' values.

In the past, most people had friends who lived in their neighborhood or city. Today, however, many people have friends who live farther away. You may have **virtual friends**, or people you meet through social media, websites, chat rooms, or gaming. True friendships can sometimes develop between virtual friends, particularly if friends share some real-life friends. You should be careful, however, about sharing information with people you have only met online (**Figure 14.24**). These people might not be representing themselves truthfully. If a virtual friend offers to meet you in person, talk about the situation with a trusted adult before agreeing to meet.

Strategies for Building Healthy Friendships

It can be hard to make friends, and arguing with friends is not unusual. Determining whether someone shares your core values and beliefs can take time, especially if you are still trying to figure out what your values and beliefs are. Even when arguments arise, however, there are ways to maintain healthy friendships over time.

Make Time for Relationships

It takes time and energy to build and maintain close relationships with friends. Even when you are busy with homework, sports, or other extracurricular activities, you should try to find time to connect and spend time with acquaintances and friends. As you build new friendships, you will need time to get to know other people and understand how their

Figure 14.24
You can form meaningful relationships online, but you should keep in mind that you cannot truly know who you are talking to. *What is the term for people you meet online and do not interact face-to-face?*

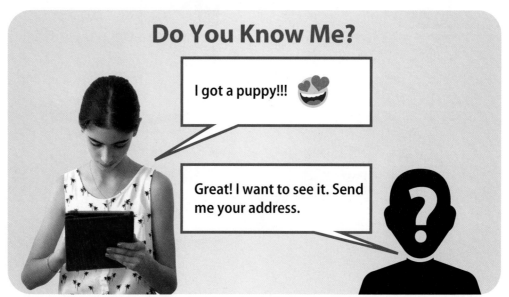

Left: Ramazan Ece/Shutterstock.com; Emoji: Dmytro Onopko/Shutterstock.com; Right: Best Vector Elements/Shutterstock.com

values and beliefs align with yours. If you want to get to know someone, you could try spending time in a group, doing an activity together, or talking throughout the day.

Step Away from the Screen

Online communication is a great way to connect with friends and get to know people. The best relationships, however, are formed and maintained through face-to-face interactions. In-person communication is an important part of having a close relationship. Make sure not to rely too much on virtual interaction, which lacks important aspects of nonverbal communication (**Figure 14.25**). One of the best ways to keep a relationship strong is to step away from the screen and make time to be physically present with someone.

Be a Good Friend

Healthy friendships are mutual, meaning that each person contributes equally to the relationship. You can be a good friend by listening carefully to what your friends are saying. Also, avoid interrupting, judging, or criticizing them when they are talking. Other strategies you can use to keep your friendships strong include the following:

- Support and encourage your friends, and celebrate their successes.
- Avoid teasing or criticizing your friends.
- Do not gossip or spread rumors about your friends. Spreading unkind words about your friends or acquaintances is hurtful and just makes others feel bad.
- Work with your friends to solve disagreements and problems.
- Express your feelings openly during conflicts, and listen carefully to your friend's point of view.
- Apologize if you hurt your friend, and try to find ways to make it better.

Figure 14.25
Online communication lacks nonverbal cues. It is difficult for the reader to tell how the person sending a text message feels. The person receiving the message cannot read the body language of the speaker, like the hunched shoulders and frown of the boy in the photo.

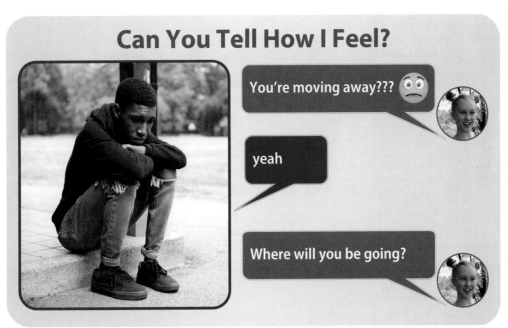

Left: iStock.com/Flamingo_Photography; Right: Tanya Po/Shutterstock.com; Emoji: 32 pixels/Shutterstock.com

Damage Control: The Negative Effects of Gossip and Rumors

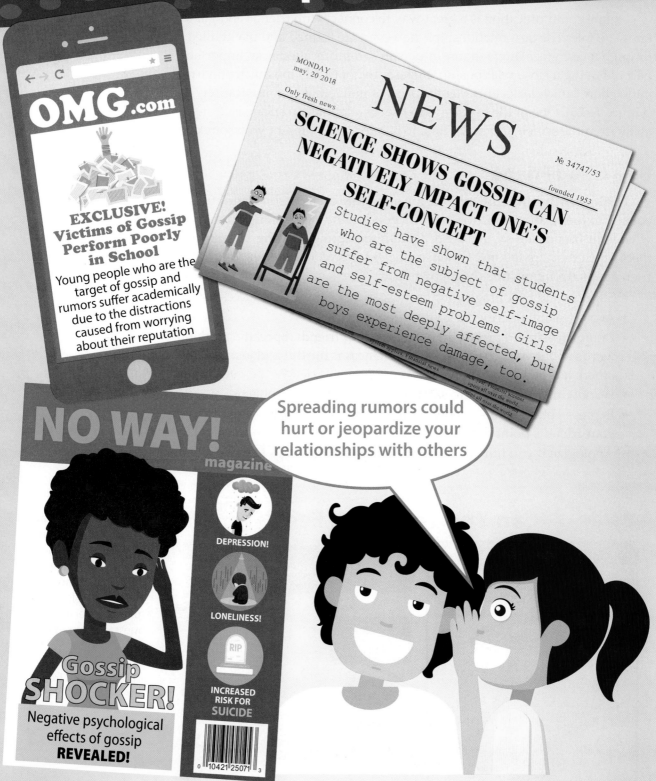

Common Problems in Friendships

Although friendships can improve your life in many ways, they can also be a source of problems. At times, even close friendships can be complicated and confusing. Cliques, jealousy, and changes over time are common problems in friendships.

Cliques

Many middle school students enjoy spending time with groups of friends. Sometimes, groups of friends exclude other people from that group, which can lead to hurt feelings (**Figure 14.26**). A **clique** is a small group of friends who deliberately exclude other people from joining or being a part of their group.

People who are part of a clique often feel pressured to act a certain way. They may feel pressured to fit in, dress a certain way, listen to a particular style of music, or adopt the attitudes and behaviors of group members. Sometimes, cliques can also pressure group members to act in ways that endanger their health and wellness. For example, a group may encourage cigarette smoking. In this way, cliques can reduce each person's individuality and compromise well-being, which is unhealthy.

Jealousy

Jealousy may sometimes occur in a friendship. You may feel jealous of your friend's achievement in a particular area, such as schoolwork, athletics, or music. You may also feel jealous of other aspects of a friend's life, such as his or her home, dating relationship, or family life. Feelings of jealousy are normal if they occur once in a while. Continuous jealous feelings, however, can harm a relationship over time.

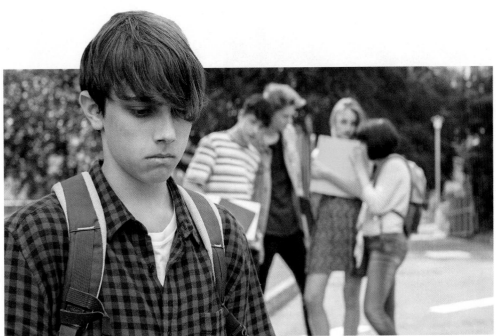

Daisy Daisy/Shutterstock.com

Figure 14.26
Purposefully excluding people from a group of friends is often considered a form of bullying and can be very hurtful. *What is the name of a group of friends who deliberately exclude others?*

Honestly expressing your emotions, including jealousy, can prevent negative feelings from building up over time and weakening your friendship. If you value your friendship and want to keep it, try to move beyond feelings of jealousy.

Changes over Time

Experiencing physical, emotional, and social changes can influence your friendships (**Figure 14.27**). This is particularly true if you and a friend change in different ways. You may no longer share the same interests with your childhood friends. You may need to stop spending time with a friend who makes unsafe or unhealthy decisions.

Sometimes, old friendships can be maintained, but change in some way. For example, you might see an old friend less frequently as your interests and peer groups change. You might find that you prefer spending time with different people if you feel less close with and less connected to your old friends.

Figure 14.27
If one friend changes physically, emotionally, or socially at a different rate or in a different way than another friend, distance between the two people can result.

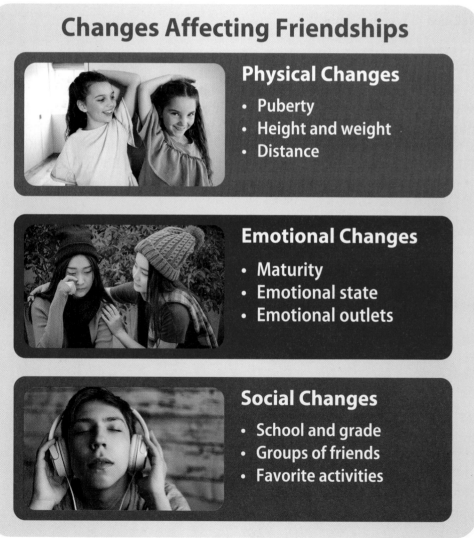

Changes Affecting Friendships

Physical Changes
- Puberty
- Height and weight
- Distance

Emotional Changes
- Maturity
- Emotional state
- Emotional outlets

Social Changes
- School and grade
- Groups of friends
- Favorite activities

Top to bottom: Monkey Business Images/Shutterstock.com; AppleZoomZoom/Shutterstock.com; Liyba Dozz/Shutterstock.com

If you feel that you and a friend are drifting apart, tell your friend how you feel. If both of you are interested in maintaining the friendship, you can work together to find ways of remaining close.

Peer Pressure

Peer pressure is a common element present in friendships. *Peer pressure* is the influence a person feels from *peers*, or people of the same age, to act or think in particular ways. Peer pressure can be positive or negative.

Positive Peer Pressure

Although people often associate peer pressure with negative activities, peer pressure can have a positive influence (**Figure 14.28**). For example, you might feel pressured to participate in community service projects with a school group or athletic team. A friend may encourage you to study harder and improve your grade in a class. In these cases, pressure from peers can help broaden your perspective of the world, help your community, or help you succeed in a certain class.

Negative Peer Pressure

In some friendships, one person pressures another to do something he or she is not comfortable doing. Friends might pressure each other to drink alcohol, skip class, or tease a classmate to fit in with a group of friends. Most people want to be liked and to fit in with a group. They may decide to go along with a certain behavior, even if they are uncomfortable with it. They may worry about being teased or excluded if they do not join in a group activity. Sometimes, young people worry that standing up for what they believe could cause them to lose a friendship.

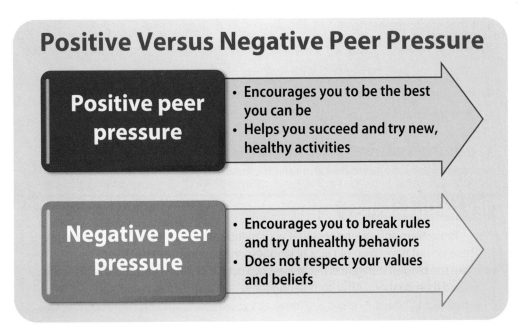

Positive Versus Negative Peer Pressure

Positive peer pressure
- Encourages you to be the best you can be
- Helps you succeed and try new, healthy activities

Negative peer pressure
- Encourages you to break rules and try unhealthy behaviors
- Does not respect your values and beliefs

Figure 14.28
Peer pressure may include encouragement of risky behaviors, but it can also include support for healthy activities.

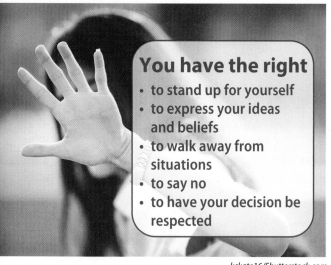

You have the right

- to stand up for yourself
- to express your ideas and beliefs
- to walk away from situations
- to say no
- to have your decision be respected

kckate16/Shutterstock.com

Figure 14.29 If a person is trying to pressure you into risky behaviors, this person is not truly your friend because he or she does not have your health and wellness at heart.

In healthy friendships, this type of negative peer pressure does not occur. True friends respect each other's choices. If you are experiencing negative peer pressure, you have the right to stand up for what you believe, and to walk away from situations that make you uncomfortable (**Figure 14.29**). If a friend ends a relationship with you over this choice, he or she does not respect you and your friendship. Standing up to peer pressure is especially important when friends are doing something that could hurt you or someone else.

What can you do to stand up to peer pressure? Strategies you can use to respond to negative peer pressure include the following:

- Focus on your own thoughts, feelings, and values, and use a good decision-making process to make sure your actions reflect your core beliefs.
- Have the strength and self-confidence to walk away from a situation or from people who make you uncomfortable.
- Refuse to join in teasing a person because he or she acts or looks different.
- Choose friends who have values similar to yours. People who share your values, goals, and beliefs will probably support the decisions you make.
- Support other people when they resist peer pressure. Sometimes, having just one other person say, "I agree, this is a bad idea," is all it takes to change a group's behavior.
- If peer pressure continues over time, talk to someone you trust—a parent or guardian, teacher, or guidance counselor.

Lesson 14.3 Review

1. What are acquaintances?
2. **True or false.** One way to be a good friend is to celebrate your friend's successes.
3. What is the best way to deal with jealousy in a friendship?
4. Pressure to _____ is an example of positive peer pressure.
   A. tease your friend
   B. smoke cigarettes
   C. skip class
   D. study for a big exam
5. **Critical thinking.** Why do you think face-to-face interactions are better than online interactions for building relationships?

Hands-On Activity

Brainstorm acts of kindness that your friends and peers would enjoy receiving. These do not have to be big acts of kindness. In relationships, little things can make the biggest difference. List at least five acts of kindness you could realistically do and then do them. After completing these acts, write a few paragraphs summarizing how they positively impacted your friendships and peer relationships.

Dating Relationships

Learning Outcomes

After studying this lesson, you will be able to

- **describe** the characteristics of a healthy dating relationship.
- **identify** strategies to set boundaries for physical intimacy before and during a dating relationship.
- **follow** strategies for forming a healthy dating relationship.
- **describe** ways to handle the end of a dating relationship.

Key Terms 🖝

casual dating way of getting to know how you interact with and feel about another person

infatuation intense romantic feelings for another person that develop suddenly and are usually based on physical attraction

passion powerful feeling based on physical attraction

exclusive committed to being romantically involved with only one dating partner

intimacy closeness

group dating going out with a group that includes the person one is interested in rather than dating as a couple

Graphic Organizer 🖝

Dating Need-to-Know

On a separate piece of paper, draw a heart like in the example below. Skim this lesson and write the main headings in a circle around the heart. As you read the lesson, take notes under each heading. Then, identify the five most important facts you learned in this lesson and write them in the middle of the heart.

Rawpixel.com/Shutterstock.com

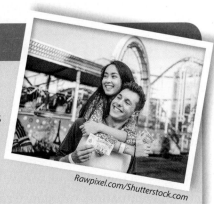

Characteristics of Healthy Dating Relationships
- *Attraction—infatuation without closeness*
- *Closeness*

1.
2.
3.
4.
5.

The End of a Dating Relationship

Strategies for Forming Healthy Dating Relationships

Heart: popular business/Shutterstock.com

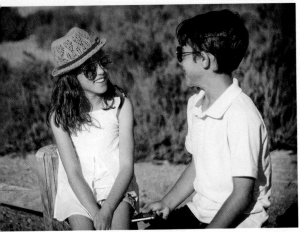

Nadia Cruzova/Shutterstock.com

Figure 14.30 Adolescents can slowly get to know one another on an individual basis without committing to a full dating relationship. *What is this informal version of dating called?*

Dating relationships are a new type of relationship for many young people. The decision to begin dating is personal, and different people feel ready to begin dating at different times. Some young people are interested in and ready for dating earlier than their peers. These people may feel attracted to a person in a romantic way and decide to act on those feelings. Other young people may not yet feel this type of attraction for someone else. Some families may have rules that limit or forbid dating until a certain age.

Remember that Kai, from the previous lessons, has a girl he likes in his class. Kai does not feel comfortable having a girlfriend yet, so his friends suggest that they go on a group date with a few other kids in his class. Kai feels like he can relax and get to know the girl he likes better in this setting.

Like Kai and the girl in his class, a couple can go out on a date without being in a dating relationship. **Casual dating** is a way of getting to know how you interact with and feel about another person (**Figure 14.30**). It can help you learn more about yourself. A *dating relationship* exists when two people date on a regular basis.

Characteristics of Healthy Dating Relationships

All types of healthy relationships share similar qualities, such as honesty and trust, mutual respect, and care and commitment. Healthy dating relationships also have the following qualities:

- **Attraction.** Attraction refers to the physical and emotional connection that draws people together. Being attracted to someone means it is exciting to be with that person. Attraction without closeness is sometimes **infatuation**, or intense romantic feelings that develop suddenly and are usually based on physical attraction.
- **Closeness.** Closeness arises because two people share personal feelings and thoughts that they do not share with others.
- **Individuality.** In healthy dating relationships, each person maintains his or her own unique identity. The relationship does not redefine a person. Each person's core values, beliefs, and sense of self remain the same.
- **Balance.** People in a healthy dating relationship see each other regularly, but make time for friends and family members. In a healthy dating relationship, people also share time and activities equally and fairly.
- **Open communication, honesty, and respect.** Both people in a relationship should feel comfortable expressing their likes, dislikes, goals, values, and thoughts (**Figure 14.31**). In a healthy dating relationship, the couple can discuss these topics openly, honestly, and with respect.
- **Support.** In a healthy dating relationship, both people should support each other's successes, happiness, talents, interests, and goals.
- **Safety.** In healthy dating relationships, each person feels safe with the other person. Each person respects the other's personal boundaries and cares for his or her well-being.

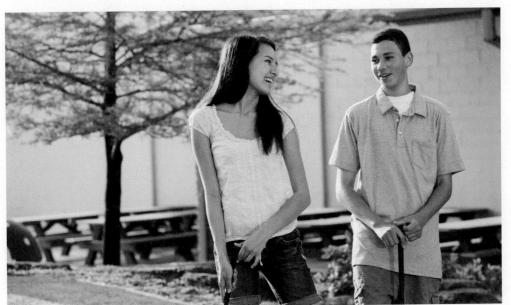

Over time, a couple in a dating relationship may develop feelings of love. Feelings of *love* describe an intense affection for and attachment to another person. Love develops gradually as people get to know each other deeply and should not be confused with feelings of passion. **Passion** can be very powerful and exciting, but is typically short-lived because it is based in physical attraction.

As love develops, commitment should become part of a healthy dating relationship. Commitment means promising to be **exclusive**, or romantically involved with only one dating partner. Commitment also means that you agree to work at maintaining the relationship.

Physical Intimacy and Abstinence

Dating relationships often include some type of physical **intimacy**, or closeness, such as holding hands and kissing. Before you start dating, you should know how you feel about being physically intimate with another person. It is better to know your limits and boundaries before you are in a situation that requires a quick decision. Be sure to enforce these personal boundaries during the relationship.

Many factors, including your values, religion, and judgment, will influence decisions you make about physical intimacy. *Abstinence*, or the commitment to refrain from sexual activity, is the healthiest decision for young people. Abstinence is the only method that is 100 percent effective in preventing sexually transmitted infections, HIV/AIDS, and pregnancy (Figure 14.32). It also prevents emotional consequences such as anxiety over a partner leaving and guilt over keeping sexual activity a secret. Finally, it avoids social consequences related to being exclusive.

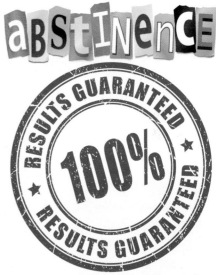

Figure 14.32 Abstinence is the best decision for young people who want to maintain good physical, mental, emotional, and social health. It prevents many health consequences, including STIs and pregnancy. *Identify three factors that can influence decisions you make about physical intimacy.*

As with physical intimacy, you should consider your own boundaries related to abstinence before starting a dating relationship. When you start dating, communicate these boundaries and stick to them (**Figure 14.33**). In a healthy dating relationship, you will not feel pressured by your partner to engage in physically intimate or sexual behavior that does not feel comfortable. Keep in mind that abstinence is a choice that will affect not just your present, but also your future. It is possible to maintain a rewarding, fun, healthy romantic relationship without engaging in sexual activity.

Strategies for Forming Healthy Dating Relationships

If you are interested in having a romantic relationship, you should take steps to ensure it is healthy. Strategies you can use for forming a healthy relationship include the following:

- Get to know the person you might want to date before dating. Talk to this person at school, during an activity, or on the phone before going out with him or her. This will help you figure out if you share common interests.
- Go out with a group that includes the person in whom you are interested. This **group dating** is a good way to get to know a possible dating partner. Being with a group reduces the pressure of having to keep a conversation going with someone you are just getting to know. Group dating is also a good way to stay safe, especially if you do not know the person very well.
- Find ways to cope with your nerves. You may feel nervous about talking to or meeting with the person you may want to date. These feelings are normal. In fact, the other person will probably be nervous, too. If talking makes you nervous, plan activities that do not require much conversation, such as seeing a movie, playing miniature golf or bowling, or going to a school dance.

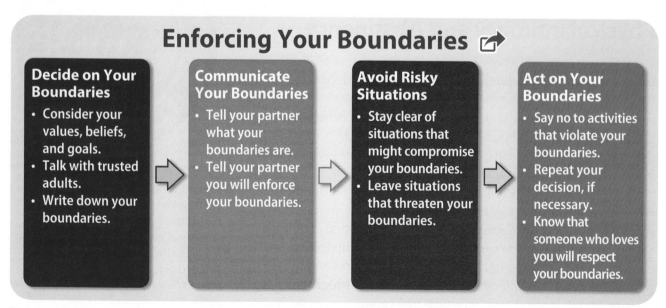

Figure 14.33 It is important to formally decide what your boundaries are before you are confronted with a risky situation because you will be more prepared to enforce these boundaries.

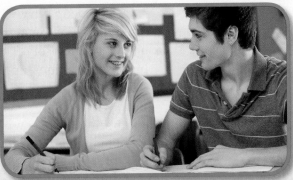

Monkey Business Images/Shutterstock.com

Travis's First Date?

Today, Travis was asked by Casey to go on a date. Travis finds Casey attractive, both in her physical appearance and personality. Travis and Casey have been in some classes together and have some mutual friends, but they did not know each other before this year. Travis is definitely interested in getting to know Casey better.

Travis's older sister has a boyfriend and seems happy about it, but Travis is not sure if he is ready for a dating relationship. Travis participates in many extracurricular activities and is still trying to make friends at his school and in his community. He worries that having a dating relationship with Casey will keep him from making more friends. Travis is not 100 percent sure how his parents would feel about him dating at his age, but he thinks they would accept it. According to Travis's classmates, Casey is very interested in having a dating relationship with Travis.

Thinking Critically

1. What factors are influencing Travis's decision to go out with Casey? Which of these factors are internal and which are external?

2. What information do you think Travis should gather before trying to make this decision? How should he go about gathering this information?

3. Imagine that Travis ultimately decides not to go out with Casey. Write a script for a healthy, realistic conversation in which Travis tells Casey about his decision.

4. Why do you think it is sometimes difficult for young people to say "no" to activities their peers want them to do?

The End of a Dating Relationship

Many dating relationships between young people eventually end. These relationships often do not last long, partly because the partners' goals and beliefs are still forming and changing during these years as partners try to figure out their own identities. These changes can lead to one partner realizing that the relationship no longer works for him or her.

Breakups can be emotionally painful, especially for the person who does not want to end the relationship. It is important, however, to recognize when a relationship is not working. Someone ready to end a relationship should talk to the other person honestly—and with understanding. It is not fair to the other person to string him or her along.

No matter how a relationship ends, both people involved will probably find it difficult to cope. When a relationship ends, people commonly feel sad, angry, lonely, and even physically ill. These feelings are a normal reaction to the end of a relationship and will heal over time.

Some people try to cope with the loss of a dating relationship by quickly beginning a new relationship. By doing this, however, they do not allow themselves time to process their feelings about the end of their previous relationship. Some of these feelings can spill over into the new relationship, which is unfair to new dating partners. New partners deserve to be with someone who is focusing on the new relationship rather than continuing to cope with the loss of a past relationship.

Moving quickly into a new relationship also does not give a person enough time to think about why the previous one did not work. Trying to understand that can help a person see if he or she needs to act differently in the next relationship.

Lesson 14.4 Review

1. What is the difference between casual dating and a dating relationship?
2. Which of the following is characteristic of a healthy dating relationship?
   A. Pressure.
   B. Individuality.
   C. Infatuation.
   D. Teasing.
3. **True or false.** Group dating can make it easier to get to know someone you do not know well.
4. Why do many dating relationships among young people eventually end?
5. **Critical thinking.** How does abstinence prevent the negative physical, emotional, and social consequences of early sexual activity?

Hands-On Activity

Even if dating is still years away for you, it is a good idea to think about what your rights and responsibilities in a dating relationship might be. For this activity, imagine that you are in a dating relationship. Complete the table below using what you learned in this lesson, your experiences, and your opinions. Reach out to trusted adults who have experience in healthy dating relationships to help you complete the table. Do you believe dating partners should have a conversation about the information contained in this table? If so, when and how should they discuss? If not, why not?

My rights in the relationship	
My responsibilities in the relationship	
My partner's rights in the relationship	
My partner's responsibilities in the relationship	

Summary

Lesson 14.1 **What Is a Healthy Relationship?**

- Relationships affect a person's health and well-being. Some relationships meet basic human needs. Relationships also meet the need to feel connected and loved.
- Healthy relationships are characterized by honesty, trust, mutual respect, care and commitment, emotional control, understanding, and good interpersonal skills.
- You can communicate effectively by using active listening, clearly expressing yourself, being assertive, using I-statements, watching your nonverbal communication, and using online communication wisely.
- Conflict is normal, even in healthy relationships. Good conflict resolution involves the negotiation process. Some schools offer peer mediation to help with this.

Lesson 14.2 **Family Relationships**

- Family relationships serve the unique functions of providing for physical needs, meeting mental and emotional needs, and educating and socializing children.
- Communities offer many resources to help families fulfill their functions.
- Good communication and conflict resolution skills can help you maintain healthy relationships with parents or guardians.
- Siblings often experience rivalry. Strategies of good communication and conflict resolution can help you maintain healthy relationships with siblings.

Lesson 14.3 **Peer Relationships**

- Friendships include close friends, casual friends, acquaintances, and virtual friends. Celebrating diversity will help you strengthen your friendships.
- Strategies for building healthy friendships include making time for relationships, stepping away from the screen, and being a good friend.
- Common problems in friendships include cliques, jealousy, and changes over time.
- Peer pressure can be positive or negative. If you encounter negative peer pressure, you can stand up to it and stick to your own beliefs and values.

Lesson 14.4 **Dating Relationships**

- Healthy dating relationships have the characteristics of attraction; closeness; individuality; balance; open communication, honesty, and respect; support; and safety.
- Before a dating relationship, you need to consider your boundaries regarding physical intimacy. Sexual abstinence is the best choice for young people in dating relationships.
- Strategies for forming healthy dating relationships include getting to know people, dating in groups, and coping with nerves.
- The end of a dating relationship is difficult for both partners. Usually, people need time to heal and examine the past relationship.

Check Your Knowledge ↗

Record your answers to each of the following questions on a separate sheet of paper.

1. What are the characteristics of a healthy relationship?
2. **True or false.** Effective communication uses you-statements to express feelings.
3. Which of the following is a good skill for conflict resolution?
   A. Behave passively.
   B. Interrupt the other person.
   C. Keep calm.
   D. Insist on your way.
4. What does it mean to socialize children?
5. Explain why parents or guardians and young people often have conflicts during adolescence.
6. Which of the following strategies would help maintain a healthy relationship with a sibling?
   A. Avoid your sibling.
   B. Do not tell your parent or guardian.
   C. Refuse to leave a heated situation.
   D. Identify a personal space for each person.
7. **True or false.** Apologizing if you hurt your friend will help keep your friendship strong.
8. What is a clique?
9. Which of the following is a good strategy for resisting negative peer pressure?
   A. Focus on your own thoughts, feelings, and values.
   B. Choose friends with different values.
   C. Join in teasing other people.
   D. Stay in uncomfortable situations.
10. **True or false.** In a dating relationship, a person's core values should change.
11. Why is sexual abstinence the best choice for young people?
12. **True or false.** Group dating can help you get to know a potential dating partner.

Use Your Vocabulary ↗

acquaintances	group dating	peer mediation
active listening	immediate family	rituals
casual dating	infatuation	sibling rivalry
clique	interpersonal skills	socialize
communication process	intimacy	stereotypes
diversity	nonverbal	traditions
exclusive	communication	verbal communication
feedback	passion	virtual friends

13. Read the text passages that contain each of the terms above. Then, write the definitions of each term in your own words. Double-check your definitions by rereading the text and using the text glossary.
14. On a separate sheet of paper, list words that relate to each of the terms above. Then, work with a partner to explain how these words are related.

Think Critically

15. **Identify.** Identify a character in a book, movie, or television show who has healthy relationships with family members and friends. What makes the character's relationships healthy? Explain.

16. **Assess.** Assess your communication skills by analyzing your communication with family members and friends. In what areas of communication are you doing well? What areas do you need to improve?

17. **Compare and contrast.** Compare and contrast positive and negative peer pressure. Explain how each type of peer pressure can cause or solve problems in a friendship.

18. **Determine.** Compare and contrast healthy friendships and healthy dating relationships. Some people say that a healthy friendship is the foundation of a healthy dating relationship. Do you agree or disagree? Why?

DEVELOP Your Skills

19. **Communication skills.** Start a conversation with your parents or another trusted adult about the expectations for relationships at this point in your life. Express your thoughts about and discuss the types of people who make good friends, appropriate and inappropriate activities to do with friends, information that should be shared with trusted adults, the appropriate time to start dating, and the characteristics of an appropriate date.

20. **Advocacy, teamwork, and technology skills.** Work with a team of your classmates to write a conversational blog post for people your age. Cover the most important topics in this chapter, according to your team, and enhance your blog post with information from valid and reliable print, digital, or in-person sources.

21. **Goal-setting skills.** Choose a relationship in your life that needs improvement. Identify what you can realistically do to improve it. Use the strategies discussed in previous chapters and set a goal for

yourself to improve, change, or end the relationship. Implement your plan and write a journal entry reflecting on what you learned about yourself and relationships.

22. **Accessing information.** Many resources are available to help young people navigate relationships. It is important that people who are struggling with relationships reach out to gain help. Spend time searching online for valid and reliable websites that help young people build healthy relationships and deal with relationship struggles. Then, identify adults in your life whom you could comfortably go to for help with improving your relationships. Finally, identify professionals in your community who help people improve and manage relationships. Make a list of all these resources and then highlight the top three you would use if you needed assistance with the relationships in your life.

Chapter 15

Understanding Violent Behavior

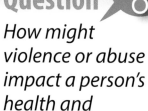

Essential Question

How might violence or abuse impact a person's health and wellness?

Video
Access the Chapter 15 video to start thinking about chapter topics.

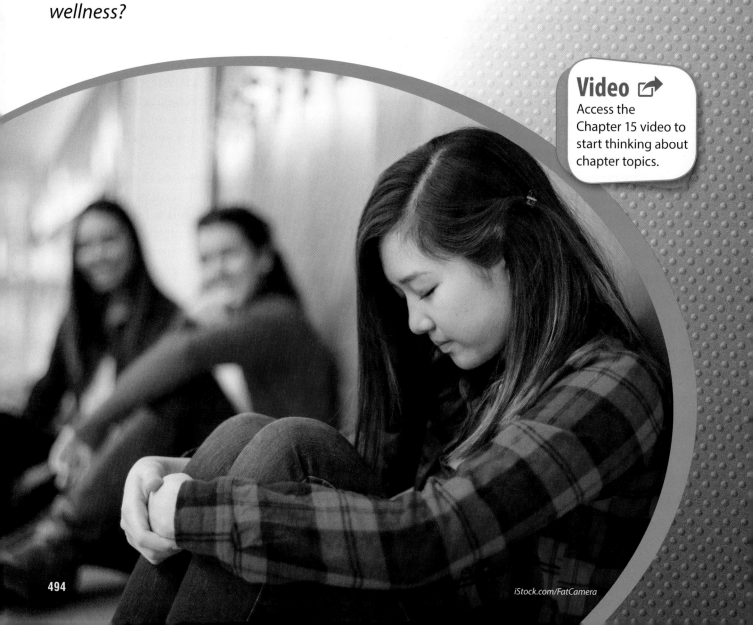

iStock.com/FatCamera

Reading Activity

As you read this chapter, write any comments or questions you may have about the content on a separate sheet of paper. After you finish reading the chapter, review your comments and questions with a partner. Try to answer each other's questions. If you have any questions you cannot answer, discuss them with the rest of the class to pursue the answers to your questions.

How **Healthy** Are You?

In this chapter, you will be learning about violent behaviors. Before you begin reading, take the following quiz to assess your current understanding of how violent behaviors affect a person's health and well-being.

Health Concepts to Understand	Yes	No
Do you consider intimidating a friend or spreading rumors about a classmate examples of violent behavior?		
Do you think harassment and hazing are types of bullying?		
Do you think there is ever a good reason to behave like a bully?		
Are you aware of strategies you can use to respond to and stop bullying?		
Do you avoid using fake screen names online?		
Do you only say things to someone online that you would be willing to say in person?		
Are you aware of strategies you can use to respond to cyberbullying?		
Do you believe that all types of abuse are wrong, no matter who is committing the abuse and who is being abused?		
If your school has a violence-prevention program, do you follow the rules of the program?		
Are you aware of community resources to help reduce gang violence?		
Do you celebrate differences in others and encourage other people to do the same?		

Count your "Yes" and "No" responses. The more "Yes" responses you have, the more you understand the effects of violent behaviors. Now, take a closer look at the questions with which you responded "No." Think about how you can increase your understanding of issues in these areas.

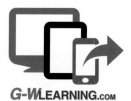

While studying this chapter, look for the activity icon to

- **practice** key terms with e-flash cards and matching activities.
- **reinforce** what you learn by completing graphic organizers, self-assessment quizzes, and review questions.
- **expand** knowledge with interactive activities and activities that extend learning.

www.g-wlearning.com/health/

Bullying and Cyberbullying

Key Terms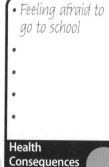

violent behavior intentional use of words or actions that cause or threaten to cause injury to someone or something

bullying repeated aggressive behavior toward someone that causes the person injury or discomfort

peer abuse violent mistreatment of one peer by another

harassment type of bullying that targets a particular part of a person's identity, such as race, religion, gender, or sexual orientation

hazing use of pressure by a group to make someone do something embarrassing or even dangerous to be accepted by a group

cyberbullying form of bullying that uses electronic means

Learning Outcomes

After studying this lesson, you will be able to

- **discuss** what violent behavior is.
- **contrast** bullying, cyberbullying, harassment, and hazing.
- **describe** the consequences of bullying.
- **evaluate** strategies for responding to bullying.
- **identify** the consequences of cyberbullying.
- **explain** ways of responding to cyberbullying.
- **list** strategies for bullying prevention.

Anita Patterson Peppers/Shutterstock.com

Graphic Organizer

Bullying Affects Your Health

Before reading this lesson, try to answer the following question: "How do you think bullying and cyberbullying affect your overall health?" In an organizer like the one shown below, list at least five predictions of bullying-related health problems based on your current knowledge and experience. After reading the lesson, write at least five bullying-related health consequences and five strategies for responding to bullying. An example is provided for you.

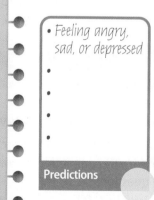

- Feeling angry, sad, or depressed

Predictions

- Feeling afraid to go to school

Health Consequences

- Tell a trusted adult

Strategies for Responding

When you think of the word *violence*, you may not think of intimidating a friend or spreading rumors about a classmate. Both of these actions, however, are examples of violent behavior. Isabela and Sofia are sisters who go to the same school. Sofia likes to play sports and is outgoing, but Isabela is quiet in class. Sofia's friends like to make fun of Isabela for being shy, and when Sofia sees them gossiping online about her sister, she feels uncomfortable. Isabela avoids many of her classmates and feels nervous going to school. Because of her anxiety, Isabela dropped out of the school play. She feels bad because she regrets her decision, but she does not want to spend more time with her classmates.

The actions of Sofia's friends are violent behavior. **Violent behavior** is the intentional use of words or actions that cause or threaten to cause injury to someone or something. An example of violent behavior might be hitting someone, forcing someone to do something, or destroying someone's belongings. Although violent behavior often involves the use of physical force, it is not always physical. Violent behavior can also refer to behavior that results in *psychological injury*, or injury to a person's social or emotional wellness. Many factors can lead to violence, but violent behavior is always a personal choice (**Figure 15.1**).

Violent behavior among peers often happens in schools and takes the form of bullying and cyberbullying or hazing. In this lesson, you will learn about these types of violent behavior and ways to respond to and prevent them.

Risk Factors for Violent Behavior

Individual risk factors

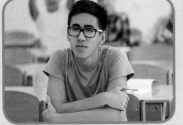
Africa Studio/Shutterstock.com

- Lack of control over behavior and anger
- History of early aggressive behavior
- Exposure to violence, abuse, and conflict in the family
- Misuse of tobacco, alcohol, or drugs
- Rejection of social values or institutions
- Immaturity
- *Prejudice*, or unfair negative beliefs about a group of people
- Discrimination and bias
- Stressful events
- Physical or mental illness

Family risk factors

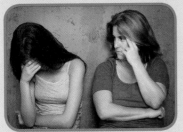
Kamira/Shutterstock.com

- Authoritarian parenting style (one that demands strict obedience)
- Discipline for breaking rules that is either too harsh, lenient, or inconsistent
- Poor supervision of children
- Low level of parental involvement and emotional attachment
- Low level of parental education and income
- Parental misuse of illegal substances
- Criminal record
- Poor family functioning
- Access to weapons

(Continued)

Figure 15.1
Several factors can affect whether a person or group chooses violence. These risk factors can be related to the individual who chooses violence, the family, peers, and the community. The presence of risk factors does not necessarily mean that a person will become violent. Still, one of the best ways to understand and prevent violence is to pay attention to its risk factors.

Risk Factors for Violent Behavior *(Continued)*	
Peer and social risk factors 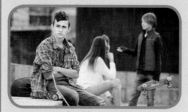 *Iakov Filimonov/Shutterstock.com*	• Rejection by peers • Peer pressure • Little interest or involvement in school • Involvement in gangs • Poor academic performance
Community risk factors 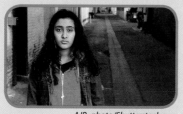 *AJR_photo/Shutterstock.com*	• Lack of economic opportunities • Poverty • Lack of community groups and social services • High crime and unemployment rates • Lack of strong families in the community • High rate of families moving out of the community

Bullying

Bullying is a type of repeated aggressive behavior toward someone that causes the person injury or discomfort. Bullying involves a power imbalance, which means the bully uses his or her power to control or harm others. Bullying is also called **peer abuse** because it involves ongoing violent behavior toward a peer. You will learn more about abuse in the next lesson.

Bullying can be physical or emotional (**Figure 15.2**). For example, a bully might hit, push, corner, or shove someone. Examples of emotional bullying include ridiculing or mocking a person, spreading rumors, making fun of someone, or taking someone's belongings. Excluding someone from a group of friends is another form of emotional bullying.

Figure 15.2
Bullying can include both physical violence and emotional violence. Both intend to cause injury or discomfort to a person. *Is forming cliques a form of emotional or physical bullying?*

Physical Versus Emotional Bullying

Physical
• Hitting or punching
• Pushing or shoving
• Kicking
• Biting
• Choking
• Physical intimidation

Emotional
• Teasing
• Gossiping
• Name-calling
• Threatening
• Mocking
• Excluding
• Embarassing
• Stealing

Left to right: Syda Productions/Shutterstock.com; Monkey Business Images/Shutterstock.com

One particular type of bullying is **harassment**. Harassment hurts another person and is a form of discrimination, making it illegal. Harassment targets a particular part of your identity, such as your race, religion, gender, or sexual orientation. **Hazing** is also a type of bullying. It is the use of group pressure to make someone do something embarrassing or even dangerous in order to be accepted. Hazing can be dangerous, which is why most states have laws against it.

BUILDING Your Skills

Rumor Has It

Rumors are (unfortunately) a common part of young people's lives. People often spread unkind gossip to gain popularity or status. Sometimes, people spread gossip just because others are doing it, even though it is hurtful to the victim. If you have ever had a rumor spread about you, then you know the pain it can cause. If you have ever spread a rumor, then you probably know the uneasy feeling that spreading it causes. Spreading rumors is a form of bullying. So, what can you do if you hear a rumor?

Strategies for Responding to Rumors

- **Just STOP it.** When you hear a rumor about another person, do not tell anyone else. Remember that this rumor is about a real person, and spreading this rumor will only hurt that person more. A rumor will only last as long as people continue to talk about it.
- **Do not be part of the audience.** Simply listening to a rumor makes you part of the rumor. If the person spreading the rumor does not get attention or a reaction, he or she will be less likely to spread rumors in the future. It can be hard to resist an interesting story, but make an effort to say, "I'm not interested in hearing mean gossip, thanks."
- **Reverse the pressure.** Ask the person who is spreading the rumor, "How do you know this is true?" or "Is this your information to spread?" This will make the person stop and hopefully quit spreading information about another person.

- **Talk with the victim of the rumor.** Find a private time and place to talk to the person about whom you heard a rumor. Tell the person what you heard. Perhaps the person can set the record straight or at least become aware of what is being said. You could offer to help the person go talk with a trusted adult to show support.

Stopping the spread of rumors is a difficult task, especially because it often feels like everyone talks about other people. You can, however, be an inspiration to others. Try practicing these strategies. You can be the first in your group of friends, and maybe even in your school, to stop the spread of rumors that harm other people.

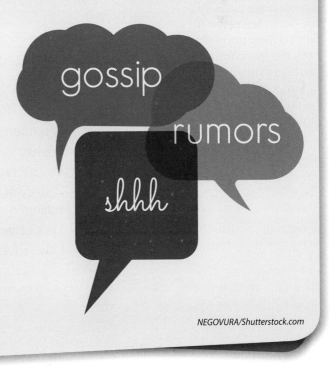

NEGOVURA/Shutterstock.com

Bullying is always the fault of the bully. Usually, the bully has personal problems that motivate him or her to hurt others. There is never a good reason to behave like a bully, even if a person acts or looks different from you (**Figure 15.3**).

Consequences of Bullying

Bullying can have severe and lasting consequences. Young people who are bullied may change their behavior, worry about going to school, or have trouble concentrating on homework. They might stop hanging out with friends after school or going to parties. They might even quit playing a sport or some other activity to avoid the bully. People who are bullied can become seriously depressed. They can have difficulty sleeping and feel fearful of other people.

Some common signs that a person is being bullied include the following:

- feeling angry, sad, lonely, and depressed
- feeling bad about one's self
- wanting to hurt someone else or one's self
- feeling helpless to stop the bullying
- feeling afraid to go to school

Bullying does not just hurt the victim. It also hurts the bully and other people. By bullying, the bully does not deal with his or her deeper problems. Young people who are not bullied do not like seeing violent, bullying behavior. They may worry that the bully will start picking on them next.

Figure 15.3
Bullying is never an appropriate behavior and will not make the bully or the victim feel better. In fact, bullying can make a bully feel even worse and can lead to more violent behavior. *Who is at fault for bullying in every situation?*

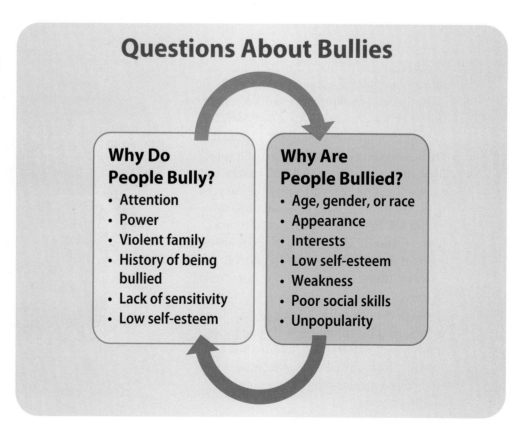

Questions About Bullies

Why Do People Bully?
- Attention
- Power
- Violent family
- History of being bullied
- Lack of sensitivity
- Low self-esteem

Why Are People Bullied?
- Age, gender, or race
- Appearance
- Interests
- Low self-esteem
- Weakness
- Poor social skills
- Unpopularity

Bullies create an environment in which stress and violence seem normal, causing harm to everyone involved.

Strategies for Responding to Bullying

Bullying is never the fault of the person being bullied. You and others have a right to feel safe at school and in the community. If you are being bullied or if you see someone being bullied, you can use the following strategies to respond to and stop the bullying:

- If you see someone bullying another person, do not participate. Instead, tell the bully to stop and ask how you can help the person being bullied (**Figure 15.4**).
- Ignore anyone who bullies you. Bullies feel more powerful when people react to their meanness. Acting like you do not even notice or care can discourage a bully's behavior.
- Stand up for yourself. Bullies often pick on people who seem scared or weak. Sometimes, simply standing up to a bully can get the bully to change his or her behavior. Tell the bully to leave you alone calmly and loudly. Then, just walk away.
- Avoid bullying back. Even if you are angry, do not respond by hitting or yelling at the bully. This can encourage the bully to continue his or her bad behavior. It can also get you in trouble.
- Tell an adult. It is important to talk to a trusted adult if you or someone you know is being bullied. Teachers, principals, school nurses, and other adults can help stop bullying. This helps keep you and other people safe.

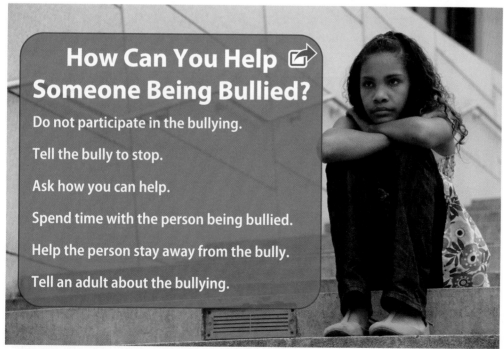

How Can You Help 🖃 Someone Being Bullied?

Do not participate in the bullying.

Tell the bully to stop.

Ask how you can help.

Spend time with the person being bullied.

Help the person stay away from the bully.

Tell an adult about the bullying.

iStock.com/RushOnPhotography

Figure 15.4
If you see someone being bullied by another person, there is almost always something you can do to help stop the bully.

Cyberbullying

Cyberbullying is a form of bullying that uses electronic communication. In some ways, cyberbullying is similar to traditional bullying. Both cause emotional harm to the victim. In other ways, cyberbullying can be worse than traditional bullying. Electronic media can spread news far and quickly. Because people hide behind fake screen names online, they can say things they would not say in person.

Sometimes, cyberbullying happens unintentionally. One person might post a joke about someone else and not realize that it was hurtful. Cyberbullying that happens repeatedly over time, however, is not accidental. Cyberbullying can involve embarrassing, harassing, or threatening peers in any of the ways shown in **Figure 15.5**.

Consequences of Cyberbullying

Cyberbullying can have serious and lasting consequences. Some of these consequences include the following:

- anxiety and depression
- loneliness and isolation
- low self-esteem
- lower grades
- aggressive actions
- withdrawal from friends and social activities
- changes in sleep, appetite, and behavior
- anxiety before, during, or after using a phone, computer, or tablet
- avoidance of phones, computers, or tablets
- suicidal thoughts and behaviors

Figure 15.5
Cyberbullying can occur in many settings, including social media, texting or e-mail, chat rooms, gaming, and websites. *In what way is cyberbullying similar to traditional bullying?*

What Is Cyberbullying?

- Sending aggressive, mean, or threatening e-mails or text messages
- Sharing hurtful messages, photos, or videos about someone on social media
- Blocking people's e-mail addresses or unfriending them on social media for no reason
- Spreading personal or embarrassing information or rumors about people
- Hacking into people's e-mail accounts or social media pages and impersonating them to others
- Creating websites or documents to ridicule or embarrass other people

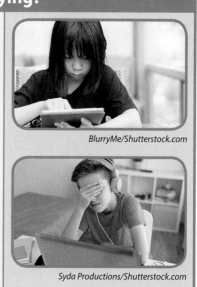

BlurryMe/Shutterstock.com

Syda Productions/Shutterstock.com

How to Spot Cyberbullying

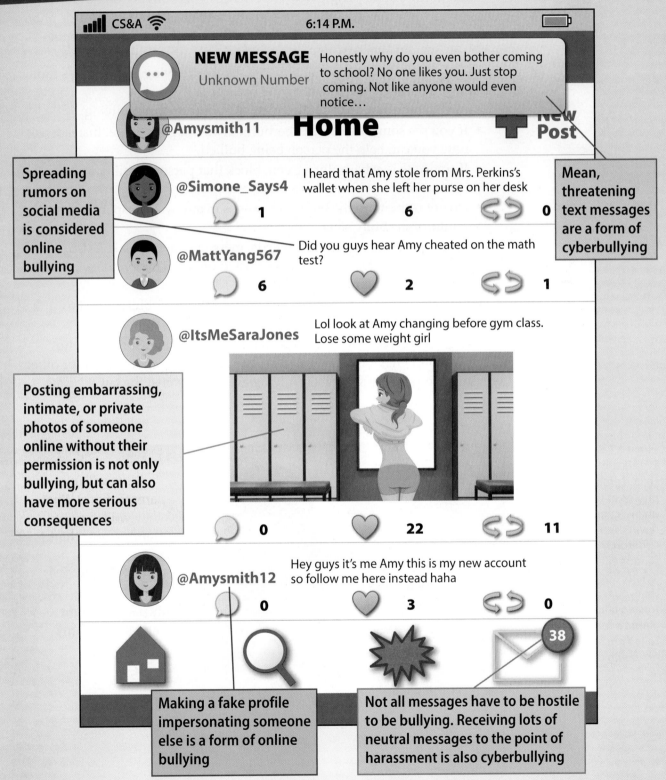

Top to bottom: Hermin/Shutterstock.com; WEB-DESIGN/Shutterstock.com; VectorZilla/Shutterstock.com; LOVIN/Shutterstock.com; maradaisy/Shutterstock.com; Peshkova/Shutterstock.com; Lorelyn Medina/Shutterstock.com

Cyberbullying is difficult to escape. Most young people spend a lot of time using their phones, computers, or tablets. Because of this, cyberbullying can happen any time of day or night.

Strategies for Responding to Cyberbullying

Sometimes, young people who experience cyberbullying do not want to tell anyone. They may feel embarrassed about the messages, videos, or photos shared about them (**Figure 15.6**). They may also worry that their parents or guardians will take away their phones, tablets, or computers. In these situations, it is important to remember that cyberbullying is the bully's fault and never the fault of the person being bullied.

The following strategies can help you respond to cyberbullying:

- If you see someone being cyberbullied, do not participate. Instead, ask how you can help the person being bullied.
- If someone is cyberbullying you, block that person's ability to contact you.
- Do not respond to the bully's messages in any way. Responding will reinforce the bully's behavior.
- Save or screenshot the bully's texts, messages, and e-mails. Also, screenshot any hurtful messages posted online. This evidence can help prove you are being cyberbullied.
- Communicate with a trusted adult about the cyberbullying. The adult can intervene and help stop this behavior.

Many school districts have rules about cyberbullying. Students who engage in this behavior can be suspended or kicked off sports teams or other activities. Certain types of cyberbullying are even against the law.

Figure 15.6
Even if someone has shared embarrassing photos or videos online, cyberbullying is never the victim's fault. Cyberbullying can have serious effects on your health. It is important that you report it to a trusted adult. *Why might young people not want to tell anyone that they are being bullied?*

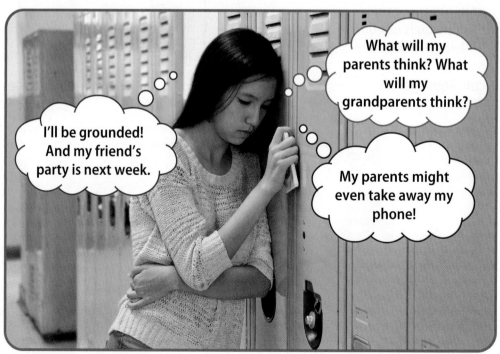

iStock.com/StphaneLemire

Bullying Prevention

Bullying is a serious problem in many schools. In addition to hurting victims, it can cause stress and fear for all students (**Figure 15.7**). Schools often have programs for preventing bullying. Participating in these programs can help you learn about bullying and ways to respond. You can also take action on your own to prevent bullying in your school and among your peers. The following strategies can help stop bullying before it begins:

- Focus on your own beliefs and build your confidence. Bullies sometimes target people who seem weak or insecure. Being comfortable with yourself can keep bullies away.
- Understand the signs of bullying behavior. If you are acting like a bully, stop and think about why. Talk to a trusted adult about your feelings.

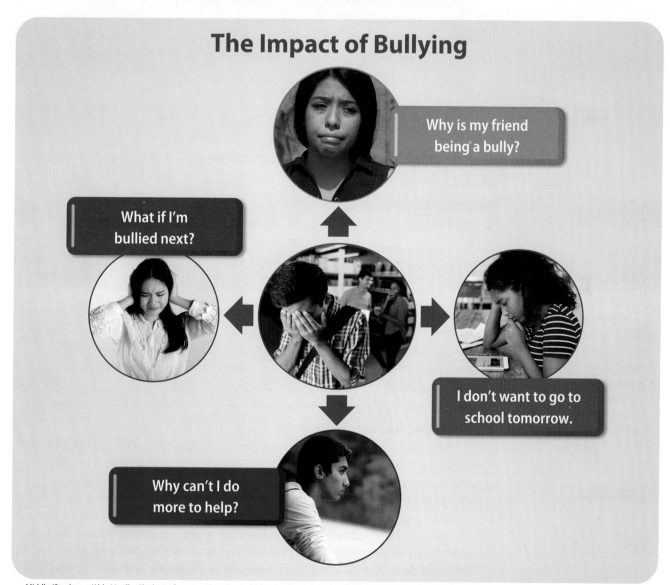

Middle: iStock.com/Aldo Murillo; Clockwise from top: cheapbooks/Shutterstock.com; Monkey Business Images/Shutterstock.com; PT Images/Shutterstock.com; Tao Jiang/Shutterstock.com

Figure 15.7   Bullying at school causes an atmosphere full of fear and stress for all students, not only the person or people being bullied.

- Celebrate your peers' differences. Appreciating differences and diversity can create a positive environment and help people feel better about themselves.
- Avoid bullies whenever possible. If a bully is nearby, sit in a different part of the cafeteria or hang out in a different place after school.
- Use the buddy system. Try to be with a friend whenever you might run into a bully. This might prevent the bully from acting.
- Never share the passwords to your computer, phone, or social media accounts with anyone. This way, bullies cannot impersonate you online.
- Do not send or post anything online that you would not want shared with others.
- If you see signs of bullying behavior, tell a trusted adult. A trusted adult can help address the situation before it gets worse.

In addition to these strategies, communicating regularly with a trusted adult can help protect you from bullying. If you tell an adult about your relationships at school and online, that adult can help you with difficult situations. The adult can also advocate for you if bullying does occur.

Lesson 15.1 Review

1. **True or false.** Violent behavior always includes the use of physical force.
2. Because it involves ongoing violent behavior toward a peer, _____ is also called *peer abuse*.
3. Which type of bullying targets a particular part of a person's identity?
4. Loneliness, lower grades, aggressive actions, and anxiety using technology are all health consequences for victims of _____.
5. **Critical thinking.** Explain why cyberbullying can sometimes be worse than traditional bullying. What can you do to respond to and prevent cyberbullying?

Hands-On Activity

On a piece of paper, draw a square and then draw something that you like inside of it. For example, you could draw your favorite animal or your favorite video game character. Then, sit in a circle with three other students. Going around the circle, describe hurtful things that you have heard said in your school or that have been said to you. Each time a hurtful statement is said, use a different-colored marker to color in the square over your drawing. Continue doing this until your time is up. What did the hurtful statements your group discussed do to your drawing? Can the layers of marker be taken back? Would apologizing to your drawing remove the layers of marker? Discuss the power of words in your group.

Abuse and Neglect

Learning Outcomes

After studying this lesson, you will be able to

- **identify** the types of abuse.
- **explain** what domestic violence is.
- **summarize** the effects of child abuse and the results of reporting it.
- **list** forms of sibling abuse and elder abuse.
- **discuss** the cycle of abuse and ways of responding to abuse.
- **identify** strategies for preventing abuse.

Graphic Organizer

Abuse and Neglect Wheel

To record your notes for this lesson, draw a wheel like the one shown below on a separate piece of paper. In the middle of the wheel, write the phrase *Abuse and Neglect*. As you read the lesson, assign a category to each section based on a different topic covered in the lesson. Write that topic at the top of each section. Fill the wheel with your notes on different types of abuse and neglect.

Dirk Ercken/Shutterstock.com

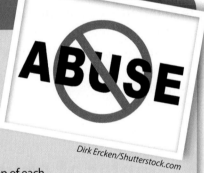

Key Terms

abuse consistent, violent mistreatment of a person

physical abuse any act that causes physical harm to a person; may involve hitting, kicking, choking, slapping, or burning

emotional abuse attitudes or controlling behaviors that harm a person's mental health; also called *verbal*, *mental*, or *psychological abuse*

sexual abuse any sexual activity to which one person does not or cannot consent

domestic violence abuse that involves couples who are married or in a romantic relationship

child abuse any act an adult commits that causes harm or threatens to cause harm to a child

neglect type of child abuse in which a child's basic physical, emotional, medical, or educational needs are not met by parents or guardians

sibling abuse violent mistreatment of one sibling by another

elder abuse mistreatment of older adults in their homes, nursing homes, or other living situations

n healthy relationships, there is no place for violent behavior or abuse. Consider, for example, Sofia and Isabela from the previous lesson. Sofia and Isabela have healthy relationships with their family. Their friend Tad, however, is always fighting with his mother. Sometimes, his mother calls him names and shoves him out of the house. Sofia and Isabela are unsure how to help their friend. Tad thinks the way his mother behaves is normal. Sofia and Isabela know, however, that all types of abuse are wrong, no matter the circumstances.

Types of Abuse

Abuse refers to the consistent, violent mistreatment of a person. For example, hitting someone whenever you are angry is abuse. Shaking a sibling is also abuse. Like violent behavior, abuse is not always physical. People can use words, attitudes, and behaviors to abuse another person (**Figure 15.8**). The following are types of abuse:

- **Physical abuse** is any intentional act that causes physical harm to another person. Physical abuse may involve hitting, kicking, choking, slapping, biting, shaking, or burning someone.
- **Emotional abuse** (also called *mental*, *verbal*, or *psychological abuse*) involves attitudes or controlling behaviors that harm a person's mental health. It includes making threats, calling someone names, delivering insults, and isolating a person.
- **Sexual abuse** is any sexual activity to which one person does not or cannot consent. Sexual abuse can include unwanted sexual activity or harassment.

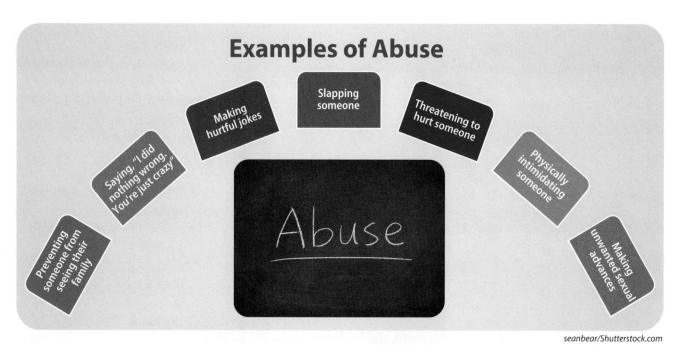

Examples of Abuse

Preventing someone from seeing their family

Saying, "I did nothing wrong. You're just crazy"

Making hurtful jokes

Slapping someone

Threatening to hurt someone

Physically intimidating someone

Making unwanted sexual advances

Abuse

seanbear/Shutterstock.com

Figure 15.8   Many different actions can be considered abuse, but all are part of a violent, consistent mistreatment of another person. *What are the three types of abuse?*

Abuse happens in unhealthy relationships. It can occur in families, between friends, among classmates, or between dating partners. In all of these settings, abuse has serious physical and emotional consequences and can sometimes be a crime (**Figure 15.9**). Often, abusers try to make victims feel responsible for the abuse. This is *never* the case. No matter the situation, the abuser is *always* responsible for the abuse. Some examples of abuse are domestic violence, child abuse, sibling abuse, and elder abuse. As you learned in the previous lesson, bullying is a type of peer abuse.

Domestic Violence

Domestic violence is abuse that involves couples who are married or in a romantic relationship. This type of abuse occurs when one person in a relationship uses abuse to try to control or dominate the other person. It also includes the threat of physical violence. Domestic violence can occur in person or electronically, and may occur between current or former partners.

Domestic violence often starts with threats and emotional abuse. Over time, harsh words lead to physical attacks. When violence occurs in a relationship, a person should leave the relationship or seek help as soon as possible. Abuse and violent behavior have no place in healthy relationships (**Figure 15.10**).

Violent Crimes Common in Abuse

Crime	Description
Assault	The threat of physical injury to another person
	The threat of forced sexual activity to another person
Battery	The physical injury of another person
Rape	Sexual activity that is forced on another person
	Sexual activity to which another person cannot consent (for example, due to age or condition)

Figure 15.9 Abuse is a criminal action and can have serious legal consequences, as with assault, battery, and rape.

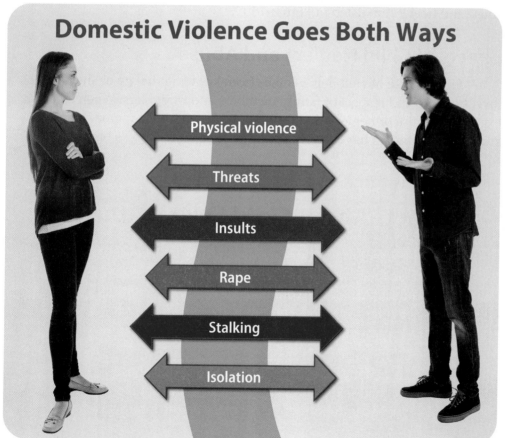

Domestic Violence Goes Both Ways

Physical violence

Threats

Insults

Rape

Stalking

Isolation

Figure 15.10
In a relationship, either member can perform acts of domestic violence. Abusers often try to make the victim feel responsible for the abuse. This is never the case. The abuser is always responsible for his or her violent behavior.

iStock.com/tetmc

Victims of domestic violence may suffer physical injuries, such as bruises or broken bones. They also suffer emotionally and may feel anxiety, fear, and shame. Abuse can lead to depression and feelings of hopelessness. Victims of domestic violence may feel socially isolated and alone. They may not want to tell anyone about the abuse.

Child Abuse

Each year in the United States, nearly 700,000 children experience some form of abuse or neglect. Nearly 1,700 children die from abuse or neglect each year. **Child abuse** refers to any intentional act an adult commits that causes harm or threatens to cause harm to a child. Child abuse can take many forms. For example, withholding love, ignoring a child, and being emotionally distant are examples of emotional abuse. *Child sexual abuse* is a specific type of abuse in which an adult engages a child in any sexual activity. This may include kissing, touching, having the child view sexual images, or looking at the child sexually (**Figure 15.11**). Child sexual abuse may involve the use of pressure, force, or deception by the adult to the child.

Another type of child abuse is neglect. **Neglect** occurs when an adult fails to meet a child's basic physical, emotional, medical, or educational needs. Neglect also includes the failure to protect a child from harm. For example, a neglected child may be supervised inadequately or exposed to a dangerous living situation. A child who does not have enough food or clothes suited to the season is a victim of neglect. Some specific risk factors related to child abuse and neglect are listed in **Figure 15.12**.

Effects of Child Neglect and Abuse

A child's sense of well-being comes from knowing that he or she has the love, support, and respect of family members and caregivers. When children experience abuse or neglect, their sense of well-being is shattered. Not surprisingly, this can have serious consequences on children's health.

Figure 15.11
Young people under a certain age cannot consent to sexual activities. This means that any adult who engages in sexual activity with a child can be charged with rape or sexual abuse.

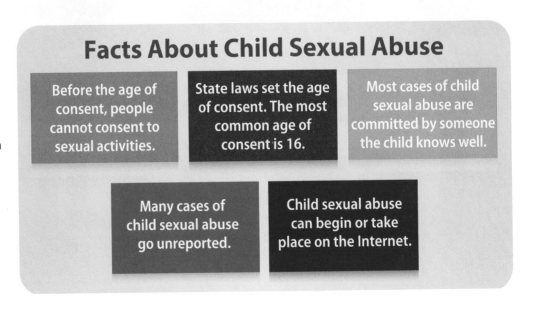

Facts About Child Sexual Abuse

Before the age of consent, people cannot consent to sexual activities.

State laws set the age of consent. The most common age of consent is 16.

Most cases of child sexual abuse are committed by someone the child knows well.

Many cases of child sexual abuse go unreported.

Child sexual abuse can begin or take place on the Internet.

Risk Factors for Child Abuse and Neglect

- Expensive or unavailable healthcare
- Unplanned pregnancy
- Teen pregnancy
- Emotional immaturity
- Marriage difficulties
- Lack of knowledge about parenting and child development
- Many children in the home or very young children
- Use of physical punishment for discipline
- Premature birth or low birthweight
- Dislike of child
- Disobedience and arguing
- Frequent crying

Figure 15.12
The risk factors for child abuse and neglect are similar to the risk factors for violent behavior, which you learned about in the previous lesson. Some additional, specific risk factors are listed here. *What is neglect?*

Physical consequences of child abuse or neglect can range from severe bruises to broken bones, burns, brain damage, and poor development. Abused children also have an increased risk of developing health problems and diseases as adults. Children who are abused or neglected are more likely to behave in unhealthy ways. Abused children have an increased risk of smoking, abusing alcohol or drugs, doing poorly in school, and committing crimes.

Children who are abused or neglected also have a greater risk of psychological problems. These problems include depression, anxiety, eating disorders, and post-traumatic stress disorder (PTSD). Ongoing abuse may cause children to develop learning, attention, and memory problems.

Child abuse or neglect can lessen a person's ability to establish and maintain healthy relationships in adulthood. People who do not experience love, trust, and support in their early years may have trouble building healthy relationships with others later.

Reporting of Child Abuse and Neglect

Paying attention to the signs of child abuse and neglect can help people identify when this violent behavior is occurring (**Figure 15.13**). Anyone who suspects that a child is the victim of abuse should report his or her concern to authorities. Many states have hotlines with staff available to take the information. People can also call the organization Childhelp (800-422-4453) any time of day to get help for a child.

Signs of Child Abuse and Neglect

Type of Abuse	Signs
Physical abuse	• Injuries, such as broken bones or severe bruises • Many injuries on different parts of the body • Several injuries that occurred at different times
Sexual abuse	• Bruises in the pelvic area • Difficulty or pain when walking or sitting • Torn clothing
Emotional abuse	• Withdrawn attitude and unwillingness to talk to others • Anxiety and worry • Difficulty sleeping • Aggressive or inappropriate behavior
Neglect	• Underweight • Poor physical development • Lack of cleanliness

Figure 15.13 Sometimes, children and young people who are abused blame themselves. It is important to remember that the victim is *never* responsible for abuse. The abuse is a result of the abuser's problems.

Some professionals are required by law to report child abuse. These workers, called *mandated reporters*, include teachers and other school personnel, social workers and child welfare workers, and healthcare professionals.

Once child abuse is reported, the state child welfare agency looks into the matter. Staffers will talk with the parents or guardians, the child, and other people who might have relevant information. If the agency finds that abuse has occurred, it may take the child away from the parents and try to find a foster home. In *foster care*, adults agree to take the role of parent for children who are not their own. Those who commit child abuse may be required to receive counseling and treatment. They may be prosecuted and, if found guilty, sent to prison.

Sibling Abuse

Sibling abuse is the mistreatment of one sibling by another. Sibling abuse can be physical, emotional, or sexual and has serious health consequences. According to some studies, sibling abuse is one of the most common types of family abuse. Sibling abuse most often occurs in families where other unhealthy relationships exist.

Some conflict or rivalry is normal between siblings, but abuse is not. Unlike rivalry, abuse is part of an ongoing, chronic pattern. Sibling abuse is typically one-sided and aims to dominate the victim.

CASE STUDY

Aarav and Rajesh: Boys Will Be Boys

Aarav is 12 years old, and he is scared of his older brother Rajesh. Rajesh always taunts Aarav about his weight, calling him "fatty" or "doughboy" and pinching the fat around his waist or on his arms. Aarav became very upset one day and told his dad about Rajesh's mean comments and actions. His father told Rajesh to stop teasing his brother, but it did not work, and Rajesh's teasing only got worse.

Often, Aarav's parents work late into the evening, which means that Rajesh is in charge at home after school. Rajesh yells at Aarav to do all of the chores, and if Aarav resists, Rajesh will hit, kick, and push him until he obeys. Aarav tries his hardest to stay out of his brother's way and not anger him. Rajesh tells Aarav that he will hurt him more if he tells anyone about their fights. A few times, Aarav has had to hide the scrapes and bruises from his parents and people at school.

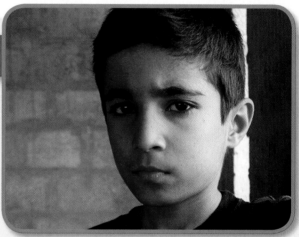

iStock.com/danishkhan

Thinking Critically

1. Are Rajesh's actions toward Aarav abuse? If yes, which type(s) of abuse?

2. What can Aarav do to stop his brother's actions? Whom should he talk to about his situation?

3. What are some possible health consequences for Aarav due to his brother's actions?

Elder Abuse

Victims of **elder abuse** are older adults who are mistreated in their homes, nursing homes, or other living situations. Typically, family members or paid caregivers commit elder abuse. This abuse can take the following forms:

- physical abuse, including inappropriate use of medications or restraints
- emotional abuse, including ignoring calls for help
- sexual abuse
- financial abuse, including the theft of money or property
- neglect, including failure to provide food, water, medications, and basic hygiene

Many cases of elder abuse go unreported. Older adults who are abused and neglected often feel helpless, lonely, and distressed. They also tend to die earlier than older adults who have not been abused (**Figure 15.14**).

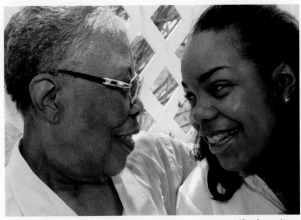

iStock.com/nano

Figure 15.14 Many older adults are dependent on their families or caregivers to help them meet their daily living needs. These older adults require the support of loved ones to help protect themselves against harm. If this care is not provided, older adults can be severely hurt by abuse or neglect. *What are the emotional consequences of elder abuse?*

Strategies for Responding to Abuse

Immediate strategies for responding to abuse should address the victim's injuries and report the abuse. For example, victims of domestic violence may need medical care or shelter for a period of time. Abused children may need foster care and counseling for dealing with emotional pain. It is also important to report abuse to the appropriate authorities. If you witness any type of abuse, you should tell a trusted adult, such as a school official, teacher, parent or guardian, or police officer. This adult can help get the victim the help he or she needs.

Because abuse is ongoing violent mistreatment, it usually follows a pattern called the *cycle of abuse*. The cycle of abuse includes four stages: tension building, incident, reconciliation, and calm (**Figure 15.15**). These four stages repeat continuously as long as abuse continues.

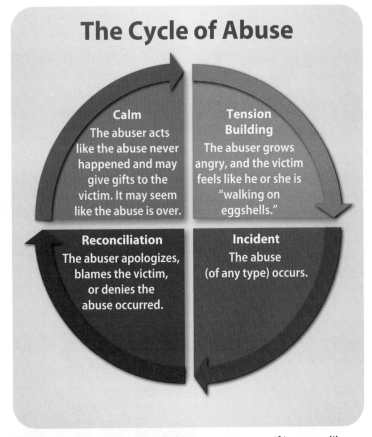

Figure 15.15 The cycle of abuse repeats even if it seems like the abuse has ended in the calm stage. The only way to stop abuse is to break the cycle.

An important step in responding to and stopping abuse is to break the cycle of abuse. Ways of breaking this cycle include the following strategies:

- Recognize the abusive situation for what it is. Do not make excuses for the abuser. There is never a good reason for engaging in abusive behavior.
- Do not try to change the abuser. You cannot change another person. Abusers need professional help.
- Leave or help someone leave the abusive situation. Crisis shelters are available to help some victims of abuse.
- Seek professional help, such as counseling. Intervention by a professional can help the abuser and the victim work through the situation.

Abuse Prevention

Many communities take steps to help prevent abuse. For example, educational programs give people the facts about abuse and help them recognize when abuse is happening. Some schools hold campaigns to educate students about and prevent peer abuse. Online resources and government agencies also share information about abusive situations and behaviors (**Figure 15.16**). You can also help prevent abuse using the following strategies:

- Learn about abusive behavior and the cycle of abuse. If you know what abuse is, you can keep yourself from acting abusively.
- Tell others about the definition of abusive behavior and the signs of abuse. This will help others recognize and avoid abuse.
- If you have been a victim of abuse, seek help in processing your experience. Victims of abuse can sometimes become abusers themselves if issues are not resolved.

Figure 15.16
Family shelters, abuse hotlines, and prevention programs are some examples of resources available to help prevent abuse. *How do educational programs help prevent abuse?*

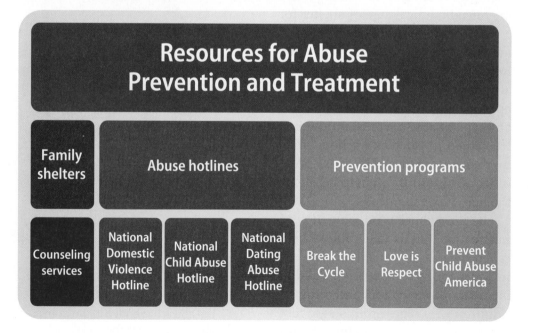

Resources for Abuse Prevention and Treatment

Family shelters	Abuse hotlines			Prevention programs		
Counseling services	National Domestic Violence Hotline	National Child Abuse Hotline	National Dating Abuse Hotline	Break the Cycle	Love is Respect	Prevent Child Abuse America

- Develop your skills in communicating effectively and resolving conflicts.
- Surround yourself with healthy relationships (**Figure 15.17**).
- Report any signs of abuse to the appropriate people. Catching abusive behavior early can help prevent abuse from getting worse.
- If a relationship shows signs of becoming abusive, leave the relationship. Abusive behavior cannot be excused.

Abuse is a serious problem, and sometimes victims have trouble recognizing when they are being abused. Sometimes, it can help to get another opinion on a difficult situation. Talking regularly with a trusted adult about your relationships can help you identify situations that may become abusive.

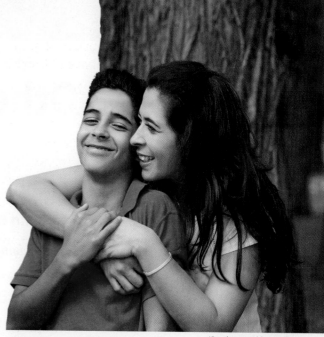

iStock.com/Aldo Marillo

Figure 15.17 Healthy relationships will help you feel connected and will give you support if you encounter abuse.

Lesson 15.2 Review

1. Making threats and calling someone names is a form of _____ abuse.
   - **A.** physical
   - **B.** emotional
   - **C.** sexual
   - **D.** sibling

2. _____ violence occurs when one person in a romantic relationship abuses, controls, or dominates the other person.

3. **True or false.** Just as some sibling rivalry is normal between siblings, so is sibling abuse.

4. What are the four stages of the cycle of abuse?

5. **Critical thinking.** List two short-term and two long-term health consequences of child abuse for children.

Hands-On Activity

Learning about abuse is often very difficult. Perhaps you have seen abuse in your own family or that of a close friend. Perhaps you have never witnessed it. Either way, information about abuse can be shocking and hard to process. On a separate piece of paper, summarize what you believe are the five most important facts from this lesson. Talk about your summary with a classmate and discuss the similarities and differences between the facts you chose. Although it is never fun, talking about abuse can make people more likely to speak up and reach out for help. If you had concerns that someone was being abused, what would you do?

Lesson 15.3

Other Types of Violence

Key Terms 📑

school violence any violent behavior that occurs on school property, at school-sponsored events, or on the way to or from school or to or from school events

gangs groups of people who carry out violent and illegal acts

human trafficking form of modern slavery in which people are forced to perform some type of job or service against their will

hate crimes threats or attacks against someone because of his or her race, ethnic origin, disability, sexual orientation, or religion

homicide crime of killing another person

terrorism use of violence and threats to frighten and control groups of people to further an ideological aim

Learning Outcomes

After studying this lesson, you will be able to

- **explain** what school violence is and how schools prevent it.
- **describe** the reasons for and consequences of people joining gangs.
- **list** ways to protect yourself from human trafficking.
- **describe** how hate crimes can be prevented.
- **discuss** the consequences of homicide.
- **identify** ways to help prevent terrorism.
- **explain** what you can do to help prevent violence.

Graphic Organizer 📑

Other Types of Violence

You learned about abuse, neglect, bullying, and cyberbullying in the previous lessons. In this lesson, you will learn about other types of violence. On a separate piece of paper, write the phrase *Other Types of Violence* in the middle of an organizer like the one below. As you read this lesson, fill in topics related to violence. Continue to categorize and explain related topics until you complete the organizer.

iQoncept/Shutterstock.com

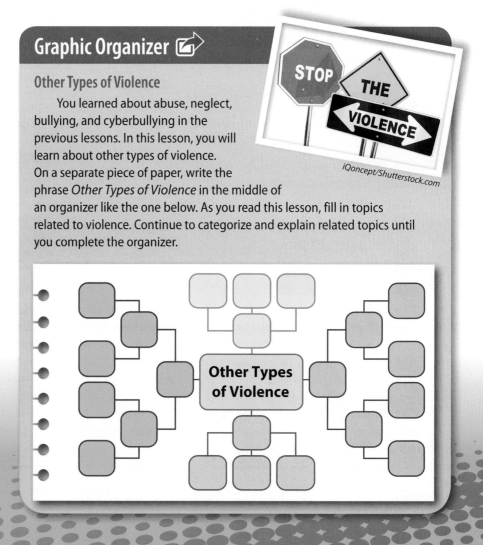

Other Types of Violence

L ately, Sofia from the previous lessons has been watching the news with her parents. The more she learns about the world, the more she fears violence that could impact her community. Stories about gang violence and terrorism sometimes make Sofia afraid of going to public events. She wishes someone would tell her how to avoid and prevent these types of violence.

Violence can occur in many places, even in places where people should feel safe. You have already learned about bullying and abuse, two types of violence. In this lesson, you will learn about other types of violent behavior and ways to respond to and prevent them.

School Violence

School violence is any emotional or physical violent behavior that occurs on school property, at school-sponsored events, or on the way to or from school or school events (**Figure 15.18**). School violence can include bullying and cyberbullying. It also includes fighting and the use of weapons at school.

School should be a safe place for all students, but school violence puts students in danger. For example, a fight might seem like it only affects two students, but if a fight gets out of control, even uninvolved students can get hurt. Even if they are not physically injured, students who are exposed to violence can feel depressed, anxious, and fearful. If a student brings a weapon to school, many people can be hurt and even die. Violent behavior in schools can also have serious school and legal consequences. Fighting with another student can lead to detention, suspension, or expulsion. Attacking another student can lead to arrest by the police.

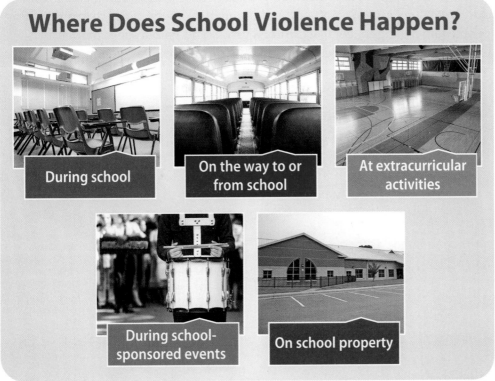

Where Does School Violence Happen?

During school

On the way to or from school

At extracurricular activities

During school-sponsored events

On school property

Figure 15.18
School violence can happen at school, but can also occur in other locations for school-related events. *Is physical violence on the school bus considered school violence? Why or why not?*

Left to right: cozyta/Shutterstock.com; Suzanne Tucker/Shutterstock.com; stockvideofactory/Shutterstock.com; Rattanapon Ninlapoom/Shutterstock.com; vincent noel/Shutterstock.com

Many schools establish violence-prevention programs to help create a culture that has *zero tolerance* for violent behaviors. This means that the school takes violence seriously and does not accept it in any form. Schools often use the following strategies to prevent and reduce violence:

- Select strong, positive, responsible student leaders who act appropriately and are not afraid to speak out against violence.
- Develop positive team-building activities, such as community service work, to forge bonds among students.
- Have a zero-tolerance policy toward violence. Any acts of violence result in serious consequences.
- Have a buddy system, with older students looking out for younger students.
- Encourage students to report any violent acts they observe immediately (**Figure 15.19**).
- Enforce rules regarding keeping school doors locked.
- Ensure a weapon-free school. Communicate rules about weapons and search students' belongings as necessary.
- Offer peer mediation programs to prevent conflicts from escalating.

To help reduce violence, students can cooperate with these programs and rules. For example, obeying rules about locking school doors can help keep dangerous people out of the building. Students have an important role in school strategies for violence prevention.

Gang Violence

Gang violence is violent behavior carried out in a gang. **Gangs** are groups of people who commit violent and illegal acts. These actions can include selling drugs, stealing, attacking others, and damaging others' property. Some young people join a gang to feel like part of a group and gain a sense of identity. Others do so because of peer pressure, the desire to make money, or the hope of protecting themselves and their families.

Figure 15.19
When young people quickly alert adults about violent behaviors, adults can prevent or stop dangerous situations.

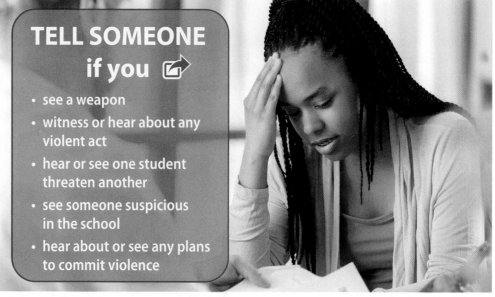

TELL SOMEONE if you ↱

- see a weapon
- witness or hear about any violent act
- hear or see one student threaten another
- see someone suspicious in the school
- hear about or see any plans to commit violence

iStock.com/Steve Debenport

People who join gangs commonly become involved in acts of violence and other crimes. Gang members are likely to drop out of school and be unable to find a job. They may also become addicted to and sell or buy drugs. As a result, gang members often go to prison or become victims of violence. Committing a crime or going to prison can severely impact a person's future.

You can help reduce gang violence by avoiding gangs and joining other groups to feel connected (**Figure 15.20**). Communities also have resources that help reduce the amount of gang violence. For example, officials in cities often take steps to limit the size and reach of gangs. To be successful, city workers and police officers have to be deeply engaged in the community and build trust.

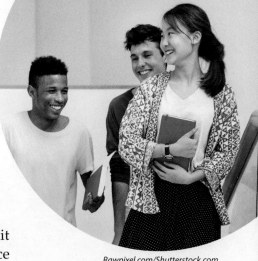

Rawpixel.com/Shutterstock.com

Figure 15.20
Often, people join gangs to feel like part of a group. To avoid gangs and other soures of violent behavior, build strong, healthy relationships with your peers. These relationships will help you feel fulfilled and accepted, so you will not have to look for these feelings in dangerous places. *What kinds of acts do people in gangs commit?*

Human Trafficking

Human trafficking is a form of modern slavery in which people are forced to perform some job or service against their will. For example, an employer may use threats of violence to make another person work. Victims may be forced to work long hours for very little money. Sometimes a human trafficker may force the victim to engage in sexual activity.

Victims of human trafficking can suffer greatly. Their physical health can decline from overwork and abuse. They suffer emotionally from worry and sometimes from separation from friends and family. Human trafficking is a serious crime, and it is important to report any suspected cases of human trafficking to the appropriate people (**Figure 15.21**).

To help reduce human trafficking in your community, pay attention to your personal safety, especially in public places and online. Walk with a friend or trusted adult in public and do not give out your personal information or talk to strangers. Always bring a trusted adult if you are meeting someone you know online.

Figure 15.21
Victims of human trafficking need the help of their communities. They need people to pay attention to signs of possible human trafficking and alert the authorities to any suspected cases.

Signs of Human Trafficking

- Unexplained, regular school absences
- Running away from home
- Regular travel
- Bruises or other physical injuries
- Lack of control over schedule
- Hunger
- Sudden changes in behavior or hygiene
- Dodging questions or lying
- Older boyfriend or girlfriend
- Lack of concentration
- Anxiety, anger, and depression

STOP HUMAN TRAFFICKING

If you know a victim of human trafficking,

talk to a trusted adult,

call the National Human Trafficking Hotline (1-888-373-7888), or

text HELP to BeFree (233733)

ria_airborne/Shutterstock.com

Hate Crimes

Hate crimes are threats or attacks against someone because of his or her race, ethnic origin, disability, sexual orientation, or religion. Hate crimes include damaging someone's property, making threats, and carrying out emotional and physical attacks.

Victims of hate crimes can suffer injury or loss of property. They may be emotionally scarred by the crime. Hate crimes also tend to hurt the victim's community. This is because people who commit hate crimes see the person they attack as a symbol of a larger group.

Most states have laws against hate crimes. These laws increase the punishment for hate crimes, such as personal violence or property damage. Committing a hate crime can result in school consequences, such as suspension or expulsion. It can also result in legal consequences such as juvenile criminal charges.

Appreciating diversity and discouraging violent behavior can help reduce hate crimes. Hate crimes are usually motivated by prejudice and bias. Do not engage in these ideas. Instead, celebrate differences and encourage others to do the same (**Figure 15.22**).

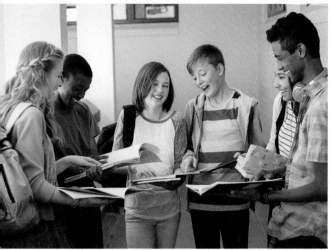

iStock.com/Wavebreakmedia

Figure 15.22 Sometimes, violence is motivated by prejudice or bias. To help prevent these types of violence, celebrate the diversity of your classmates. Celebrating your differences can help encourage understanding and kindness. *When violence is motivated by a person's race, ethnic origin, disability, sexual orientation, or religion, what kind of crime is this?*

Homicide

Killing someone is an extremely serious crime called a **homicide**. Homicides occur through physical injury. For example, attacking another student and causing death can lead to homicide. So can using a weapon at school. Whether intentional or unintentional, homicides lead to serious, lasting consequences.

Homicide robs another person of his or her life. It devastates families, friends, and communities. No one deserves to be a victim of homicide, and homicide only makes the problems in a person's life worse. Homicide leads to serious criminal charges. In some states, young people who commit homicide are treated as adults. These young people can be sentenced to life in prison.

The most important step in preventing homicide is reporting violent behavior to trusted adults. If a person threatens to kill someone, take this seriously and tell a school official, teacher, or other adult. You should also immediately report any weapons or violent situations you see at school or in your community. Reporting these situations can allow an adult to intervene before a homicide can occur.

Terrorism

Terrorism is the use of violence and threats to frighten and control groups of people. Terrorism is ideologically motivated. This means it aims to punish people for or convince people of certain ideas. Some examples of terrorism are killing or injuring people to promote a political or religious view.

Terrorism often leads to the loss of many lives and creates fear in communities. It is a serious crime that does nothing to validate the terrorist's viewpoint.

Most terrorism is a result of violent extremism. *Violent extremism* refers to beliefs that support the use of violence to promote an idea. For example, a violent extremist view might support hurting people who practice a particular religion.

The best way to prevent terrorism is to report any suspicious activity to the police (**Figure 15.23**). If you report suspicious activity, you should describe what you saw, when and where you saw it, and why it is suspicious. Another way to prevent terrorism is to celebrate the differences among people. Celebrating differences and encouraging others to do the same can reduce violent extremism.

What to Do If You Are a Victim of Violence

Unfortunately, violence sometimes occurs. In these situations, knowing how to respond is important. Violence can have serious physical and emotional effects, such as physical injuries and feelings of helplessness. Your actions immediately following violent behavior can affect your well-being and the well-being of others. The following strategies can help you respond to violent behavior:

- If someone in a relationship uses or threatens you with violence, tell a trusted adult and get out of that relationship as soon as possible. There is no excuse for violent behavior.
- If you witness or suspect violence of any kind, tell a trusted adult.
- If you are tempted to act violently, get out of the situation and talk to a trusted adult. You may need professional help to work through your feelings.
- If you are a victim of violence, get medical help for any physical injuries. Report the violence to a trusted adult, such as a parent or guardian, school official, or the police. Seek professional help for dealing with the emotional impact of the violence.

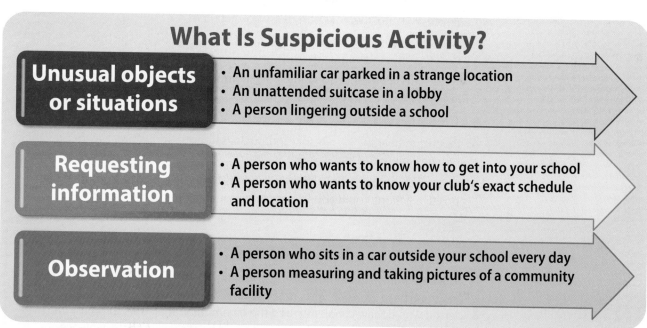

Figure 15.23 There are certain activities that make people suspects for terrorism. If you witness a person doing anything suspicious, such as the examples listed here, immediately report this to the police.

Violence Prevention

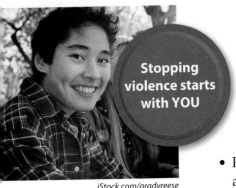

iStock.com/gradyreese

Stopping violence starts with YOU

Figure 15.24
By behaving in a nonviolent way and inspiring others to do so, by standing up against violence, and by practicing healthy conflict resolution, you can help reduce and prevent violent behaviors in your community. *What should you do if you witness any threats or violent behavior?*

Everyone in a community has a role in reducing and preventing violent behavior. This includes you. Behaving in a nonviolent way is one way you can reduce violence (**Figure 15.24**). You can also recognize the signs of violence and reduce risk factors. The following strategies are ways you can help prevent and reduce violence:

- Resist the pressure to hurt others or join gangs. Focus on your values and beliefs and find healthy ways to feel good about yourself.
- Practice healthy conflict resolution. Use the negotiation process and keep calm.
- Give support to others who resist the pressure to act violently.
- Learn self-control to prevent yourself from becoming violent. Encourage others to use self-control, too.
- Choose your friends carefully. Build healthy relationships that are free from violence.
- Do not pick up a gun or other weapon. Report unsecure guns to a trusted adult.
- Practice safety when home alone and in public places. For example, lock the doors and windows at home. Do not give out your personal information.
- If you are tempted to act violently, seek help from a trusted adult.
- Talk to a trusted adult if you witness any threats or violent behavior.

Taking these personal steps to prevent violence can help build a community in which violence is less common. This type of community is better for you and others.

Lesson 15.3 Review

1. Which of the following is part of school violence?
   A. Teasing from a sibling at home.
   B. A parent neglecting a child.
   C. Bullying on the bus.
   D. All of the above.

2. What form of violence could include an employer forcing employees to work long hours for very little money?

3. **True or false.** Hate crimes are threats or attacks against someone for no reason.

4. Practicing healthy _____ resolution, such as negotiating, is one way to prevent or reduce violence.

5. **Critical thinking.** People often join gangs to feel like part of a group. What positive actions could young people take instead to get this feeling?

Hands-On Activity

Search online for a reliable article about an act of violence that influenced your community. Read the article and identify the risk factors that led to violence and the type of violence. Also, describe how the violence affected the victim, the person who behaved violently, and the community. Share this summary with the class and lead a discussion about what could have prevented the violence.

Summary

Lesson 15.1 Bullying and Cyberbullying

- Violent behavior is the intentional use of words or actions that cause or threaten to cause injury to someone or something. Violent behavior results in physical or psychological injury.
- Bullying is repeated aggressive behavior that causes a person physical or emotional injury or discomfort. It includes harassment and hazing.
- If you witness bullying, do not participate, tell the bully to stop, and avoid bullying back. Tell an adult if you or someone you know is being bullied.
- Cyberbullying is a form of bullying that uses electronic communication. Since young people spend so much time online, cyberbullying can be difficult to escape.
- Schools often have programs to teach you how to respond to bullying and prevent it.

Lesson 15.2 Abuse and Neglect

- The consistent, violent mistreatment of a person is abuse. Abuse can be physical, emotional, or sexual. Abusers often try to make their victims feel responsible for the abuse, but this is never the case.
- Domestic violence involves couples who are married or in a romantic relationship. Child abuse refers to intentional acts that cause harm or threaten to cause harm to a child.
- Sibling abuse is the mistreatment of one sibling by another. This can be physical, emotional, or sexual, and is one of the most common types of family abuse. Older adults who are mistreated are victims of elder abuse.
- If you witness any type of abuse, tell a trusted adult. Abuse typically follows a pattern called the cycle of abuse, which includes four stages that repeat as abuse continues.

Lesson 15.3 Other Types of Violence

- Any emotionally or physically violent behavior that occurs in locations or events related to school is school violence. Many schools establish a zero-tolerance policy for violence due to its harmful effects on students.
- Gang violence is carried out by groups of people who commit violent and illegal acts. Human trafficking involves forcing people to perform a job or service against their will. Threats or attacks against someone because of race, ethnic origin, disability, sexual orientation, or religion are hate crimes.
- Killing someone is called *homicide* and can be punished with life in prison, even for adolescents. The use of violence and threats to frighten or control groups of people is terrorism.
- If you are a victim of violence or if you witness violence, tell a trusted adult. Get professional help for physical or emotional injuries from the impact of violence. To help reduce and prevent violent behavior, practice healthy conflict resolution and build healthy relationships free from violence.

Check Your Knowledge ⤤

Record your answers to each of the following questions on a separate sheet of paper.

1. A(n) _____ injury harms a person's social or emotional wellness.

2. What kind of violent behavior includes hazing, harassing, spreading rumors, and forming cliques?

3. Which of the following is *not* a sign that a person is being bullied?
   - **A.** Feeling angry, sad, or lonely.
   - **B.** Wanting to hurt someone else or one's self.
   - **C.** Having improved self-esteem.
   - **D.** Feeling helpless to stop the bullying.

4. _____ is a form of bullying that uses electronic communication.

5. _____ abuse is *not* a type of abuse.
   - **A.** Physical
   - **B.** Nonviolent
   - **C.** Sexual
   - **D.** Emotional

6. **True or false.** A child who does not have enough food or clothes suited to the season may be a victim of neglect.

7. Giving an older adult an inappropriate amount of medications is one form of _____ _____.

8. **True or false.** Victims of abuse can become abusers if they do not resolve their emotional issues.

9. Most schools aim to create a culture that has _____ tolerance for violent behaviors.

10. What are groups of people who commit violent and illegal acts?

11. Which form of violence aims to punish people for or convince people of certain ideas?

12. **True or false.** There are sometimes acceptable excuses for violent behavior in a relationship.

Use Your Vocabulary ⤤

abuse	gangs	peer abuse
bullying	harassment	physical abuse
child abuse	hate crimes	school violence
cyberbullying	hazing	sexual abuse
domestic violence	homicide	sibling abuse
elder abuse	human trafficking	terrorism
emotional abuse	neglect	violent behavior

13. With a partner, choose two words to compare from the list above. Create a Venn diagram to compare your words and identify differences. Write one term under the left circle and the other term under the right. Where the circles overlap, write three characteristics the terms have in common. For each term, write a difference of the term for each characteristic in its respective outer circle.

14. For each of the terms above, identify a word or group of words describing a quality of the term—an *attribute*. Pair up with a classmate and discuss your list of attributes.

Think Critically

15. **Determine.** Is spreading rumors a form of violence? Why or why not?

16. **Compare and contrast.** Describe the similarities and differences between bullying and cyberbullying. What are the effects of each?

17. **Cause and effect.** Why do you think experiencing abuse makes a person more likely to become an abuser? How can abuse be a cycle over generations?

18. **Draw conclusions.** Often, people remain silent about difficult situations that involve abuse. How can silence about abuse in relationships allow the abuse to keep happening?

19. **Identify.** Why is it important to report any suspicious activity you witness?

DEVELOP Your Skills

20. **Goal-setting skills.** Review the risk factors for violent behavior in Figure 15.1. What risk factors are present in your life? in your family and community? Identify two risk factors you want to reduce and set SMART goals for changing them.

21. **Accessing information skills.** Working with a partner, choose one type of violence discussed in this chapter. Using reliable online and print resources, research the type of violence and its legal consequences in your state. Include information about whether the violence can lead to arrest, fines, or time in prison. Write a blog post summarizing what you learned and share it with your classmates.

22. **Communication, conflict resolution, and teamwork skills.** Working in a team, plan and script a role-play about standing up to violence or abuse. Your role-play should end healthfully and should include the use of assertive communication skills. It should confront and address the violence in a way that ensures everyone's safety physically, socially, and mentally. As you develop the role-play, pay attention to each team member's verbal and nonverbal communication. If someone is uncomfortable, show empathy and rework the role-play. Enlist the help of your teacher, if needed, and perform the role-play for the class.

23. **Advocacy and accessing information skills.** Identify 10 agencies in your community that assist people affected by violent behavior. These can be victims of violence, abusers, or family members. Create a resource list with each agency's name, mission, and contact information.

24. **Advocacy and teamwork skills.** Working in a team, choose one type of violence discussed in this chapter. Then, review the information in this chapter about avoiding and preventing this type of violence. Take notes about this information and do additional research to learn about avoidance and prevention strategies. Using what you learn, design a campaign to reduce this type of violence in your community. Put the campaign into action and summarize how successful it was.

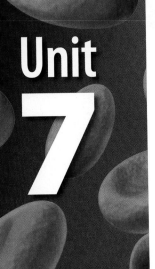

Unit 7

The Body and How It Develops

Warm-Up Activity

Ask Angelique: Going to the Doctor

Angelique is a popular social media presence in your community and age group. She focuses on helping teenagers through tough stuff. One of the ways she connects with her audience is through a Question and Answer blog. Angelique posts questions or situations that teenagers send her and asks other teenagers to provide advice based on their own experiences.

Read the post below and respond to Anonymous on a separate sheet of paper. Find a partner and review each other's responses.

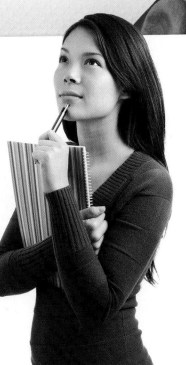

Maridav/Shutterstock.com

> Dear Angelique,
>
> How old does someone need to be to go into a doctor's appointment alone, without parents? I am 14 and I feel like I want to talk to my doctor about issues without my parents hearing. I trust my parents and they are great, but I worry that they might react strongly and embarrass me in front of my doctor. I know that I can talk with my parents, but sometimes I just want to be independent. If it is OK for me to go into my appointments alone, how do I tell my parents that is what I want?
>
> Thanks,
> Anonymous

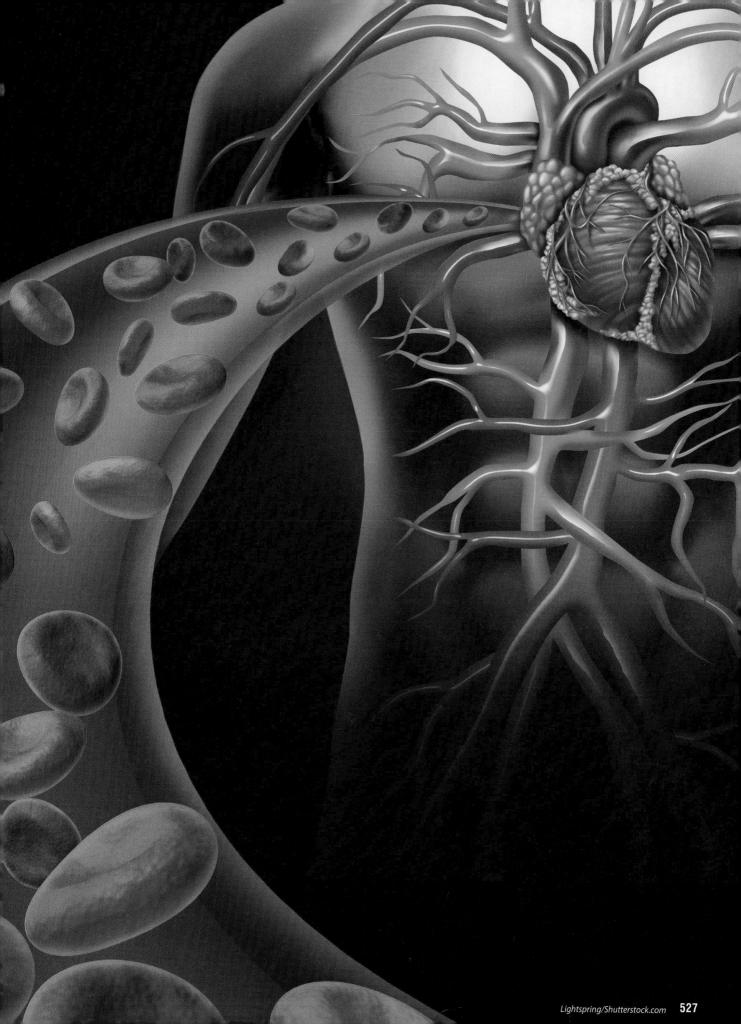

527

Chapter 16

Human Development

Essential Question

What intellectual, emotional, and social developments occur during each stage of the life span?

Video

Access the Chapter 16 video to start thinking about chapter topics.

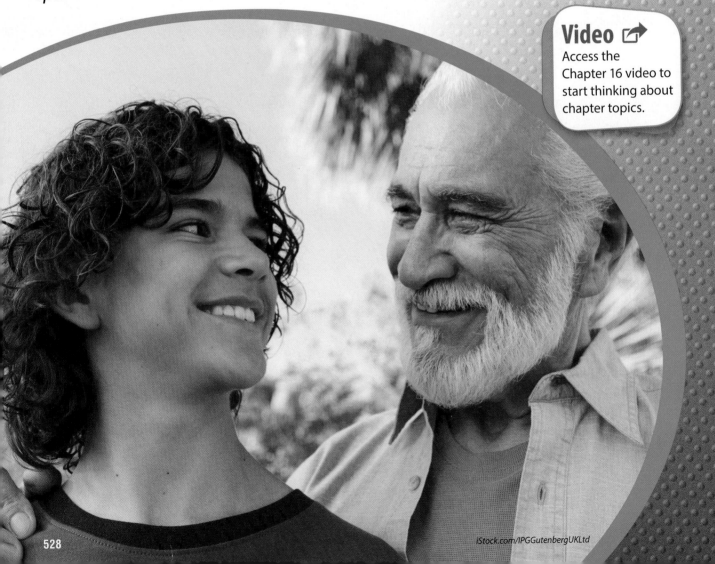

iStock.com/IPGGutenbergUKLtd

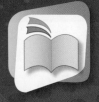

Reading Activity

Before reading this chapter, scan the chapter title. Write a paragraph describing what you know about this topic. As you are reading the chapter, compare and contrast the information in the chapter with the information you already know about the human life cycle. After reading, consider how the information in this chapter supports or contradicts your understanding of the subject matter.

How Healthy Are You?

In this chapter, you will be learning about human development. Before you begin reading, take the following quiz to assess your understanding of human development, and how health needs change throughout the life span.

Health Concepts to Understand	Yes	No
Do you understand the functions of the male and female reproductive systems?		
Do you know the differences among the germinal stage, embryonic stage, and fetal stages of pregnancy?		
Can you name each of the developmental stages of a person?		
Can you name the milestones typical in the infancy, toddler, preschool, and middle childhood life stages?		
Do you know the physical changes that accompany puberty in males and females?		
Do you understand how the adolescent brain can be more susceptible to risky behaviors?		
Do you understand that as teens grow, so does their need to establish independence and rely on their own judgment?		
Do you understand how the body and a person's health needs change during adulthood?		
Do you understand what it means to grieve the loss of a loved one?		

Count your "Yes" and "No" responses. The more "Yes" responses you have, the more you understand human development. Now, take a closer look at the questions with which you responded "No." Think about how you can increase your understanding of issues in these areas.

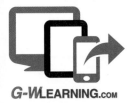

While studying this chapter, look for the activity icon **to**

- **practice** key terms with e-flash cards and matching activities.
- **reinforce** what you learn by completing graphic organizers, self-assessment quizzes, and review questions.
- **expand** knowledge with interactive activities and activities that extend learning.

www.g-wlearning.com/health/

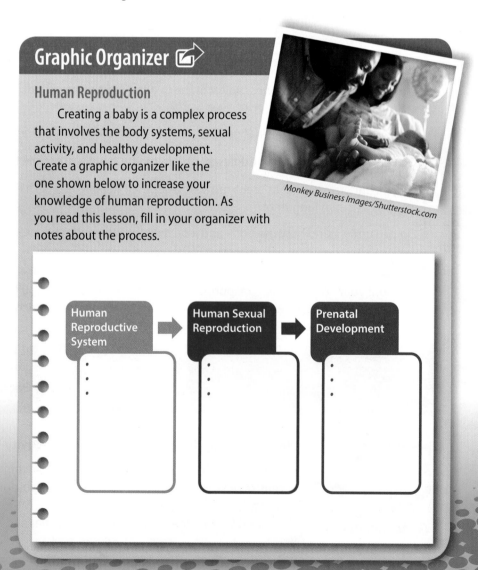

Lesson 16.1

The Beginning of Life

Key Terms 🔗

reproductive system body system that consists of a group of organs working together to make the creation of new life possible

ovulation release of an egg from one of the follicles into the uterus

menstruation discharge of some blood and tissues from the uterus

fertilization process by which the sperm and egg combine to create a zygote

zygote egg that has been fertilized by a sperm

obstetrician/gynecologist (OB/GYN) type of doctor who specializes in pregnancy, labor, and delivery

prenatal development period of growth that occurs from conception to birth

embryo term that describes a developing baby during the embryonic stage of prenatal development

fetus term that describes a developing baby during the fetal stage of prenatal development

Learning Outcomes

After studying this lesson, you will be able to

- **describe** the male and female reproductive systems.
- **explain** what the menstrual cycle is.
- **explain** what causes fertilization to take place.
- **summarize** the changes in a pregnant woman's body.
- **describe** what happens to the developing child in the three stages of fetal development.

Graphic Organizer 🔗

Human Reproduction

Creating a baby is a complex process that involves the body systems, sexual activity, and healthy development. Create a graphic organizer like the one shown below to increase your knowledge of human reproduction. As you read this lesson, fill in your organizer with notes about the process.

Monkey Business Images/Shutterstock.com

Human Reproductive System	Human Sexual Reproduction	Prenatal Development
• • •	• • •	• • •

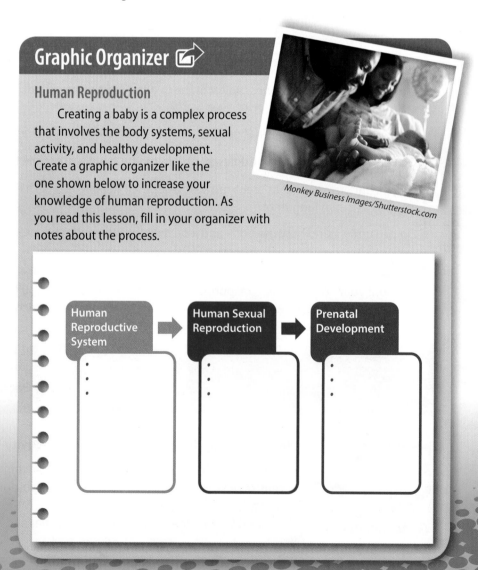

The story of your life began as a single cell. This cell was created from the merging of two cells. One cell was from your father and one cell was from your mother. The combination of these two cells produced you—a unique human being unlike any that has ever been or ever will exist. One such unique human being is 10-year-old Xavier. He was created from the merging of one cell from his biological father and one cell from his biological mother (**Figure 16.1**). In this lesson, you will learn how this amazing process works.

The Human Reproductive System

The human **reproductive system** is a body system in which organs work together to make the creation of new life possible. An *organ* is a body part with a specific function. The heart is the organ that pumps blood throughout the body. Unlike other body systems, the reproductive system does not begin to work at birth. It does not become capable of working until *puberty*, which is when the body reaches sexual maturity. Also unlike other body systems, the reproductive system is different in males and females. (You will learn more about puberty and care of the reproductive systems later in this chapter.)

The Male Reproductive System

The male organs of reproduction produce and transport hormones and *sperm*, or male sex cells (**Figure 16.2**). Male sex organs include the testes and penis, seminal vesicles, prostate, and vas deferens. These organs grow and mature as boys enter puberty. The *testes* produce sperm and the hormone *testosterone*. The *scrotum*, a saclike structure, holds the testes.

Figure 16.1 A human person is created from a combination of a female's egg and the sperm of a male. *Which body system works to create a human life?*

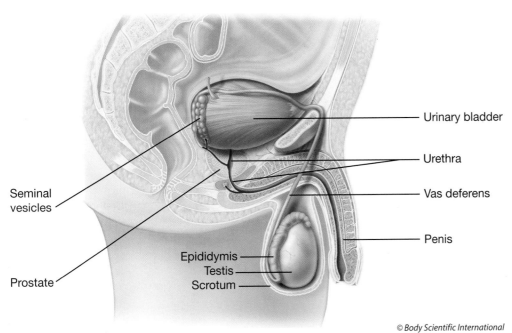

Figure 16.2 This illustration shows the side view of the male reproductive organs. Sperm form in the testes (one *testis* shown) and are carried to the penis by the vas deferens. The seminal vesicles and prostate secrete a fluid that mixes with sperm, called *semen*.

Seminal vesicles

Prostate

Epididymis

Testis

Scrotum

Urinary bladder

Urethra

Vas deferens

Penis

© Body Scientific International

As the sperm mature, they enter the *epididymis*. This structure is a coiled tube along the outer wall of the testes. It leads into another tube, the *vas deferens*. This tube carries sperm to the *penis*, the male organ used in sexual intercourse.

The penis contains tissues that can fill with blood. When that happens, the penis becomes stiff. This is called an *erection* and happens when a male is sexually excited. Intense stimulation causes the epididymis and vas deferens to contract and send sperm into the urethra. The *urethra* is a tube within the penis that has an opening at the outer end.

Before sperm leave the body, the *seminal vesicles* and *prostate* secrete a fluid called *semen*. Semen protects and nurtures sperm. *Ejaculation* occurs when more contractions force the semen out through the opening of the urethra.

The Female Reproductive System

The female reproductive organs have several functions (**Figure 16.3**). The *ovaries* produce female sex cells, or eggs (*ova*), and the hormones *progesterone* and *estrogen*. There are two ovaries, which are small, almond-shaped organs in the lower abdomen. Each ovary contains thousands of immature eggs. A *follicle*, which is a single layer of nurturing cells, surrounds each egg.

Once a female reaches sexual maturity, a single egg and its follicle grow toward maturity each month. They leave the ovary and enter the nearby opening of the fallopian tube. One *fallopian tube* leads from each ovary to one side of the *uterus*. That structure is a hollow organ lined with a tissue called *endometrium*. The walls of the uterus contain strong muscles and many blood vessels. During pregnancy, a baby develops within the uterus.

The *vagina* is a tube-like structure lined with a moist membrane. It leads from the uterus to an outer opening between the female's legs. A baby is delivered by leaving the uterus and passing through the vagina.

When females reach puberty, they begin to have a menstrual cycle each month. At the start of the cycle, a follicle develops within an ovary.

Figure 16.3
This illustration shows the side view of the female reproductive organs. Female sex organs include the ovaries, fallopian tubes, uterus, and vagina. *What term describes the release of an egg from a follicle into the uterus?*

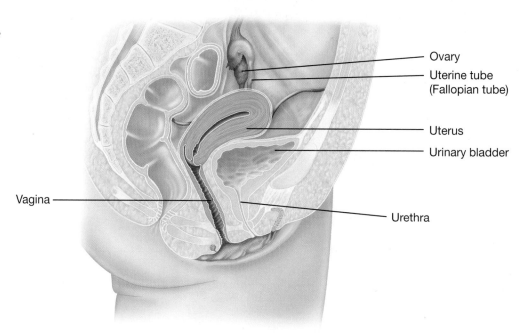

Ovary
Uterine tube (Fallopian tube)
Uterus
Urinary bladder
Vagina
Urethra

© *Body Scientific International*

The follicle grows and develops with its egg. At the midpoint of the menstrual cycle, ovulation occurs. **Ovulation** is the release of an egg from a follicle into the uterus. When this happens, the lining of the uterus thickens. This change prepares the uterus to accept a fertilized egg. If that does not occur, menstruation begins. **Menstruation** is the discharge of some blood and tissues from the uterus (**Figure 16.4**). It marks the end of a menstrual cycle, and is followed by the beginning of a new menstrual cycle.

Women have menstrual cycles each month for many years. They do not have a cycle during pregnancy, however. Each menstrual cycle lasts around 28 days. That time span can vary from person to person and even from month to month for the same person. Just before or during menstruation, a female may feel some discomfort, called *cramps*. How much discomfort is felt also varies from female to female.

Human Sexual Reproduction

Humans reproduce through sexual intercourse. For pregnancy to take place, a male's sperm must enter the female's vagina. The sperm then swim from the vagina to the fallopian tube, where an egg may be located. There, one sperm and the mature egg combine in a process called **fertilization**.

When fertilization takes place, a single sperm breaks through the outer layers of the egg. The fertilized egg is called a **zygote** (**Figure 16.5**). At that point, pregnancy begins.

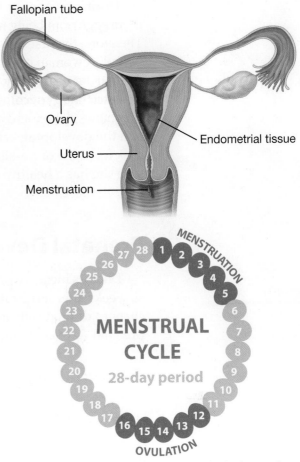

Top to bottom: © Body Scientific International; Photoroyalty/Shutterstock.com

Figure 16.4   Eggs are produced in the ovaries and are then released into the uterus. If a pregnancy does not occur during ovulation, menstruation begins. This is the discharge of some blood and tissues from the uterus. *How long does one menstrual cycle last?*

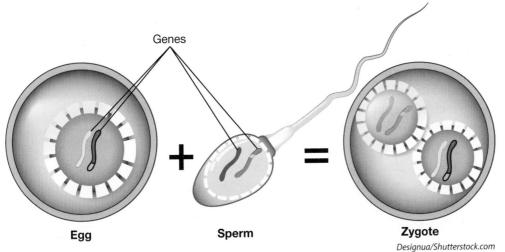

Figure 16.5
Since a zygote is formed from both a sperm and an egg, it includes the genes from both the mother and father. *What is the process called during which one sperm and one mature egg combine to form a zygote?*

Designua/Shutterstock.com

During pregnancy, the woman's body releases hormones. They stop any more eggs from being released. They also prevent menstruation from occurring. Therefore, the first sign that a woman is pregnant is often a missed menstrual period. A woman can confirm she is pregnant by having a pregnancy test.

During pregnancy, a mother should make regular visits to an **obstetrician/gynecologist (OB/GYN)**. This type of doctor specializes in pregnancy, labor, and delivery. The doctor helps the mother ensure that she and the developing baby are both healthy during pregnancy. He or she can look for signs of possible difficulties. An OB/GYN can help the mother make sure she has a healthy diet. It is very important for a pregnant woman to receive this care.

Prenatal Development

Doctors measure pregnancies in weeks. Most babies are born 36 to 40 weeks after fertilization. During a pregnancy, the developing baby changes dramatically and rapidly. This period of change is known as **prenatal development**. It consists of three stages.

Germinal Stage

The *germinal stage* of prenatal development begins at fertilization and lasts about two weeks. In this phase, the single-celled zygote goes through a process of dividing itself into many cells. First, the single cell divides into two. These two cells then each divide, producing four cells. Those cells also divide, and so on. In five days, the zygote divides seven times, forming a ball of 128 cells. Meanwhile, this ball of cells has traveled to the uterus. After eight to ten days, it implants itself in the lining of the uterus. This implanted mass of cells is called an **embryo**.

Embryonic Stage

The *embryonic stage* of prenatal development lasts about six weeks. It is a critical period. During this time, the embryo begins to form the various tissues and organs that make a human. Systems that will help the embryo develop also take shape during this stage (**Figure 16.6**). They include the following:

- A membrane grows and surrounds the embryo implanted in the uterus.
- An organ called the *placenta* forms in the uterus. Rich in blood vessels, it helps support the embryo. The placenta removes waste products of the embryo and supplies needed hormones to the embryo. It also prevents bacteria from reaching the embryo. The placenta blocks some—but not all—harmful substances from reaching the embryo as well. Chemicals such as alcohol, nicotine, and many drugs can still pass from the mother to the developing baby. The placenta cannot block them. These substances can be very harmful to the baby.
- The *umbilical cord* also forms. This tube is full of blood vessels. It connects the placenta to the developing baby at its abdomen. The cord carries food and oxygen from the mother to the embryo.

During the embryonic stage, the body's major organs also begin to take form. Around three weeks, heartbeat begins.

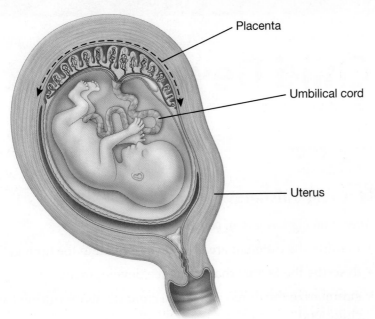

Placenta

Umbilical cord

Uterus

Figure 16.6
After the ball of cells implants itself in the lining of the uterus, the embryo begins to form the various tissues and organs that make a human. *Which stage of prenatal development involves this formation of tissues and organs?*

Fetal Stage

The ninth week of pregnancy marks the beginning of the *fetal stage*. At this stage, the baby is now called a **fetus**. This stage lasts until the baby is born. During the fetal stage, the fetus grows considerably. By the fourth month, the fetus has grown enough that the mother has a bump in her abdomen that makes her look pregnant. After nine months, most of the organs, bones, and muscles of the fetus have completed their development. When that occurs, the baby is ready to be born.

Lesson **16.1** Review

1. When does the reproductive system become capable of working?
2. In the female reproductive system, _____ is the release of an egg into the uterus.
3. **True or false.** The placenta and umbilical cords are formed during the germinal stage of pregnancy.
4. Which stage of pregnancy starts at the ninth week and lasts until the baby is born?
5. **Critical thinking.** Explain the process of human sexual reproduction, from sexual intercourse to pregnancy.

Hands-On Activity

It can be uncomfortable to talk about reproduction, especially when using words that you do not use in "normal conversation." The best way to become more comfortable talking about human development and sexual health is through practice. Using appropriate vocabulary and maturity, explain how life begins to a classmate. Start with ovulation and end with the birth of the baby. As you describe this process, your classmate should listen carefully and ask questions when something does not make sense or whenever appropriate.

Child Development

Key Terms 👉

human life cycle sequence of developmental stages a person experiences from birth through adulthood

milestones important events that occur in each of the developmental stages of the human life cycle

life span actual number of years a person lives

life expectancy estimate of how long a person in a particular society is likely to live

early childhood period of time from infancy through the preschool years

temper tantrum toddler's episode of emotional upset that often includes yelling, crying, hitting, kicking, or even biting

gross-motor skills movements that use the large muscles of the body

fine-motor skills movements that use the small muscles of the body

middle childhood period of time when children are between five and 12 years of age; also called the *school-age years*

Learning Outcomes

After studying this lesson, you will be able to

- **identify** the different areas of development in the human life cycle.
- **describe** the factors that influence development.
- **summarize** the different ways a child develops during early childhood.
- **explain** the different ways a child develops during middle childhood.

Graphic Organizer 👉

The Developing Child

Throughout the human life cycle, a person will experience physical, intellectual, emotional, and social changes. As you read this lesson, use an organizer like the one shown below to take notes about the various developments that occur during a person's early childhood years and his or her middle childhood years. Examples are provided for you.

Tanya Little/Shutterstock.com

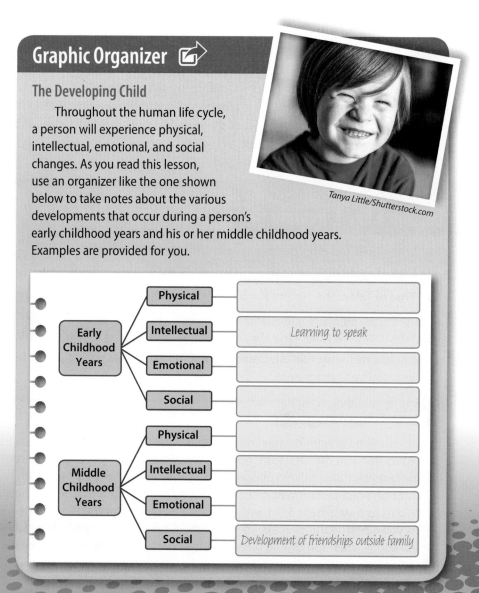

Early Childhood Years
- Physical
- Intellectual — *Learning to speak*
- Emotional
- Social

Middle Childhood Years
- Physical
- Intellectual
- Emotional
- Social — *Development of friendships outside family*

human life is made up of stages like a book is made up of chapters. The opening chapter of a book sets the stage for the following chapters. The story of a life unfolds in the same way that chapters build on each other. Each new chapter brings new elements to the plot. In this lesson, you will learn about the many changes that occur during the first chapters, or the early years, of life.

For example, Xavier from the first lesson remembers watching his little brother grow from an infant into a toddler and learn how to walk and talk. Xavier also recognizes the changes that he has gone through himself in middle childhood. He has grown several inches, learned how to be a good friend, and started to build his self-esteem.

The Human Life Cycle

When a baby is born, the **human life cycle** begins. This cycle carries a person through a series of developmental stages. With each new stage, the person begins a new phase of life. The human life cycle includes four developmental stages (**Figure 16.7**).

Each developmental stage of the human life cycle includes **milestones**, or important events. Some people reach a milestone earlier or later than others in the same stage. For example, a major developmental milestone of childhood is learning how to walk. The exact age at which a child begins to walk, however, differs from one child to the next. You will learn about adolescence and adulthood in the last two lessons of this chapter. This lesson will focus on early childhood and middle childhood.

Not all people experience every stage in the human life cycle. Some people have a much shorter life span than others. A person's **life span** is the actual number of years he or she lives. Each person's life span depends on his or her family background, environment, and lifestyle. People age at different rates, which can affect their life spans. This is because aging carries with it risks for disease and disability that can shorten a life span.

Stages of the Human Life Cycle	
Stage	**Description**
Early childhood *Tatiana Chekryzhova/Shutterstock.com*	Infancy (from birth to one year of age), the toddler years (from one to three years of age), and the preschool years (from three to five years of age)
Middle childhood *Africa Studio/Shutterstock.com*	Five to 12 years of age
Adolescence *Kseniia Perminova/Shutterstock.com*	Twelve to 19 years of age
Adulthood *RossHelen/Shutterstock.com*	Twenty years of age and older

Figure 16.7 Looking at your baby pictures and school photos together will show how dramatically you changed throughout childhood.

As the health of a society improves, so does the life expectancy of its people. **Life expectancy** is an estimate of how long a person in a particular society is likely to live. In the United States, the average life expectancy is 76.3 years for males and 81.2 years for females. Life expectancy differs from one country to another. It can also differ for groups in the same country (**Figure 16.8**).

Types of Human Development

People develop physically, intellectually, emotionally, and socially. These types of development are related and affect each other. Following are descriptions of the types of development:

- *Physical development* includes growth of the body and body parts. The other aspects of human development build on the basis of these physical changes. For instance, the brain develops and grows more complex in structure. These changes allow a child to process information, learn, and think in more complex ways.
- *Intellectual development* describes the growth of a person's ability to think. This includes how a person processes information and responds to the world. This type of development also includes learning to speak.
- *Emotional development* refers to a person's ability to form his or her own identity and personality. It includes the ability to act and react independently and to have self-esteem.
- *Social development* refers to the ability to interact with others in acceptable ways. Social and interpersonal skills develop throughout a person's life. Much of the foundation for these skills is laid in childhood.

Influences on Development

Many factors influence how a person develops. Some are internal, meaning they come from the person himself or herself. Others are external, or outside the person (**Figure 16.9**).

Figure 16.8
Certain factors can change a person's life expectancy. *What is the average life expectancy for males and females in the United States?*

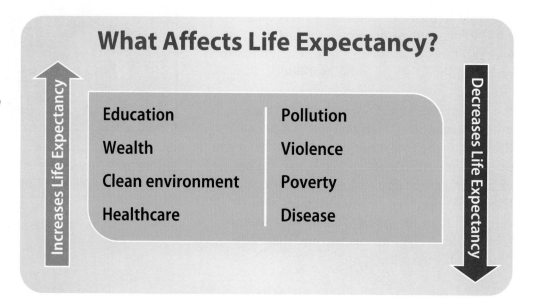

What Affects Life Expectancy?

Increases Life Expectancy		Decreases Life Expectancy
Education	Pollution	
Wealth	Violence	
Clean environment	Poverty	
Healthcare	Disease	

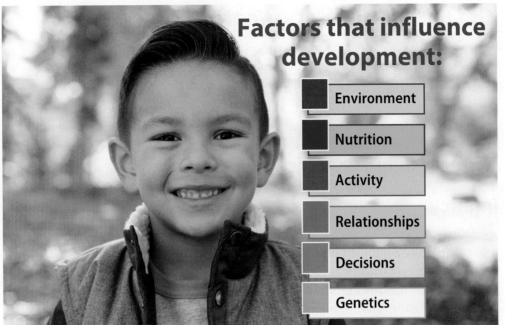

Factors that influence development:

- Environment
- Nutrition
- Activity
- Relationships
- Decisions
- Genetics

iStock.com/monkeybusinessimages

Figure 16.9 A person's level of physical activity, his or her behavior, and his or her family environment are all examples of influences that can affect how a person develops.

One key factor that influences development is the person's genetic makeup. A person's genetic makeup is the special combination of characteristics that come from his or her biological parents. Each person's genetic makeup is unique, except in the case of identical twins, who have the same genetic makeup. A person's genetic makeup sets many physical traits, such as hair and eye color. It also gives a person certain tendencies, such as whether he or she is likely to be tall or short.

Genetic makeup is not the only influence on physical appearance, however. The food a child eats when developing can affect his or her height, for instance. A childhood illness can affect physical development as well.

Family is one of the most important influences on development and health. This influence is seen in a person's genetic makeup. People in some families are at greater risk to develop certain diseases, for instance. The childhoods that parents had can influence how they raise their children. That can affect the development of those children.

The environment a person lives in also affects development and health. Growing up in a small town is different from growing up in a large city. Each type of place provides a different set of experiences. Those experiences can influence how a child develops. The healthcare that a person receives is an important part of the environment, too.

The decisions that a person makes have a major impact on his or her development. How a person talks and acts with other people shapes the friendships he or she can form. The friends a person chooses to spend time with can have an impact, too. Friends who are responsible, caring people will influence a person to be that way also (Figure 16.10). People who make risky choices can influence someone to make similar unwise choices.

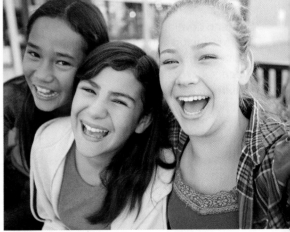

iStock.com/bowdenimages

Figure 16.10 The people you choose to spend your time with can influence you to engage in either risky or healthy behaviors.

The Early Childhood Years

The term **early childhood** describes the period of time from infancy through the preschool years. During this time, infants learn many new skills. They then become toddlers, who are always on the move. Toddlers next turn into engaging and curious preschoolers. During the preschool years, children immerse themselves in life, soaking up everything they encounter, learning and growing faster than ever before. Throughout the magical years of early childhood, children reach many milestones.

Infancy

During the first year of life, *infants* learn how to adapt to life. Infants rely completely on their parents or caregivers to meet all of their needs. As caregivers respond promptly to an infant's smiling, crying, or other attempts to communicate, they reassure the baby that he or she is safe and loved. As a result, infants form a strong attachment to their caregivers.

As infants grow, they achieve many milestones. They learn how to roll over, explore and grasp objects, and respond to voices. By the end of infancy, some children will say their first recognizable words. Others may not speak until they are toddlers. Even children who do not speak can show signs that they understand many words and phrases. When children do say their first words, they have reached a major developmental milestone.

The Toddler Years

Toddlers are one to three years of age. The growth and development that occurs in these years is amazing (**Figure 16.11**).

Figure 16.11
Learning to walk, talk, and become more independent are milestones that humans typically experience during development in the toddler years. *What is the term for negative behavior that tests the limits of a toddler's independence?*

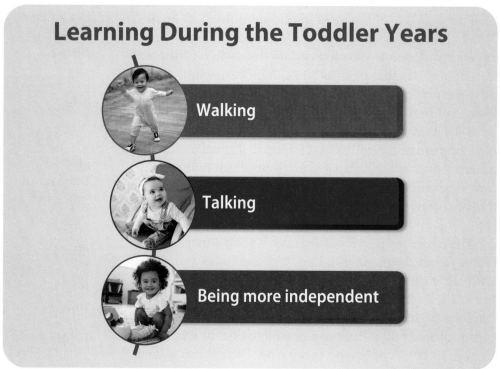

Learning During the Toddler Years

Walking

Talking

Being more independent

Top to bottom: Bplanet/Shutterstock.com; Dusan Petkovic/Shutterstock.com; Monkey Business Images/Shutterstock.com

Physically, toddlers begin to lose some of the baby fat they had as infants. They also develop more teeth, which helps them feed themselves. A major physical milestone of toddlers is taking their first steps. Once toddlers learn how to walk, they are constantly on the go and exploring everything.

A toddler's language skills are a sign of his or her intellectual growth and development. A child's first words are typically simple ones like *dada* or *mama*. Once children begin to speak, their language skills grow quickly. By the end of the toddler years, children can often say several hundred words.

Toddlers become more independent, and they often focus on doing what they want to do. If parents or caregivers prevent them from doing what they want, toddlers often react with frustration and anger. This is called a **temper tantrum**, and it includes yelling, crying, hitting, kicking, or even biting. These reactions are normal and are simply the way toddlers test limits. Temper tantrums usually occur less frequently as children learn those limits.

The Preschool Years

Preschoolers are children between three and five years of age. During this stage of development, children are usually very active. They show rapid development of two kinds of motor skills, which include the following:

- **Gross-motor skills** involve movements that use the large muscles of the body. Running, hopping, and climbing are just a few examples of preschoolers' activities that require gross-motor skills (**Figure 16.12**).
- **Fine-motor skills** involve movements that use the body's small muscles. Preschoolers can use these skills to copy letters of the alphabet, put jigsaw puzzles together, or build a tower of blocks.

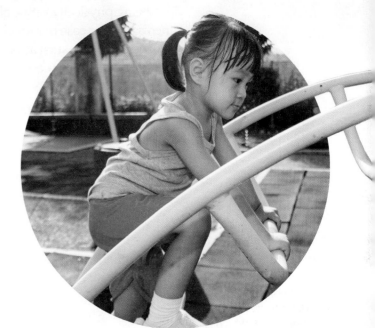

iStock.com/kiankhoon

Figure 16.12
Skills involving large muscle movements like climbing, running, and hopping are developed during the preschool years. *What are these large muscle movement skills called?*

Because of preschoolers' improved motor skills, they can interact with more objects and engage in more activities than toddlers. Brain development enables preschoolers to observe more and develop more ideas about their world. Language skills also continue to improve at a rapid rate among preschoolers.

In the preschool years, children engage in more social activities than ever before. This enables preschoolers to form relationships with new adults and friends. Preschoolers seek to please others, especially parents, caregivers, family members, familiar adults, and friends. Children this age are forming their first friendships. Preschoolers also begin to develop empathy. *Empathy* is a sense of how another person may be feeling. This is an emotional milestone because it prepares children to form healthy, close relationships.

The Middle Childhood Years

Middle childhood, or the school-age years, refers to the period of time when children are between five and 12 years of age. This stage includes another major milestone—children begin going to school. During these years, important physical, intellectual, emotional, and social growth and development take place.

Physical Development

Children tend to grow at a slow and steady pace during the school-age years. By the end of this period, though, growth may alternate between periods of quick development and slow change. This is why the height and weight of children who are the same age can be very different (**Figure 16.13**).

Children who eat too many calories and are not active enough physically can become overweight. Children who become overweight or obese often have a difficult time losing weight as they mature. Establishing healthful habits of eating and physical activity can help children be healthy throughout their lives.

Being physically active also helps children improve their motor skills. It increases their ease of movement as well. Many school-age children enjoy playing organized sports, such as baseball or soccer. Children who are active develop muscle strength and coordination faster than children who are less active.

Intellectual Development

Children encounter many new learning opportunities in the school years. Schoolwork increases their language and problem-solving skills. Advances in brain development enable school-age children to become logical thinkers who learn from their previous experiences. Children apply knowledge they have gained in the past to solve current problems.

Figure 16.13
Toward the end of middle childhood, children gain weight and develop at different rates, which is why few children are the same height and weight.

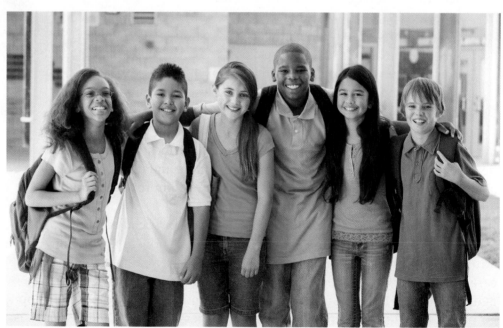

iStock.com/monkeybusinessimages

During the school-age years, children think about their world in a concrete way. This means that they think about the present and generally do not think about the future. School-age children often do not link today's actions to future effects. They have not yet developed the skill of planning because they cannot think abstractly (Figure 16.14).

In addition, school-age children generally think about issues in either-or terms. They seek answers that are simple and straightforward, and do not yet see the complexity of problems very easily.

Emotional and Social Development

School-age children have an expanding social network. These years are characterized by the development of friendships and other relationships outside the family. Children learn how to be a good friend.

During the school-age years, children also develop their *self-esteem*. This is a person's sense of worth, purpose, security, and confidence. Healthy self-esteem develops by having supportive family and friends. It also develops from having accomplishments. When children successfully deal with mistakes and accomplish projects at school, they learn to feel confident about their abilities. Handling arguments with friends and adapting to changes at home can also build self-esteem.

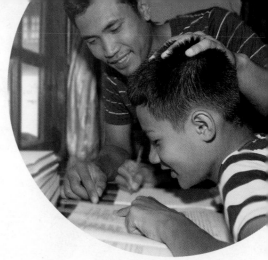

i am way/Shutterstock.com

Figure 16.14
Since school-age children have difficulty planning in a concrete way, parents and guardians should help their children plan for future needs and consequences.

Lesson 16.2 Review

1. Important events in the development of a human life, like learning how to walk, are called _____.
2. What are the four types of human development?
3. What is the difference between gross-motor skills and fine-motor skills?
4. What is a major milestone of middle childhood?
5. **Critical thinking.** What developments occur for children during middle childhood? Explain physical, intellectual, social, and emotional developments.

Hands-On Activity

Talk with your parents, guardians, or other trusted adults about your childhood, from infancy through your middle childhood years. Ask about your milestones as well as all aspects of your development (physical, intellectual, emotional, and social). Combine the information from this conversation with your memories to create a timeline of your childhood so far. Use images and pictures if you can. Are there times that are harder for you to remember? What about for the adults in your life? How do your memories compare to theirs?

Adolescence and Puberty

Learning Outcomes

After studying this lesson, you will be able to

- **describe** the physical changes that occur in males during puberty.
- **explain** the physical changes that occur in females during puberty.
- **summarize** the intellectual, emotional, and social growth and development that occurs during adolescence.
- **identify** common health and wellness issues that affect adolescents.

Graphic Organizer 🖝

Adolescent Development

On a separate sheet of paper, create a graphic organizer like the one shown below. As you read this lesson, take notes on each type of development that humans experience during adolescence. List as many details as you need to fill out the organizer. An example is provided for you.

antoniodiaz/Shutterstock.com

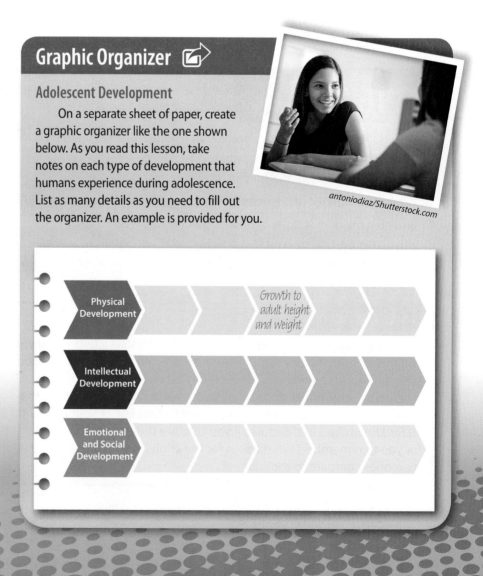

Physical Development — Growth to adult height and weight

Intellectual Development

Emotional and Social Development

A child's body and mind transform during adolescence. No longer children, but not yet adults, adolescents undergo changes that prepare their minds and bodies for adulthood. On their way to adulthood, adolescents experience many physical, intellectual, emotional, and social changes. These changes begin with puberty, when the reproductive system starts to mature.

Xavier looks forward to becoming a teenager. He hopes that he will grow taller and grow a beard. He is excited to go to high school, get a job, and learn how to drive. You will learn about these changes and other aspects of adolescence in this lesson.

Physical Development and Puberty

Physical changes are the trademark of **adolescence**, or the period of development between 12 and 19 years of age. During this time, males and females complete most of their physical growth. They achieve their adult height and weight. Their sexual organs also mature, which means they become capable of sexual reproduction. **Puberty** is the period of time during which all of these physical changes are taking place. Everyone goes through puberty, so it helps to know what changes to expect during this time (**Figure 16.15**).

Sex hormones drive the physical and emotional changes of puberty. Puberty is triggered when brain hormones affect the testes in males and the ovaries in females.

Puberty in Males

Puberty begins in males around 10 to 14 years of age. The hormone **testosterone** triggers growth and development of the male sex organs. These hormones also cause the development of male secondary sexual characteristics, which include the following:

- pubic, facial, and body hair
- deep voice
- broad shoulders
- muscle mass

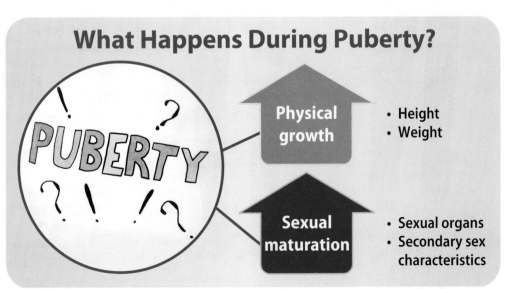

Figure 16.15
Both males and females will experience physical growth and sexual maturation during puberty. *During which stage of the life span does puberty begin?*

designer491/Shutterstock.com

Puberty: What to Expect

Males:
Starts between ages 10–14

Females:
Starts between ages 8–14

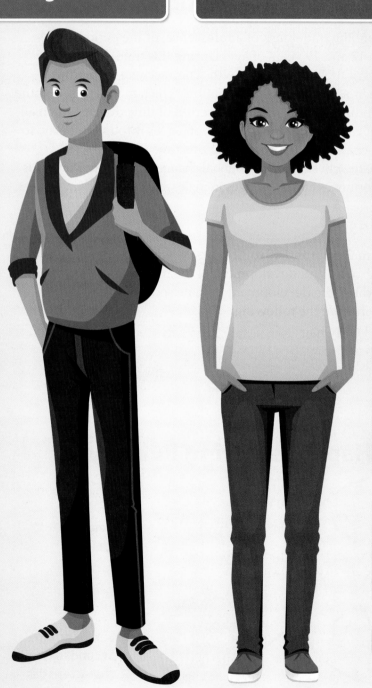

Males:
- Voice deepens, but may crack occasionally
- Shoulders broaden
- Facial, body, pubic hair growth begins
- Muscle mass increases
- Increase in height up to 4 inches per year
- Weight gain
- Acne breakouts may appear on face, shoulders, and back

Females:
- Increased oil production in skin and scalp may lead to acne
- Breasts develop
- Underarm, leg, and pubic hair growth begins
- Menstruation begins
- Increase in height up to 3 inches per year
- Weight gain, and additional fat concentrated in hips, thighs, and buttocks
- Hips widen

Boy: Jemastock/Shutterstock.com; Girl: Volhah/Shutterstock.com

During puberty, males also grow taller and gain weight quickly. Their growth rate may even double, and males can grow 4 inches in one year. By the time puberty ends, a male may have grown 14 inches and gained 40 pounds.

Another change that happens during puberty is increased oil production on the skin and scalp. This extra oil can lead to acne on the face, shoulders, back, and chest. Sometimes, males experience swelling in their breasts. This development can be upsetting to some boys. It is normal, however, and usually goes away as adolescence continues.

Males experience erections and sexual desires during puberty. As their reproductive systems develop, they should start paying attention to possible problems and important care procedures (**Figure 16.16**). Males also become curious about sex. They may feel sexually attracted to another person.

Caring for the Male Reproductive System

Problems	Care
Hernia	Get medical care.
Sexually transmitted infections (STIs)	Practice abstinence and get medical care.
Testicular cancer	Check the testes for any swelling or lumps.
Testicular injury	Wear protective equipment.
Testicular torsion	Seek emergency care.

Figure 16.16 Listed are possible problems of the male reproductive system and care procedures. In addition to these care procedures, males should practice good reproductive hygiene. They should keep the organs of the reproductive system clean and protected.

CASE STUDY

Akiko Feels Left Behind

"Why does everyone look and act so much older than me?" Akiko asks her older sister. Akiko is in eighth grade and feels like the other kids, especially the other girls, are all getting a lot taller and more mature than she is. Akiko thinks she still looks like a little kid. There are girls in her class who have started wearing bras and shaving under their arms. Some of her friends have even gotten their periods already. Akiko feels like her body looks the same as it has for years, except maybe she is a little taller.

Akiko is not ready to be an adult yet. She likes the freedom of being a kid, but she does not want to be left behind. Some of her friends have started to ask boys out on dates. There is someone Akiko thinks she likes, but she does not really know what that means. Akiko thinks maybe she just likes this person because her friends do. She might want to have a boyfriend, but she is also kind of grossed out by the idea, especially the idea of kissing a boy. Akiko is pretty sure she would rather just hang out with her friends watching videos, creating new and

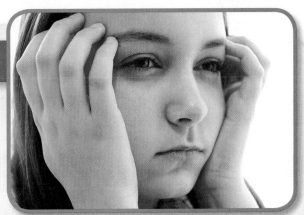

Monkey Business Images/Shutterstock.com

amazing food dishes, and playing outside. Akiko is so confused about life right now that she does not know what she really wants. She thinks being in middle school is tough, and she is not even talking about SCHOOL!

Thinking Critically

1. If you were Akiko's older sister, what would you say to Akiko? How would you say it? When would be the best time and place to have this conversation?

2. Is Akiko's social-emotional development abnormal? What about her physical development? Explain.

Puberty in Females

Females begin puberty earlier than males. The first sign of puberty in females is breast development, which occurs around 8 to 14 years of age. In females, the hormone **estrogen** triggers growth and development of the female sex organs. Estrogen also causes development of female secondary sexual characteristics. These include breast development and growth of pubic, underarm, and leg hair. During puberty, a girl's hips also widen, and fat is added to the hips and buttocks.

During puberty, a female's body grows quickly as well. Girls can grow up to 3 inches per year. By the end of puberty, a female may have grown 10 inches and gained 25 pounds.

Females also begin menstruating during puberty. The *menarche*, or first menstrual period, may be upsetting to a young female. Parents or a doctor can help an adolescent girl understand what menstruation means and how to prepare for this monthly cycle. As their reproductive systems develop, females should start paying attention to possible problems and important care procedures (**Figure 16.17**).

Like males, females experience increased oil secretion on the skin and scalp. They may also develop acne. With these physical changes, females also grow curious about sex and may experience sexual attraction.

Intellectual Development

During adolescence, the brain is still developing. Young adolescents think in concrete terms, as they did in childhood. They often view the world in black-and-white terms and may fail to see the complexity of many situations. Adolescents may be unable to imagine future consequences that could arise from their actions. As a result, young adolescents may act without thinking and take risks that can harm their health, such as experimenting with alcohol or drugs.

As adolescents mature, they develop the ability to think more abstractly and to see more than two sides of issues. This ability permits them to handle more challenging situations or problems. They can think through issues that are more complex. They can understand different points of view.

Figure 16.17
Listed are possible problems of the female reproductive system and care procedures. *How can a girl better understand and prepare for her monthly period?*

Caring for the Female Reproductive System	
Problems	**Care**
Breast cancer	Check the breasts for any lumps or swelling.
Ovarian cysts	Get medical care.
Premenstrual syndrome (PMS)	Treat cramps with medication, if necessary.
Sexually transmitted infections (STIs)	Practice abstinence and get medical care.
Toxic shock syndrome	Change tampons every four hours.
Yeast infection	Keep the reproductive area clean, change sanitary napkins every four hours, and get medical care.

Over time, adolescents gain the ability to think about more abstract concepts. Even older adolescents, however, may occasionally fail to predict the consequences of their actions (Figure 16.18). They may still take risks. They can participate in risky behaviors when they ignore what they have learned intellectually and focus on what they see as emotional and social needs. For example, adolescents sometimes engage in risky behavior in the hopes of winning the acceptance or respect of peers.

Emotional and Social Development

Adolescents feel the need to establish their independence, to be on their own, and to rely on their own judgment. School activities and friends offer plenty of opportunities to gain independence. The chance to make independent decisions and explore life is important for adolescents' emotional growth.

Some adolescents emphasize their independence by distancing themselves from their parents or guardians. They might not be as affectionate as they were in childhood. This change can be upsetting to parents. Some adolescents say less to their parents or guardians about their day at school than they did when younger. They often do this out of a desire to maintain privacy and to show their independence.

While adolescents seek independence, they also have a strong need to feel that they belong. The social world becomes increasingly important to them. Adolescents' relationships will include new friends, friends of the opposite sex, boyfriends or girlfriends, teachers, and coaches. As their social life grows, adolescents get a taste of what adult life is like.

Adolescents are typically concerned about being accepted by their peers. They may seek their peers' approval and try to fit into a group of peers at school or in the neighborhood (Figure 16.19). Peers can be a source of support and fun. Unfortunately, adolescents can also be negatively influenced by peers. That influence may cause them to engage in behaviors they might not otherwise choose.

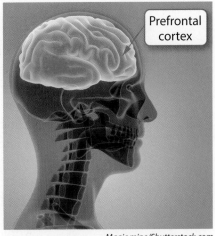

Magic mine/Shutterstock.com

Figure 16.18 One of the last portions of the brain to fully develop is the prefrontal cortex, which is responsible for rational thinking and decision making. The prefrontal cortex usually has not fully developed until age 25. Because of this, young people may have trouble practicing good judgment.

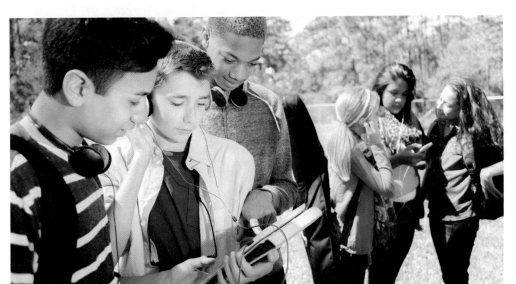

iStock.com/fstop123

Figure 16.19
After valuing family relationships for most of their lives, adolescents typically begin to value peer relationships as well. *What health and wellness issue can result from a desire to fit in with peers?*

Another important change in adolescence is development of a sense of personal identity. Adolescents ask questions like "Who am I?" and "What am I really like?" They may act, talk, and relate to others in different ways over time. These changes are often an attempt to try out different personalities. Adolescents are looking for the one that feels right, when they feel true to themselves. Over time, adolescents come to have a surer sense of who they are. They can base that sense of identity on the values they hold, the goals they have, and the ways of acting that feel most right to them.

Health and Wellness Issues

Adolescents face health and wellness issues that are not common in childhood. They also face issues not usually seen in adulthood. Some of these issues arise because of newly acquired independence. For instance, having the ability to drive means they now face decisions about how to drive safely.

BUILDING Your Skills

Peer Pressure Throughout the Life Span

During childhood and adolescence, peers become a major source of stress. (Remember, the stress from peers can be good!) Peers are people around the same age and they have a big influence on a person's decisions, behaviors, and life, especially through childhood and adolescence, but even throughout adulthood.

Sometimes, peers will explicitly ask or tell another person to do something (external peer pressure). Other times, the pressure is internal, meaning the individual wants to do something that others are doing because they want to fit in. The desire to fit in and belong with others is a natural and powerful feeling. Both types of peer pressure (internal and external) can be positive and persuade people to do great things. Both can also be negative, however, and push people to behave in ways that do not promote physical, social, or mental health.

Role-Play: Positive and Negative

In small groups, choose a stage of life to focus on: early childhood, middle childhood, adolescence, or adulthood. Then, plan and perform two role-play situations, both based on the stage of life you chose. The first role-play situation should involve the person dealing healthfully with positive peer pressure. The second role-play situation should involve the person dealing healthfully with negative peer pressure. Once you have performed your role-play situations, answer the following questions:

1. What similarities in peer pressure across life stages are present? What differences?

2. What strategies are effective at dealing with peer pressure? Are these the same for both positive and negative peer pressure? Explain.

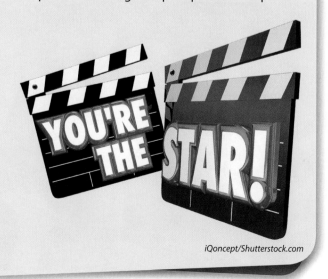

iQoncept/Shutterstock.com

Handling Peer Pressure

Some health and wellness issues result from new pressures from peers. Adolescents might see someone being bullied. Then, they face the choice between standing up for the person being bullied or being a bystander. To make this choice, they need to call on their sense of what is right. They may also have to take safety into account. Adolescents not sure of how to handle situations like this can talk to a trusted adult.

Adolescents can also be pressured to join with others in risky behaviors. Adolescents who think about their own identity and values can resist this kind of negative peer pressure. Thinking about the consequence of these risky behaviors can help as well.

Using a decision-making process can help adolescents prepare for resisting peer pressure (**Figure 16.20**). Good decision making starts with identifying the issue or problem. Then you need to identify all the choices you can make. Once you identify your choices, you weigh the costs and benefits of each option. Use your values and goals to help you analyze these costs and benefits. Then choose the option that has the best balance of costs and benefits. Taking this approach can help you resist negative peer pressure.

Teen Pregnancy

One possible consequence of giving in to negative peer pressure is becoming a parent. Since adolescents have reached sexual maturity, they run the risk of pregnancy if they engage in sexual behavior.

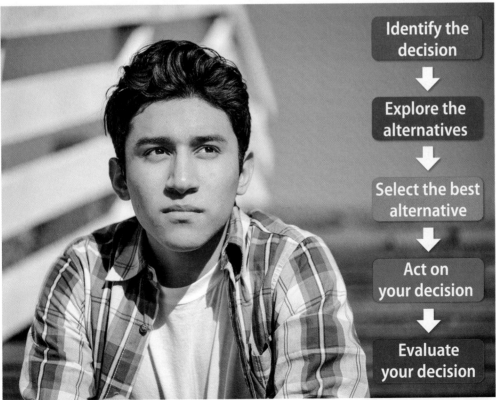

Figure 16.20
Using the decision-making process can help young people, who are learning what they think is right and wrong, stand up for their beliefs and values.

Identify the decision
↓
Explore the alternatives
↓
Select the best alternative
↓
Act on your decision
↓
Evaluate your decision

mdurson/Shutterstock.com

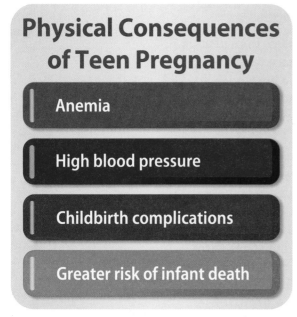

Physical Consequences of Teen Pregnancy

- Anemia
- High blood pressure
- Childbirth complications
- Greater risk of infant death

Figure 16.21 Adolescent girls, in particular, are at an increased risk of physical complications and illnesses during pregnancy. *What kind of medical care is important for adolescent girls who become pregnant?*

Pregnancy can cause serious problems for adolescent girls since their bodies are still developing (**Figure 16.21**). The demands of a growing fetus can interfere with growth during puberty. It is very important that a pregnant adolescent get good prenatal care.

Being a parent poses other challenges to adolescents, too. Adolescent parents are at risk of dropping out of school. This can rob them of the chance to build the future they want for themselves. Adolescent parents are at risk of living in poverty as well.

Adolescent parents also face emotional difficulties. Parenting is hard work, full of responsibilities. Adolescents who are still trying to sort out their own lives can feel overwhelmed by meeting the demands of a baby. They can feel depressed and alone. Adolescent parents also face changes to relationships that can cause difficulties. Some experience strained relations with family members. Others find that they no longer see their friends because they have to spend so much time caring for a child or because they are no longer in school.

Some adolescents who become pregnant choose to give their babies up for adoption. They feel unable to meet the demands of parenting. State agencies can help a teen with that choice. For instance, California has a *Safely Surrendered Baby Law* that helps adolescent mothers give up their child while ensuring that the baby's health and safety are protected.

Lesson 16.3 Review

1. What is the time period in adolescence during which physical growth and sexual development occur?

2. The hormone _____ causes the development of male sex organs and secondary sexual characteristics, like facial hair and a deep voice.

3. **True or false.** Relationships including friends, coaches, boyfriends or girlfriends, and teachers, help adolescents feel that they belong.

4. Thinking about their values and identity can help adolescents resist negative _____ _____.

5. **Critical thinking.** How can emotional and social development during adolescence cause conflict between the adolescent and his or her parents or guardians? What changes are occurring?

Hands-On Activity

Create a Venn diagram to compare and contrast puberty and adolescence in females and males. Be sure to include all aspects of health and development as you complete the diagram. After it is complete, draw conclusions about puberty and adolescence for teenagers in general.

Adulthood and Aging

Learning Outcomes

After studying this lesson, you will be able to

- **identify** and **describe** the stages of adulthood.
- **describe** how people can adapt to the changes that occur during aging.
- **summarize** types of care people may need as they approach the end of life.
- **explain** the stages of grief and how people can cope with grief and loss.

Key Terms 🔗

young adulthood stage of human development that occurs from 20 to 40 years of age

middle adulthood stage of human development that occurs from 40 to 65 years of age

older adulthood stage of human development that begins at 65 years of age

sandwich generation adults who care for their parents as well as their own children

hospice care type of care given to people who are dying that provides comfort and support to them and their families

Graphic Organizer 🔗

The Effects of Aging

As you learned earlier in the chapter, growth and development begins before a baby is even born. Once a baby is born, growth and development occur rapidly throughout childhood and into adolescence when puberty begins. In this lesson, you will learn that development continues into adulthood. As you are reading this lesson, use an organizer like the one shown below to take notes about the development and changes that occur during adulthood.

India Picture/Shutterstock.com

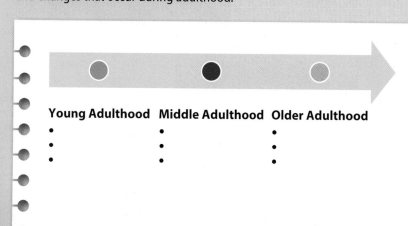

Young Adulthood	Middle Adulthood	Older Adulthood
•	•	•
•	•	•
•	•	•

How do you know when you have become an adult? Do you become an adult when you reach a certain age—18 or 21, for example? Does a particular event such as getting a driver's license, graduating from high school or college, or getting married make you an adult? Do you become an adult when your body is fully developed and capable of reproduction?

Xavier, from the previous lessons, wonders about adulthood. His older cousins are in their 20s, his parents are in their 40s, and his grandparents are in their 60s. Xavier is curious about what to expect as he grows older.

In this lesson, you will learn about the different stages of adulthood (**Figure 16.22**). You will also learn about changes that occur during each of these stages and how these changes affect health. Some health changes that occur in adulthood are inevitable. Others can be avoided by making healthful choices today and throughout life.

The Mature Adult

Adulthood is defined in many different ways. In the United States, state and federal governments see most people as adults when they become 18 years old. In most states, people are able to vote and marry without their parents' permission once they reach that age. When a person turns 18, he or she can also be treated as an adult in a court of law.

Figure 16.22
Humans continue to develop beyond childhood and adolescence, growing from young adults, to middle adults, and finally older adults.

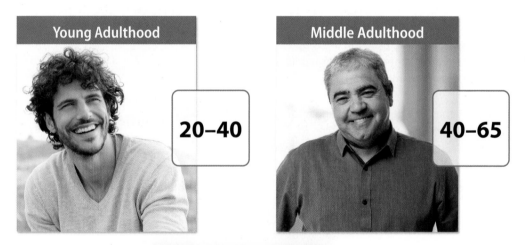

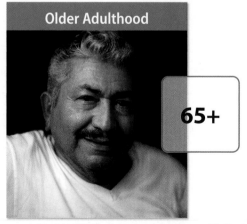

Left to right: Rido/Shutterstock.com; Asier Romero/Shutterstock.com; Joseph/Shutterstock.com

Another definition of adulthood is based on physical maturity. As you read in the previous lesson, adolescents develop mature reproductive systems. They become physically able to have children. Adolescents must mature in many other ways, however, to be considered adults. Perhaps most importantly, they must gain intellectual, emotional, and social maturity (Figure 16.23).

Stages of Adulthood

Adults continue to change and develop through various stages of adulthood. **Young adulthood** occurs from 20 to 40 years of age, **middle adulthood** occurs from 40 to 65 years of age, and **older adulthood** is considered 65 years of age and older. Adults in each stage share many experiences, rewards, and challenges.

Young Adulthood

People achieve full physical maturity in young adulthood. Adults who are 20 to 40 years of age possess their greatest strength, endurance, and cognitive abilities. Their sensory organs and reflexes have reached peak performance. As a group, young adults are healthy and active.

There are benefits to reaching adulthood. Many young adults get jobs and enjoy having an income. That income allows them to buy goods and services they want. Many begin to set up their own homes and live independently.

Of course, living independently carries responsibilities as well. Young adults who rent an apartment sign a legal agreement called a *lease*. By signing it, they promise to make rental payments on time. Those who borrow money to buy a car are responsible for making regular payments.

There is no typical young adult in the United States. Young adults may be single, married, or divorced. Some have children, and some do not. Some live alone, some live with their parents, and some live with other young adults.

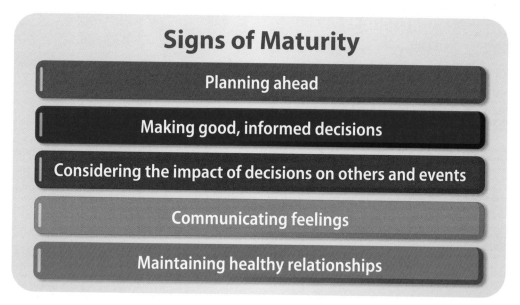

Signs of Maturity

Planning ahead

Making good, informed decisions

Considering the impact of decisions on others and events

Communicating feelings

Maintaining healthy relationships

Figure 16.23
Certain character traits, like good communication and decision making, are signs that a person has reached full maturity and would be considered an adult.

Marriage and divorce are major life-changing events for young adults. In the United States, the age of marriage has risen steadily. Today, many adults are not married. Those who do marry often wait until they are older and more mature (**Figure 16.24**).

Divorce can occur during any stage of adulthood. Some 40 to 50 percent of marriages end in divorce. A divorce profoundly changes a person's life. It affects income, living arrangements, and home ownership. Divorce also causes relationships with children, other family members, and friends to change. Divorce has a major effect on a person's emotions and sense of self. Unmarried young adults with long-term relationships may experience breakups that can cause as many changes as a divorce.

Middle Adulthood

In the United States, adults who are 40 to 65 years of age tend to be fairly healthy. As a group, middle-aged adults remain active. Their physical strength and coordination, however, gradually go down over time. So does their *endurance*, or the ability to keep doing physical activities for a long period of time. Their reflexes slow, but their thinking skills and memory remain intact. Some loss of hearing and vision occurs during middle adulthood.

Many middle-aged adults have adolescent or adult children. Meeting their needs, or helping them out, may cause financial and emotional stress. Middle-aged adults often have increased responsibilities at work that can add to the stress they feel.

Figure 16.24
Fewer Americans today are getting married, and more people are waiting to do so until they are older, more financially stable, and more mature. ***What percent of marriages end in divorce?***

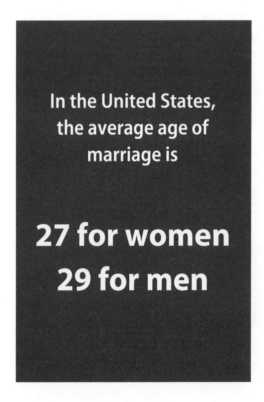

In the United States, the average age of marriage is

27 for women
29 for men

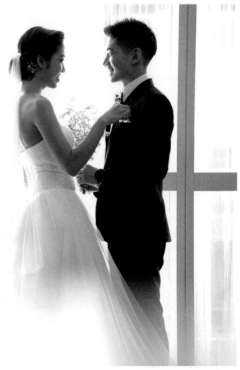

In recent years, the number of older adults has increased. As a result, more middle-aged adults—and some younger adults—find themselves caring for aging parents. Balancing personal and professional responsibilities can be a source of stress for these caregivers. This burden is even greater for adults who also have children. Adults who care for their parents as well as their own children are called the **sandwich generation** (Figure 16.25).

Older Adulthood

Advancing age brings joy and new ways of life. It can also bring loss and grief. When older adults retire from work, they find time to start new jobs, pursue hobbies, and make new friends. Many older adults enjoy the company of grandchildren and begin new relationships with their own adult children. Many older adults, however, also experience worsening health and loss of independence. They may have lower incomes and have to face the loss of friends and family.

To maintain their health, older adults need to maintain a social life, feel productive, and remain active. This is especially true for older adults who have lost their spouse and live alone. Many retired adults meet these needs by working part-time jobs. Others volunteer at schools, hospitals, or other settings that provide education or care to others. Still others take courses to learn new skills or explore new subjects.

Adaptations to Aging

A number of changes can be expected during aging. These changes are not necessarily the result of diseases or disorders. It is normal for many body functions to decline as the body grows older (**Figure 16.26** on the next page).

By adapting to the changes caused by aging, adults can maintain an active, healthy life. Some older adults use technologies that make up for reduced abilities. Hearing aids help older adults with hearing loss. Bifocals, a type of eyeglasses with extra lenses, and large fonts improve reading. Engaging in meaningful activities can help keep the mind sharp.

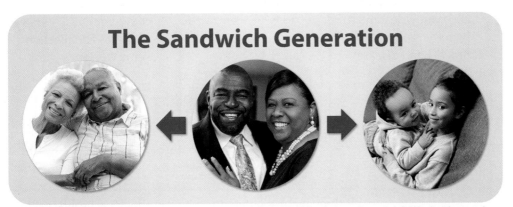

The Sandwich Generation

Left to right: Monkey Business Images/Shutterstock.com; pixelheadphoto digitalskillet/Shutterstock.com; Lightfield Studios/Shutterstock.com

Figure 16.25
People in middle adulthood are frequently faced with having to care for their own children as well as their aging parents. This is known as being in the sandwich generation.

Health Changes During Adulthood

Body System	Health Changes	Body System	Health Changes
Sensory organs 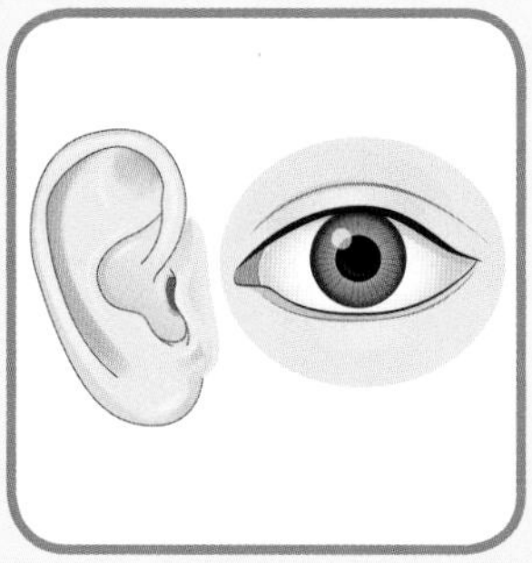 *solar22/Shutterstock.com*	• Wrinkles, age spots, and skin tags develop. • Older adults find it difficult to focus on close objects or read small print. • Hearing loss occurs.	**Respiratory system** 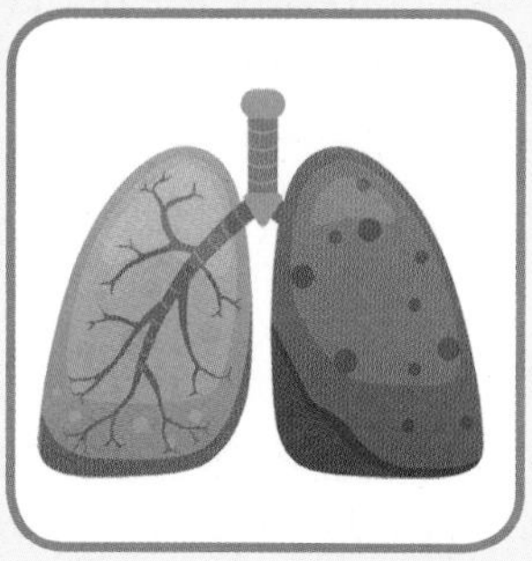 *Gaidamashchuk/Shutterstock.com*	• Chest and rib muscles weaken, leading to shortness of breath. • Risk of lung infection increases.
Digestive system 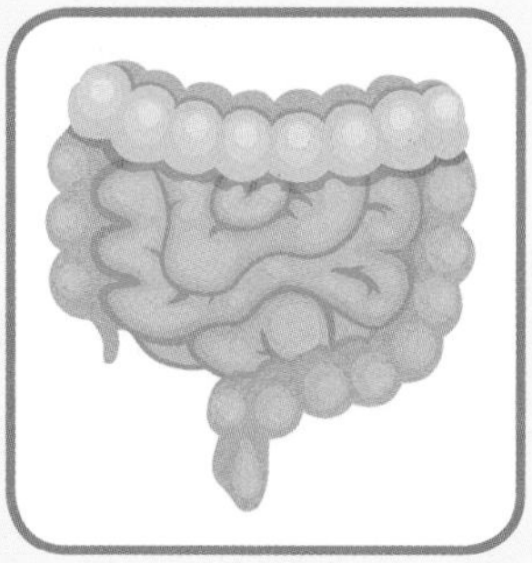 *Gaidamashchuk/Shutterstock.com*	• The mouth becomes dry, and cavities are more common. • Intestinal linings thin, slowing digestion. • Liver function decreases, increasing medication side effects.	**Reproductive system** 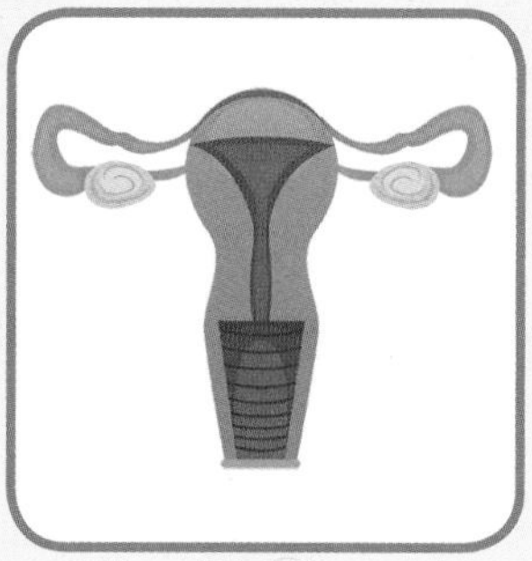 *Gaidamashchuk/Shutterstock.com*	• Women enter menopause, the end of the reproductive years. • The prostate can grow larger, causing infection.
Urinary system 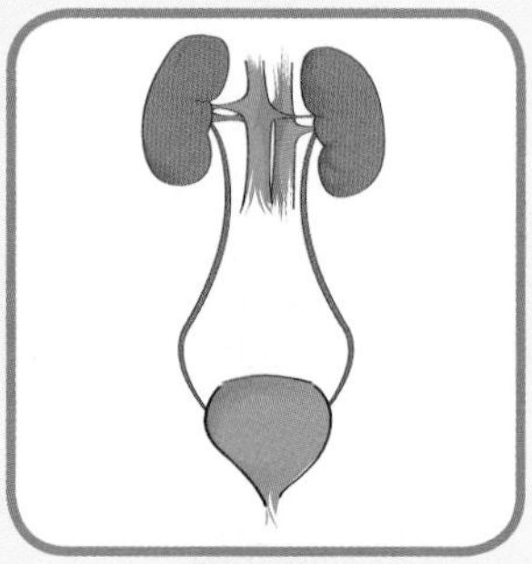 *Kateriz/Shutterstock.com*	• Kidney function decreases, leading to dehydration. • Incontinence, or the inability to control urination, sometimes develops. • The risk of urinary tract infections increases.	**Muscles and bones** 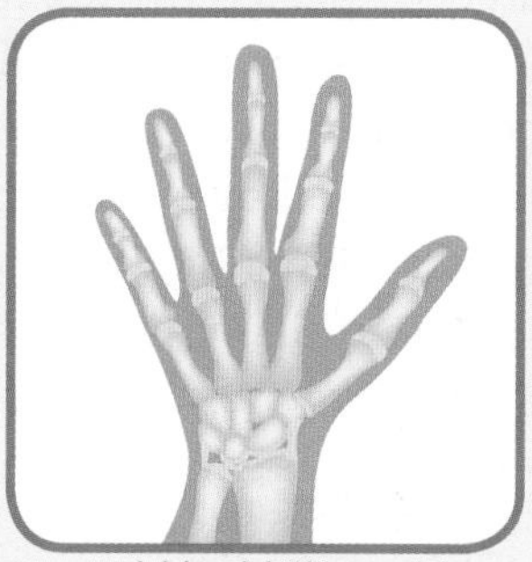 *gritsalak karalak/Shutterstock.com*	• Muscle mass and strength decrease. • Bones lose density, strength, and mass. • Joints become stiff and sometimes painful.
Circulatory system 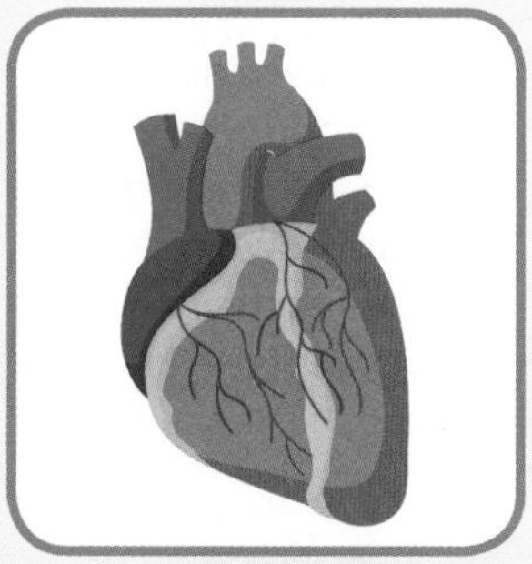 *EgudinKa/Shutterstock.com*	• Blood vessels stiffen and narrow, leading to hypertension. • Risk of heart disease increases.	**Nervous system** 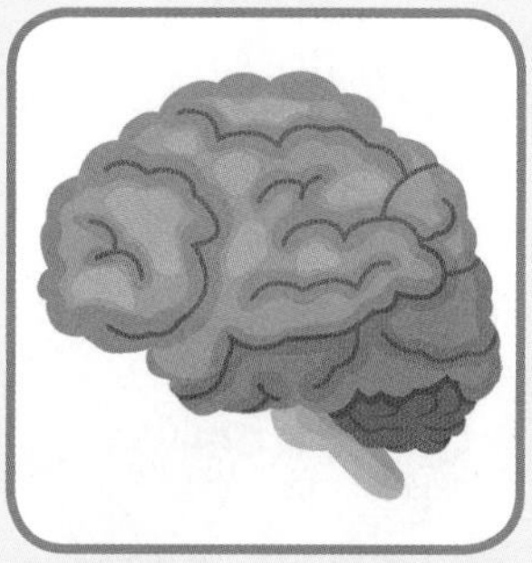 *Gaidamashchuk/Shutterstock.com*	• Memory may deteriorate. • Reflexes and reaction time worsen.

Figure 16.26   Each of the body systems slowly declines throughout adulthood, resulting in additional health changes for older adults to consider. *What is an example of a device that an older adult can use to adapt to reduced mobility, strength, and balance?*

Older adults can also adapt to reduced mobility, strength, and balance. Canes, wheelchairs, and other devices help adults to remain mobile. At home, ramps can be built to replace steps to make going up or down a level easier. The home can be modified to reduce the risk of falls.

Adults can continue to be physically active by adapting as they age. Instead of running, older adults can walk, bike, or swim. These activities keep them active while lowering the impact on their joints and bones. There is an option if endurance becomes a problem as well. Older adults can do activities more often, but for shorter periods of time.

Many older adults can live independently as long as they remain healthy. Some older adults need small amounts of help. They may be unable to drive and need someone to take them places. Adults with serious health problems, however, require a great deal of care. This can include daily care like dressing, eating, bathing, and using the bathroom. It can also mean the need for healthcare. Older adults who need a great deal of care often cannot live alone. Luckily, there are housing options such as the following to help take care of these older adults (**Figure 16.27**).

The End of Life

The human life cycle ends in death. Death can occur at any time and can be sudden or expected. When it is expected, a person may receive hospice care in the months leading up to death. The goal of **hospice care** is to provide comfort for people who are dying and their families. During hospice care, a dying person does not receive treatment for his or her disease. Instead, patients receive pain relief and emotional support and comfort.

The end of the human life cycle is often accompanied by grief. *Grief* is a complex emotional experience that includes a profound sense of loss and sadness.

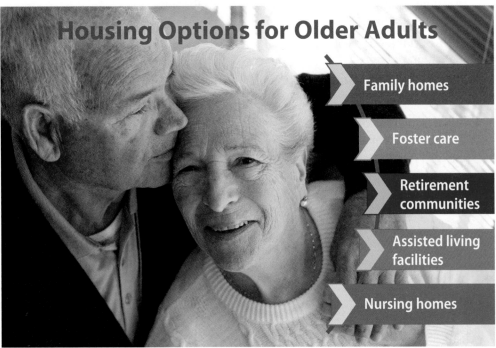

Housing Options for Older Adults

Family homes

Foster care

Retirement communities

Assisted living facilities

Nursing homes

La Vieja Sirena/Shutterstock.com

Figure 16.27
Different settings for older adult housing can provide different types of care. A nursing home, for example, can provide medical care, while assisted living facilities can provide relative independence for older adults.

As you learned in Chapter 5, a grieving person has many feelings following the death of a family member, spouse, or friend (**Figure 16.28**).

Grieving is a normal and healthy process. People should be allowed to grieve through whatever means they feel is right. They might need to feel very sad and cry for a long time. They might also need to mark the loss with a ritual, such as a funeral. During the grieving process, people can practice the following healthy behaviors:

- Avoid isolation. Instead, share feelings with trusted people.
- Do not make difficult decisions or major life changes. If major decisions must be made, discuss with close family members.
- Seek help with personal care tasks. Get professional help for coping, if necessary. Not getting necessary help can lead to depression.
- Get good nutrition, physical activity, and adequate sleep.

Figure 16.28
When a loved one dies, it is normal to experience grief. Not everyone experiences all the stages of grief, and not in a precise order, but these are the general emotions associated with the grieving process.

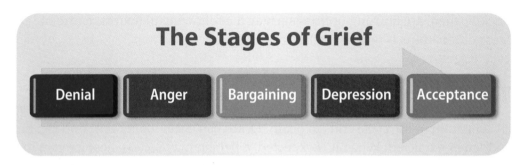

The Stages of Grief

Denial — Anger — Bargaining — Depression — Acceptance

Lesson 16.4 Review

1. Which of the following is a developmental stage of adulthood?
   A. Older adulthood.   C. Parenthood.
   B. Early adulthood.   D. All of the above.

2. **True or false.** A typical young adult is married, has children, and lives in his or her own home.

3. Adults who care for their parents as well as their own children are called the _____ generation.

4. What is the type of care given to people who are dying that provides comfort and support to them and their families?

5. **Critical thinking.** What are some examples of changes that occur throughout older adulthood? What are some ways that older adults can adapt to these changes to maintain an active, healthy life?

Hands-On Activity

Think about how you want your adulthood to look—consider all stages of adulthood. Draw, write, or create something that displays the picture in your mind. Include what health and behavioral choices you can and will make to promote health and wellness throughout adulthood. Share your drawing, writing, or creation with a classmate and with your family.

Summary

Lesson 16.1 The Beginning of Life

- The human reproductive system consists of a group of organs that begins working at puberty, when the body reaches sexual maturity. Male reproductive organs include the testes and penis, seminal vesicles, prostate, and vas deferens. Female reproductive organs include ovaries (which produce ova), uterus, and vagina.
- The male reproductive organs produce and transport sperm. The female reproductive organs produce eggs. For pregnancy to occur, the sperm enters the vagina. There, one sperm and one egg form a zygote in a process called *fertilization*.
- Prenatal development refers to the developments of a baby during pregnancy. This consists of the germinal stage, embryonic stage, and fetal stage.

Lesson 16.2 Child Development

- The human life cycle carries a person through the developmental stages. Important events that occur throughout the life cycle are called *milestones*. A person's life span is the actual number of years lived. The estimate of life span is known as *life expectancy*.
- Human development includes physical, intellectual, emotional, and social development. Many factors influence human development. The early childhood years include the infant, toddler, and preschooler stages. Children between five and 12 years of age are in middle childhood.

Lesson 16.3 Adolescence and Puberty

- Young people between 12 and 19 years of age are in *adolescence*. During adolescence, people undergo significant physical changes as they enter puberty. Some of the changes during puberty include growth in height and weight, acne, sexual attraction, and sexual curiosity for both males and females.
- During adolescence, people develop the ability to handle challenging situations and more complex issues. Adolescents want to establish independence, rely on their own judgment, and maintain privacy. Social relationships become increasingly important. This means that peer pressure can become more of an issue.

Lesson 16.4 Adulthood and Aging

- People achieve their greatest strength and cognitive abilities in young adulthood (20 to 40 years old). There are benefits to this stage, such as a job and house, and responsibilities.
- In middle adulthood (40 to 65 years old), people remain healthy. Their strength and coordination, however, begin to decline.
- Older adulthood (65 years and older) brings joys as well as loss and grief. Older adults adapt to the decline in their bodies' functions, such as mobility and strength.
- The human life cycle ends in death. If a death is not unexpected, a person may receive hospice care to provide comfort. Grief involves a profound sense of loss and sadness.

Check Your Knowledge ⤴

Record your answers to each of the following questions on a separate sheet of paper.

1. What are the names of male and female sex cells?
2. A(n) _____ is a doctor who specializes in pregnancy, labor, and delivery.
3. What are the three stages of prenatal development?
4. What is the difference between life span and life expectancy?
5. **True or false.** The early childhood stage begins after infancy and ends after preschool.
6. Which stage of development involves children beginning to go to school?
7. Which of the following is *not* a symptom of *both* male and female puberty?
   A. Growth of pubic hair.   C. Acne.
   B. Broadened shoulders.   D. Sexual attraction and curiosity.
8. **True or false.** During adolescence, people gain the ability to think about abstract concepts, which means they will no longer participate in risky behaviors.
9. Why can pregnancy cause serious physical problems for adolescent girls?
10. Which stage of adulthood involves a person's greatest strength, endurance, and cognitive abilities?
    A. Young.   C. Older.
    B. Middle.   D. None of the above.
11. Identify three things older adults can do to maintain their health.
12. List the stages of grief.

Use Your Vocabulary ⤴

adolescence	life expectancy	prenatal
early childhood	life span	development
embryo	menstruation	puberty
estrogen	middle adulthood	reproductive system
fertilization	middle childhood	sandwich generation
fetus	milestones	temper tantrum
fine-motor skills	obstetrician/gynecologist	testosterone
gross-motor skills	(OB/GYN)	young adulthood
hospice care	older adulthood	zygote
human life cycle	ovulation	

13. In teams, create categories for the terms above and classify as many of the terms as possible. Then, share your ideas with the remainder of the class.
14. Classify the list of terms above into the following categories: sexual reproduction and human development. Find a classmate to partner with and then together compare how you classified the terms. How were your lists similar? How were they different? Discuss your lists with the class.

Think Critically

15. **Identify.** Compare the structures in male and female reproductive systems and describe how each perform similar functions.

16. **Draw conclusions.** Can anyone with a uterus get pregnant the first time she has sexual intercourse? Can anyone with a penis get someone pregnant the first time he has sexual intercourse? Explain.

17. **Make inferences.** What stage of life do you believe is the most difficult? Which is the easiest? Explain your reasoning based on the information in this chapter.

18. **Predict.** "With freedom comes responsibility." How does this quote by Eleanor Roosevelt relate to your life right now? How will it relate to your life as you move through adolescence and all stages of adulthood?

DEVELOP Your Skills

19. **Access information.** What are the main questions that most people your age have about puberty, adolescence, reproduction, or the life span? What do you wish you understood better? What rumors have you heard that you are not sure are correct? Write your questions and then find correct answers from reliable sources. List the sources you used.

20. **Literacy and communication skills.** Interview a trusted older adult about human development and the human life span. Develop at least five questions about adulthood that interest you and be prepared to ask them, using proper vocabulary and maturity. Write an essay to report the results of your interview. What have you learned about adulthood? Before turning your essay in to your teacher, be sure to have the person you interviewed review it.

21. **Decision-making and goal-setting skills.** What is most important to you? What do you value? What do you believe?

Who are you, to your core? Are you able to answer these questions easily? It is all right if you cannot, but these are important questions to think about as a young person. Take some time to think about the answers to these questions and create a mission statement for your life. Post this mission statement in your locker, on the wall by your bed, on your mirror, or any place where you will see it every day. Let this serve as a reminder of who you are and what you want out of life. How can knowing your values and your self-identity improve your ability to resist negative peer pressure?

22. **Teamwork skills.** Working with a partner, draw a timeline that portrays the life span of a human. Start with prenatal development and continue all the way to the end of life. At various ages on the timeline, mark as many milestones and aspects of development as you can. Write a short explanation that describes the human development portrayed in your timeline.

Chapter 17

The Body Systems

Video ↗
Access the Chapter 17 video to start thinking about chapter topics.

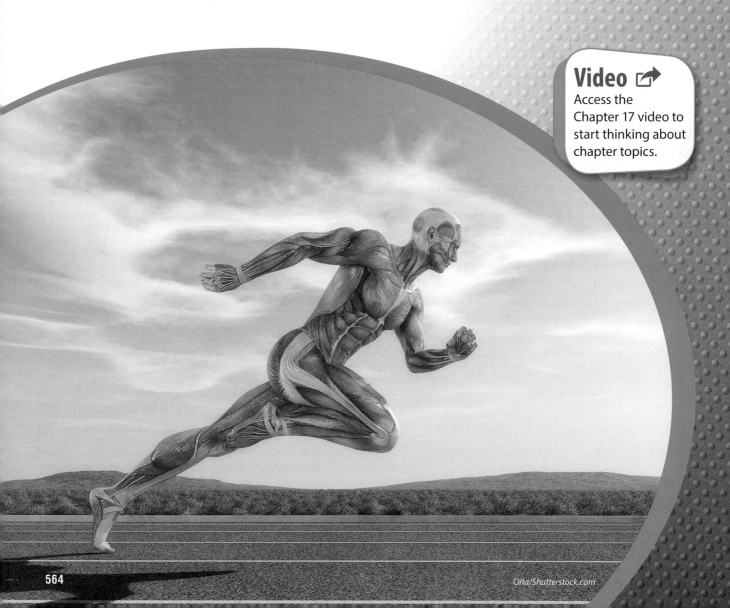

Orla/Shutterstock.com

Reading Activity

Before you read the chapter, look at the list of key terms for each lesson and create a list of any key terms with which you are not familiar. Look up these terms in a dictionary. Write down the definitions of these terms in your own words. As you read the chapter, revise your definitions as needed.

How Healthy Are You?

In this chapter, you will be learning about the human body and its systems. Before you begin reading, take the following quiz to assess your current understanding of the human body systems, and how each system affects your health and wellness.

Health Concepts to Understand	Yes	No
Do you know what is the basic unit of life?		
Can you name the body system that includes the skin, hair, and nails?		
Do you know which body system is made of 206 bones that provide structure, shape, and protection to the body?		
Can you name the three types of muscle tissue in the muscular system?		
Do you know which body system moves blood throughout the body to provide oxygen, nutrients, and energy?		
Do you know which body system exchanges oxygen and carbon dioxide through inhaling and exhaling?		
Can you name the body system that brings food into the body and breaks it down?		
Do you understand which organs are involved in the removal of liquid waste from the body in the urinary system?		
Do you know which body system removes foreign substances from the body?		
Can you name the body system that involves the brain, spinal cord, and nerves?		
Do you understand how the endocrine system uses hormones to control the body?		

Count your "Yes" and "No" responses. The more "Yes" responses you have, the more you understand human body systems. Now, take a closer look at the questions with which you responded "No." Think about how you can increase your understanding of issues in these areas.

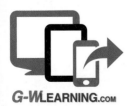

While studying this chapter, look for the activity icon to

- **practice** key terms with e-flash cards and matching activities.
- **reinforce** what you learn by completing graphic organizers, self-assessment quizzes, and review questions.
- **expand** knowledge with interactive activities and activities that extend learning.

G-WLEARNING.com

Supporting and Moving the Body

Key Terms

tissue collection of similar cells that do a certain job for the body

gland group of cells that produce and release substances into the body

organ collection of tissues that perform a specific job

body system collection of organs that work together

integumentary system body system that covers and protects the entire body

skeletal system body system made up of 206 bones that provides structure, shape, and protection to the body

joint location in the body where two or more bones meet and are held together

ligaments strong bands of tissue that hold together bones at joints to allow movement

muscular system body system that helps the body move and aids other body systems

tendons structures made of tough tissue that connect muscle to bone

Learning Outcomes

After studying this lesson, you will be able to

- **describe** the structures of the integumentary system and what they do.
- **describe** the parts of the skeletal system and what they do.
- **describe** the structures of the muscular system and what they do.
- **explain** how bones, joints, and muscles work together.

Graphic Organizer

Support and Movement

As you read through this lesson, use a graphic organizer like the one below to take notes on each system of the body that helps with the support and movement functions of humans. Make sure to note the structures, body parts, and organs involved in each body system. For each system, answer the question "what does this system allow my body to do?"

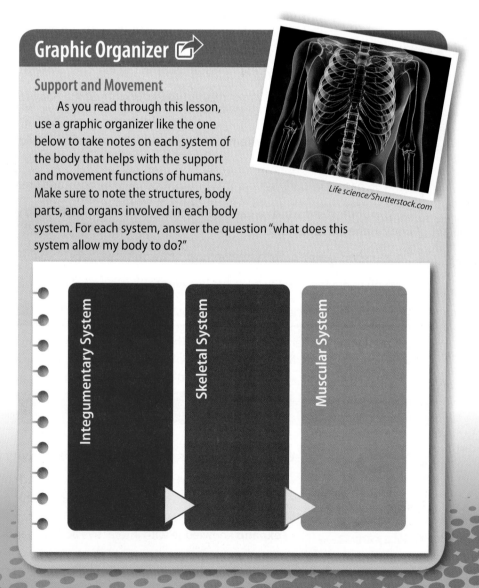

Life science/Shutterstock.com

Integumentary System

Skeletal System

Muscular System

Have you ever wondered why you sweat when you play sports, or why your skin gets darker after being in the sun? Do you know what parts of your body allow you to sit, stand upright, walk, or run? These are just a few examples of tasks your body accomplishes every day. Each task requires the cooperation of cells, tissues, and systems throughout your body. The integumentary, skeletal, and muscular systems, discussed in this lesson, provide support and movement for the body.

Organization of the Body

The body is organized into cells, tissues, organs, and body systems (**Figure 17.1**). *Cells* are the basic unit of life. All living things, including the human body, are made of cells. In the body, cells are organized as tissues. A **tissue** is a collection of similar cells that do a certain job for the body. For example, muscle tissue is made of muscle cells. Muscle tissue can contract and shorten, enabling muscles to move.

Some tissues form glands. A **gland** is a group of cells that produce and release substances into the body. For example, the salivary glands in the mouth release saliva. This liquid breaks down food so that it can be swallowed.

Tissues work together to form organs. An **organ** is a collection of tissues that perform a specific job. For example, the stomach is an organ. Its job is to store and digest food. The stomach is made of several kinds of tissue, including muscle, connective tissue, and nerve tissue.

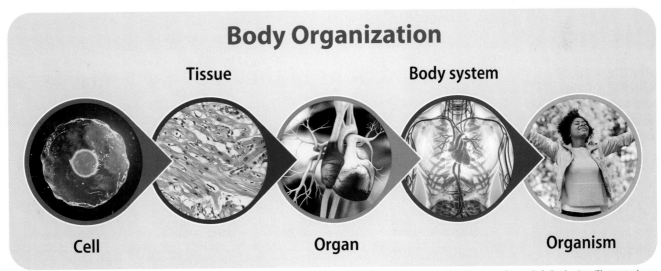

Body Organization

Tissue   Body system

Cell   Organ   Organism

Figure 17.1 At the cellular level, different cells perform functions in the body. These cells form tissues, and different tissues form organs, which carry out specific jobs. Organs make up body systems, and body systems combine to make the human organism. *What is the basic unit of life that makes up everything in the human body?*

Organs work with other organs. A collection of organs that works together is a **body system**. You learned about the male and female reproductive systems in Chapter 16. This chapter reviews the other major body systems. Each of these systems performs a set of important functions and makes up the human organism (**Figure 17.2**).

Some body systems work very closely together. For example, the skeletal and muscular systems work together so you can walk and run and move your arms. The respiratory and circulatory systems work closely together to bring air into the body and move it through the blood.

Integumentary System

The **integumentary system** is one of three systems that support and move the body. The integumentary system includes the skin, hair, and nails. It covers and protects the entire body and may be the most familiar body system. You see the integumentary system as you look at another person and when you look in the mirror. It is the only body system completely exposed to the world outside the body.

Skin

The *skin* is the largest organ in the human body. If spread flat, the skin would cover 17 to 20 square feet, about the size of a bedsheet.

Skin protects the body and does a surprising number of important jobs. Skin keeps out germs that could infect the body. Skin removes some waste and makes vitamin D, which the body needs to build strong bones. Skin also contains nerve endings that are part of the nervous system. These nerve endings allow people to sense pain, touch, and pressure.

Figure 17.2
The different body systems perform different functions. The reproductive system, which you learned about in Chapter 16, is responsible for reproducing human life. *Which body systems are responsible for moving and exchanging substances?*

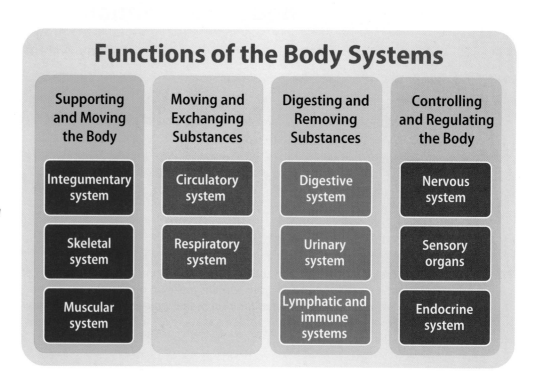

Functions of the Body Systems

Supporting and Moving the Body	Moving and Exchanging Substances	Digesting and Removing Substances	Controlling and Regulating the Body
Integumentary system	Circulatory system	Digestive system	Nervous system
Skeletal system	Respiratory system	Urinary system	Sensory organs
Muscular system		Lymphatic and immune systems	Endocrine system

As you learned in Chapter 2, skin is made of three layers: the epidermis, the dermis, and the hypodermis (**Figure 17.3**). The dermis contains a variety of glands. *Oil glands* make an oily substance called *sebum*. These glands are on all of the body except the palms and the soles of the feet. Sebum keeps the skin soft and moist and prevents hair from becoming brittle. These glands become more active at puberty. They can sometimes become blocked and infected with bacteria, causing pimples.

Sweat glands are found all over the body. *Sweat glands* release watery, salty sweat onto skin surfaces. As sweat evaporates, skin temperature drops and cools the body. Special sweat glands located in the armpit and genital areas begin to work at puberty. This type of sweat, when combined with bacteria, can result in body odor.

Hair and Nails

Hair and nails are made by cells in the skin. Both hair and nails are made of the protein keratin. Hair grows on all skin surfaces except the palms, soles, lips, nipples, and some areas of the genitals. Each hair grows from a specialized cell called a *hair follicle*. Hair, like the skin, helps protect the body. For example, eyelashes and eyebrows shield the eyes. Nose hair prevents dust and particles from entering the airways. Head hair helps regulate temperature and protects the head from sunlight.

Nails protect the ends of fingers and toes. They grow on the upper sides of fingers and toes near the ends. As they grow, the older cells are pushed out, making the nails longer.

Skeletal System

The **skeletal system** (**Figure 17.4** on the next page) is made up of 206 bones. Bones provide structure, shape, and protection. For example, you can stand upright because of your sturdy and flexible backbone.

Layers of the Skin	
Layers	**Functions**
Epidermis	• Forms the skin's outer layer and protects against foreign substances. • Continually sheds and replaces the outer layer of skin cells. • Contains *keratin*, which protects the skin from drying out and from minor cuts and scratches. • Contains *melanin*, which gives the skin pigment.
Dermis	• Contains nerve endings that sense heat, cold, pain, and pressure. • Contains *collagen*, which strengthens skin and helps hold skin to the body. • Contains *elastin*, which allows skin to stretch and return to its original shape. • Contains hair follicles, oil glands, and sweat glands.
Hypodermis	• Contains cells that store fat and help the body keep a steady temperature. • Connects the skin to underlying bone and muscle.

Figure 17.3
The three layers of skin contain keratin, melanin, nerve endings, collagen, elastin, and fat cells. Together, they form the largest organ in the human body. *Which type of gland found in the dermis keeps skin soft and hair strong, but can also cause acne?*

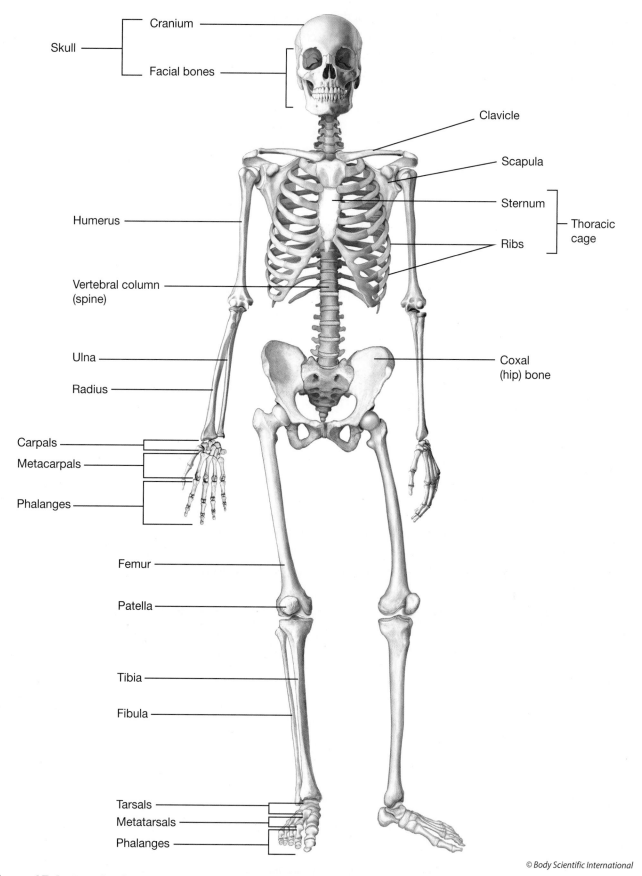

Skull ⎰ Cranium
       ⎱ Facial bones

Clavicle

Scapula

Sternum ⎱ Thoracic
Ribs   ⎰ cage

Humerus

Vertebral column
(spine)

Ulna

Radius

Coxal
(hip) bone

Carpals

Metacarpals

Phalanges

Femur

Patella

Tibia

Fibula

Tarsals

Metatarsals

Phalanges

© Body Scientific International

Figure 17.4   In red is the axial skeleton, which forms the trunk of the body. The appendicular skeleton, or bones of the arms and legs, are white. *How many bones are in the skeletal system?*

You can walk because your leg bones are strong and movable. The ribs protect the heart, lungs, and other internal organs. The skull and backbone protect the brain and spinal cord. Bones also make movement possible when they are attached to muscles.

Bone Tissue

Bones develop, grow, and change throughout life. They are made of minerals, proteins, and living cells. Bone hardness comes from the minerals *calcium* and *phosphate*. Bone flexibility comes from the protein *collagen*. To envision bone tissue, think of a gelatin dessert with marbles in it. The marbles represent the hard minerals. The firm, flexible gelatin represents collagen. Together, the gelatin and marbles have hardness and flexibility, like bones.

Bones can grow and change because they contain living bone cells. Some bone cells can make more bones. Other cells dissolve bones. Weight-bearing exercise, such as running and lifting weights, puts stress on bones. That stress pushes bone-making cells to make more bone tissue.

Bone Structure

Bones come in many shapes and sizes (**Figure 17.5**). For example, bones of the arms and legs are long. Bones of the skull, hip, and backbone are flat or have an irregular shape. Most bones have a dense outer tissue. Inside that dense tissue is a softer, spongy bone tissue. This spongy tissue contains cells that can make blood cells. The long bones of the arms and legs also have a hollow space filled with fat.

The ends of some bones are covered with *cartilage*, which is not as hard as bone. The cartilage slowly turns into bone tissue until it is all used up, causing growth. This growth stops at different ages in different people. Some people stop growing in their mid-teens. Others continue growing into their mid-twenties.

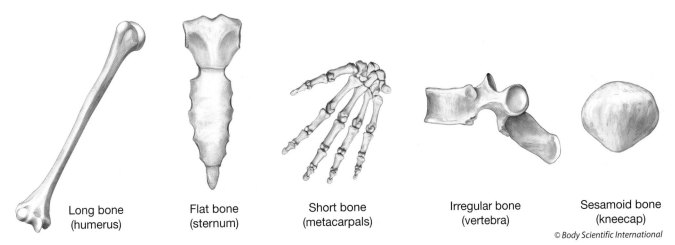

Long bone
(humerus)

Flat bone
(sternum)

Short bone
(metacarpals)

Irregular bone
(vertebra)

Sesamoid bone
(kneecap)

© *Body Scientific International*

Figure 17.5 Bones found in the body include long bones, flat bones, short bones, irregular bones, and sesamoid bones. *Which shape are the bones of the arms and legs?*

Joints

The skeletal system can move because of joints. A **joint** is a location where two or more bones meet. Some joints, such as those in the shoulder, move a great deal. Other joints, such as those in the skull, do not allow bones to move.

In joints that allow movement, bones are held together by strong bands of tissue called **ligaments**. For example, the tibia, or lower leg bone, and the femur, or large thighbone, meet at the knee joint. Ligaments hold the femur and tibia together.

The knee joint and other moving joints are kept moist by a special fluid. This fluid reduces the amount of friction between moving bones. It also cushions the bones that meet in the joint. In a joint that moves, cartilage covers the bones' surfaces. This tissue absorbs shock in the joint and protects the ends of the bones.

Muscular System

The **muscular system** helps the body move and plays important parts in other body systems. For example, the skeletal and muscular systems work together to move the body. Muscles are made of specialized tissue that can shorten and stretch. When muscle tissue shortens, or *contracts*, it pulls its ends closer. If the muscle is attached to a bone, this motion can make the bone move (**Figure 17.6**). A bone can move when a muscle stretches, too. Nerves from the brain or spinal cord stimulate muscles to contract or stretch.

Muscles are connected to bones by **tendons** made of tough tissues. Like muscles, tendons can shorten or lengthen. Muscles, bones, and tendons work closely together.

Muscle Tissue

Muscles are built from bundles of muscle cells. Different muscle cell arrangements create different types of muscle. There are three types of muscle tissue: skeletal muscle, smooth muscle, and cardiac muscle (**Figure 17.7**).

Figure 17.6
When muscles contract, they can move bones. For example, when the biceps on the front of your arm contracts, it pulls your lower arm toward your upper arm. *What is the name of the tough tissue that connects muscles to bones?*

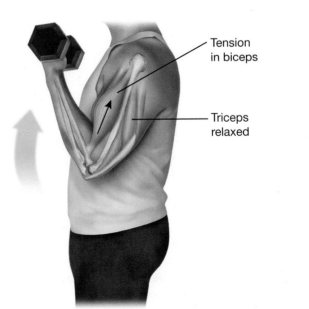

Tension in biceps

Triceps relaxed

Skeletal muscles are attached to bones. They are voluntary, which means you can control them. For example, you can choose to move your legs to walk or move them faster to run. You choose to use your hand muscles to type.

Smooth muscles cannot be controlled. These muscles work without you realizing it. They do very important work, however. For example, the smooth muscles in your intestines digest food. *Cardiac muscle* is involuntary muscle found in the heart. This muscle pumps blood through the body.

Muscle Pairs

Muscles can contract and relax. Most skeletal muscles contract to move the bones of the body. They can also relax, allowing body parts to return to an original state. Throughout the body, most skeletal muscles work in pairs to move certain body parts. Some examples of muscle pairs are the following:

- The biceps muscle contracts to bend the arm at the elbow. The triceps muscle contracts to straighten the arm at the elbow.
- The hamstring muscle contracts to bend the leg at the knee. The quadricep muscle contracts to extend the leg at the knee.
- The gluteus medius muscle contracts to bend the leg at the hip. The gluteus maximus muscle contracts to extend the leg at the hip.

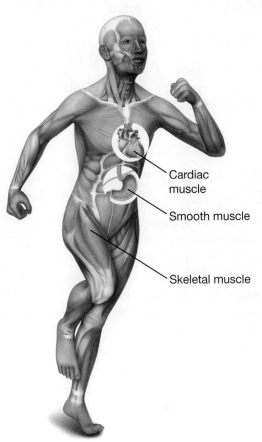

Cardiac muscle

Smooth muscle

Skeletal muscle

© Body Scientific International

Figure 17.7 You can control the skeletal muscles in your body. For example, you can raise your arm or extend your leg. You cannot control the smooth and cardiac muscles in your body. These muscles work without you knowing.

Lesson 17.1 Review

1. A body system is a collection of _____ that work together to perform a set of important functions.
2. **True or false.** The integumentary system includes the skin, hair, and nails.
3. What is a joint?
4. Which type of muscle is voluntary?
5. **Critical thinking.** Explain how the skeletal and muscular systems work together to cause movement.

Hands-On Activity

Have a classmate outline your entire body on large paper. Add drawings to "your body" of the organs and structures from this lesson (skin, glands, hair, nails, bones, muscles, joints). What behaviors will keep these structures and organs healthy? Save this drawing for use in the other lessons.

Moving and Exchanging Substances

Key Terms 🔗

circulatory system body system formed by all the structures that move blood through the body

heart hollow, muscular organ located in the center of the chest; pumps blood into the circulatory system

arteries blood vessels that carry oxygen-rich blood

capillaries small arteries that deliver oxygen and nutrients to cells and pick up cells' waste

veins blood vessels that carry oxygen-poor blood

plasma watery part of blood

respiratory system body system of organs that obtain vitally important oxygen from the outside world

bronchi two air passages, each of which connects the trachea to a lung

respiration exchange of oxygen and carbon dioxide between the body and the air around it

diaphragm sheet of muscle beneath the lungs and above the abdomen that contracts and relaxes to help the chest expand so a person can inhale or shrink so a person can exhale

Learning Outcomes

After studying this lesson, you will be able to

- **identify** the organs of the circulatory system.
- **describe** what the circulatory system does.
- **identify** the organs of the respiratory system.
- **describe** functions of the organs of the respiratory system.

Graphic Organizer 🔗

Movement and Exchange of Substances

Before you read this lesson, create a table like the one shown below. Write down three predictions about the circulatory and respiratory systems. Base these predictions on your current knowledge of the human body. As you read the lesson, make any corrections necessary to the predictions you made and include as many notes as needed to fill the table.

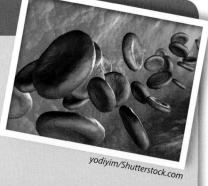

yodiyim/Shutterstock.com

Body Systems	Predictions	Notes
Circulatory system	1. 2. 3.	• • •
Respiratory system	1. 2. 3.	• • •

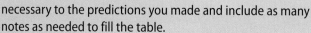

T wo body systems do the work of exchanging substances with the outside world and moving them through the body. The circulatory system moves substances through the blood. The respiratory system brings air into and out of the body. These two body systems will be explained in this lesson.

Circulatory System

The body must have a continual supply of oxygen, nutrients, and energy. Several organs work together to move the blood that contains these substances throughout the body. These organs are part of the **circulatory system**.

The circulatory system includes the heart, arteries, veins, and capillaries (**Figure 17.8**). Laid end to end, the arteries, veins, and capillaries in one adult's body would reach more than 62,000 miles. This is long enough to go around Earth's equator two and one-half times. Arteries, veins, and capillaries make it possible for blood to reach every area of the body. Blood carries oxygen, nutrients, waste, cells, and other substances throughout the body.

Heart

The **heart** is a hollow, muscular organ located in the center of the chest. The heart is a steadily working muscle. It beats around 30 million times per year and pumps about 4,000 gallons of blood each day.

The heart contains four hollow spaces called *chambers*. The top two chambers are called *atria*. The bottom two chambers are called *ventricles*. Valves control the direction of blood flow in the heart. Like doors that open only one way, the valves make sure blood flows in the right direction. For example, one valve makes sure that blood flows from an atrium to a ventricle. It will not let blood flow from a ventricle to an atrium. Other valves make sure that blood leaving a ventricle does not flow backward into the ventricle.

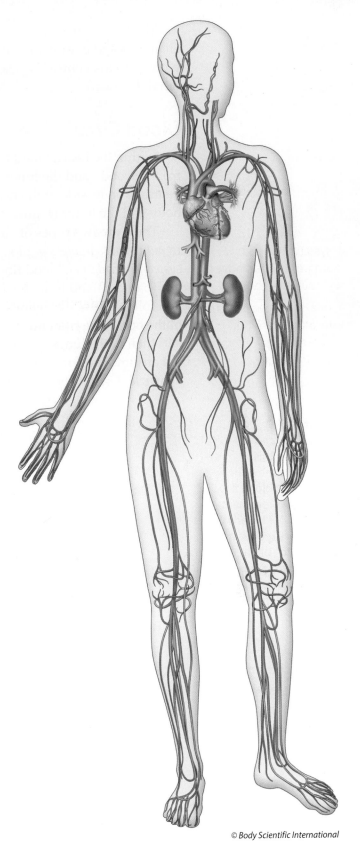

© Body Scientific International

Figure 17.8   The heart is located in the center of the chest. In this illustration, the arteries are red, and the veins are blue. As you can see, blood vessels travel throughout the body. *Which organ pumps blood through the circulatory system?*

The heartbeat you feel and hear is caused by the contraction of the heart chambers and closing of valves. The first heart sound is the atria squeezing blood into the ventricles. The second sound is the ventricles pumping blood out of the heart.

Blood Circulation

Within the heart, blood follows a specific path. The two atria receive blood from the body and the lungs. Each atrium passes this blood down to the ventricle on its side of the heart. The two ventricles pump blood back to the body and the lungs (**Figure 17.9**).

There are two types of circulation between the heart and other organs. In *pulmonary circulation*, blood flows between the heart and the lungs. In *systemic circulation*, blood flows between the heart and the rest of the body.

To understand how this works, start with the right atrium in Figure 17.9 and follow along. Oxygen-poor blood enters the right atrium from the rest of the body. The right atrium pumps the blood down into the right ventricle and then to the lungs. The lungs fill the blood with oxygen and return it to the left atrium. The left atrium then pumps oxygen-rich blood down into the left ventricle. Finally, the left ventricle pumps blood out to the rest of the body.

Figure 17.9
The arrows and the numbers in this illustration show the direction of blood flow. Blue arrows represent oxygen-poor blood. Red arrows represent oxygen-rich blood. *What are the two types of circulation between the heart and other organs?*

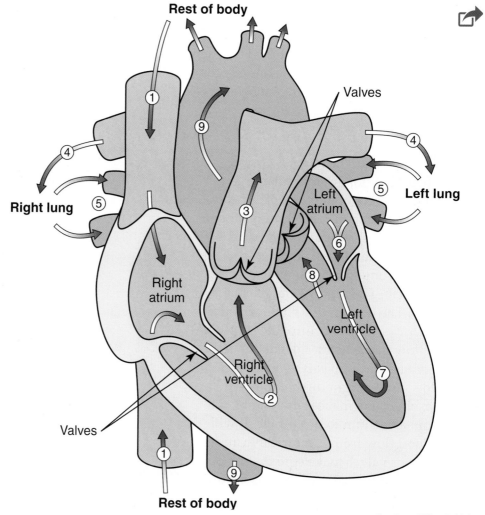

Goodheart-Willcox Publisher

Blood Vessels

Blood vessels carry blood throughout the body. **Arteries** carry oxygen-rich blood. For example, *coronary arteries* bring oxygen and nutrients to the heart muscle. If these arteries become too narrow or blocked, a heart attack can occur. The largest artery is the *aorta*, which carries blood from the left ventricle of the heart to other arteries. Most arteries carry blood from the heart to the rest of the body. These arteries have muscular walls that can handle the pressure created by the heart's pumping. Arteries branch into smaller blood vessels, and these branch into even smaller ones.

The smallest arteries are the **capillaries**. Capillaries have very thin walls with no muscle. They deliver oxygen and nutrients to body cells and pick up cells' waste. Capillaries lead into tiny veins, which lead into larger veins **(Figure 17.10)**. **Veins** carry oxygen-poor blood. Two large veins, called the *vena cavae*, carry blood into the right atrium of the heart. One vena cava brings blood from the head and upper body. The other brings blood from the lower body.

Blood

The adult body holds 5 to 6 liters (about 5.3 to 6.3 quarts) of blood. Blood transports oxygen, water, and nutrients throughout the body. It also carries other substances cells need, like proteins, hormones, and special cells. Blood also moves waste to the kidneys.

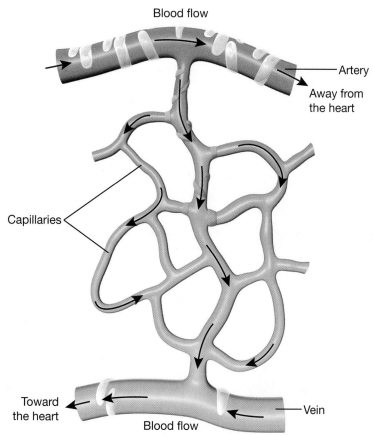

Blood flow

Artery

Away from the heart

Capillaries

Toward the heart

Vein

Blood flow

Figure 17.10
Blood flows through capillaries to deliver oxygen to body tissues. Arteries deliver oxygen-rich blood to capillaries. Once oxygen has been taken out of the blood, the blood returns to the heart through veins. *Capillaries, arteries, and veins are three types of what body part?*

iStock.com/7activestudio

Blood is mostly water. The watery portion of blood, called **plasma**, transports all the substances carried by blood. Blood also contains the following cells:

- *Red blood cells* make up one-half the blood's volume. Red blood cells contain a red substance called *hemoglobin*, which can carry and release oxygen. As a result, red blood cells transport oxygen throughout the body. Red blood cells have certain sugars that determine a person's blood type (**Figure 17.11**).
- *White blood cells* move through the blood and live in various organs of the body. They help defend the body against infections.
- *Platelets* are responsible for blood clotting. Clotting stops blood from flowing outside the wall of a blood vessel. This action helps prevent blood loss when blood vessels are injured.

All three types of blood cells are made in the *bone marrow* (a tissue inside bones).

Respiratory System

The circulatory system cannot deliver oxygen to the body's cells without the help of the respiratory system. The **respiratory system** includes organs that obtain vitally important oxygen from the outside world. This body system draws oxygen into the lungs and delivers it to blood vessels. It also takes carbon dioxide—another gas—out of the blood and sends it outside the body. Respiratory organs can be divided into the upper and lower respiratory systems.

Figure 17.11
People with type A blood have cells with type A sugar. People with type B blood have type B sugar on their red blood cells. Those with type AB blood have both A and B sugars. Type O blood has blood cells with neither kind of sugar. The type of sugar determines which blood types are compatible for donation.

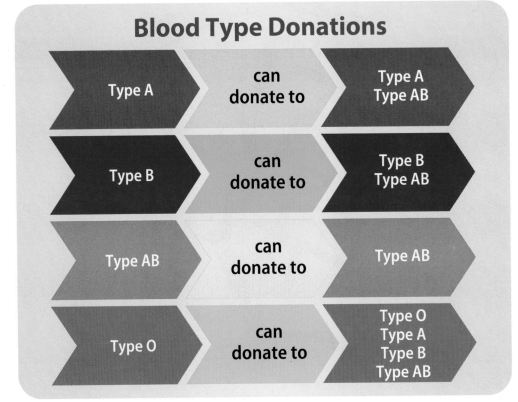

Blood Type Donations

Type A	can donate to	Type A Type AB
Type B	can donate to	Type B Type AB
Type AB	can donate to	Type AB
Type O	can donate to	Type O Type A Type B Type AB

Upper Respiratory System

The upper respiratory system allows air containing oxygen to enter the body. Air enters the nose and mouth and passes down through the throat to the *larynx* and then through the *trachea* to the lungs (**Figure 17.12**). You can feel the larynx as a bump in the front of your throat. It vibrates when you speak, as air passes across the vocal cords. A small structure covers the larynx when you swallow and prevents food from entering the trachea.

The walls of the respiratory passages make a sticky substance called *mucus*. This mucus traps bacteria and dust particles so they cannot enter the lungs. Extra mucus is made when someone has an infection or an allergic reaction. The passage behind the nose is also lined with mucus and with blood vessels that warm and moisten air. You see evidence of this on cold days when you exhale. The warm, exhaled air forms water vapor as it contacts the cold outside air.

Lower Respiratory System

The trachea branches into two **bronchi**, air passages that lead to each lung. The bronchi branch into smaller passages called *bronchioles* inside the lungs. These smaller airways end as sacks called *alveoli*. When you inhale, air fills the alveoli. The alveoli are important for oxygen exchange in the lungs. If they fill with fluid, as in pneumonia, air and oxygen cannot enter them. This can disrupt the vital process of respiration.

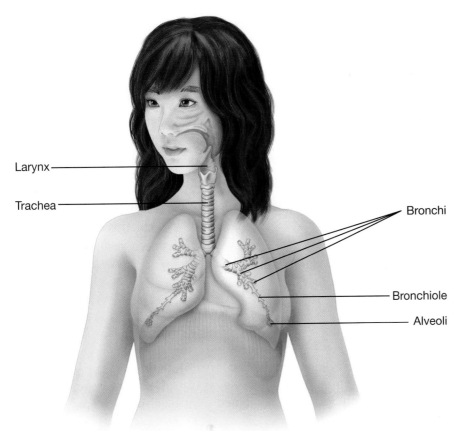

Larynx

Trachea

Bronchi

Bronchiole

Alveoli

Figure 17.12
Air enters the body through the nose or mouth and travels through the larynx and trachea to the lungs. *What sticky substance prevents dust and bacteria from entering through the nose or mouth with the air you breathe?*

© Body Scientific International

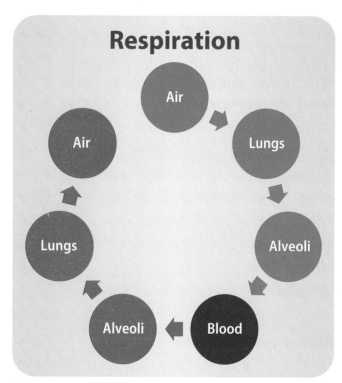

Respiration

Respiration

Figure 17.13 In respiration, the body takes in air and directs it to the alveoli. In the alveoli, oxygen (blue) leaves the air and enters the blood. Carbon dioxide (red) leaves the blood and enters the air. Air is then exhaled outside the body. *What is the main muscle doing the work of inhalation and exhalation?*

Respiration is the exchange of oxygen and carbon dioxide in the respiratory system. It includes two steps: inhaling and exhaling. When you inhale, you take in air, which reaches the lungs. Air fills the alveoli, and oxygen moves into the blood in tiny capillaries. These capillaries then deliver oxygen-rich blood to the heart.

At the same time, carbon dioxide moves from the blood into the alveoli. This air travels back into the respiratory passages. When you exhale, you push the air with carbon dioxide out of the body (**Figure 17.13**).

Muscles help the lungs take in and push out air. During inhalation, muscles enlarge the chest. This draws air in through the mouth and nose. The chief muscle doing this work is the **diaphragm**. The diaphragm is a sheet of muscle beneath the lungs and above the abdomen. As the diaphragm moves down, the chest expands. Other muscles of the chest, especially those between the ribs, also help the chest expand. Exhalation happens when these muscles relax. The chest collapses and squeezes air out the mouth and nose.

Lesson 17.2 Review

1. Which heart chamber pumps oxygen-rich blood out to the rest of the body?
2. **True or false.** Capillaries are blood vessels with very thin walls.
3. Which of the following blood cells are responsible for blood clotting?
   A. Red blood cells.
   B. Platelets.
   C. White blood cells.
   D. Plasma.
4. Explain what happens during respiration.
5. **Critical thinking.** Which type of circulation turns oxygen-poor blood into oxygen-rich blood?

Hands-On Activity

Pull out your drawing from the first lesson. Add drawings to "your body" of the organs and structures from this lesson (heart, blood vessels, lungs, nose, mouth, diaphragm, etc.). What medical specialists help care for these body systems?

Digesting and Removing Substances

Learning Outcomes

After studying this lesson, you will be able to

- **describe** the structures of the digestive system and what they do.
- **describe** the structures of the urinary system and what they do.
- **identify** the structures of the lymphatic and immune systems and explain what they do.

Graphic Organizer

Digest and Remove

On a separate sheet of paper, create a graphic organizer like the one shown below. As you read this lesson, fill in the organizer with the bodily processes involved in bringing substances into the body, digesting them, and removing them from the body. Make sure to note body parts and organs involved in the digestive, urinary, lymphatic, and immune systems.

Magic mine/Shutterstock.com

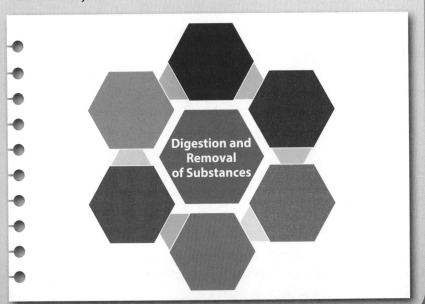

Digestion and Removal of Substances

Key Terms

digestive system body system that breaks down food to provide nutrients and energy; also removes solid waste from the body

pancreas fish-shaped organ behind the stomach that makes many kinds of enzymes needed for digestion

liver large brown organ to the right of the stomach that has many jobs, including making bile

gallbladder organ in which bile is stored until needed to digest food

appendix finger-shaped organ attached to the large intestine; made of lymphatic tissue

urinary system body system that removes liquid waste from the body

kidneys two bean-shaped organs that filter blood and make urine

bladder organ that stores urine until it can be pushed out of the body

lymphatic system body system of organs and tissues that help fight infections

spleen organ filled with white blood cells; filters blood

hree body systems help digest and remove substances. The digestive system brings food into the body. It also breaks down food to provide nutrients the body needs and removes waste. The urinary system takes liquid waste out of the body. The lymphatic and immune systems help the body fight disease. In this lesson, you will learn about the digestive, urinary, and lymphatic and immune systems.

Digestive System

The **digestive system** brings food into the body and breaks it down to provide nutrients and energy the body needs. It also removes solid waste from the body. The digestive system begins at the mouth and continues through the throat, esophagus, and stomach. It also includes the small and large intestines, liver, gallbladder, pancreas, appendix, rectum, and anus (**Figure 17.14**).

Mouth and Teeth

Digestion, or the process of breaking down food, begins in the mouth. Here, teeth break down food into a soft mass that can be swallowed.

Figure 17.14
Food travels through the digestive system from the mouth all the way to the anus. *What is the name of the process that occurs in this system and what does it do?*

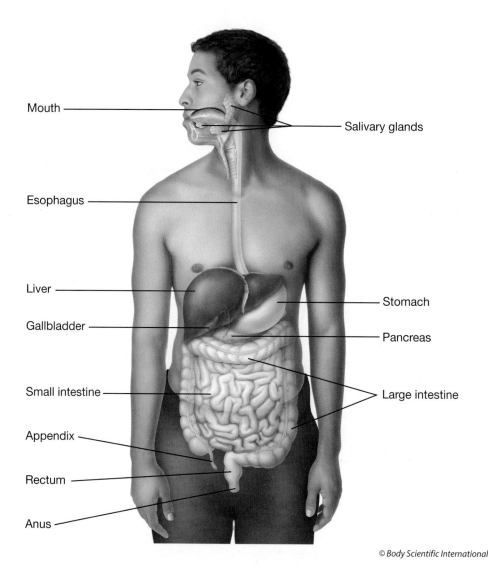

Mouth

Salivary glands

Esophagus

Liver

Stomach

Gallbladder

Pancreas

Small intestine

Large intestine

Appendix

Rectum

Anus

© Body Scientific International

Teeth have different shapes because they do different jobs. The teeth in the front, which are more pointed, tear food. The flatter, larger teeth toward the back crush food.

Salivary glands are found in and around the mouth. These glands produce a liquid called *saliva*, which moistens food. Saliva also contains substances called *enzymes* that help digest food. Enzymes use chemical reactions to break down food into nutrients and energy.

The tongue is also part of the digestive system. It pushes chewed food into the throat. Food passes from the throat into the esophagus.

Esophagus

The *esophagus* is a muscular tube that connects the throat to the stomach. Chewed food moves down the esophagus during digestion. A small, donut-shaped muscle called a *sphincter* joins the esophagus to the stomach and opens to let food pass into the stomach. The sphincter closes after food enters the stomach to prevent backflow into the esophagus.

Stomach and Small Intestine

The *stomach* is a muscular bag slightly left of the center of the body and below the ribcage. The stomach makes a mixture of enzymes and a powerful acid. Muscles of the stomach wall mix digesting food with chemicals to break it down further.

Food passes from the stomach into the *small intestine*. Another sphincter controls the flow of food from the stomach into the small intestine. Once food is in the small intestine, muscles in the walls of the small intestine contract rhythmically. These movements push the food along the small intestine. In the small intestine, nutrients are also absorbed into the blood (**Figure 17.15**).

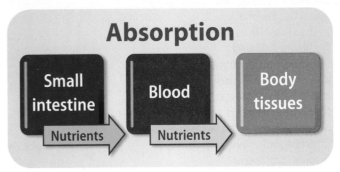

Figure 17.15 In absorption, nutrients move from food in the small intestine into the blood. Blood carries nutrients to other body tissues. Nutrients that are not absorbed into the blood travel into the large intestine. *Which organs release substances to help aid this process?*

The walls of the small intestine make enzymes needed to digest food. Most digestion happens in the first part of the small intestine. The pancreas and liver release substances to help this process.

Pancreas and Liver

The **pancreas** is a fish-shaped organ behind the stomach. It connects to the small intestine and makes many kinds of enzymes needed for digestion. These enzymes pass into the small intestine through a thin tube.

The **liver** is a large brown organ to the right of the stomach that has many jobs in the body. It helps digestion by making bile. *Bile* breaks down large fat droplets into very small fat particles that can be digested and transported through the body.

Bile is stored in the **gallbladder**. The gallbladder is a small, pear-shaped bag under the liver. It squeezes bile through a tube into the small intestine.

Large Intestine

Nutrients and materials that are not absorbed into the blood pass into the *large intestine*. This part of the digestive system prepares solid food waste for removal from the body.

Some water and minerals from food are absorbed into the blood from the large intestine. The remaining material is eliminated as *feces*. It takes about six to eight hours for food to move from the stomach to the large intestine. Undigested food spends 24 to 48 hours in the large intestine. The exact time depends on the kind of food eaten. Protein meals, such as meat and fish, take longer to digest. Time in the digestive system also varies from person to person.

Feces are stored in a part of the large intestine called the *rectum*. They are eliminated from the body when large intestine muscles push them out through an opening called the *anus* (**Figure 17.16**).

Figure 17.16
Review the steps of digestion using this illustration. Food enters the mouth and travels down the esophagus to the stomach. In the small intestine and large intestine, nutrients, water, and minerals are absorbed into the blood. Material that is not absorbed becomes feces in the large intestine and is removed through the anus.

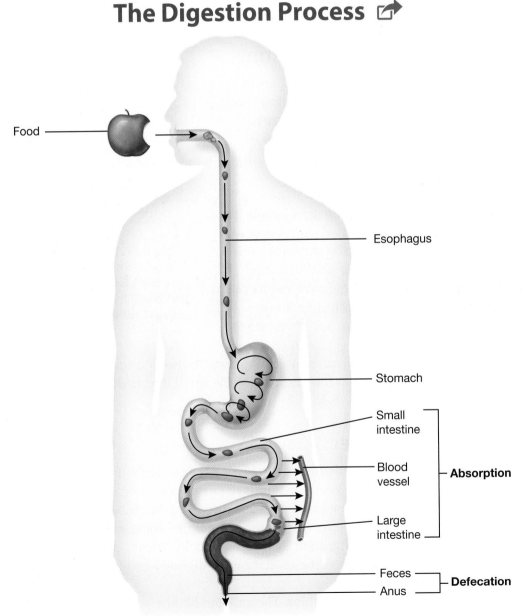

The Digestion Process

Food

Esophagus

Stomach

Small intestine

Blood vessel

Absorption

Large intestine

Feces

Anus

Defecation

© Body Scientific International

The **appendix** is attached to the large intestine, but it does not play a role in digesting food. The appendix is a finger-shaped organ made of lymphatic tissue, which you will learn about later in this lesson. The job of the appendix is unclear, but it might help protect the digestive tract from infections.

Sometimes the appendix gets infected by bacteria in the colon. Such an infection—a condition called *appendicitis*—is dangerous. An infected appendix swells as it fills with bacteria and pus. If it swells and bursts, bacteria will infect the body cavity and circulatory system. An infected appendix must be removed by surgery.

Urinary System

The **urinary system** removes liquid waste from the body. The kidneys play an important role in this system. The urinary system includes two kidneys and ureters, the bladder, and the urethra (**Figure 17.17**).

Kidneys

Two bean-shaped **kidneys** begin the process of urine production by filtering blood. Both kidneys lie against the lower back wall of the body. The left kidney is behind the spleen. The right kidney is smaller than the left kidney and lies behind and below the liver.

Kidneys remove waste from the blood. Kidneys also control the amount of water, minerals, and acid in blood. As blood moves through the kidneys, the waste that is filtered out becomes *urine*. Urine exits the kidney through a ureter. Cleansed and filtered blood returns to the circulatory system.

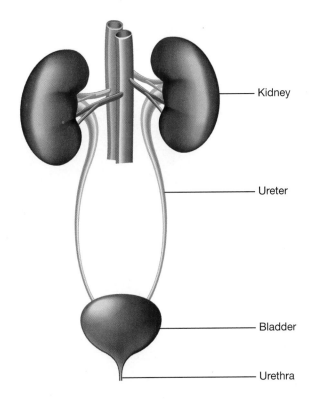

Kidney

Ureter

Bladder

Urethra

Figure 17.17
The urinary system includes two kidneys, two ureters, the bladder, and the urethra. *Which part of the urinary system stores urine?*

iStock.com/andregro4ka

Though kidneys are smaller than the stomach, they receive an enormous amount of blood. The body sends up to 25 percent of its blood to the kidneys. Kidneys must continually filter waste from blood and form urine. You would not live long if your kidneys stopped working. Waste and toxins would build up in blood quickly and soon poison every organ, including the brain.

Ureters, Bladder, and Urethra

A *ureter* is a tube that carries urine from a kidney to the bladder. Each ureter enters the top of the bladder.

The bladder is a muscular bag that sits at the level of the pubic area above the genitals. The **bladder** stores urine. When the bladder is full, the bladder muscle squeezes urine into the urethra. Two sphincters join the urethra to the bladder (**Figure 17.18**). The outermost sphincter gives you some control over urination. During toilet training, small children learn how to control this sphincter.

The *urethra* is a small tube that transports urine out of the body. The urethra exits males at the tip of the penis. The urethra is shorter in females. It exits females above the vagina.

Lymphatic and Immune Systems

The **lymphatic system** is responsible for removing foreign substances from the body. This body system includes the *immune system* and has organs and tissues that help fight infections. The main organs of the lymphatic and immune systems include lymphatic vessels, lymph nodes, tonsils, the spleen, the thymus, and white blood cells.

Figure 17.18
The internal and external urethral sphincters control the flow of urine out of the body. The internal urethral sphincter is involuntary. The external urethral sphincter is voluntary. *Which sphincter gives some control over urination?*

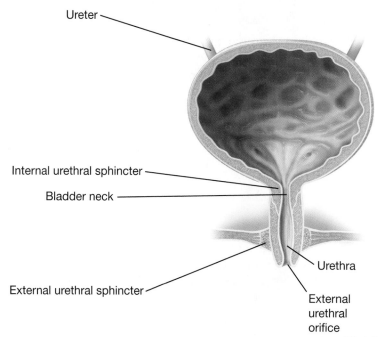

Ureter

Internal urethral sphincter

Bladder neck

External urethral sphincter

Urethra

External urethral orifice

© Body Scientific International

Lymphatic Vessels and Lymph Nodes

The *lymphatic vessels* are similar to blood vessels, but they do not carry blood. Instead, they carry fluid that builds up in tissues of the body. This fluid comes from the body's millions of tiny capillaries. Each time the heart beats, it creates blood pressure in capillaries. This pressure pushes fluid out of the capillaries and into tissues. This fluid becomes *lymph* when it enters the lymphatic capillaries and flows into other lymphatic vessels (**Figure 17.19**). Lymphatic vessels collect and transport lymph to the chest. There, lymph rejoins the blood.

Lymph is filtered by *lymph nodes* before it reenters the blood. Inside the lymph nodes, lymph contacts white blood cells. These cells remove bacteria and viruses from the fluid. They can also grow and reproduce to fight infections. In some infections, lymph nodes become swollen because of the buildup of extra white blood cells. For this reason, swollen lymph nodes are a sign that the body is fighting an infection.

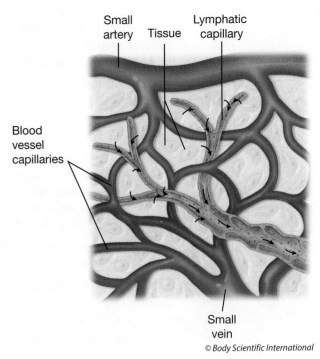

Small artery Tissue Lymphatic capillary

Blood vessel capillaries

Small vein

© Body Scientific International

Figure 17.19 Lymphatic capillaries (green) collect lymph from the fluid pushed out of blood vessel capillaries. Lymph travels through lymphatic vessels in the body. *While blood vessels carry blood, what do lymphatic vessels carry?*

CASE STUDY

Fighting Off Infections: Brian Gets a Cold

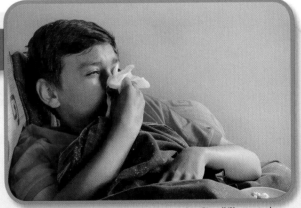

Ben Gingell/Shutterstock.com

Brian is 12 years old, and last month he had a fever and a terrible sore throat that lasted for a few days. His parents took him to the doctor, who said that Brian's lymph nodes and tonsils in his throat were both swollen from infection, which is why it hurt.

His parents never seem to get colds, but Brian gets one at least once a year. His baby sister, who is 3, gets sick even more often. Brian asked his dad about it, and he told Brian that bodies can fight off infections better as they develop. Children get sick less often as they grow up and their body systems mature.

Brian does not want to get sick anymore. It is not fun and he does not like missing school. At his next regular checkup with his doctor, he asks her what he can do to keep from getting sick. She tells Brian that he should minimize stress, get regular exercise, sleep well, and eat nutritious foods. According to her, Brian can also avoid getting sick with respiratory etiquette, such as washing his hands.

Thinking Critically

1. Which body system, when weak or underdeveloped, is the cause of infections?

2. Why are the recommendations of Brian's doctor helpful for not getting sick?

Tonsils are lymph nodes that guard the throat from infection. They are located on the sides and top of the back of the throat. The tonsils also contain white blood cells. When the throat is infected, tonsils enlarge and become red. Swollen tonsils are a sign that your body is fighting a throat infection.

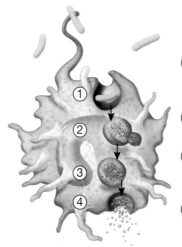

① White blood cell engulfs enemy cell (bacteria, dead cells)

② Enzymes start to destroy enemy cell

③ Enemy cell breaks down into small fragments

④ Indigestible fragments are discharged

© Body Scientific International

Figure 17.20 White blood cells can engulf and destroy enemy cells such as bacteria. *What are the proteins made by white blood cells that help protect against viruses and bacteria?*

Spleen and Thymus

The **spleen** is an organ that is filled with white blood cells and filters blood. The spleen is located to the left of the stomach and is shaped like a flattened bean. The spleen also removes dead red blood cells.

The *thymus* is a lymphatic organ located over the large blood vessels in the upper chest. In the thymus, certain kinds of white blood cells learn how to recognize and attack bacteria and viruses.

White Blood Cells

A variety of white blood cells are part of the lymphatic system. Some take in and destroy bacteria (**Figure 17.20**). Others specialize in controlling viruses. Some white blood cells make antibodies. *Antibodies* are proteins that stick to bacteria and viruses and help destroy these invaders. All these white blood cells are a vital part of the body's immune system.

Lesson 17.3 Review

1. Which of the following connects the throat to the stomach?
   A. Esophagus.
   B. Small intestine.
   C. Salivary glands.
   D. Large intestine.
2. **True or false.** In the small intestine, nutrients are absorbed into the blood.
3. Which organ removes waste from the blood and produces urine?
4. Lymphatic organs that filter lymph before it reenters the blood are called _____ _____.
5. **Critical thinking.** What would happen if your kidneys stopped working?

Hands-On Activity

Pull out your body systems drawing from the first lessons. Add drawings to "your body" of the organs and structures from this lesson (teeth, salivary glands, esophagus, stomach, intestines, liver, kidneys, bladder, etc.). What behaviors will keep these structures and organs healthy?

Controlling and Regulating the Body

Learning Outcomes

After studying this lesson, you will be able to

- **identify** the cells and structures of the nervous system.
- **explain** what the nervous system does.
- **list** the sensory organs and their functions.
- **identify** the structures of the endocrine system and describe what they do.

Graphic Organizer

Nervous and Endocrine Systems

The body systems involved in the control and regulation of the body involve many different structures and organs. On a separate sheet of paper, create a graphic organizer like the one shown below. As you read this lesson, fill in the organizer with notes on each body system, the body parts involved, and what each system does. Examples are provided for you.

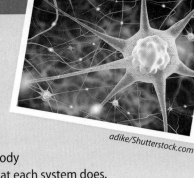

adike/Shutterstock.com

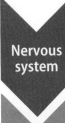

Nervous system
- *The nervous system allows a person to think, use the senses, send signals to the body to move, and control important body processes.*
-
-

Endocrine system
- *The endocrine system controls the body using hormones.*
-
-

Key Terms

nervous system body system that allows people to think, use the senses, move, and maintain important body processes

neuron cell that is specialized to receive and send signals

cerebrum largest part of the brain, which interprets information from the sensory organs; controls muscle actions and is responsible for intelligence, memory, and personality

cerebellum part of the brain that controls coordinated, smooth muscle activity

brain stem part of the brain that controls the heartbeat and breathing rate

spinal cord part of the nervous system that carries nerve signals between the brain and the body

endocrine system body system that produces chemical messengers called *hormones*, which regulate body processes

pituitary gland master gland of the body, which releases hormones to control other endocrine organs

thyroid hormone substance produced in the thyroid that increases the rate at which the body uses energy

The nervous system, sensory organs, and endocrine system help regulate the body's function internally and with the outside world. They allow the body to function smoothly and efficiently and do many complicated things. For example, the nervous system helps the body remember and perform complex tasks such as playing the piano. The nervous and endocrine systems both guide the female body through labor and the birth of a baby. In this final lesson, you will learn about the nervous system, sensory organs, and endocrine system.

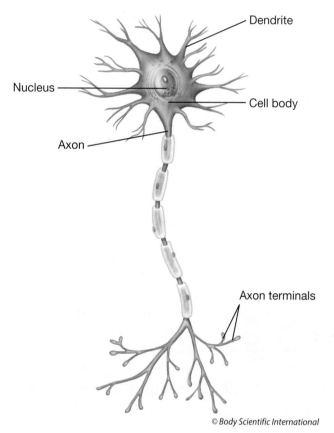

Nucleus — Dendrite — Cell body — Axon — Axon terminals

© Body Scientific International

Figure 17.21 A neuron is a special type of cell that conducts signals. In a neuron, a signal is received by the dendrites and travels to the cell body. Then, the signal travels along the axon. The axon terminals send the signal to another cell. *Neurons are the building blocks of which body system?*

Nervous System

The **nervous system** is organized into two parts. The first is the *central nervous system (CNS)*, which includes the brain and spinal cord. The second is the *peripheral nervous system (PNS)*, which includes the nerves and sensory organs. Together, these two parts of the nervous system allow people to think, use the senses, move, and maintain important body processes.

Neurons

Neurons are the building blocks of the nervous system. A **neuron** is a cell specialized to receive and send signals (**Figure 17.21**). Neurons make up the brain, spinal cord, and nerves. In addition to neurons, the nervous system has millions of other cells that protect and support them.

There are three types of neurons. Some neurons carry signals from the body to the CNS. These are *sensory neurons*. In contrast, *motor neurons* carry information from the CNS to the body. Motor neurons control the body's glands and tell muscles to contract or relax. A third type of neuron is the *interneuron*. Interneurons carry signals between neurons.

Brain

The brain controls nearly all body functions. For example, to bend the knee, the brain tells muscles on the back of the thigh to contract. At the same time, the brain tells muscles on the front of the thigh to relax. The brain also stores information and makes sense of signals coming from the sensory organs.

The brain is protected by the bones of the skull. Under the skull, layers of tissues cover and also protect the brain. A fluid flows over the brain and cushions it.

Brain Powers: The Different Abilities of the Left and Right Brain

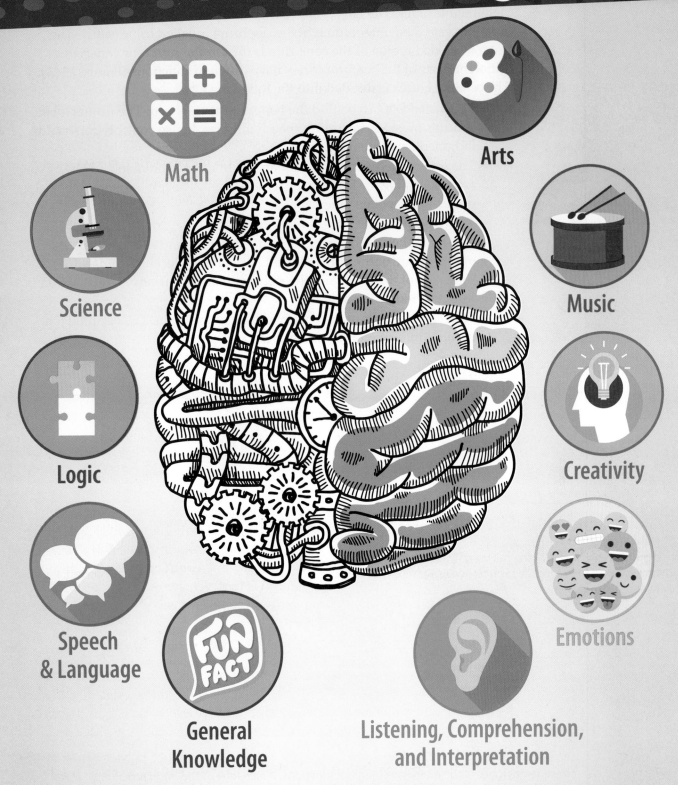

Math

Arts

Science

Music

Logic

Creativity

Speech & Language

Emotions

General Knowledge

Listening, Comprehension, and Interpretation

The largest part of the brain is the **cerebrum**. The cerebrum performs important functions. It interprets information coming to the brain from the sensory organs. It also controls muscle actions. The cerebrum is responsible for intelligence, memory, and personality.

The cerebrum is divided into two nearly equal halves—the left and right hemispheres. The halves are connected by nerves that allow them to communicate. The inner region of the cerebrum is called *white matter*. The outer, wrinkled region of the cerebrum is the *cerebral cortex*, or *gray matter*. Different parts of the cerebral cortex have different functions (**Figure 17.22**). The cerebral cortex is divided into the following *lobes*:

- The *frontal lobe* lies behind the bones of the forehead. The frontal lobe controls muscles, including speech muscles. It also controls personality, judgment, and memory.
- The *temporal lobes* are to the left and right of the frontal lobe. These areas are responsible for hearing, taste, and smell. The left temporal lobe helps understand spoken language.
- The two *parietal lobes* are behind the frontal lobe, under the top of the skull. They decode signals from the senses and muscles from the opposite side of the body. The left parietal lobe receives signals from the right side of the body, and the right parietal lobe receives information from the body's left side.
- The *occipital lobe* is at the back and base of the brain. The occipital lobe decodes information from the eyes.

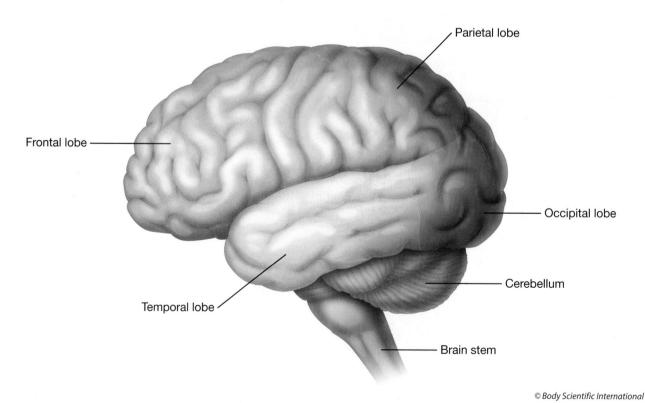

© *Body Scientific International*

Figure 17.22 The different lobes of the brain have different functions. *Which lobe of the brain is responsible for controlling personality, judgment, and memory?*

The base of the brain includes the **cerebellum** and the brain stem. The cerebellum lies below the occipital lobe. The cerebellum controls coordinated, smooth muscle activity. The **brain stem** connects the brain to the spinal cord. It controls heartbeat and breathing rate.

The brain also includes several other structures. The *thalamus* lies below the cerebrum. It sends information from sensory organs to the cerebral cortex, where the brain decodes these signals. Below the thalamus lies the hypothalamus. The *hypothalamus* regulates vital body functions. For example, it acts like a thermostat. It senses and maintains the body's temperature, at 98.6°F (37°C). The hypothalamus also helps control appetite and the cycle of waking and sleeping. In addition, the hypothalamus makes some hormones and controls the endocrine system.

Spinal Cord

The **spinal cord** carries nerve signals between the brain and the body (**Figure 17.23**). The spinal cord is protected by bones of the spine called *vertebrae*. Tissues and fluid also cover the spinal cord.

Many nerves run up and down the spinal cord. The nerves branch from the spinal cord and run to the left and right sides of the body. Some nerves control the muscles. Other nerves carry sense information from the sensory organs to the brain.

The spinal cord also controls some reflexes. A *reflex* is an automatic response to a sensation. For example, if extreme heat is sensed at the fingertips, the spinal cord sends a signal to arm muscles to contract and move the arm away from the source of heat. This response does not involve the brain. That is why a reflex can be so fast. This type of response helps keep the body safe from dangers in the environment.

Sensory Organs

Senses allow the body to know about itself and the environment outside it. You are probably familiar with the five senses of sight, sound, hearing, taste, and touch. Other senses include pressure, pain, and temperature.

Senses are possible because of nerve endings on sensory nerves. Nerve endings are specialized for detecting certain kinds of information. For example, the eye contains nerve endings that sense light. In the case of eyes and ears, nerve endings are helped by numerous other structures. The eyes and ears are sensory organs.

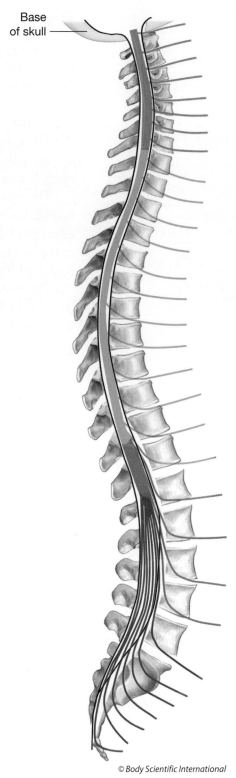

Base of skull

© Body Scientific International

Figure 17.23 The spinal cord is housed inside the vertebrae. *What is the function of the spinal cord?*

Eye

The eyes and brain work together to make vision possible. The eyes detect light with nerve endings. Nerves then carry this information to the occipital lobe of the brain, which forms images from the information it receives. Numerous structures help the eye capture light and send signals to the brain.

The eyeball is protected by the bones of the skull. A strong tissue gives the eye its spherical shape. A firm gel fills the inside of the eye to help keep the eyeball's shape.

The inner, back layer of the eyeball is the *retina* (**Figure 17.24**). The retina is made of nerve endings that are very receptive to light. These nerve endings allow the brain to see color, black and white, and shades of gray. In the center of the retina is an area rich in nerve endings. This area is responsible for forming sharp images.

The front of the eyeball's surface is covered by the *cornea*. Light enters the cornea and passes through a *lens*. The lens focuses light on the retina. The *iris*, the colored part of the eye, lies in front of the lens, under the cornea. The iris appears round and has a black, circular opening called the *pupil*. The pupil allows light into the eyeball. The iris can change the pupil's size. For example, in darkness, the iris widens the pupil to let in more light.

In front of the eyeball are *eyelids*, skin-covered flaps that can close and protect the eye. Tear glands are located above each eye. The tears lubricate and clean the eye's outer surface.

Ear

The ear is responsible for the senses of hearing and balance. The *outer ear* is shaped by cartilage and helps collect sound. Sound travels along the *auditory canal*, which ends at the eardrum.

Figure 17.24
Light enters the eye through the pupil and is focused on the retina by the lens. *What are the skin-covered flaps that can close and protect the eye?*

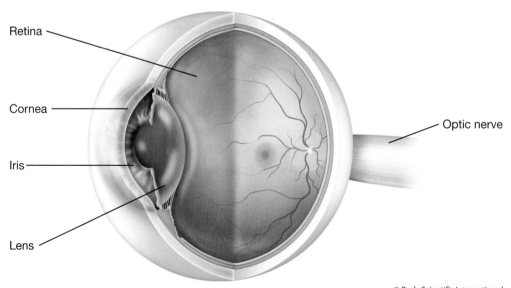

Retina

Cornea

Iris

Lens

Optic nerve

© Body Scientific International

The *middle ear* begins at the eardrum. The *eardrum* is a thin sheet of connective tissue that covers the end of the auditory canal. Sound that enters the middle ear causes the eardrum to vibrate. The eardrum rests against three tiny middle ear bones, called the *malleus, incus,* and *stapes.* These bones detect the vibrations made by the eardrum. In response, they vibrate against the cochlea, a structure in the *inner ear.* The *cochlea* is a snail-shaped organ that detects sound and sends information to the brain.

Vibrations from the middle ear bones enter the cochlea and stimulate nerve endings called *hair cells.* The hair cells send information about the vibrations along a nerve to the brain. The brain's cerebrum interprets this information as different types of sound (**Figure 17.25**).

The inner ear also contains the organs of balance. These detect the head's position and movement.

Endocrine System

The **endocrine system** produces chemical messengers called *hormones,* which regulate body processes. The organs that produce these hormones are part of the endocrine system. These organs release hormones into the blood, which carries them all over the body. Certain organs respond to certain hormones. They respond by growing or developing or by making other hormones and products.

The body makes hormones as needed. For example, insulin helps remove sugar from the blood. Insulin is produced when blood sugar rises above a certain level. When sugar returns to a healthy level, insulin production shuts off.

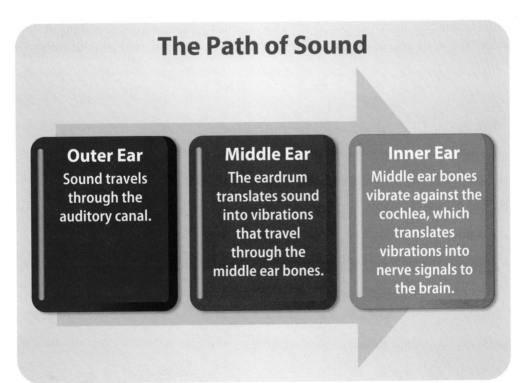

The Path of Sound

Outer Ear
Sound travels through the auditory canal.

Middle Ear
The eardrum translates sound into vibrations that travel through the middle ear bones.

Inner Ear
Middle ear bones vibrate against the cochlea, which translates vibrations into nerve signals to the brain.

Figure 17.25
Sound travels through the outer, middle, and inner ear. It is translated into vibrations and then into nerve signals. *What are the names of the three tiny middle ear bones that detect the vibrations made by the eardrum?*

Pituitary Gland

The **pituitary gland** is called the *master gland* of the endocrine system and is located beneath the hypothalamus in the brain (**Figure 17.26**). The pituitary gland uses hormones to control other endocrine organs. For example, the pituitary gland makes hormones that control growth, birth, puberty, and other activities. The pituitary gland itself is controlled by the brain's hypothalamus.

Thyroid

The *thyroid* is a gland located on the front of the neck, just below the larynx. It makes thyroid hormone. **Thyroid hormone** increases the rate at which the body uses energy. This also controls the body's temperature.

Parathyroid Glands

The *parathyroid glands* are four tiny glands located on the back of the thyroid gland. These glands make *parathyroid hormone (PTH)*. The parathyroid glands raise the blood levels of calcium and phosphate. Calcium and phosphate are minerals important for bone growth and the growth of all the body's cells.

Adrenal Glands

The *adrenal glands* are located on top of each kidney. These glands produce several hormones that control the blood levels of minerals and salts. Adrenal hormones also control how the body uses energy sources such as carbohydrates.

During stress, the adrenal glands make adrenaline. *Adrenaline* prepares the body to cope with stress by increasing the heart rate and breathing rate. Adrenaline also increases blood flow to the muscles, heart, lungs, and brain. The adrenal glands also make *cortisol*, which prepares the body to deal with stress.

Figure 17.26
The pituitary gland, which hangs beneath the hypothalamus, is controlled by the hypothalamus and regulates all other endocrine glands.

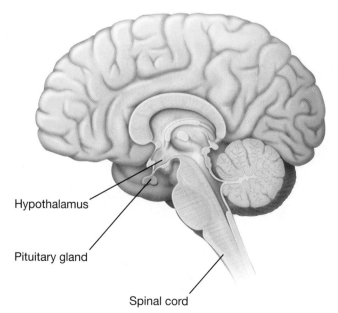

Hypothalamus

Pituitary gland

Spinal cord

Pancreas

The *pancreas* is an endocrine organ as well as part of the digestive system. As part of the endocrine system, the pancreas makes the hormones insulin and glucagon. Insulin and glucagon have opposite effects on blood sugar. *Insulin* lowers blood sugar, and *glucagon* elevates blood sugar.

BUILDING Your Skills

Reproduction and the Body Systems

In Chapter 16, you learned about the reproductive systems, which create new life. The reproductive systems are different between males and females. In males, the reproductive system includes the testes, scrotum, vas deferens, penis, urethra, seminal vesicles, and prostate. In females, it includes the ovaries, fallopian tubes, uterus, and vagina.

Some reproductive organs are shared with other body systems. For example, the urethra is also part of the urinary system. In males, the urethra carries both urine and semen. The testes and ovaries are also part of the endocrine system. The ovaries produce estrogen and progesterone and release eggs. The testes produce testosterone and sperm.

Review the Reproductive Systems

Go back to Chapter 16 and reread information about the reproductive systems in the first lesson. Review your notes about the reproductive system in males and females and identify the organs in Figure 16.2 and Figure 16.3. Then, create a cheat sheet of the most important facts about the male and female reproductive systems. Your cheat sheet should include the following information:

- major organs of the reproductive systems
- function of each organ in the reproductive systems
- production and transport of sperm and eggs
- process of fertilization

Organize your cheat sheet so it is colorful, interesting, and easy to follow. File your cheat sheet with your notes about the other body systems in this chapter. Then, in a small group, discuss how the reproductive systems are similar to and different from other body systems.

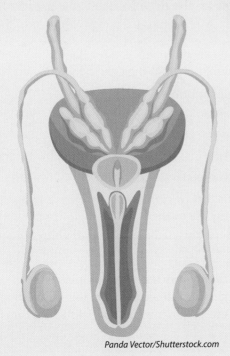

Panda Vector/Shutterstock.com

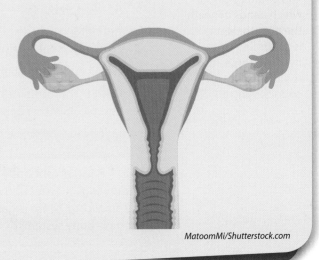

MatoomMi/Shutterstock.com

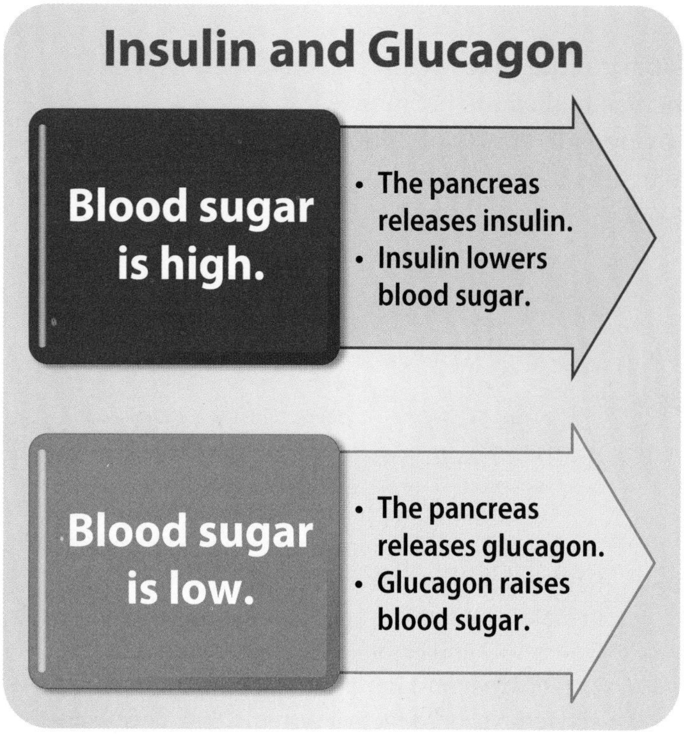

Insulin and Glucagon

Blood sugar is high.
- The pancreas releases insulin.
- Insulin lowers blood sugar.

Blood sugar is low.
- The pancreas releases glucagon.
- Glucagon raises blood sugar.

Figure 17.27 Together, insulin and glucagon keep blood sugar steady. The pancreas releases them when blood sugar becomes too high or too low. *Which disease can develop if insulin and glucagon do not work properly in the body?*

Together, these hormones keep blood sugar at a healthy level (**Figure 17.27**). If they do not work properly, a person can develop the disease *diabetes*. Diabetes results in abnormally high blood sugar. Untreated diabetes leads to kidney and eye damage. Diabetes can also cause heart disease.

Ovaries and Testes

The *ovaries* and *testes* are part of the endocrine system as well as part of the reproductive system. As you read in Chapter 16, the ovaries produce the hormones estrogen and progesterone. These hormones regulate the sexual development of females, female sex characteristics, and the female reproductive cycle.

The testes produce testosterone. This hormone controls the sexual development of males and male sex characteristics.

Lesson 17.4 Review

1. Which type of neuron carries information from the CNS to the body?
2. The _____ lobe of the brain decodes information from the eyes.
   - **A.** temporal
   - **B.** parietal
   - **C.** occipital
   - **D.** frontal
3. **True or false.** The pituitary gland is the master gland of the endocrine system.
4. Which endocrine gland produces adrenaline and cortisol?
5. **Critical thinking.** Are the neurons that carry information from the eyes and ears to the CNS motor or sensory neurons? Explain.

Hands-On Activity

Pull out your body systems drawing from the previous lessons. Add drawings to "your body" of the organs and structures from this lesson (brain, spinal cord, sense organs, glands, etc.). What medical specialists help care for these body systems?

Summary

Lesson 17.1 Supporting and Moving the Body

- Cells are the basic unit of life. A tissue is a collection of similar cells that do a certain job. An organ is a collection of tissues that perform a specific job.
- The integumentary system includes the skin, hair, and nails. It covers and protects the body, keeps out germs, and makes vitamin D.
- The skeletal system is made of 206 bones that provide structure, shape, and protection. At joints, bones are held together by ligaments.
- The muscular system helps the body move as muscle tissue contracts. There are three types of muscle tissue: skeletal muscles, smooth muscles, and cardiac muscle.

Lesson 17.2 Moving and Exchanging Substances

- The circulatory system is responsible for the flow of blood and substances through the body. Arteries carry oxygen-rich blood while veins carry oxygen-poor blood. Capillaries deliver oxygen and nutrients to body cells and pick up cell waste.
- Blood transports oxygen, water, nutrients, proteins, hormones, and special cells throughout the body and moves waste to the kidneys.
- The respiratory system delivers oxygen to blood vessels, then sends carbon dioxide out of the body. This exchange is called *respiration*.

Lesson 17.3 Digesting and Removing Substances

- The digestive system breaks down food to provide nutrients and energy for the body. It also removes waste from the body.
- Undigested food passes into the large intestine, where it is removed from the body as feces. The urinary system removes liquid waste from the body using the kidneys, ureters, bladder, and urethra.
- The lymphatic system, including the immune system, is responsible for removing foreign substances from the body. The main organs of this system are the lymphatic vessels, lymph nodes, tonsils, spleen, thymus, and white blood cells.

Lesson 17.4 Controlling and Regulating the Body

- The nervous system contains the brain, spinal cord, nerves, and sensory organs. The brain controls body functions, stores information, and makes sense of signals coming from sensory organs. The spinal cord carries nerve signals between the brain and the body.
- Senses allow the body to know about itself and the surrounding environment.
- The endocrine system uses hormones to control the body. This system uses the pituitary gland, thyroid, parathyroid glands, and adrenal glands to produce various hormones. The pancreas, ovaries, and testes also produce hormones for the endocrine system.

Check Your Knowledge ⤴

Record your answers to each of the following questions on a separate sheet of paper.

1. **True or false.** A tissue is a collection of organs that works together.

2. Which of the following is a function of the skin?
   A. Keep out germs.
   B. Provide structure and shape.
   C. Enable movement.
   D. Circulate blood.

3. Which muscle contracts to bend the arm at the elbow?

4. **True or false.** Arteries carry oxygen-rich blood, and veins carry oxygen-poor blood.

5. What is the name of the watery portion of blood?

6. The _____ is the site of oxygen and carbon dioxide exchange in the lungs.

7. Which organ of the digestive system makes bile?

8. **True or false.** Ureters carry urine from the bladder out of the body.

9. Why do the lymph nodes swell when the body is fighting infections?

10. **True or false.** In a reflex, the spinal cord signals the body to move without involving the brain.

11. Explain how the ear converts sounds into vibrations.

12. Which of the following hormones lowers blood sugar?
    A. Glucagon.
    B. Thyroid hormone.
    C. Parathyroid hormone.
    D. Insulin.

Use Your Vocabulary ⤴

appendix	gallbladder	pancreas
arteries	gland	pituitary gland
bladder	heart	plasma
body system	integumentary system	respiration
brain stem	joint	respiratory system
bronchi	kidneys	skeletal system
capillaries	ligaments	spinal cord
cerebellum	liver	spleen
cerebrum	lymphatic system	tendons
circulatory system	muscular system	thyroid hormone
diaphragm	nervous system	tissue
digestive system	neuron	urinary system
endocrine system	organ	veins

13. Choose one of the terms on the list above. Then, use the Internet to locate photos that visually show the meaning of the term you chose. Share the photo and meaning of the term in class. Ask for clarification if necessary.

14. Work with a partner to write the definitions of the terms above based on your current understanding. Then, team up with another pair to discuss your definitions and any discrepancies. Finally, discuss the definitions with the class.

Think Critically

15. **Make inferences.** Each body system performs essential functions. Choose one body system and summarize why it is important to keep its organs in good working order.

16. **Compare and contrast.** List the body systems discussed in this chapter and their major functions. Then, compare and contrast the functions. Note any functions that body systems have in common.

17. **Identify.** Health behaviors can affect the health and functionality of all body systems. Identify five physical, mental, or social health behaviors that would improve health. Explain how the behaviors would help each body system.

18. **Predict.** Choose one body system and predict how its failure would affect the body.

DEVELOP Your Skills

19. **Teamwork and communication skills.** Working in a small group, choose one lesson from this chapter. Review the lesson and your notes and create a digital presentation summarizing the most important information. Then, reteach the lesson to your peers using the presentation and at least two activities.

20. **Accessing information and literacy skills.** Visit a library and find a children's book about the human body. Read the children's book and compare the information in the book to the information in this chapter. How accurate is the children's book? To which age group would the children's book appeal? What would you change about the book to make it more accurate or engaging?

21. **Accessing information and communication skills.** Talk with a trusted adult about your most recent physical examination at the doctor. Review what happened during the examination and identify all the body systems and organs that the doctor evaluated. Did the doctor focus on one system more than the others? Why do you think the doctor did this? Discuss any questions or comments you have about the physical examination with the trusted adult.

22. **Teamwork, accessing information, and communication skills.** Working with a partner, create a list of professionals who specialize in keeping the body functioning. Then, identify one profession you would like to explore more deeply. Create a list of 5 to 10 interview questions for a person in your chosen profession. Reach out to someone who has this job and ask your questions during an interview (in person, via video conferencing, or on the phone). Report the results of your interview to the class in a creative way.

23. **Research skills.** Choose one body system and research online about ways to keep it healthy. Be sure to use only reliable websites and resources. Keep track of your sources and take notes about the information you find. Then, identify 10 things you can do today to keep the body system healthy. Share these 10 things with the class.

Body Mass Index-for-Age Percentiles

Body Mass Index for Boys

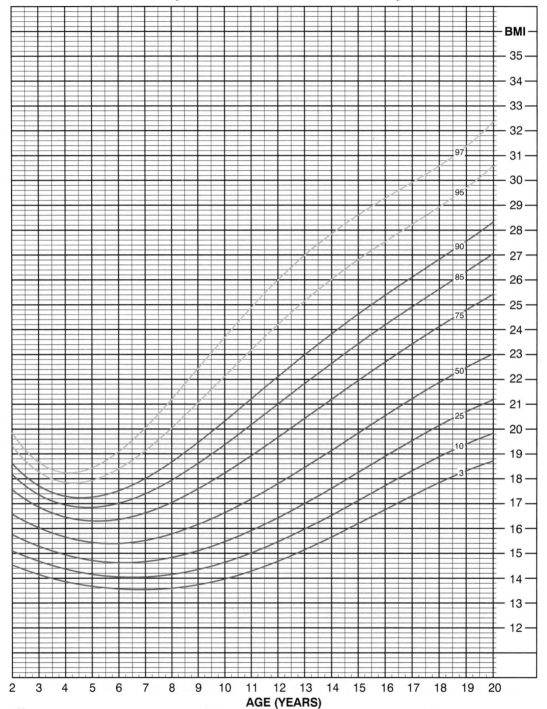

Key

Weight Status Category	Percentile Range
Underweight	Less than the 5th percentile
Healthy weight	5th percentile to less than the 85th percentile
Overweight	85th to less than the 95th percentile
Obese	Equal to or greater than the 95th percentile

SOURCE: Developed by the National Center for Health Statistics in collaboration with the National Center for Chronic Disease Prevention and Health Promotion

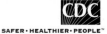

SAFER · HEALTHIER · PEOPLE™

Copyright Goodheart-Willcox Co., Inc.

Body Mass Index for Girls

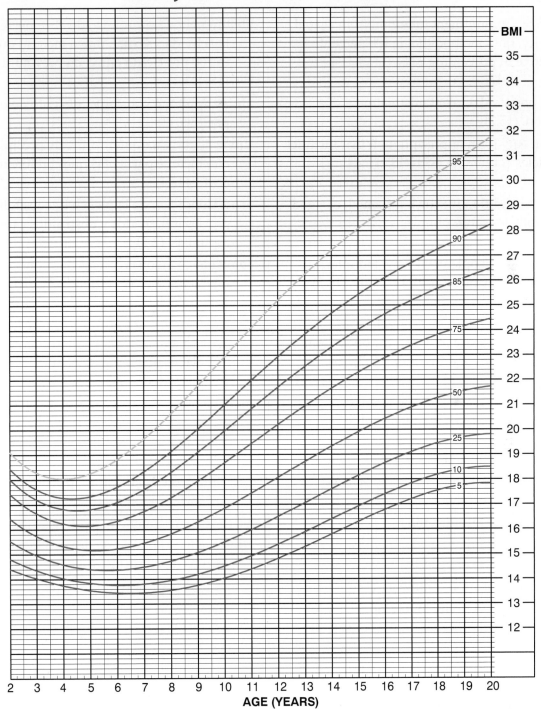

BMI

| 35 |
| 34 |
| 33 |
| 32 |
| 31 |
| 30 |
| 29 |
| 28 |
| 27 |
| 26 |
| 25 |
| 24 |
| 23 |
| 22 |
| 21 |
| 20 |
| 19 |
| 18 |
| 17 |
| 16 |
| 15 |
| 14 |
| 13 |
| 12 |

95
90
85
75
50
25
10
5

AGE (YEARS)

Key

Weight Status Category	Percentile Range
Underweight	Less than the 5th percentile
Healthy weight	5th percentile to less than the 85th percentile
Overweight	85th to less than the 95th percentile
Obese	Equal to or greater than the 95th percentile

SOURCE: Developed by the National Center for Health Statistics in collaboration with the National Center for Chronic Disease Prevention and Health Promotion

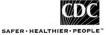

SAFER · HEALTHIER · PEOPLE™

Glossary/Glosario

English

Español

A

abstinence. Commitment to refrain from sexual activity; only method that is 100 percent effective in preventing STIs. (11.2)

abstinencia. Compromiso de abstenerse de la actividad sexual; único método que es 100 por ciento eficaz en prevenir los ITS. (11.2)

abuse. Consistent, violent mistreatment of a person. (15.2)

abuso. Maltrato constante, violento de una persona. (15.2)

acid rain. Any form of precipitation that includes particles containing acid. (13.1)

lluvia ácida. Cualquier forma de precipitación que incluye partículas que contienen ácido. (13.1)

acne. Skin condition in which inflamed, clogged hair follicles cause pimples. (2.1)

acné. Condición de la piel en que los folículos pilosos inflamados y obstruidos causan espinillas. (2.1)

acquaintances. People you know and interact with, but may not consider friends. (14.3)

conocidos. Personas con las que conoce e interactúa, pero no puede considerar amigos. (14.3)

acquired immunodeficiency syndrome (AIDS). Often fatal disease in which the body cannot fight infections and diseases. (11.3)

síndrome de inmunodeficiencia adquirida (SIDA). Enfermedad, con frecuencia fatal, en que el cuerpo no pueda combatir infecciones y enfermedades. (11.3)

active listening. Way of paying attention to spoken messages with the goal of understanding the message and the speaker's feelings about it. (14.1)

escuchar activamente. Manera de prestar atención a los mensajes hablados con la meta de entender el mensaje y los sentimientos sóbrelo del orador. (14.1)

addiction. Physical and psychological need for a substance or behavior. (8.2)

adicción. Necesidad física y psicológica para una sustancia o comportamiento. (8.2)

addictive. Habit-forming. (8.1)

adictivo. Que genera dependencia. (8.1)

adolescence. Period of development between 12 and 19 years of age. (16.3)

adolescencia. Período de desarrollo entre 12 y 19 años de edad. (16.3)

advocate. Support or recommend. (1.3)

proponer. Soportar o recomendar. (1.3)

aerobic exercise. Activity involving the use of oxygen to fuel processes in the body. (7.2)

ejercicio aeróbico. Actividad que consiste en el uso de oxígeno para alimentar procesos en el cuerpo. (7.2)

air quality index (AQI). Number that communicates to the public the level of pollutants in the air. (13.2)

índice de calidad del aire (AQI). Número que comunica al público el nivel de los contaminantes en el aire. (13.2)

The numbers in parentheses following definitions represent the lesson in which the terms appear.

English

Al-Anon Family Groups. Support group where family members and friends who have loved ones with an alcohol-use disorder come together to share their experiences, receive encouragement, and learn ways to cope with the problem. (9.2)

Alateen. Support group where young people who have loved ones with an alcohol-use disorder come together to share their experiences and learn ways to cope with problems. (9.2)

alcohol. Type of drug (known as a *depressant*) found in drinks—such as beer, wine, and liquor—that can cause a person to act and feel differently. (9.1)

Alcoholics Anonymous (AA). Self-help program for people with alcohol-use disorders to help them change how they think about drinking. (9.2)

alcohol-use disorders. Conditions that occur when the recurrent use of alcohol causes problems that interfere with a person's health and responsibilities at school, home, or work. (9.1)

anabolic steroids. Artificial hormones used to treat certain types of muscular disorders that can have harmful side effects. (6.4)

anaerobic exercise. Activity involving the use of energy stored in the muscles to supply the body with the fuel it needs. (7.2)

anaphylaxis. Allergic response in which fluid fills the lungs and air passages narrow, restricting breathing. (12.3)

anorexia nervosa. Eating disorder in which people have an intense fear of gaining weight and lose far more weight than is healthy. (6.4)

Español

Grupos de Familia Al-Anon. Grupo de apoyo donde familiares y amigos quien tienen seres queridos con un trastorno por consumo de alcohol se une para compartir sus experiencias, recibir ánimo, y aprender maneras para enfrentarse con el problema. (9.2)

Alateen. Grupo de apoyo donde los jóvenes quien tienen seres queridos con un trastorno por consumo de alcohol se une para compartir sus experiencias y aprender maneras para enfrentarse con problemas. (9.2)

alcohol. Tipo de droga (llamado un *depresor*) se encuentra en bebidas—tal como cerveza, vino, y licor—que pueden causar una persona se actúa y siente diferente. (9.1)

Alcohólicos Anónimos (AA). Programa de auto-ayuda para personas con trastornos por consumo de alcohol para ayudarles a cambiar como piensan en beber. (9.2)

trastornos por consumo de alcohol. Condiciones que ocurren cuando el uso de alcohol recurrente causa problemas que interfieren con la salud de una persona y sus responsabilidades en escuela, en casa, o en el trabajo. (9.1)

esteroides anabólicos. Hormonas artificiales utilizadas para tratar algunos tipos de trastornos musculares que pueden tener efectos secundarios dañinos. (6.4)

ejercicio anaeróbico. Actividad que consiste en el uso de energía almacenado en los músculos para proveer el cuerpo con el combustible se necesité. (7.2)

anafilaxia. Reacción alérgica en la que fluidos llenan los pulmones y las vías aéreas estrechas, restringiendo la respiración. (12.3)

anorexia nerviosa. Trastorno alimenticio en que personas tienen un miedo intenso a aumentar de peso y pierden mucho más peso de lo que es saludable. (6.4)

English

antibiotics. Substances that target and kill pathogenic bacteria. (11.1)

antidepressants. Medications that treat depression by making certain chemicals in the brain more available. (5.2)

antiperspirant. Product designed to stop or dry up sweat. (2.1)

antipsychotics. Medications that manage the symptoms of schizophrenia. (5.2)

anti-retroviral therapy (ART). Treatment for HIV/AIDS in which a cocktail of three drugs is given to interfere with HIV reproduction. (11.3)

antisocial personality disorder. Condition identified by ignoring social rules and engaging in impulsive behavior. (5.1)

anxiety disorder. Condition in which someone responds with extreme or unrealistic fear and dread to certain situations, experiences, or objects. (5.1)

appendix. Finger-shaped organ attached to the large intestine; made of lymphatic tissue. (17.3)

arteries. Blood vessels that carry oxygen-rich blood. (17.2)

arthritis. Condition that results in inflammation of the joints, causing pain and stiffness. (11.4)

asthma. Chronic disease caused by blockages of airflow to and from the lungs. (8.1)

astigmatism. Condition in which the eye does not focus light evenly onto the retina; objects appear blurry and stretched out. (2.2)

attention deficit hyperactivity disorder (ADHD). Condition in which a person has difficulty paying attention and controlling behavior. (5.1)

attitudes. Set ways a person thinks or feels about someone or something. (4.1)

Español

antibióticos. Sustancias que ataca y destruye las bacterias patógenas. (11.1)

antidepresivos. Medicaciones que tratan la depresión por hacer que ciertas sustancias químicas en el cerebro están más disponibles. (5.2)

antitranspirante. Producto diseñado para detener o secar el sudor. (2.1)

antipsicóticos. Medicaciones que controlan los síntomas de la esquizofrenia. (5.2)

terapia antirretroviral (TARV). Tratamiento para el VIH/SIDA en el que se administra un coctel de tres drogas para interferir en la reproducción del VIH. (11.3)

trastorno de personalidad antisocial. Condición identificada por ignorando normas sociales y exhibiendo comportamiento impulsivo. (5.1)

trastorno de ansiedad. Condición en que alguien responde con temor y miedo extremo o poco realista a algunas situaciones, experiencias, u objetos. (5.1)

apéndice. Órgano con forma de dedo adjunto al intestino grueso; hecho de tejido linfático. (17.3)

arterias. Vasos sanguíneos que llevan la sangre rica en oxígeno. (17.2)

artritis. Condición que resulta en la inflamación de las articulaciones, causando dolor y rigidez. (11.4)

asma. Enfermedad crónica causada por bloqueos de la circulación del aire a y de los pulmones. (8.1)

astigmatismo. Condición en que el ojo no enfoca la luz uniformemente a la retina; los objetos aparecen nublados y estirados. (2.2)

síndrome de déficit atencional (ADHD). Condición en que una persona tiene dificultad prestando atención y controlando comportamiento. (5.1)

actitudes. Maneras fijas en que una persona piensa o siente sobre alguien o algo. (4.1)

English

autoimmune disease. Condition that causes the body's immune system to attack and damage the joints. (11.4)

automated external defibrillator (AED). Rescue device that delivers a controlled, precise shock to the heart. (12.3)

AWARxE Prescription Drug Safety Program. Organization that spreads awareness of the growing prescription drug abuse problem. (10.3)

B

beliefs. Things a person knows to be true, based on real experiences, scientific facts, or what a person has learned from others. (4.1)

binge drinking. Consuming four drinks for women and five drinks for men on the same occasion. (9.1)

binge-eating disorder. Eating disorder characterized by people eating very large amounts of food with no control. (6.4)

biodegradable. Able to break down without causing harm when thrown out. (13.2)

bipolar disorder. Condition identified by periods of intense depression that alternate with periods of manic moods. (5.1)

bladder. Organ that stores urine until it can be pushed out of the body. (17.3)

blood alcohol concentration (BAC). Percentage of alcohol that is in a person's blood. (9.1)

body art. Permanent decorations that are applied to the body; examples include tattoos and piercings. (2.1)

body composition. Ratio of the various components—fat, bone, and muscle—that make up a person's body. (6.3)

body image. Person's thoughts and feelings about how he or she looks. (6.4)

Español

enfermedad autoinmune. Condición que causa el sistema inmunológico del cuerpo a atacar y dañar las articulaciones. (11.4)

desfibrilador automático externo (DEA). Dispositivo de rescate que ofrece una descarga controlada, precisa al corazón. (12.3)

programa de seguridad AWARxE de medicamentos recetados. Organización que concientiza del problema en crecimiento del abuso de medicamentos recetados. (10.3)

creencias. Cosas una persona sabe que es cierto, basado en experiencias auténticos, hechos científicos, o que una persona he aprendido de otros. (4.1)

consumo excesivo de alcohol. Consumiendo cuatro bebidas para mujeres y cinco bebidas para hombres en la misma ocasión. (9.1)

trastorno por atracón. Trastorno alimenticio caracterizada por personas comiendo cantidades muy grandes de comida sin dominio. (6.4)

biodegradable. Capaz de descomponer sin causar daño cuando tirado. (13.2)

trastorno bipolar. Condición identifica por periodos de depresión intenso que alternan con períodos de estados maníacos. (5.1)

vejiga. Órgano que almacena la orina hasta puede ser empujado fuera del cuerpo. (17.3)

concentración de alcohol en la sangre (BAC). Porcentaje de alcohol que está en la sangre de una persona. (9.1)

arte corporal. Decoraciones permanentes que se aplican al cuerpo; ejemplos incluyen tatuajes y *piercings*. (2.1)

composición corporal. Proporción de los componentes varios—grasa, hueso, y músculo—que forman el cuerpo de una persona. (6.3)

imagen corporal. Pensamientos y sentimientos de una persona sobre cómo él o ella se ve. (6.4)

English

body mass index (BMI). Measure used to estimate whether a person is a healthy weight for his or her height. (6.3)

body system. Collection of organs that work together. (17.1)

borderline personality disorder (BPD). Condition identified by unstable identity and interpersonal relationships. (5.1)

brain stem. Part of the brain that controls the heartbeat and breathing rate. (17.4)

bronchi. Two air passages, each of which connects the trachea to a lung. (17.2)

brownfield site. Land, such as an old factory or gas station, that contains hazardous waste. (13.2)

bulimia nervosa. Eating disorder in which a person has recurrent episodes of binge eating followed by purging. (6.4)

bullying. Repeated aggressive behavior toward someone that causes the person injury or discomfort. (15.1)

bystander. Someone who is at an event or incident, but is not directly involved. (12.3)

C

caffeine. Substance that produces a temporary increase in activity in the body, making it difficult to sleep. (3.3)

cancer. Complex disease that typically involves an uncontrolled growth of abnormal cells. (11.4)

capillaries. Small arteries that deliver oxygen and nutrients to cells and pick up cells' waste. (17.2)

carbohydrates. Major source of energy for the body; found in fruits, vegetables, grains, and milk products. (6.1)

carcinogens. Cancer-causing agents. (8.1)

cardiopulmonary resuscitation (CPR). Emergency procedure that uses chest compressions to restore heartbeat; may also involve mouth-to-mouth breathing. (12.3)

Español

índice de masa corporal (IMC). Medida utilizada para estimar si una persona tiene un peso saludable para su estatura. (6.3)

sistema corporal. Colecciones de órganos que funcionan juntos. (17.1)

trastorno de personalidad limítrofe (BPD). Condición identifica por identidad y relaciones interpersonales inestables. (5.1)

tallo cerebral. Parte del cerebro que controla el latido y la frecuencia respiratoria. (17.4)

bronquios. Dos vías aéreas, cada uno de los cuales conecta la tráquea a un pulmón. (17.2)

sitio previamente urbanizado. Tierra, tal como una fábrica o gasolinera, que contiene residuos peligrosos. (13.2)

bulimia nerviosa. Trastorno alimenticio en que una persona tiene episodios recurrentes de atracón seguido por vómitos. (6.4)

intimidación. Comportamiento repetido y agresivo hacia alguien que causa herida o incomodidad de la persona. (15.1)

transeúnte. Alguien que está en un evento o incidente, pero no está involucrado directamente. (12.3)

cafeína. Sustancia que fabrica un aumento temporal de actividad en el cuerpo, que complique el sueño. (3.3)

cáncer. Enfermedad compleja que típicamente consiste en crecimiento incontrolado de células anormales. (11.4)

capilares. Arterias pequeñas que entrega el oxígeno y los nutrientes a las células y recoge los residuos de las células. (17.2)

carbohidratos. Fuente importante de energía para el cuerpo; se encuentra en frutas, verduras, granos, y productos lácteos. (6.1)

cancerígenos. Agentes que causan cáncer. (8.1)

reanimación cardiopulmonar (RCP). Procedimiento emergencia que utiliza compresiones del pecho para devolver el latido; puede también consiste en respiración boca a boca. (12.3)

English

casual dating. Way of getting to know how you interact with and feel about another person. (14.4)

cavities. Holes in the teeth that occur when plaque eats into a tooth's enamel. (2.2)

cerebellum. Part of the brain that controls coordinated, smooth muscle activity. (17.4)

cerebrum. Largest part of the brain, which interprets information from the sensory organs; controls muscle actions and is responsible for intelligence, memory, and personality. (17.4)

child abuse. Any act an adult commits that causes harm or threatens to cause harm to a child. (15.2)

chlamydia. Bacterial infection known as a "silent" disease because it has few or no symptoms. (11.2)

chronic bronchitis. Ongoing condition in which small tubes in the lungs become swollen and irritated. (8.1)

circadian rhythms. Naturally occurring physical, behavioral, and mental changes in the body that typically follow the 24-hour cycle of the sun. (3.1)

circulatory system. Body system formed by all the structures that move blood through the body. (17.2)

clique. Small group of friends who deliberately exclude other people from joining or being a part of their group. (14.3)

club drugs. Several different types of drugs that young people may abuse at parties, bars, and concerts. (10.2)

cocaine. Drug that usually comes in the form of white powder made from the leaves of the coca plant. (10.2)

collaborate. Work together. (1.3)

communicable disease. Condition someone can develop after coming into contact with humans, animals, or plants infected with the disease; also called *infectious disease*. (11.1)

Español

citas casuales. Manera de conocer cómo se interactúa con y se siente sobre otra persona. (14.4)

caries. Orificios en los dientes que ocurren cuando la placa carcome el esmalte de un diente. (2.2)

cerebelo. Parte del cerebro que controla la actividad de los músculos coordinados, lisos. (17.4)

cerebro. Parte más grande del cerebro, que interpreta información de los órganos sensoriales; controla acciones musculares y es responsable por la inteligencia, memoria, y personalidad. (17.4)

abuso infantil. Cualquier acción que un adulto comete que causa daño o amenaza causar daño a un niño. (15.2)

clamidia. Infección bacteriana conocido como una enfermedad "silencioso" porque tiene pocos o no síntomas. (11.2)

bronquitis crónica. Condición en curso en que tubos pequeños en los pulmones se hinchan y se irritan. (8.1)

ritmos circadianos. Cambios físicos, conductuales, y mentales que ocurren naturalmente en el cuerpo que típicamente sigue el ciclo de 24 horas del sol. (3.1)

sistema circulatorio. Sistema corporal formada por todas las estructuras que mueven la sangre por el cuerpo. (17.2)

camarilla. Grupo pequeño de amigos que excluya deliberadamente otras personas de unirse o ser un parte de su grupo. (14.3)

drogas de club. Varios tipos diferentes de drogas que jóvenes pueden abusar en fiestas, bares, y conciertos. (10.2)

cocaína. Droga que usualmente proviene en la forma de polvo blanco hecho de las hojas de las plantas de coca. (10.2)

colaborar. Trabajar juntos. (1.3)

enfermedad transmisible. Condición alguien puede contraiga después de entrar en contacto con humanos, animales, o plantas infectados con la enfermedad; también llamada *enfermedad infeccioso*. (11.1)

English

communication process. Exchange of messages and responses between two or more people. (14.1)

composting. Process of gathering food scraps and yard waste into a bin and letting it decompose and then adding it to soil to help plants grow. (13.2)

concussion. Type of brain injury that results from a blow or jolt to the head or upper body. (7.3)

conflict resolution skills. Strategies that can help you deal with arguments in a positive, respectful way to promote healthy relationships. (1.3)

conjunctivitis. Viral or bacterial infection that causes inflammation of part of the eye; also known as *pinkeye*. (11.1)

culture. Beliefs, values, customs, and arts of a group of people. (1.2)

cyberbullying. Form of bullying that uses electronic means. (15.1)

D

dandruff. Dead skin that flakes off the scalp due to dryness, infrequent shampooing, or irritation. (2.1)

decision-making skills. Tools a person uses to make good choices about health and wellness. (1.3)

delayed sleep phase syndrome (DSPS). Condition that results from a delay in the sleep-wake cycle that affects a person's daily activities. (3.2)

deodorant. Product designed to cover up body odor. (2.1)

dependence. Effect that occurs when the body needs an addictive substance in its system to function "normally" or feel "normal." (8.2)

dermis. Middle layer of the skin, which contains hair follicles. (2.1)

Español

proceso de comunicación. Intercambio de mensajes y respuestas mientras dos o más personas. (14.1)

compostaje. Proceso de recolectar restos de comida y residuo de la yarda en un recipiente y dejarlo descomponer y después añadirlo la tierra para ayudar a las plantas a crecer. (13.2)

contusión cerebral. Tipo de lesión cerebral resultado de un golpe o impresión a la cabeza o cuerpo superior. (7.3)

habilidades de resolución de conflictos. Estrategias que pueden ayudarse resolver disputas en una manera positiva, respetuosa para promover relaciones sanas. (1.3)

conjuntivitis. Infección vírica o bacteriana que causa inflamación en parte del ojo; también conocido como *pinkeye*. (11.1)

cultura. Creencias, valores, costumbres, y artes de un grupo de personas. (1.2)

ciberacoso. Forma de intimidación que utiliza medios electrónicos. (15.1)

caspa. Piel muerta que desprende del cuero cabelludo por la resequedad, el champú poco frecuente, o la irritación. (2.1)

capacidad para tomar decisiones. Herramientas una persona utiliza para tomar decisiones buenas acerca de su salud y bienestar. (1.3)

síndrome de la fase de sueño retrasada (DSPS). Condición que resulta de un retraso en el ciclo sueño-vigilia que afecta las actividades diarias de una persona. (3.2)

desodorante. Producto diseñado para cubrir el olor corporal. (2.1)

dependencia. Consecuencia que ocurre cuando el cuerpo necesita una sustancia adictiva en su sistema para funcionar "normalmente" o para sentir "normal." (8.2)

dermis. Capa intermedia de la piel, que contiene folículos pilosos. (2.1)

English

detoxification. Process of completely stopping all alcohol use to remove the substance from the body. (9.2)

diabetes mellitus. Disease resulting from the body's inability to regulate glucose; commonly known as *diabetes*. (11.4)

diaphragm. Sheet of muscle beneath the lungs and above the abdomen that contracts and relaxes to help the chest expand so a person can inhale or shrink so a person can exhale. (17.2)

dietary fiber. Tough, complex carbohydrate that the body is unable to digest. (6.1)

Dietary Guidelines. United States government recommendations for forming patterns of eating that will promote health. (6.2)

digestive system. Body system that breaks down food to provide nutrients and energy; removes solid waste from the body. (17.3)

dislocation. Serious injury in which bones move out of their normal position. (7.3)

diversity. Inclusion of people with different backgrounds. (14.3)

domestic violence. Abuse that involves couples who are married or in a romantic relationship. (15.2)

drug abuse. Continued use of a drug despite negative or harmful outcomes. (10.2)

drug addiction. Complete dependence on a drug. (10.2)

drugs. Medications and other substances that change the way the body or brain functions. (10.1)

E

early childhood. Period of development from infancy through the preschool years. (16.2)

eating disorder. Serious illness that causes major disturbances in a person's daily diet. (6.4)

Español

desintoxicación. Proceso de parar completamente todo uso de alcohol para quitar la sustancia del cuerpo. (9.2)

diabetes mellitus. Enfermedad resultante de la incapacidad del cuerpo a regular la glucosa; comúnmente conocido como *diabetes*. (11.4)

diafragma. Chapa de músculo bajo los pulmones y arriba del abdomen que contrae y relaja para ayudar el pecho expande para que una persona puede inhalar o encoge para que una persona puede exhalar. (17.2)

fibra dietética. Un carbohidrato complejo y duro que el cuerpo es incapaz de digerir. (6.1)

Lineamientos Dietéticos. Recomendaciones del gobierno de los Estados Unidos para formar patrones de comer que promoverá la salud. (6.2)

sistema digestivo. Sistema corporal que descompone la comida para proveer las nutrientes y la energía; quita los residuos sólidos del cuerpo. (17.3)

dislocación. Lesión grave en que huesos mueven afuera de sus posiciones normales. (7.3)

diversidad. Inclusión de personas con orígenes diferentes. (14.3)

violencia doméstica. Abuso que consiste en parejas que están casadas o en una relación romántica. (15.2)

abuso de drogas. Uso continuado de una droga a pesar de resultados negativos o dañinos. (10.2)

drogadicción. Dependencia completa en una droga. (10.2)

drogas. Medicinas y otras sustancias que cambian la manera en que el cuerpo o cerebro funciona. (10.1)

primera infancia. Período de desarrollo desde la infancia hasta los años preescolares. (16.2)

trastorno alimenticio. Enfermedad grave que provoca perturbaciones grandes en la dieta diaria de una persona. (6.4)

English

economic environment. Person's level of education and income level. (1.2)

eczema. Chronic condition that causes swollen, red, dry, and itchy patches of skin on one or more parts of the body. (2.1)

elder abuse. Mistreatment of older adults in their homes, nursing homes, or other living situations. (15.2)

embryo. Term that describes a developing baby during the embryonic stage of prenatal development. (16.1)

emergency preparedness. Knowing how to respond to a specific type of emergency. (12.1)

emotional abuse. Attitudes or controlling behaviors that harm a person's mental health; also called *verbal, mental,* or *psychological abuse.* (15.2)

emotional awareness. Skill of knowing which emotions you feel, and why. (4.2)

emotional intelligence (EI). Skill of understanding, controlling, and expressing your emotions and sensing the emotions of others. (4.2)

emotions. Moods or feelings you experience. (4.2)

empathy. Ability to put yourself in someone else's shoes, and to understand someone else's wants, needs, and viewpoints. (4.2)

emphysema. Disease that causes the airways in the lungs to become permanently enlarged. (8.1)

enabling. Encouraging a person's unhealthy behaviors, either intentionally or unintentionally. (9.2)

endocrine system. Body system that produces chemical messengers, called *hormones,* which regulate body processes. (17.4)

endurance. Ability to continue an activity over a period of time without tiring. (7.2)

Español

entorno económico. Nivel de educación y de ingresos de una persona. (1.2)

eczema. Condición crónica que causa parches de piel hinchados, rojas, secas, y pruritos en uno o más partes del cuerpo. (2.1)

abuso de ancianos. Maltrato de adultos mayores en sus casas, hogares de ancianos, u otras situaciones de vida. (15.2)

embrión. Término que describe un bebé en desarrollo durante la etapa embrionaria del desarrollo prenatal. (16.1)

preparación ante emergencias. Saber cómo responder a un tipo específico de emergencia. (12.1)

abuso emocional. Actitudes o comportamientos dominantes que dañan la salud mental de una persona; también llamada *abuso verbal, mental,* o *psicológico.* (15.2)

conciencia emocional. Habilidad de comprender cuales emociones se siente y por qué. (4.2)

inteligencia emocional (EI). Habilidad de comprender, controlar, y expresar sus emociones y sentir las emociones de otras personas. (4.2)

emociones. Estados de ánimo y sentimientos experimenta. (4.2)

empatía. Capacidad de ponerse en los zapatos de otra persona, y comprender los deseos, necesidades, y puntos de vista de otra persona. (4.2)

enfisema. Enfermedad que causa las vías respiratorias en los pulmones a ser aumentados para siempre. (8.1)

posibilitar. Incentivando los comportamientos de mal salud, ya sea intencional o no accidental. (9.2)

sistema endocrino. Sistema corporal que produce los mensajeros químicos, llamadas *hormonas,* que controlan los procesos corporales. (17.4)

resistencia. Capacidad de continuar una actividad durante un periodo de tiempo sin ser cansado. (7.2)

English

environment. Circumstances, objects, or conditions that surround a person in everyday life. (1.2)

epidermis. Outermost layer of the skin. (2.1)

escape plan. Strategy that outlines safe routes and procedures for leaving the house in the event a fire occurs. (12.1)

estrogen. Hormone that triggers growth and development of the female sex organs. (16.3)

eustress. Positive stress. (4.3)

exclusive. Committed to being romantically involved with only one dating partner. (14.4)

exercise. Type of planned, structured, and purposeful physical activity. (7.1)

extinguish. Put out. (12.1)

F

fad diets. Weight-loss plans that often forbid eating certain types of food groups and may require the purchase of special, and often costly, prepared meals. (6.3)

family history. Record of a disease's presence and impact within a family. (1.2)

family therapy. Type of therapy in which all family members meet together with a therapist to build positive, healthy relationships. (5.2)

farsightedness. Condition in which distant objects are seen more clearly than nearby objects. (2.2)

fasting. Not eating any food or drink except water for an entire day. (6.3)

fats. Type of nutrient largely made up of fatty acids, which provide a valuable source of energy. (6.1)

feedback. Constructive response to a message to communicate that it was received and understood. (14.1)

fertilization. Process by which the sperm and egg combine to create a zygote. (16.1)

Español

entorno. Circunstancias, objetos, o condiciones que rodean una persona en la vida diaria. (1.2)

epidermis. Capa más externa de la piel. (2.1)

plan de escape. Estrategia que resume las rutas seguras y procedimientos para salir la casa en el evento que ocurra un fuego. (12.1)

estrógeno. Hormona que provoque el crecimiento y desarrollo de los órganos sexuales femeninas. (16.3)

eustress. Estrés positiva. (4.3)

exclusivo. Comprometido a ser involucrada románticamente con solamente uno pareja de citas. (14.4)

ejercicio. Tipo de actividad física que se planifica, estructurada, y con un propósito. (7.1)

extinguir. Apagar. (12.1)

dieta relámpago. Plan de pérdida de peso que a menudo prohíbe algunos tipos de grupos alimenticios y puede que demandar la compra de comida especial, y a menudo es costoso, preparada. (6.3)

historia familiar. Historia de la presencia y el impacto de una enfermedad dentro de una familia. (1.2)

terapia familiar. Tipo de terapia en que todos los miembros de la familia se reúnen juntos con una terapeuta para construir relaciones positivas y sanas. (5.2)

vista cansada. Condición en que objetos alejados se los ven con más claridad que objetos cercas. (2.2)

ayuno. No comer ninguna comida o bebida excepto de agua para un día entero. (6.3)

grasas. Tipo de nutrientes compuesto en gran parte de ácidos grasos, que provee una fuente de energía. (6.1)

contestación. Respuesta constructiva a un mensaje para comunicar que fue recibido y entendido. (14.1)

fertilización. Proceso por el cual el espermatozoide y el óvulo combinan para crear un cigoto. (16.1)

English

fetus. Term that describes a developing baby during the fetal stage of prenatal development. (16.1)

fight-or-flight response. Body's impulse to either fight off or flee from threatening situations. (4.3)

fine-motor skills. Movements that use the small muscles of the body. (16.2)

fire triangle. Model to help you remember the elements that are needed for a fire to occur; elements include fuel, heat, and oxygen. (12.1)

first aid. Treatment given in the first moments of an accident or injury—usually before medical professionals arrive on the scene. (12.3)

first-aid kit. Container that includes the supplies needed to treat most types of minor injuries. (12.3)

fitness. Body's ability to meet daily physical demands. (7.1)

FITT. Acronym used to focus on the key fitness factors of frequency, intensity, time, and type. (7.4)

flammable. Easily set on fire. (12.1)

food sanitation. Food safety practices that maintain the safety of food you handle and eat; includes refrigerating and freezing certain foods, cooking meat thoroughly, and washing vegetables and fruits. (11.5)

fossil fuels. Natural forms of energy, such as oil, natural gas, and gas, that were formed a very long time ago, when dinosaurs lived on Earth. (13.2)

fracture. Broken bone. (7.3)

frostbite. Injury caused by the freezing of skin and body tissues. (7.3)

G

gallbladder. Organ in which bile is stored until needed to digest food. (17.3)

Español

feto. Término que describe un bebé en desarrollo durante la etapa fetal del desarrollo prenatal. (16.1)

respuesta de lucha o huida. Impulso del cuerpo para ya sea a combatir o huir de situaciones amenazantes. (4.3)

habilidades de motricidad fina. Movimientos que utilizan los músculos pequeños del cuerpo. (16.2)

triangulo del fuego. Modelo para ayudarle a recordar los elementos necesarios para que ocurra un fuego; los elementos incluyen combustible, calor, y oxígeno. (12.1)

primeros auxilios. Tratamiento dado en los primeros momentos de un accidente o lesión—a menudo antes de que los profesionales médicos lleguen a la escena. (12.3)

botiquín. Recipiente que incluye las provisiones necesarias para tratar la mayoría de tipos de lesiones menores. (12.3)

buena forma. Capacidad del cuerpo para satisfacer las demandas físicas diarias. (7.1)

FITT. Acrónimo usado para concentrarse en los factores claves de buena forma de frecuencia, intensidad, tiempo, y tipo. (7.4)

inflamable. Incendiado fácilmente. (12.1)

saneamiento de alimentos. Prácticas de seguridad de alimentos que mantienen la seguridad de la comida se maneja y se come; incluye refrigerar y congelar algas comidas, cocinar bien la carne, y lavar verduras y frutas. (11.5)

combustibles fósiles. Formas naturales de energía, tal como petróleo, gas natural, y gas, que fueran formados hace mucho tiempo, cuando los dinosaurios vivían en la Tierra. (13.2)

fractura. Rotura de un hueso. (7.3)

congelación. Lesión resultada de la congelación de la piel y el tejido del cuerpo. (7.3)

vesícula. Órgano en que la bilis se almacena hasta que necesitan para digerir los alimentos. (17.3)

English

gangs. Groups of people who carry out violent and illegal acts. (15.3)

genes. Segments of DNA that determine the structure and function of a person's cells and affect his or her development, personality, and health. (1.2)

genital herpes. Viral infection that results in sores on the genitals. (11.2)

gingivitis. Inflammation of the gums. (2.2)

gland. Group of cells that produce and release substances into the body. (17.1)

goal. Plan of action that will guide someone in achieving something he or she wants to reach. (1.3)

gonorrhea. Bacterial infection that primarily affects the genitals, rectum, and throat. (11.2)

gratitude. Emotion that means being thankful or grateful. (4.2)

green products. Goods that have a less harmful impact on the environment than traditional products. (13.2)

gross-motor skills. Movements that use the large muscles of the body. (16.2)

group dating. Going out with a group that includes the person one is interested in rather than dating as a couple. (14.4)

H

hackers. People who illegally access data in your computer. (12.2)

hallucinogens. Drugs that alter the way people view, think, and feel about things, causing hallucinations. (10.2)

harassment. Type of bullying that targets a particular part of a person's identity, such as race, religion, gender, or sexual orientation. (15.1)

hate crimes. Threats or attacks against someone because of his or her race, ethnic origin, disability, sexual orientation, or religion. (15.3)

Español

pandillas. Grupos de personas que llevar a cabo acciones violentos e ilegales. (15.3)

genes. Segmentos de ADN que determinan la estructura y la función de las células de una persona y afectan su desarrollo, la personalidad, y la salud. (1.2)

herpes genital. Infección vírica que resulta en llagas en los genitales. (11.2)

gingivitis. Inflamación de las encías. (2.2)

glándula. Grupa de las células que produce y emite sustancias en el cuerpo. (17.1)

meta. Plan de acción que le guiará alguien en logrando algo que él o ella quiere lograr. (1.3)

gonorrea. Infección bacteriana que afecta principalmente los genitales, el recto, y la garganta. (11.2)

gratitud. Emoción que significa ser agradecido. (4.2)

productos verdes. Bienes que tienen un impacto menos dañino por el ambiente que productos tradicionales. (13.2)

habilidades de motricidad gruesa. Movimientos que utilizan los músculos grandes del cuerpo. (16.2)

citas en grupo. Salir con un grupo que incluye la persona uno está interesado en vez de salir en citas como pareja. (14.4)

hacker. Personas que accedan ilegalmente a los datos en su computadora. (12.2)

alucinógenos. Drogas que alteran la manera en que personas ven, piensan, y sienten sobre cosas, causando alucinaciones. (10.2)

acoso. Tipo de intimidación que dirigir una parte particular de la identidad de una persona, tal como raza, religión, sexo, u orientación sexual. (15.1)

crímenes de odio. Amenazas o ataques contra alguien porque su raza, origen étnico, discapacidad, orientación sexual, o religión. (15.3)

English

hazing. Use of pressure by a group to make someone do something embarrassing or even dangerous to be accepted by a group. (15.1)

health. Absence of physical illness and disease. (1.1)

healthcare. Treatment and prevention of illnesses, injuries, or diseases to improve wellness. (1.1)

health literacy. Person's ability to locate, interpret, and apply information as it relates to his or her health. (1.3)

health-related fitness. Type of fitness a person needs to perform daily activities with ease and energy. (7.2)

heart. Hollow, muscular organ located in the center of the chest; pumps blood into the circulatory system. (17.2)

heart attack. Medical emergency in which flow of blood to the heart is restricted, causing the heart to beat irregularly and inefficiently. (11.4)

heavy drinking. Consuming eight or more drinks for women and 15 or more drinks for men in one week; can lead to alcohol dependence. (9.1)

heroin. Drug similar to painkillers that has dangerous side effects and is very addictive. (10.2)

HIV-positive. Status determined by a laboratory test that indicates the presence of HIV antibodies in a person's blood. (11.3)

homicide. Crime of killing another person. (15.3)

hospice care. Type of care given to people who are dying that provides comfort and support to them and their families. (16.4)

human immunodeficiency virus (HIV). Virus that infects and kills cells, weakening the body's immune system; leads to AIDS. (11.3)

Español

novatadas. Uso de presión por un grupo a hacer que alguien haga algo embarazoso o hasta peligroso para ser aceptado por un grupo. (15.1)

salud. Falta de padecimiento física y enfermedad. (1.1)

asistencia médica. Tratamiento y la prevención de los padecimientos, heridas, o enfermedades a mejorar el bienestar. (1.1)

conocimientos de salud. Capacidad de una persona de localizar, interpretar, y aplicar información en relación con su salud. (1.3)

buena forma relacionada con la salud. Tipo de buena forma una persona necesita realizar actividades diarias con facilidad y energía. (7.2)

corazón. Órgano hueco, muscular localizado en el centro del pecho; bombea la sangre en el sistema circulatorio. (17.2)

ataque cardíaco. Emergencia médica en que el flujo de la sangre al corazón se restringe, causando el corazón a batir irregularmente y de forma ineficiente. (11.4)

consumo pesado de alcohol. Consumiendo ocho o más bebidas para mujeres y quince o más bebidas para hombres en una semana; puede llevar dependencia de alcohol. (9.1)

heroína. Droga similar a los analgésicos que tiene efectos secundarios peligrosos y es muy adictivo. (10.2)

VIH-positivo. Situación determinada por una prueba de laboratorio que indica la presencia de anticuerpos del VIH en la sangre de una persona. (11.3)

homicidio. Crimen de matar otra persona. (15.3)

cuidado de hospicio. Tipo de asistencia dado a las personas que están muriendo que provee comodidad y apoyo a ellos y sus familias. (16.4)

virus de la inmunodeficiencia humana (VIH). Virus que infecta y destruye las células, debilitando así el sistema inmunológico del cuerpo; lleva al SIDA. (11.3)

English

human life cycle. Sequence of developmental stages a person experiences from birth through adulthood. (16.2)

human papillomavirus (HPV). Most commonly contracted STI that causes genital infections and sometimes cancer. (11.2)

human trafficking. Form of modern slavery in which people are forced to perform some type of job or service against their will. (15.3)

hyperthermia. Serious condition that results when the heat-regulating mechanisms of the body are unable to deal with the heat from the environment, which results in a very high body temperature. (7.3)

hypodermis. Innermost layer of the skin, which contains fat, blood vessels, and nerve endings; attaches to underlying bone and muscle. (2.1)

hypothermia. Serious condition that results when a person's body loses heat faster than it can produce it. (7.3)

I

identity. Who you are, which includes your physical traits, activities, social connections, and internal thoughts and feelings. (4.1)

identity theft. Stealing and using someone's personal identifying information, often for financial gain. (12.2)

illegal drugs. Substances that are against the law to use because they can be harmful to a person's health. (10.2)

immediate family. Person's parents or guardians and siblings. (14.2)

individual therapy. Type of therapy that involves a one-on-one meeting with a therapist to discuss feelings and behaviors. (5.2)

infatuation. Intense romantic feelings for another person that develop suddenly and are usually based on physical attraction. (14.4)

Español

ciclo de la vida humana. Secuencia de las etapas de desarrollo una persona experimenta desde el nacimiento hasta la adultez. (16.2)

virus del papiloma humano (VPH). ITS más comúnmente contratado que causa infecciones genitales y a veces cáncer. (11.2)

trata de personas. Forma de la esclavitud moderna en que personas se fuerzan a desempeñar algún tipo de trabajo o servicio contra de su voluntad. (15.3)

hipertermia. Condición grave que resulta cuando los mecanismos del cuerpo por la regulación del calor no pueden resolver el calor del ambiente, que resulta en una temperatura corporal muy alta. (7.3)

hipodermis. Capa más interna de la piel, que contiene grasa, vasos sanguíneos, y terminaciones nerviosas; se une al hueso subyacente y al músculo. (2.1)

hipotermia. Condición grave que resulta cuando el cuerpo de una persona pierde el calor más rápido que puede producirlo. (7.3)

identidad. Quien es, que incluye sus características físicas, actividades, relaciones sociales, y pensamientos y sentimientos internos. (4.1)

usurpación de identidad. Robar y utilizar la información personal de identificación de alguien, a menudo por ganancias financieras. (12.2)

drogas ilegales. Sustancias que son contra la ley para usar porque pueden ser dañinos para la salud de una persona. (10.2)

familia inmediata. Los padres o guardianes y hermanos de una persona. (14.2)

terapia individual. Tipo de terapia que consiste en una reunión uno a uno con una terapeuta para discutir los sentimientos y comportamientos. (5.2)

infatuación. Sentimientos intensos románticos por otra persona que desarrollan bruscamente y son por lo general basado en atracción física. (14.4)

English

influenza. Viral infection of the respiratory system; also known as *the flu*. (11.1)

inhalants. Chemicals that people breathe in to experience some type of high. (10.2)

inhibition. Self-control that keeps people from taking dangerous risks. (9.1)

inpatient treatment. Type of treatment that involves staying in a healthcare facility for a period of time. (5.2)

insomnia. Trouble falling or staying asleep. (3.2)

integumentary system. Body system that covers and protects the entire body. (17.1)

intensity. Measure of how much energy is used during exercise. (7.4)

interpersonal skills. Abilities that help people communicate and relate in positive ways with others. (14.1)

intimacy. Closeness. (14.4)

J

jet lag. Fatigue that people feel after changing time zones when they travel. (3.1)

joint. Location in the body where two or more bones meet and are held together. (17.1)

K

kidneys. Two bean-shaped organs that filter blood and make urine. (17.3)

L

latex condom. Device that provides a barrier to microorganisms that cause STIs. (11.2)

legal drugs. Medications that can treat health conditions to improve a person's health and enhance wellness. (10.1)

Español

influenza. Infección vírica del sistema respiratorio; también conocido como *la gripe*. (11.1)

inhalantes. Productos químicos que las personas inhalan para experimentar algún tipo de colocón. (10.2)

inhibición. Autocontrol que prevenir personas a tomando riesgos peligrosos. (9.1)

tratamiento hospitalario. Tipo de tratamiento que consiste en quedarse en un centro de servicios médicos para un periodo de tiempo. (5.2)

insomnio. Dificultad de quedarse o permanecer dormido. (3.2)

sistema integumentario. Sistema corporal que cubre y protege todo el cuerpo. (17.1)

intensidad. Medida de cuanta energía es usado durante ejercicio. (7.4)

habilidades interpersonales. Habilidades que ayudan a personas comunicar y relacionar en maneras positivas con otros. (14.1)

intimidad. Cercanía. (14.4)

jet lag. Fatiga que las personas experimentan después de cambiar zonas de tiempo durante un viaje. (3.1)

articulación. Localización en el cuerpo donde dos o más huesos se unen y se mantienen juntos. (17.1)

riñones. Dos órganos con forma de frijol que filtran la sangre y hacen la orina. (17.3)

condón de látex. Dispositivo que proporciona una barrera para microorganismos que causan los ITS. (11.2)

drogas legales. Medicinas que pueden tratar condiciones de salud para mejorar la salud de una persona y aumentar bienestar. (10.1)

English

lice. Tiny insects that attach to hair and feed on human blood. (2.1)

life expectancy. Estimate of how long a person in a particular society is likely to live. (16.2)

life span. Actual number of years a person lives. (16.2)

ligaments. Strong bands of tissue that hold together bones at joints to allow movement. (17.1)

liver. Large brown organ to the right of the stomach that has many jobs, including making bile. (17.3)

long-term non-progressors. HIV-positive people whose infection progresses to AIDS slowly. (11.3)

lymphatic system. Body system of organs and tissues that help fight infections. (17.3)

M

major depression. Condition identified by intense negative feelings that do not go away and negatively affect daily life; also known as *clinical depression*. (5.1)

marijuana. Drug made up of dried parts of the cannabis plant. (10.2)

maximum heart rate. Number of beats per minute a person's heart can achieve when working its hardest; varies by age. (7.4)

mediation. Method of resolving conflict that involves a third, neutral party. (1.3)

mediator. Neutral third party who helps resolve conflicts by listening carefully to each person's point of view. (1.3)

medical emergency. Urgent, life-threatening situation. (12.3)

medication abuse. Intentionally taking a drug in a way other than its intended use. (10.1)

Español

piojos. Minúsculos insectos que se adhieren al pelo y se alimentan de la sangre humana. (2.1)

esperanza de vida. Estimación de cuánto tiempo una persona en una sociedad particular es probable a vivir. (16.2)

período de vida. Número real de años una persona vive. (16.2)

ligamentos. Bandas fuertes de tejido que mantienen juntos los huesos a las articulaciones para permitir el movimiento. (17.1)

hígado. Órgano marrón grande al derecho del estómago que tiene muchos trabajos, incluyendo hacer la bilis. (17.3)

no progresores a largo plazo. Personas VIH-positivas cuyas infecciones progresa lentamente al SIDA. (11.3)

sistema linfático. Sistema corporal de órganos y tejidos que ayudan combatir las infecciones. (17.3)

depresión grave. Condición identifica por sentimientos intensos negativos que no se van y afectan negativamente la vida diaria; también llamado *depresión clínica*. (5.1)

marihuana. Droga hecha de partes secos de la planta cannabis. (10.2)

ritmo cardiaco máximo. Número de latidos por minuto el corazón de una persona puede lograr cuando trabajando más duro; varía en edad. (7.4)

mediación. Método de resolución de conflictos que involucra a un tercero neutral. (1.3)

mediador. Tercero neutral quien ayuda a resolver los conflictos por escuchando atentamente a las perspectivas de cada persona. (1.3)

emergencia médica. Situación urgente, mortal. (12.3)

abuso de medicinas. Intencionalmente tomando una droga en una manera otra del uso previsto. (10.1)

English

medication misuse. Taking medication in a way that does not follow the medication's instructions; often unintentional. (10.1)

medications. Drugs and medicines used to treat symptoms of an illness or to cure, manage, or prevent a disease. (10.1)

meditation. Strategy of clearing negative thoughts from your mind and relaxing your body to relieve stress. (4.3)

melatonin. Hormone that increases feelings of relaxation and sleepiness and signals that it is time to go to sleep. (3.1)

menstruation. Discharge of some blood and tissues from the uterus. (16.1)

mental and emotional health. Aspect of health that has to do with a person's thoughts and feelings. (1.1)

mental illness. Mental or emotional condition so severe that it interferes with daily functioning; also known as *mental disorder*. (5.1)

methamphetamine. Stimulant that speeds up brain functions. (10.2)

method of transmission. Way a disease gets from one organism to another; may be direct or indirect. (11.1)

middle adulthood. Stage of human development that occurs from 40 to 65 years of age. (16.4)

middle childhood. Period of time when children are between five and 12 years of age; also called the school-age years. (16.2)

milestones. Important events that occur in each of the developmental stages of the human life cycle. (16.2)

mindfulness. Strategy that involves being present in the moment and paying attention to thoughts and feelings in a nonjudgmental way. (4.3)

minerals. Inorganic elements found in soil and water that the body needs in small quantities. (6.1)

Español

mal uso de medicinas. Tomando medicina en una manera que no siga las instrucciones de la medicina; a menudo accidental. (10.1)

medicamentos. Drogas y medicinas utilizados para tratar síntomas de una dolencia o curar, manejar, o prevenir una enfermedad. (10.1)

meditación. Estrategia de despejar los pensamientos negativos de su mente y relajar su cuerpo para aliviar el estrés. (4.3)

melatonina. Hormona que aumenta las sensaciones de relajación y cansancio y hace señales que es tiempo a dormir. (3.1)

menstruación. Emisión de algún sangre y tejidos del útero. (16.1)

salud mental o emocional. Aspecto de salud que refiere a los pensamientos y sentimientos de una persona. (1.1)

enfermedad mental. Condición mental o emocional tan grave que interfiere con el funcionamiento diario; también llamado *trastorno mental*. (5.1)

metanfetamina. Estimulante que acelera las funciones cerebrales. (10.2)

método de transmisión. Manera en que una enfermedad transfiera de un organismo a otro; pueda ser directa o indirecta. (11.1)

adultez media. Etapa de desarrollo humano que ocurre desde 40 hasta 65 años de edad. (16.4)

niñez media. Período de tiempo cuando niños tienen entre cinco y doce años; también llamado los años de la edad escolar. (16.2)

hitos. Eventos importantes que ocurren en cada de las etapas de desarrollo del ciclo de la vida humana. (16.2)

concienciación. Estrategia que consiste en ser presente en el momento y prestar atención a los pensamientos y sentimientos en una manera no crítico. (4.3)

minerales. Elementos inorgánicos que se encuentran en el suelo y el agua que el cuerpo necesita en cantidades pequeños. (6.1)

English

moderate drinking. Consuming no more than one drink per day for women and no more than two drinks per day for men; also called *social drinking*. (9.1)

mononucleosis. Common viral infection that spreads through kissing or by sharing certain objects; also known as *mono* and *the kissing disease*. (11.1)

muscular system. Body system that helps the body move and aids other body systems. (17.1)

MyPlate food guidance system. United States government system that helps people put the *Dietary Guidelines* into practice. (6.2)

N

narcolepsy. Disorder that affects the brain's ability to control the sleep-wake cycle. (3.2)

natural disasters. Events or forces of nature that usually cause great damage. (12.1)

nearsightedness. Condition in which objects close to the eye appear clear, while objects farther away appear blurry. (2.2)

neglect. Type of child abuse in which a child's basic physical, emotional, medical, or educational needs are not met by parents or guardians. (15.2)

nervous system. Body system that allows people to think, use the senses, move, and maintain important body processes. (17.4)

neuron. Cell that is specialized to receive and send signals. (17.4)

nicotine. Toxic chemical in tobacco leaves that makes tobacco products addictive. (8.1)

nicotine replacement. Smoking cessation technique that involves the use of nicotine gum or the nicotine patch to lessen withdrawal symptoms. (8.3)

Español

consumo moderado de alcohol. Consumiendo no más de una bebida por día para mujeres y no más de dos bebidas por día para hombres; también llamado *consumo social de alcohol*. (9.1)

mononucleosis. Infección vírica común que propague mientras besando o compartiendo ciertos objetos; también conocido como *mono* y *enfermedad del beso*. (11.1)

sistema muscular. Sistema corporal que ayuda al cuerpo a mover y ayuda otros sistemas corporales. (17.1)

sistema de guía de comida MiPlato. Sistema del gobierno de los Estados Unidos que ayuda personas a poner en práctica los *Lineamientos Dietéticos*. (6.2)

narcolepsia. Trastorno que afecta la habilidad del cerebro a controlar el ciclo sueño-vigilia. (3.2)

desastres naturales. Eventos o fuerzas de la naturaleza que por lo general causan grandes daños. (12.1)

miopía. Condición en que los objetos cercas del ojo aparecen claros, mientras objetos más alejados aparecen nublados. (2.2)

negligencia. Tipo de abuso infantil en que los necesidades físicos, emocionales, médicos, o educativos básicos de un niño no se cumplen por los padres o guardianes. (15.2)

sistema nervioso. Sistema corporal que permite a las personas pensar, usar los sentidos, mover, y mantener procesos corporales importantes. (17.4)

neurona. Célula que está especializada por recibir y enviar señales. (17.4)

nicotina. Sustancia química en las hojas de tabaco que hacen adictivos los productos del tabaco. (8.1)

reemplazo de la nicotina. Técnica de dejar de fumar que consiste en el uso del chicle de nicotina o el parche de nicotina para disminuye los síntomas de abstinencia. (8.3)

English

night-light. Small lamp, often attached directly to an electrical outlet, that provides dim light during the night. (3.3)

noncommunicable diseases. Medical conditions that cannot be spread through person-to-person contact, but develop as a result of heredity, environment, and lifestyle factors; also known as *noninfectious diseases*. (11.4)

nonverbal communication. Sending of messages through facial expressions, body language, gestures, tone and volume of voice, and other signals that do not involve the content of words. (14.1)

nutrient-dense foods. Foods that are rich in needed nutrients and have little or no solid fats, added sugars, refined starches, and sodium. (6.2)

nutrients. Chemical substances that give your body what it needs to grow and function properly. (6.1)

O

obesity. Having a considerable excess of body weight from fat. (6.3)

obstetrician/gynecologist (OB/GYN). Type of doctor who specializes in pregnancy, labor, and delivery. (16.1)

older adulthood. Stage of human development that begins at 65 years of age. (16.4)

opportunistic infections. Conditions that occur when pathogens take advantage of a weakened body; the cause of death in HIV/AIDS cases. (11.3)

optimism. Ability to keep a positive outlook and focus on the good aspects of stressful situations. (4.2)

organ. Collection of tissues that perform a specific job. (17.1)

orthodontist. Dental specialist who prevents and corrects teeth misalignments. (2.2)

Español

luz de noche. Lamparilla, a menudo unido directamente a una toma de corriente, que provee luz débil durante la noche. (3.3)

enfermedades no transmisibles. Condiciones médicas que no puedan propagar mientras contacto persona a persona, pero contraigan como resultado de la herencia, la ambiente, y factores del estilo de vida; también conocido como *enfermedades no infecciosas*. (11.4)

comunicación no verbal. Envió de mensajes mientras expresiones del rostro, lenguaje corporal, gestos, tono y volumen de voz, y otras señales que no involucran el contenido de las palabras. (14.1)

alimentos ricos en nutrientes. Alimentos que son ricos en nutrientes necesarias y tienen pequeño o no grasas sólidas, azucares agregadas, almidones refinados, y sodio. (6.2)

nutrientes. Sustancias químicas que le dan al cuerpo lo que necesita para crecer y funcionar correctamente. (6.1)

obesidad. Teniendo un exceso considerable de peso corporal de grasa. (6.3)

obstetra/ginecólogo. Tipo de médico que se especializa en el embarazo, el parto, y el alumbramiento. (16.1)

adultez más vieja. Etapa de desarrollo humano que comienza a 65 años de edad. (16.4)

infecciones oportunistas. Condiciones que ocurran cuando agentes patógenos se aprovecha de un cuerpo debilitado; causa de la muerte en casos de VIH/SIDA. (11.3)

optimismo. Capacidad de mantener una actitud positiva y concentrarse en los aspectos buenos de situaciones estresantes. (4.2)

órgano. Colección de tejidos que realiza un trabajo específico. (17.1)

ortodoncista. Especialista dental quien previene y corrige las desalineaciones de los dientes. (2.2)

English

outpatient treatment program. Provides drug education or counseling without requiring a hospital stay. (10.3)

overdose. Taking too much of a medication; often causes dangerous, life-threatening consequences. (10.1)

overnutrition. Condition that results from people eating too many foods that contain high amounts of added sugar, solid fat, sodium, refined carbohydrates, or too many calories. (6.2)

over-the-counter (OTC) medications. Medicines people can purchase without a doctor's written order or prescription to treat the symptoms of many minor health conditions. (10.1)

overweight. Having excess body weight from fat. (6.3)

ovulation. Release of an egg from one of the follicles into the uterus. (16.1)

ozone. Gas made up of oxygen that naturally exists high above Earth's atmosphere. (13.1)

P

pancreas. Fish-shaped organ behind the stomach that makes many kinds of enzymes needed for digestion. (17.3)

parasomnia. Term for sleep disorders that occur when people are partially, but not completely, awoken from sleep. (3.2)

passion. Powerful feeling based on physical attraction. (14.4)

pathogens. Microorganisms that cause communicable diseases. (11.1)

pedestrians. People walking, running, or bicycling along a road. (12.2)

peer abuse. Violent mistreatment of one peer by another. (15.1)

peer mediation. Process in which specially trained students work with other students to resolve conflicts. (14.1)

peer pressure. Influence that people your age have on your actions. (8.2)

Español

programa de tratamiento ambulatorio. Provee educación o terapia sobre las drogas sin requiere una estancia hospitalaria. (10.3)

sobredosis. Tomando demasiado mucho de una medicina; a menudo causa consecuencias peligrosas y fatales. (10.1)

sobrealimentación. Condición que resulta de personas comer demasiados alimentos que contienen cantidades altas de azúcar agregada, grasa sólida, sodio, carbohidratos refinados, o demasiado calorías. (6.2)

medicinas sin receta. Medicinas que personas puedan comprar sin un orden escrito del doctor o una receta para tratar los síntomas de muchas condiciones minores de la salud. (10.1)

con sobrepeso. Teniendo un exceso de peso corporal de grasa. (6.3)

ovulación. Liberación de un óvulo de uno de los folículos en el útero. (16.1)

ozono. Gas hecho de oxígeno que naturalmente existe alto sobre la atmosfera de la Tierra. (13.1)

páncreas. Órgano con forma de pescado detrás del estómago que hace muchos tipos de enzimas necesarias para la digestión. (17.3)

parasomnia. Término para trastornos del sueño que ocurren cuando la gente está parcialmente, pero no completamente, despierto del sueño. (3.2)

pasión. Sentimiento fuerte basado en atracción física. (14.4)

agentes patógenos. Microorganismos que causan enfermedades transmisibles. (11.1)

peatones. Personas caminando, corriendo, o yendo en bicicleta por la calle. (12.2)

abuso de pares. Maltrato violento de un par por un otro. (15.1)

mediación entre pares. Proceso en que estudiantes especialmente entrenados trabajan con otros estudiantes a resolver los conflictos. (14.1)

presión social. Influencia que la gente a su edad tiene sobre sus acciones. (8.2)

English

peers. People who are similar in age to one another. (1.2)

periodontitis. Infection caused by bacteria getting under the gum tissue and destroying the gums and bone. (2.2)

physical abuse. Any act that causes physical harm to a person; may involve hitting, kicking, choking, slapping, or burning. (15.2)

physical activity. Broad term that describes structured exercise as well as other activities that use energy. (7.1)

Physical Activity Guidelines for Americans. Resource health professionals use to provide guidance on how people can improve their health through physical activities. (7.1)

physical environment. Places where a person spends his or her time, such as school, home, or workplace; the region in which a person lives; the air a person breathes; and the water a person drinks. (1.2)

physical health. Aspect of health that refers to how well a person's body functions. (1.1)

pituitary gland. Master gland of the body, which releases hormones to control other endocrine organs. (17.4)

plaque. Sticky, colorless film that coats the teeth and dissolves their protective enamel surface. (2.2)

plasma. Watery part of blood. (17.2)

poisonous. Able to cause illness or death upon entering the body. (12.1)

pollutants. Substances that contaminate the environment and can harm people. (13.1)

precautions. Actions you take to prevent something bad from happening. (12.1)

prenatal development. Period of growth that occurs from conception to birth. (16.1)

presbyopia. Condition beginning in middle age in which the lens of the eye loses its elasticity and it becomes harder to see close objects clearly. (2.2)

Español

pares. Personas quienes son similares en edad al otro. (1.2)

periodontitis. Infección debido a bacterias metiendo debajo del tejido de las encías y destruyendo las encías y el hueso. (2.2)

abuso físico. Cualquier acción que causa daño físico a una persona; puede implicar golpear, patear, ahogar, abofetear, o quemar. (15.2)

actividad física. Termino general que describe el ejercicio estructurado, así como otras actividades que utilizan energía. (7.1)

Directrices de Actividad Física para los Americanos. Recurso que profesionales de salud utilizan para proveer guía en como personas pueden mejorar sus saludes mientras actividades físicas. (7.1)

alrededores. Sitios donde una persona pasa su tiempo, tal como la escuela, la casa, o el lugar de trabajo; la región en que una persona vive; el aire una persona respira; y el agua una persona bebe. (1.2)

salud física. Aspecto de salud que refiere a como bien el cuerpo de una persona funciona. (1.1)

glándula pituitaria. Glándula maestra del cuerpo, que emite hormonas para controlar otros órganos endocrinos. (17.4)

placa. Capa pegajosa, incolora que cubre los dientes y disuelve su superficie de esmalte. (2.2)

plasma. Parte acuoso de la sangre. (17.2)

venenoso. Capaz de causar una dolencia o la muerte al entrar en el cuerpo. (12.1)

contaminantes. Sustancias que contaminan el ambiente y puede dañarse a las personas. (13.1)

precauciones. Acciones se toma para prevenir algo malo suceda. (12.1)

desarrollo prenatal. Período de crecimiento que ocurre desde la concepción hasta el nacimiento. (16.1)

presbicia. Condición que empieza en la media edad en que la lente del ojo se pierde su elasticidad y se vuelve más difícil ver los objetos cercas con claridad. (2.2)

English

prescription medications. Medicines that people can only purchase with a doctor's written order for the treatment of a specific illness or condition. (10.1)

preventive healthcare. Going to the doctor when you are well to help you stay healthy; involves getting an annual physical exam, regular checkups, and screenings for conditions like hearing or vision loss. (1.1)

primary care physician. Regular doctor who provides checkups, screenings, treatments, and prescriptions. (1.1)

progressive muscle relaxation. Strategy of tensing and then relaxing each part of your body and breathing deeply to relieve stress. (4.3)

protein. Nutrient the body uses to build and maintain all of its cells and tissues. (6.1)

puberty. Stage of life when the body reaches sexual maturity. (16.3)

public service announcement (PSA). Message that is shown in the media to support public health. (10.3)

pulse. Person's heart rate. (7.4)

R

recycling. Process in which used materials are turned into new products. (13.2)

refusal skills. Strategies you can use to stand up to pressures and influences that want you to engage in unhealthy behaviors. (1.3)

rehabilitation program. Treatment for drug addiction that may involve detoxification, medications, or time spent in a rehabilitation facility. (10.3)

relapse. Occurrence when a person takes a drug again after deciding to stop. (10.3)

Español

medicamentos recetados. Medicinas que personas solamente puedan comprar con un orden escrito del doctor para el tratamiento de una dolencia o condición especifica. (10.1)

cuidados saludes preventivos. Ir al médico cuando está bien para ayudarse mantiene la salud; consiste en recibiendo un examen físico anual, chequeos regulares, y proyecciones para condiciones como la pérdida de audición o visión. (1.1)

médico de atención primaria. Médico de cabecera que ofrece chequeos, proyecciones, tratamientos, y recetas. (1.1)

relajación muscular progresiva. Estrategia de tensar y luego relajar cada parte de su cuerpo y respirar profundamente para aliviar el estrés. (4.3)

proteína. Un nutriente que el cuerpo utiliza para construir y mantener todo tipo de células y tejidos. (6.1)

pubertad. Etapa de la vida cuando el cuerpo alcanza la madurez sexual. (16.3)

anuncio de servicio público. Mensaje que se muestra en la media para apoyar la salud pública. (10.3)

pulso. Latido del corazón de una persona. (7.4)

reciclaje. Proceso en que materiales usados se conviertan en productos nuevos. (13.2)

habilidades de rechazo. Estrategias puede utilizar para enfrentarse a presiones e influencias que quieren envolverse en conducta de mala salud. (1.3)

programa de rehabilitación. Tratamiento para drogadicción que pueda involucrar la desintoxicación, medicinas, o tiempo pasado en un centro de rehabilitación. (10.3)

relapso. Incidencia cuando una persona toma una droga de nuevo después de decidirse a parar. (10.3)

English

REM sleep. Active stage of sleep during which your breathing changes, your heart rate and blood pressure rise, and your eyes dart around rapidly. (3.1)

renewable energy. Type of energy that cannot be used up, such as wind, water, or solar power. (13.2)

reproductive system. Body system that consists of a group of organs working together to make the creation of new life possible. (16.1)

residential treatment program. Plan for helping people get through the early stages of breaking an addiction in an inpatient environment with lots of support and few distractions. (10.3)

resilience. Ability to bounce back from traumatic or stressful events. (4.2)

resistance. Opposition. (7.2)

respiration. Exchange of oxygen and carbon dioxide between the body and the air around it. (17.2)

respiratory etiquette. Practice of covering your mouth and nose with a tissue while coughing or sneezing, or sneezing into your sleeve. (11.5)

respiratory system. Body system of organs that obtain vitally important oxygen from the outside world. (17.2)

response substitution. Smoking cessation technique that involves responding to difficult feelings and situations with behaviors other than smoking. (8.3)

risk factors. Aspects of people's lives that increase the chances that they will develop a disease or disorder. (1.2)

rituals. Series of actions performed as part of a ceremony. (14.2)

S

sandwich generation. Adults who care for their parents as well as their own children. (16.4)

Español

sueño REM. Etapa activa de sueño mientras que su respiración cambie, su ritmo cardiaco y presión sanguínea suben, y sus ojos lanzan rápidamente por todo. (3.1)

energía renovable. Tipo de energía que no puede ser agotado, como tal la energía eólica, del agua, y solar. (13.2)

sistema reproductivo. Sistema corporal que consiste en un grupo de órganos trabajando juntos para hacer posible la creación de una vida nueva. (16.1)

programa de tratamiento residencial. Plan para ayudar a personas a superar las primeras etapas de romper una adicción en un ambiente hospitalario con mucho apoyo y pocas distracciones. (10.3)

resistencia. Capacidad de recuperarse de eventos traumáticos o estresantes. (4.2)

resistencia. Oposición. (7.2)

respiración. Intercambio del oxígeno y el dióxido de carbono entre el cuerpo y el aire alrededor de ello. (17.2)

etiqueta respiratoria. Práctica de cubrir su boca y nariz con un pañuelo mientras tose o estornuda, o estornuda en su manga. (11.5)

sistema respiratorio. Sistema corporal de órganos que obtienen oxígeno de la vital importancia del mundo exterior. (17.2)

sustitución de respuesta. Técnica de dejar de fumar que consiste en contestando a sentimientos y situaciones difíciles con comportamientos aparte de fumar. (8.3)

factores de riesgo. Aspectos de las vidas de personas que aumentan las oportunidades que desarrollarán una enfermedad o trastorno. (1.2)

rituales. Serie de acciones realizan como parte de una ceremonia. (14.2)

generación de sándwiches. Adultos que cuidan a sus padres además de sus propios hijos. (16.4)

English

saturated fats. Type of fat found mainly in animal-based foods, such as meat and dairy products. (6.1)

schizophrenia. Condition identified by irregular thoughts and delusions, hearing voices, and seeing things that are not there. (5.1)

school violence. Any violent behavior that occurs on school property, at school-sponsored events, or on the way to or from school or to or from school events. (15.3)

secondhand smoke. Tobacco smoke released into the environment by smokers, which other people nearby inhale. (8.1)

sedentary. Inactive. (7.1)

self-esteem. How you feel about yourself. (4.1)

self-image. Your mental picture of yourself, which includes how you look, how you act, your skills and abilities, and your weaknesses; also called *self-concept*. (4.1)

sets. Anaerobic exercises done in groups of repetitions followed by rest. (7.4)

sexual abuse. Any sexual activity to which one person does not or cannot consent. (15.2)

sexually transmitted infections (STIs). Communicable diseases spread from one person to another during sexual activity. (11.2)

short sleepers. People who can function well on less sleep than other people. (3.1)

sibling abuse. Violent mistreatment of one sibling by another. (15.2)

sibling rivalry. Competition with a brother or sister. (14.2)

side effect. Unpleasant and unwanted symptom that occurs from taking a medication. (10.1)

skeletal system. Body system made up of 206 bones that provides structure, shape, and protection to the body. (17.1)

skill-related fitness. Type of fitness that improves a person's performance in a particular sport. (7.2)

Español

grasas saturadas. Tipo de grasa se encuentra principalmente en alimentos de origen animal, tal como carne y productos lácteos. (6.1)

esquizofrenia. Condición identifica por pensamientos irregulares y delirios, escuchando voces, y viendo cosas que no están presentes. (5.1)

violencia escolar. Cualquier comportamiento violento que ocurre en la propiedad escolar, en eventos patrocinadas por la escuela, o de camino a o de escuela o de eventos escolares. (15.3)

humo de segunda mano. Humo de tabaco liberado en el ambiente por fumadores, que otras personas ciertas inhalan. (8.1)

sedentario. Inactivo. (7.1)

autoestima. Como se siente sobre sí mismo. (4.1)

imagen de sí mismo. Su imagen mental de usted mismo, que incluye como se ve, como se comporta, sus habilidades y talentos, y sus debilidades; también llamado *concepto de sí mismo*. (4.1)

series. Ejercicios anaeróbicos hecho en grupos de repeticiones antes de reposo. (7.4)

abuso sexual. Cualquier actividad sexual cuál una persona no consiente o no puede consentir. (15.2)

infecciones de transmisión sexual (ITS). Enfermedades transmisibles propagada de una persona a otro durante la actividad sexual. (11.2)

personas que duermes poco. Personas quienes pueden funcionar bien con dormir menos que otros. (3.1)

abuso de hermano. Maltrato violento de un hermano por un otro. (15.2)

rivalidad entre hermanos. Competencia con un hermano o una hermana. (14.2)

efecto secundario. Síntoma desagradable y no deseado que resulta de tomar medicina. (10.1)

sistema esquelético. Sistema corporal hecho de 206 huesos que proviene estructura, forma, y protección al cuerpo. (17.1)

condición física relacionada a la habilidad. Tipo de gimnasia que mejora el rendimiento de una persona en un deporte en particular. (7.2)

English

skills-training program. Plan that teaches people skills for dealing with peer pressure and for handling stressful life events without relying on drugs. (10.3)

sleep apnea. Potentially serious disorder in which a person stops breathing for short periods of time during sleep. (3.2)

sleep deficit. Condition that occurs when people frequently get less sleep than they should. (3.1)

sleep deprived. Term used to describe a person who gets inadequate amounts of sleep. (3.1)

sleep-wake cycle. Pattern of sleeping in a 24-hour period. (3.1)

sleep-wake schedule. Routine for going to bed at about the same time each night and getting up at about the same time each morning. (3.3)

SMART goals. Plan of action that is specific, measurable, achievable, relevant, and timely. (1.3)

smog. Fog that has mixed with smoke and chemical fumes. (13.1)

smoking cessation. Quitting smoking. (8.3)

sober living communities. Alcohol- and drug-free living environments that reduce some of the temptation and pressure people may feel to use alcohol and drugs. (10.3)

social environment. People with whom a person interacts, such as family members, friends, peers, teachers, coaches, neighbors, and coworkers. (1.2)

social health. Aspect of health that involves interacting and getting along with others in positive, healthy ways. (1.1)

socialize. Teaching children to behave in socially acceptable ways. (14.2)

spinal cord. Part of the nervous system that carries nerve signals between the brain and the body. (17.4)

spleen. Organ filled with white blood cells; filters blood. (17.3)

Español

programa de capacitación de habilidades. Plan que aprenda a personas las habilidades para lidiar con presión social y para manejar eventos estresantes de vida sin depender de las drogas. (10.3)

apnea del sueño. Trastorno potencialmente grave en que una persona deja de respirar por periodos breves durante el sueño. (3.2)

déficit de sueño. Condición que ocurre cuando la gente frecuentemente recibe menos sueño que deben. (3.1)

con falta de sueño. Término usado por describir una persona que recibe cantidades deficientes del sueño. (3.1)

ciclo sueño-vigilia. Patrón de sueño en un periodo de 24 horas. (3.1)

plan de sueño-vigilia. Rutina para dormirse casi al mismo tiempo cada noche y despertarse casi al mismo tiempo cada mañana. (3.3)

metas SMART. Plan de acción que es específico, medible, pertinente, y oportuno. (1.3)

smog. Niebla que se ha mezclado con humo y vapores químicos. (13.1)

dejar de fumar. Dejando de fumar. (8.3)

comunidades de vida sobria. Ambientes libres de alcohol y drogas que reduzcan un poco de la tentación y presión personas pueden sentir a utilizar alcohol y drogas. (10.3)

entorno social. Personas con quien alguien interactúa, tal como familiares, amigos, pares, maestros, entrenadores, vecinos, y compañeros. (1.2)

salud social. Aspecto de salud que consiste en interactuando y llevando bien con otras personas en maneras positivas y sanas. (1.1)

socializar. Enseñar a los niños comportarse en maneras socialmente aceptables. (14.2)

médula espinal. Parte del sistema nervioso que lleva señales nerviosas entre el cerebro y el cuerpo. (17.4)

bazo. Órgano lleno de glóbulos blancos; filtra sangre. (17.3)

English

sprain. Common sports injury involving the stretching or tearing of ligaments (tissues that hold joints together). (7.3)

standard precautions. Infection control practices that apply when giving first aid to any person under any circumstances. (12.3)

stereotypes. Oversimplified ideas about a group of people. (14.3)

stigma. Mark of shame or embarrassment that is usually unfair. (5.2)

stimulus control. Smoking cessation technique that involves avoiding tempting situations and managing feelings that lead to nicotine use. (8.3)

strangers. People whom you do not know. (12.2)

stress. Physical, mental, and emotional reactions of your body to the challenges you face. (4.3)

stressor. Any factor that causes stress. (4.3)

stroke. Medical emergency in which blood flow to part of the brain is interrupted, injuring or killing brain cells. (11.4)

suicide. Act of taking one's own life. (5.3)

suicide clusters. Series of suicides in a particular community that occur in a relatively short period of time. (5.3)

suicide contagion. Term that describes the copying of suicide attempts after exposure to another person's suicide. (5.3)

support groups. Gatherings in which a therapist meets with a group of people who share a common problem. (5.2)

survivors. People who lose a loved one to suicide. (5.3)

sustainability. Actions that maintain the natural resources in the environment. (13.2)

Español

esguince. Herida de deportes común que consiste en el estirando o desgarrando de los ligamentos (tejidos que integran juntos las articulaciones). (7.3)

precauciones estándares. Prácticas de control de infecciones que aplican cuando se dé primeros auxilios a cualquier persona bajo cualquier circunstancia. (12.3)

estereotipos. Ideas demasiadas simplificadas sobre un grupo de personas. (14.3)

estigma. Marca de desgracia o vergüenza que es generalmente injusto. (5.2)

control de estímulos. Técnica de dejar de fumar que consiste en evitar situaciones tentadoras y manejar sentimientos que provocar al uso de la nicotina. (8.3)

desconocidos. Personas a las que no conoce. (12.2)

estrés. Reacciones físicas, mentales, y emocionales de su cuerpo a los retos que se enfrenta. (4.3)

estresor. Cualquier factor que causa el estrés. (4.3)

derrame cerebral. Emergencia medical en que el flujo sanguíneo a parte del cerebro se interrumpe, hiriendo o matando las células cerebrales. (11.4)

suicidio. La acción de quitarse la vida a sí mismo. (5.3)

grupos de suicidios. Series de suicidios en una comunidad particular que ocurren en un periodo de tiempo relativamente corto. (5.3)

contagio de suicidio. Termino que describe la copia de intentos de suicidio después de exposición al suicidio de otra persona. (5.3)

grupos de apoyo. Reuniones en que una terapeuta encuentra con un grupo de personas quienes comparten un problema común. (5.2)

sobrevivientes. Personas que pierden un ser querido por suicidio. (5.3)

sostenibilidad. Acciones que mantienen los recursos naturales en el ambiente. (13.2)

English

syphilis. Bacterial infection divided into stages that causes extremely serious health problems and disability. (11.2)

T

tar. Residue produced by burning tobacco; consists of small, thick, sticky particles. (8.1)

target heart rate. Heart rate to aim for while performing aerobic exercise to get the best results from a workout; varies by age. (7.4)

temper tantrum. Toddler's episode of emotional upset that often includes yelling, crying, hitting, kicking, or even biting. (16.2)

tendons. Structures made of tough tissue that connect muscle to bone. (17.1)

terrorism. Use of violence and threats to frighten and control groups of people to further an ideological aim. (15.3)

testosterone. Hormone that triggers growth and development of the male sex organs. (16.3)

therapist. Professional who diagnoses and treats people with mental health conditions. (5.2)

thyroid hormone. Substance produced in the thyroid that increases the rate at which the body uses energy. (17.4)

tinnitus. Pain or ringing in the ears after exposure to excessively loud sounds. (2.2)

tissue. Collection of similar cells that do a certain job for the body. (17.1)

tobacco. Plant used to create tobacco-related products, such as cigarettes and chewing tobacco. (8.1)

tolerance. Effect that occurs when the body needs more and more of a substance to experience the desired effects. (8.2)

tonsillitis. Bacterial or viral infection that affects the tonsils. (11.1)

Español

sífilis. Infección bacteriana se divide en etapas que causa problemas de salud extremadamente grave y discapacidad. (11.2)

alquitrán. Residuo producido por la combustión del tabaco; consiste en partículas pequeñas, espesas, y pegajosas. (8.1)

meta de ritmo cardíaco. La frecuencia cardíaca deseada para el desempeño de ejercicio aeróbico que conduce a los resultados mejores de un entrenamiento; varía según la edad. (7.4)

rabieta. Episodio de un niño pequeño de trastorno emocional que a menudo incluye gritar, llorar, golpear, patear, o aún morder. (16.2)

tendones. Estructuras hechas de tejido duro que conectan musculo al hueso. (17.1)

terrorismo. Uso de violencia y amenazas para asustar y controlar grupas de personas para promover un objetivo ideológico. (15.3)

testosterona. Hormona que provoque el crecimiento y desarrollo de los órganos sexuales masculinos. (16.3)

terapeuta. Profesional que diagnostica y trata las personas con condiciones de salud mental. (5.2)

hormona tiroidea. Sustancia producida en la glándula tiroidea que aumenta la tasa a la que el cuerpo usa la energía. (17.4)

tinnitus. Dolor o acúfeno en las orejas después de exposición a sonidos excesivamente ruidosos. (2.2)

tejido. Colección de las células similares que hacen un trabajo similar para el cuerpo. (17.1)

tabaco. Planta utilizada para crear productos relatados al tabaco, tal como cigarrillos y tabaco de mascar. (8.1)

tolerancia. Consecuencia que ocurre cuando el cuerpo necesita más y más de una sustancia para experimenta los efectos deseados. (8.2)

amigdalitis. Infección bacteriana o vírica que afecta las amígdalas. (11.1)

English

toxic. Poisonous. (8.1)

traditions. Specific patterns of behavior passed down in a culture. (14.2)

trans fats. Type of fat found in food from animals, such as cows and goats; used to be found in many processed foods, such as packaged cookies and chips. (6.1)

trichomoniasis. Curable infection caused by protozoa that is more common among young women than men. (11.2)

triggers. Reminders that cause people to feel a strong desire for a substance. (8.2)

tryptophan. Substance that helps the body make chemicals that help you sleep. (3.3)

tumor. Mass of abnormal cells. (11.4)

U

undernutrition. Condition that results from people not receiving all the nutrients they need from the foods they eat. (6.2)

underweight. Having less body fat than what is considered healthy. (6.3)

unsaturated fats. Type of fat found in plant-based foods, such as vegetable oils, some peanut butters and margarines, olives, salad dressing, nuts, and seeds. (6.1)

urinary system. Body system that removes liquid waste from the body. (17.3)

V

vaccine. Substance that contains a dead or nontoxic part of a pathogen that is injected into a person to train his or her immune system to eliminate the live pathogen. (11.5)

veins. Blood vessels that carry oxygen-poor blood. (17.2)

Español

tóxico. Venenoso. (8.1)

tradiciones. Patrones específicos de comportamiento transmitido en una cultura. (14.2)

grasas trans. Tipo de grasa se encuentra en alimentos de origen animal, tal como vacas y cabras; solía ser encuentra en muchas comidas precocinadas, tal como galletas y papas fritas empacados. (6.1)

tricomoniasis. Infección curable causada por protozoos que es más común entre mujeres jóvenes que en hombres. (11.2)

desencadenantes. Recuerdos que causan a personas sentirse un deseo fuerte para una sustancia. (8.2)

triptófano. Sustancia que ayuda al cuerpo producir los químicos que ayudan dormirse. (3.3)

tumor. Masa de células anormales. (11.4)

desnutrición. Condición que resulta de personas no recibir todas las nutrientes necesarias de los alimentos que comen. (6.2)

bajo peso. Teniendo menos grasa corporal que es considerada saludable. (6.3)

grasas insaturadas. Tipo de grasa se encuentra en alimentos de origen vegetal, tal como aceite vegetal, algunas mantequillas de maní y margarina, olivas, arreglos de ensalada, nueces, y pepitas. (6.1)

sistema urinario. Sistema corporal que quita los residuos líquidos del cuerpo. (17.3)

vacuna. Sustancia que contiene un parte muerte o no tóxico de un agente patógeno en una persona para entrenar su sistema inmunológico a eliminar el agente patógeno vivo. (11.5)

venas. Vasos sanguíneos que llevan la sangre pobre en oxígeno. (17.2)

English

verbal communication. Use of words to send a spoken or written message. (14.1)

violent behavior. Intentional use of words or actions that cause or threaten to cause injury to someone or something. (15.1)

virtual friends. People you meet through social media, websites, chat rooms, or gaming. (14.3)

visualization. Strategy of imagining a pleasant environment when faced with stress. (4.3)

vitamins. Substances that come from plants or animals that are necessary for normal growth and development. (6.1)

W

well-being. State of health and wellness in which people generally feel good about their present conditions. (1.1)

wellness. Balance of all aspects of health—physical, mental and emotional, and social. (1.1)

withdrawal. Unpleasant symptoms that occur when someone addicted to a substance tries to stop using that substance. (8.2)

Y

young adulthood. Stage of human development that occurs from 20 to 40 years of age. (16.4)

Z

zero-tolerance policy. Rule that results in punishment of young people caught driving with any level of alcohol in their system. (9.1)

zygote. Egg that has been fertilized by a sperm. (16.1)

Español

comunicación verbal. Uso de las palabras para enviar un mensaje hablado o escrito. (14.1)

comportamiento violento. Uso deliberado de las palabras o acciones que causan o amenazan a causar herida a alguien o algo. (15.1)

amigos virtuales. Personas que conoce mientras la media social, sitios web, salas de chat, o los videojuegos. (14.3)

visualización. Estrategia de imaginarse un ambiente agradable cuando se enfrenta con el estrés. (4.3)

vitaminas. Sustancias de origen vegetal o animal que se necesita para crecimiento y desarrollo normal. (6.1)

bienestar. Estado de salud y bienestar en el que personas generalmente se sienten bien sobre sus condiciones presentes. (1.1)

bienestar. Equilibrio de todos los aspectos de salud—físico, mental y emocional, y social. (1.1)

abstinencia. Síntomas desagradables que ocurren cuando alguien adicto a una sustancia trata a dejar usando esa sustancia. (8.2)

adultez joven. Etapa de desarrollo humano que ocurre desde 20 hasta 40 años de edad. (16.4)

política de tolerancia cero. Regla que resulta en el castigo de jóvenes pillado manejando con cualquier nivel de alcohol en sus sistemas. (9.1)

cigoto. Ovulo que ha sido fecundado por un espermatozoide; también llamada *zigoto*. (16.1)

Index

cardiac muscle, 573
cardio. *See* aerobic exercise
cardiopulmonary resuscitation (CPR), 417–418
cartilage, 571
casual dating, 486
C.A.U.T.I.O.N. system for cancer detection, 364
cavities, 53
CD4 cells, 353
cells, 567
central nervous system (CNS), 275, 590
cerebellum, 593
cerebral cortex, 592
cerebrum, 592
chambers, 575
chemicals, 431–434, 437
    Resource Conservation and Recovery Act, 437
    safe use, 433–434
    toxic, 431–433
chemotherapy, 364
child abuse and neglect, 510–512
    effects and health consequences, 510–511
    reporting, 511–512
Childhelp, 511
childhood, 470, 540–543
    early, 540–541
    family educates and socializes children, 470
    middle, 542–543
child sexual abuse, 510
chlamydia, 342–343
choking, 415–416
cholesterol, 163, 166
chromosomes, 16
chronic bronchitis, 246
chronic diseases, 277, 365–366
chronic obstructive pulmonary disease (COPD), 365
    cigarettes, 244, 264. *See also* tobacco use
circadian rhythms, 69
circulation, 576–577
circulatory system, 245, 360–362, 575–578
    blood, 577–578
    blood vessels, 577
    common diseases, 360–362
    heart, 575–576
    tobacco use's effects, 245
cirrhosis, 277
Clean Air Act, 436–437
clean energy. *See* renewable energy
clinical depression, 135
cliques, 481
club drugs, 312
CNS. *See* central nervous system
cocaine, 309–310
cochlea, 59, 595
cocktail of drugs, 356
cold sores, 54
collaborate, 24

collagen, 40, 571
color blindness, 57
combustion triangle, 388
communicable diseases, 335–340, 342–348, 371–376
    common, 338–340
    methods of transmission, 337–338
    pathogens, 335–337
    preventing, 371–376
    sexually transmitted infections (STIs), 342–348
    treating, 340
communication, 30–32, 458–463
    nonverbal, 459, 463
    process, 458
    skills, 30–32
    verbal, 458
    ways to be effective, 459–463
communication process, 458
communication skills, 30–32
community, 398–406, 471
complex carbohydrates, 162
composting, 445
compromise, 26, 466
concussion, 226
condoms, 348
cones, 57
conflict management. *See* conflict resolution
conflict resolution, 25–26, 464–467
conflict resolution skills, 26, 465–467
conflicts, 464
conjunctivitis, 339–340
consent, obtaining before giving first aid, 410
constrict, 245
contaminants, 182
cooldowns, 234
coordination, 220
COPD (chronic obstructive pulmonary disease), 365
cornea, 56, 594
coronary arteries, 577
cortisol, 596
CPR (cardiopulmonary resuscitation), 417–418
crack cocaine (crack), 309
cramps, 533
crystal meth, 310
culture, 20
cuts, 411–412
cyberbullying, 502–504
    impact, 502
    responding to, 504
    spotting different forms, 503
cycle of abuse, 513–514

D

dairy group, 173
dandruff, 47
date rape drugs, 312

dating, 486–490
    abstinence during, 487–488
    characteristics of healthy relationships, 486–487
    end of a relationship, 489–490
    forming a healthy relationship, 488
    physical intimacy, 487–488
dating relationship, 486
death, 559–560
decibels, 60
decision making, 23–24, 288
decision-making skills, 23
deep breathing, 122
dehydration, 169
delayed sleep phase syndrome (DSPS), 76–77
dental caries. *See* cavities
deodorant, 40
dependence (dependency stage), 256, 274, 282
depressant, 273
depression, 135
dermatitis. *See* eczema
dermatologist, 42
dermis, 40
detoxification, 290
development
    adolescence, 545–550
    adulthood, 554–559
    areas of, 538
    early childhood, 540–541
    influences, 538–539
    middle childhood, 542–543
    prenatal, 534–535
developmental stages. *See* human life cycle
diabetes (diabetes mellitus), 366–368, 380, 598
    reducing risk, 380
    statistics, 367
    type 1, 368
    type 2, 368, 380
diaphragm, 580
dietary fiber, 163
Dietary Guidelines for Americans, 171–172
dietary supplements, 196
diets. *See* fad diets; weight management
digestion, 582
digestive system, 582–585
direct transmission, 338
discrimination, protecting HIV-positive individuals
    from, 355
diseases
    chronic, 246, 277, 365–366
    communicable, 335–340
    noncommunicable, 358–369
    preventing and reducing risk, 371–380
    sexually transmitted infections (STIs), 342–348
dislocation, 226
disposal of hazardous substances, 440
distraction strategies, 121

diversity, 477
DNA, 16
domestic violence, 509–510
dosage, 300
dose, 300
dreaming, 71–72
drinking. *See* alcohol use; underage drinking
driving under the influence (DUI), 280
driving while intoxicated (DWI), 280
drug abuse
    definition, 315
    education campaigns, 319–320, 322
    health and life consequences, 315–316
    preventing, 319–320, 322–323
    treating, 323–325
    See also illegal drugs
drug addiction, 317, 319–320, 322–326
    advocating for a drug-free life, 322
    definition, 317
    education campaigns, 319–320, 322
    helping someone who is addicted, 325–326
    preventing, 319–320, 322–323
    treating, 323–325
drug interactions, 302
drugs, 299. *See also* drug abuse; drug addiction;
    illegal drugs
drunk, 275
drunk driving, 280
drying out. *See* detoxification
DSPS (delayed sleep phase syndrome), 76–77
DUI (driving under the influence), 280
dust mites, 427
DWI (driving while intoxicated), 280
dysentery, 337

E

ear canal. *See* auditory canal
eardrum, 59, 594–595
early childhood, 540–541
ears, 58–60, 594–595
    common problems, 60
    parts and functions, 59, 594–595
    protecting, 60
Earth Day, 438
eating disorders, 198–202
    anorexia nervosa, 198–199
    binge-eating disorder, 200
    bulimia nervosa, 199–200
    prevalence, 201
    prevention, 200, 202
    seeking professional help, 202
    treatment, 202
eating plan, 171–182
    breakfast's importance, 178
    calories, 179–180

family relationships, 469–475
    common problems, 472–473
    coping with changes, 475
    functions unique to families, 469–470
    maintaining, 472–474
    parents or guardians, 471–473
    rules, 472–473
    siblings, 473–474
Family Smoking Prevention and Tobacco Control Act, 262–263
family therapy, 141
farsightedness, 58
FASD (fetal alcohol spectrum disorder), 277
fasting, 192
fats, 165–166
fat-soluble vitamins, 167
FDA, 166, 262
feedback, 458
feelings. *See* emotions
female reproductive system, 532–533
fertilization, 533
fetal alcohol spectrum disorder (FASD), 277
fetal stage, 535
fetus, 249, 535
fever blisters. *See* cold sores
fight-or-flight response, 118
fine-motor skills, 541
fire prevention and safety, 388–391
    escape plan, 390–391
    fire triangle, 388
    inspection checklist, 390
fire triangle, 388
first aid, 408–418
    cardiopulmonary resuscitation (CPR), 417–418
    choking victims, 415–416
    determining if you can help, 410
    kit, 408
    medical emergencies, 414–418
    obtaining consent, 410
    treating common injuries, 411–414
first-aid kit, 408
fitness
    definition, 209
    health-related, 215–219
    personal plan, 228–234
    physical activity, 210–213
    safety precautions, 222–225
    skill-related, 218–220
    SMART goals, 229
    treating injuries, 225–226
fitness safety, 222–225
    drinking water during physical activity, 224
    injury prevention, 222–223
    protective equipment, 222
    weather-related injuries and conditions, 224–225
FITT (frequency, intensity, time, and type), 230–231

five-and-five method, 416
flammable, 388
flashbacks, 134, 311
flexibility, 217
flu. *See* influenza
follicle, 532
food
    breakfast's importance, 178
    calories, 172, 179–180
    choices, 177–182
    groups, 172–174
    nutrient-dense, 171, 178
    nutrition information, 178–179
    preparation methods, 182
    recommended amounts, 175
    reducing waste, 443
    safety, 182
    sanitation, 374
food groups, 172–174
food safety, 182
food sanitation, 374
fossil fuels, 439
foster care, 512
fracture, 226
frequency, intensity, time, and type (FITT), 230–231
friendships, 477–484
    building and maintaining, 478–479
    changes over time affect, 482–483
    common problems, 481–482
    gossip and rumors can impact, 480
    peer pressure, 483–484
frontal lobe, 592
frostbite, 225
fruits group, 172
fungi, 336–337

G

gaining weight, 193
gallbladder, 583
gangs, 518
gang violence, 518–519
generalized anxiety disorder, 132
genes, 16
genetic risk factors, 16, 18
genital herpes, 345
germinal stage, 534
germs. *See* pathogens
GHB, 312
gingivitis, 53
glands, 567
glucagon, 597
glucose, 163, 366
goals, 24, 55, 188–190, 229–231
gonorrhea, 343
gossip, 480, 499

grains group, 172
gratitude, 112–113
gray matter, 592
green living, 441–446
    away from home, 445–446
    energy conservation, 442–443
    planting trees, 445
    product choices, 443
    reducing food waste, 443
    transportation choices, 446
green products, 443
grief, 152, 559–560
grinding of teeth, 54, 80–81
gross-motor skills, 541
group dating, 488
guardians, 471–473
gum disease, 53
gums, 53
guns. *See* weapons safety

H

hackers, 401
hair, 42, 47–48, 569
hair cells, 595
hair follicles, 40, 569
halitosis. *See* bad breath
hallucinations, 310
hallucinogens, 310–311
Hands-Only™ CPR, 417
hand washing, 372–374
hangover, 276
harassment, 499
hate crimes, 520
hay fever, 366
hazing, 499
health, 7–13, 15–21, 23–32
    advocating for self, family, and community,
        30–32
    aspects, 7–8
    differs from wellness, 7
    healthcare's role, 10–13
    improving through lifestyle choices, 15
    mental and emotional, 8–9
    physical, 8
    risk factors, 16–21
    skills and resources for maintaining, 23–32
    social, 8
    well-being, 8, 10
health and wellness continuum, 15
healthcare, 10–13
    insurance, 12–13
    preventive, 10
    services, 11–12
    settings, 12
health insurance, 12–13

*Health Insurance Portability and Accountability Act
    (HIPAA)*, 354
health literacy, 26–29, 42
    evaluating claims, 28–29, 42
    locating reliable information, 27–28
health maintenance organization (HMO), 12
health-related fitness, 215–219, 228
    body composition, 217–218
    checking your level, 228
    endurance, 216–217
    flexibility, 217
    heart and lung strength, 215–216
    muscle strength, 216
hearing, 60, 434
heart, 215–216, 245, 575–576
heart attack, 361
heart disease, 360–362, 377–378
heart rate, 233
heavy drinking, 274
Heimlich maneuver, 416
hemorrhoids, 164
heredity, 359
heroin, 311–312
herpes, 345
HHS (United States Department of Health and
    Human Services), 171
high, 307
high self-esteem, 102, 104
*HIPAA (Health Insurance Portability and
    Accountability Act)*, 354
HIV, 351–356
    confidentiality of test results, 354
    preventing and treating, 355–356
    protecting HIV-positive individuals from
        discrimination, 355
    signs and symptoms of infection, 352–353
    testing, 354–355
    transmission, 352
hives, 413
HIV-positive, 351, 355
HMO (health maintenance organization), 12
homicide, 520
hormones, 595
hospice care, 559
HPV (human papillomavirus), 345–346
huffing. *See* inhalants
human body. *See* body systems; development;
    human life cycle
human immunodeficiency virus. *See* HIV
human life cycle, 537
    adolescence, 545–552
    adulthood, 554–559
    death, 559–560
    definition, 537
    early childhood, 540–541
    middle childhood, 542–543

microorganisms, 335
middle adulthood, 556–557
middle childhood, 542–543
middle ear, 595
milestones, 537
mindfulness, 124
minerals, 168–169
miscarriage, 249
moderate drinking, 274
moderate intensity, 232
mononucleosis (mono), 338–339
mood disorders, 134–136
    bipolar disorder, 135
    depression, 135
    self-harm, 135–136
motor neurons, 590
motor vehicle accidents, alcohol use and, 280–281
mouth, 51–56, 80–81, 582–583
    bad breath, 54
    care and hygiene, 54, 56
    cold sores, 54
    digestion process, 582–583
    grinding of teeth, 54, 80–81
    gum disease, 53
    misaligned and impacted teeth, 54
    tooth decay, 53
mucus, 579
muscle endurance, 217
muscles, 216, 572–573
muscular system, 572–573
myopia. *See* nearsightedness
MyPlate food guidance system, 172–176, 178
    food group proportions, 172–174
    nutritional needs during pregnancy, 175
    recommended food amounts, 175

N

nails, 48–49, 569
naps, 84, 86
narcolepsy, 82
Narcotics Anonymous, 325
National Institute on Drug Abuse (NIDA), 320
natural disasters, 392
nearsightedness, 58
needs, 23, 469–470
neglect, 510
negotiation, 26, 465–466
nervous system, 590–595
neurons, 590
nicotine, 243
nicotine addiction, 260
nicotine replacement, 260
NIDA (National Institute on Drug Abuse), 320
night-light, 90
nightmares, 78–79

"night owl" syndrome. *See* delayed sleep phase syndrome
noise pollution, 434
noncommunicable diseases, 358–369
    arthritis, 369
    cancer, 362–364
    diabetes (diabetes mellitus), 366–368
    heart disease, 360–362
    reducing risk, 376–380
    respiratory, 365–366
    risk factors, 359–360
noninfectious diseases. *See* noncommunicable diseases
nonverbal communication, 459, 463
nurse practitioner, 11
nutrient-dense foods, 171, 178
nutrients, 161–169, 175, 178–179
    carbohydrates, 162–163
    fats, 165–166
    minerals, 168–169
    needed for body to function properly, 161–162
    needs during pregnancy, 175
    protein, 164–165
    reliable information sources, 178–179
    vitamins, 166–167
    water, 169
nutrition
    eating plan, 171–182
    needs during pregnancy, 175
    nutrients, 161–169
    reliable information sources, 178–179
Nutrition Facts label, 178–179

O

obesity, 186–188
OB/GYN (obstetrician/gynecologist), 534
obsessive-compulsive disorder (OCD), 134
obstetrician/gynecologist (OB/GYN), 534
obtaining consent, 410
occipital lobe, 592
OCD (obsessive-compulsive disorder), 134
oil glands, 569
oils, 174
older adulthood, 557
online communication, 463
online privacy and safety, 400–401
opioids, 301, 305, 311–312
opportunistic infections, 353
optimal health, 15
optimism, 111, 120
oral health, 51–56
organisms, 335
organs, 531, 567
orthodontist, 54
osteoarthritis, 369
OTC (over-the-counter) medications, 300

outer ear, 594
outpatient facilities, 12
outpatient treatment programs, 324
ova, 532
ovaries, 532, 598
overbite, 54
overdose, 304
overnutrition, 176–177
over-the-counter (OTC) medications, 300
overweight, 186–188
ovulation, 533
ozone, 428

P

PACT (Prevent All Cigarette Trafficking) Act, 262
pancreas, 583, 597–598
panic attacks, 132
panic disorder, 132
paranoia, 137
parasomnia, 77–81
    bed-wetting, 78
    nightmares, 78–79
    restless legs syndrome (RLS), 80
    sleepwalking, 78, 80
    teeth grinding, 80–81
parathyroid glands, 596
parathyroid hormone (PTH), 596
parents, 471–473
parietal lobes, 592
particulate matter, 427
passion, 487
passive communication, 460
pathogens, 335–337
    bacteria, 335–336
    fungi, 336–337
    preventing communicable diseases, 371–376
    protozoa, 337
    viruses, 336
pedestrians, 403–404
peer abuse, 498
peer mediation, 467
peer pressure, 252–253, 287, 314, 483–484, 551
    resisting through refusal skills, 265–266, 289, 322–323, 347
    role-playing exercise, 550
peers, 19, 197, 252, 287, 314, 477–484
    definition, 19
    influence on alcohol use, 287
    influence on body image, 197
    influence on drug use, 314
    influence on tobacco use, 252
    relationships, 477–484
pelvic inflammatory disease (PID), 343
penis, 532
periodontitis (periodontal disease), 53

peripheral nervous system (PNS), 590
personal fitness plan, 228–234
    checking your health-related fitness level, 228
    FITT, 230–231
    setting goals, 229–231
    workouts, 231–234
personal hygiene. *See* hygiene
personality disorders, 136–137
pesticides, 432
pharmacy, 301
phobias, 132, 134
physical abuse, 508
physical activity, 190–191, 209–213, 222–226
    benefits, 210–212
    choosing, 212–213
    drinking water during, 224
    guidelines, 212
    injury prevention, 222–223
    protective equipment, 222
    safety precautions, 222–225
    treating injuries, 225–226
    weather-related injuries and conditions, 224–225
Physical Activity Guidelines for Americans, 212
physical dependence, 256, 274
physical development, 538, 540–542, 545–548
physical environment, 18
physical fitness. *See* fitness
physical health, 8, 120
physical identity, 100
physical intimacy, 487–488
physical needs, 469–470
physician assistant, 11
PID (pelvic inflammatory disease), 343
piercings, 46
pimples. *See* acne
pinkeye. *See* conjunctivitis
pinna, 59
pituitary gland, 596
placenta, 534
plant-based protein sources, 165
plaque
    fatty deposits in blood vessels, 360
    film on teeth, 53
plasma, 578
platelets, 578
PNS (peripheral nervous system), 590
Poison Control Center, 388, 433
poisoning prevention, 387–388
poisonous, 387
pollutants, 426
pollution, 426–434, 436–437
    air, 426–428, 436–437
    chemicals, 431–434, 437
    environmental protection laws, 436–437
    noise, 434
    water, 429–430, *437*

pores, 41
positive outlook, 111, 120, 191
post-traumatic stress disorder (PTSD), 134
power, 220
PPO (preferred provider organization), 12
precautions, 387. *See also* safety precautions
pre-exposure prophylaxis (PrEP), 356
preferred provider organization (PPO), 12
pregnancy
    adolescent, 551–552
    alcohol use during, 277
    changes to a woman's body, 534
    difficulties of adolescent and teen pregnancies,
      551–552
    nutritional needs during, 175
    teen, 551–552
    tobacco use during, 249
prenatal development, 534–535
PrEP (pre-exposure prophylaxis), 356
presbyopia, 58
preschoolers, 541
prescription medications, 301
    AWARxE Prescription Drug Safety Program, 320
    facts about misuse and abuse, 321
Prevent All Cigarette Trafficking (PACT) Act, 262
preventive healthcare, 10
primary care physician, 11
priorities, 23
products, green, 443
progesterone, 532
prognosis, 359
progressive muscle relaxation, 122
prostate, 532
protein, 164–165
    plant-based sources for vegetarians, 165
protein foods group, 174
protozoa, 337
PSA (public service announcement), 320
psychological abuse. *See* emotional abuse
psychological dependence, 256, 274
psychological identity, 100
psychological injury, 497
PTH (parathyroid hormone), 596
PTSD (post-traumatic stress disorder), 134
puberty, 531, 545–548
public service announcement (PSA), 320
pulmonary circulation, 576
pulse, 228
puncture wounds, 411–412
pupil, 56, 594
purging, 200

R

rabies virus, 413
radiation therapy, 364

range of motion, 217
rapid eye movement (REM) sleep, 71
reaction time, 220
recommended food amounts, 175
rectum, 584
recycling, 439–440
red blood cells, 578
reduction, 438–439
refined grains, 172
reflex, 593
refusal skills, 24–25, 265–266, 289, 322–323, 347
regular use stage, 255, 282
Rehabilitation Act of 1973, 355
rehabilitation programs, 324
rejuvenate, 68
relapse, 324, 359
relationships
    communication, 458–463
    community, 471
    conflict resolution, 464–467
    dating, 486–490
    family, 469–475
    friendships, 477–484
    healthy versus unhealthy, 456–458
    importance, 455–456
    peer, 477–484
relaxation techniques, 87–88, 122–124
remission, 359
REM (rapid eye movement) sleep, 71
renewable energy, 439
reproduction, 533–534, 597
reproductive systems, 531–533, 597
    female, 532–533
    male, 531–532
rescue breaths, 417
residential treatment programs, 324
resilience, 114
resistance, 216
resistance stage, 118
Resource Conservation and Recovery Act, 437
respiration, 580
respiratory allergies, 366
respiratory etiquette, 374
respiratory system, 245–246, 365–366, 380, 578–580
response substitution, 261
restless legs syndrome (RLS), 80
retina, 57, 594
retrovirus, 356
rheumatoid arthritis, 369
R.I.C.E. treatment, 225
risk factors, 16–21, 359–360
    environmental, 18–20
    genetic, 16, 18
    lifestyle choices, 17, 20–21
    for noncommunicable diseases, 359–360
    of suicide, 147–149

rituals, 470
RLS (restless legs syndrome), 80
rods, 57
Rohypnol®, 312
rumors, 480, 499
runoff, 429

S

SAD (seasonal affective disorder), 135
Safe Drinking Water Act, 437
Safely Surrendered Baby Law, 552
safety equipment, 222
safety precautions, 387–396, 398–406, 408–418
    emergency preparedness, 392–394
    fall prevention, 387
    fire prevention and safety, 388–391
    first-aid basics, 408–418
    home, 387–396
    Internet, 400–401
    poisoning prevention, 387–388
    public places, 399
    school, 398–399
    traffic and vehicle, 403–405
    water activities, 405–406
    weapons, 388
saliva, 583
salivary glands, 583
SAMHSA (Substance Abuse and Mental Health Services Administration), 325
sandwich generation, 557
saturated fats, 165
schizophrenia, 137
school
    advocating for health, 30
    environment, 30
    safety precautions, 398–399
school-age years. *See* middle childhood
school violence, 517–518
science, 27
scrapes, 411–412
scrotum, 531
seasonal affective disorder (SAD), 135
sebum, 569
secondhand smoke, 248–249
sedentary, 212
self-concept. *See* self-image
self-discovery, 99–104
    identity, 100
    self-esteem, 101–104
    self-image, 100–101
self-esteem, 101–104, 543
    building, 102
    factors, 102
    high, 102, 104
    low, 104

self-harm, 135–136
self-image, 100–101
self-management skills, 260–261, 291
self-worth, 99
semen, 532
semicircular canals, 59
seminal vesicles, 532
senses, 593–595
sensory neurons, 590
sensory organs, 593–595
sets, 234
sexual abuse, 508
sexual activity
    resisting through refusal skills, 347
    setting boundaries before dating, 487–488
sexually transmitted infections (STIs), 342–348
    common, 342–346
    help available from community resources, 348
    how contracted, 342
    preventing, 346–348
    treating, 348
sexual reproduction, 533–534, 597
shock
    electrical, 414
    medical condition, 410
short sleepers, 69
short-term goal, 24
sibling abuse, 512
sibling rivalry, 473
siblings, 473–474
side effects, 142, 301–302
sidestream smoke, 248
SIDS (sudden infant death syndrome), 249
simple carbohydrates, 162
skeletal muscles, 573
skeletal system, 569–572
    bones, 569–571
    joints, 572
skill-related fitness, 218–220
    agility, 218
    balance, 218
    coordination, 220
    power, 220
    reaction time, 220
    speed, 218
skills
    communication, 30–32, 458–463
    conflict resolution, 25–26
    decision-making, 23
    goal-setting, 24
    health literacy, 26–29
    interpersonal, 457
    refusal, 24–25
    self-management, 260–261, 291
skills-training programs, 324

sun protection factor (SPF), 44
support groups, 141, 291–292, 325
survivors, 151
susceptible, 338
sustainability, 441
sweat glands, 569
syphilis, 344
systemic circulation, 576

T

tar, 246
target heart rate, 233
tattoos, 46
TBI (traumatic brain injury), 138
teen pregnancy, 551–552
teeth, 51–56, 582–583
    care and hygiene, 54, 56
    digestive process, 582–583
    grinding, 54, 80–81
    gum disease, 53
    misaligned and impacted, 54
    parts, 51–52
    tooth decay, 53
    wisdom, 54
teeth grinding, 54, 80–81
temper tantrum, 540–541
temporal lobes, 592
tendons, 572
terminal, 359
terrorism, 520–521
testes, 531, 598
testosterone, 312, 531, 545
tetanus, 412
thalamus, 593
thankfulness, 112–113
THC, 307–308
THC extraction, 308
T-helper cells, 353
therapist, 141
therapy, 141
thrush, 353
thymus, 588
thyroid, 596
thyroid hormone, 596
time management, 120
tinnitus, 60
tissues, 567
tobacco, 243–245, 261–263
    advertising and labeling laws, 262–263
    definition, 243
    pledging freedom from, 261
    products, 243–245
    sales restrictions, 262
    smokeless, 244
Tobacco Control Act, 262–263

Tobacco Rule, 262
tobacco use
    cancers caused, 247
    government efforts to limit, 262–265
    health hazards, 245–247
    impact on user's appearance, 248
    pledging freedom from, 261
    prevention, 262–266
    products and methods, 243–244
    quitting, 259–261
    reasons young people try smoking, 251–254
    resisting through refusal skills, 265–266
    secondhand smoke, 248–249
    stages of addiction, 255–256
    state smoking bans, 263–264
    why quitting is difficult, 254–256
    withdrawal symptoms, 256
toddlers, 540–541
tolerance stage, 255–256, 282
tonsilitis, 339
tonsils, 588
tooth decay, 53
topical, 300
total color blindness, 57
toxic, 244
trachea, 579
traditions, 470
traffic safety, 403–404
trans fats, 165–166
transportation, green choices, 446
traumatic brain injury (TBI), 138
treatment of hazardous substances, 440
trees, planting, 445
trichomoniasis, 344–345
triggers, 256, 261
Truvada, 356
tryptophan, 86–87
tuberculosis, 353
tumor, 246, 362
type 1 diabetes mellitus, 368
type 2 diabetes mellitus, 368, 380

U

ultraviolet (UV) light, 40, 43–45
umbilical cord, 534
unconscious, 67
underage drinking, 278–279
underbite, 54
undernutrition, 176
underweight, 186–187
United States Department of Agriculture (USDA), 171
United States Department of Health and Human Services (HHS), 171
United States Food and Drug Administration. *See* FDA
unsaturated fats, 165

upper respiratory system, 579
ureters, 586
urethra, 532, 586
urinary system, 585–586
urine, 585
USDA (United States Department of Agriculture), 171
uterus, 532
UV. *See* ultraviolet light

V

vaccines, 375–376
vagina, 532
values, 23, 100
vaping, 244
vas deferens, 532
vegetables group, 173
vegetarians, 165
vehicle safety, 405
veins, 577
vena cavae, 577
ventricles, 575
verbal abuse. *See* emotional abuse
verbal communication, 458
vertebrae, 593
vigorous intensity, 232
violence, 282, 497–507, 508–515, 517–522
    abuse, 508–515
    alcohol use and, 282
    bullying, 498–501, 505–506
    cyberbullying, 502–504
    gang, 518–519
    hate crimes, 520
    homicide, 520
    human trafficking, 519
    preventing, 521
    school, 517–518
    terrorism, 520–521
    what to do if you are a victim, 521
violent behavior, 497
violent extremism, 521
virtual friends, 478
viruses, 336
vision, 56–58, 594
visualization, 122
vitamins, 166–167
voluntary muscles. *See* skeletal muscles

W

wants, 23
warm-ups, 232
water, 169
    drinking during physical activity, 224
water activity safety, 405–406
water pollution, 429–430, 437

water-soluble vitamins, 167
water treatment, 430
weapons safety, 388
weather-related injuries and conditions, 224–225
weight
    body composition and, 185–187
    determining healthy, 184–187
    health consequences of underweight and
        overweight, 187–188
    management, 184–193
weight management, 184–193
    body composition, 185–187
    determining a healthy weight, 184–187
    gaining weight, 193
    goals, 188–190
    health consequences of underweight and
        overweight, 187–188
    help from a healthcare professional, 192
    physical activity, 190–191
    positive thinking, 191
    strategies, 188–193
    support of friends and family, 191
    unhealthy strategies, 192–193
well-being, 8, 10
wellness, 7–13
    aspects, 7–8
    differs from health, 7
    healthcare's role, 10–13
    improving through lifestyle choices, 15
    mental and emotional health, 8–9
    physical health, 8
    risk factors, 16–21
    skills and resources for maintaining, 23–32
    social health, 8
    well-being, 8, 10
white blood cells, 578, 588
whitehead, 41
white matter, 592
whole grains, 172
wisdom teeth, 54
withdrawal, 256
workouts, 231–234
    aerobic, 232–233
    anaerobic, 233–234
    maximizing, 232–234
    tracking, 231

Y

yoga, 122–123
young adulthood, 555–556

Z

zero-tolerance policy, 281, 518
zygote, 533